TRAUMATIC BRAIN INJURY

Volume II
Recovery and
Rehabilitation

TRAUMATIC BRAIN INJURY

Volume II
Recovery and Rehabilitation

RALPH M. REITAN

DEBORAH WOLFSON
Neuropsychology Laboratory
Tucson, Arizona

Keith Kasnot
Medical Illustrator

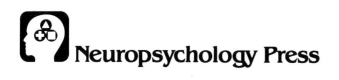
Neuropsychology Press

Neuropsychology Press
1338 East Edison Street
Tucson, Arizona 85719

Made in the United States of America.

ISBN 0-934515-07-7
Library of Congress Card Number: 86-060952

Great care has been taken to maintain the accuracy of the information contained in the volume. However, Neuropsychology Press cannot be held responsible for errors or for any consequences arising from the use of the information contained herein.

PREFACE

The principal focus of this book is on recovery and rehabilitation of persons who have sustained cerebral damage as a result of a traumatic injury. Our review of this topic includes a description of traumatic tissue damage and biological methods of repair; conventional prognostic indicators; outcome studies; neuropsychological evaluation of spontaneous recovery; and methods for retraining impaired neuropsychological functions. A special chapter is devoted to the various theories of brain-behavior relationships because of the importance of understanding the entire recovery process within an integrated framework.

Finally, we have presented neuropsychological test results of individual patients who have been tested at specified intervals in order to assess and evaluate the recovery (and sometimes deterioration) process. We believe that careful review and study of these case presentations is essential for the practicing clinical neuropsychologist who wishes to gain further expertise not only in evaluating subjects with traumatic brain injury but in clinical neuropsychological assessment more generally.

The clinical presentation of case material gives the reader an opportunity to consider the data of the Halstead-Reitan Battery not only in terms of the range of measurements employed but also with respect to the methodological organization of the tests. We have had an opportunity recently to review clinical interpretations done by well-known neuropsychologists who have specialized in the area of traumatic brain injury. In many instances the approach to neuropsychological examination is represented only by administration of a series of tests. These tests are interpreted according to the adequacy of performance of the individual subject and an assessment of performance is based on comparisons with normative data. To some extent comparisons may be made between various tests in order to determine whether the individual performed as well as might be expected on all of the measures. In this respect the most common approach is to compare performances on neuropsychological tests with results on general intelligence measures and conclude that the individual is impaired if certain test scores are lower than others.

Obviously, the range of variability that occurs among normal subjects creates a significant problem in using this particular methodological approach. For example, many individual subjects show considerable variability between Verbal and Performance IQ values. Silverstein (1987) estimates that 5% of the time normal individuals with a Verbal IQ of 115 will have a Performance IQ that is either below 88 or above 134 points.

Nevertheless, the approach in clinical interpretation often is to administer an extensive series of neuropsychological tests and identify those tests which were done most poorly. These tests in turn serve as the focus for attention and the basis for interpretation of neuropsychological deficits without taking into consideration the fact that every individual, when given an extensive series of tests, is going to do somewhat poorly on some of them.

When this method is applied in a research context, using summary measures such as the Halstead Impairment Index, the results make this quite clear. For example, the normal range for the Impairment Index is 0.0 to 0.3, indicating that up to 30% of the tests may have scores in the impaired range. An Impairment Index of 0.4 (40% of the test scores are impaired) constitutes a borderline normal score. Only when the Impairment Index is 0.5 or greater (indicating that 50% of the tests have scores in the impaired range) is the variable considered to be suggestive of brain damage.

It should be remembered that although the Impairment Index is based upon tests which have been identified through careful research as being sensitive to cerebral damage, normal subjects perform somewhat poorly (i.e., in the brain-damaged range) on a substantial proportion of these tests. Therefore, any approach that depends exclusively (or even heavily) on identification of neuropsychological tests on which the individual performs poorly as a basis for determining whether brain damage is present is subject to serious methodological criticism. Obviously, it is not satisfactory to merely give an extensive series of neuropsychological tests and identify acquired deficits as being represented by the tests on which the individual happened to perform poorly.

The solution to this problem resides in using not only an interpretive framework based on level of performance (how well the subject has done), but additional methodological approaches to evaluation of the data as well (Reitan, 1966a; Reitan & Wolfson 1985a, 1986b). In essence, the Halstead-Reitan Battery is organized so that the results can be evaluated in four successive steps: (1) according to *level of performance,* (2) with relation to *patterns and relationships among the test results* that reflect the biological status of various areas within the cerebral hemispheres, (3) according to the occurrence of *specific deficits* that occur almost exclusively with persons having cerebral damage, and (4) with relation to *comparative performances on the two sides of the body* as they relate to the differential status of the contralateral cerebral hemisphere.

The complementary value of these approaches is expressed in an integrated interpretation of the results for the individual subject. Thus, the fundamental difference between using only a series of tests and using the Halstead-Reitan Battery is that the latter procedures require that explicit criteria be met, within an organized methodological framework, to draw conclusions about cerebral damage in the individual case.

These comments prompt a brief reference to the use of "fixed" batteries as contrasted with "flexible" batteries. The Halstead-Reitan Battery is frequently cited as an example of a "fixed" battery and is so identified because the tests included are represented by a standard battery.

Supposed advantages of the "flexible" battery include the prerogative to select certain tests to evaluate specific areas of function that accord with the patient's complaints. Of course, such a procedure might be quite circular in nature if the end result is only to document through psychological testing the patient's own initial self-examination (self-diagnosis). Further, if the complaints are not sufficiently comprehensive, or if the patient is not able to offer an adequate and complete self-diagnosis, the resulting test battery may totally fail to recognize and evaluate significant areas of dysfunction. In any case, the resulting series of tests will show a range of scores. Some tests will have been performed more poorly than others and consequently will be selected as indications of neuropsychological deficits.

In contrast, the "fixed" battery approach is not prejudiced in its selection of tests. Instead, the Halstead-Reitan Battery has been developed to reflect impaired brain functions as manifested by thousands of individual patients with brain damage. In this sense, the Halstead-Reitan Battery might be thought of as a comprehensive battery, having been validated on thousands of patients in order to be certain that all relevant areas of brain functions were not only included in the assessment, but that they also provided a balanced representation of the various neuropsychological functions subserved by the brain.

Finally, the tests included in the Halstead-Reitan Battery (as contrasted with tests in a "flexible" battery devised for each patient in accordance with the individual's complaints) have been subject to rigorous research in order to validate each instrument as a neuropsychological test. Various tests included in the Battery have been further validated in terms of their complementary significance and interpretation for assessment of the individual.

It would seem that a "fixed" battery of tests is necessary in order to achieve a balanced interpretation of brain-behavior relationships, using tests that have been validated as a Battery for interpretation of results for the individual subject. In contrast, the "flexible" battery, to the degree that it represents a unique battery for each individual subject, has been less carefully validated in terms of either formal research effort or individual interpretation. In fact, even some of the most commonly used individual tests that are frequently included in "flexible" batteries have scarcely any validating information in the literature to indicate that they have been shown, through formal controlled research studies, even to be sensitive to cerebral damage.

Results of the Halstead-Reitan Battery obtained on individual subjects regularly demonstrate the advantage of an approach in which a standard and comprehensive battery of tests is used. For example, from the tests alone it is often possible to determine that cerebral damage has been sustained, to judge the area or location of principal involvement, and to assess whether the injury is recent or whether the brain has had a chance to stabilize. Further, from the point of view of rehabilitation it is imperative to have a balanced representation of the nature and degree of neuropsychological deficit.

Considering the extensive research that undergirds the tests included in the Halstead-Reitan Battery, and the degree of clinical experience that supports the use of these individual tests as a cohesive battery, it would seem that the term "fixed battery," as it applies to the Halstead-Reitan Battery, implies a standardized, validated and clinically-tested battery. In contrast, the term "flexible battery," at least as applied to many instances we have recently observed in clinical practice, implies a series of tests that sometimes have not even been validated as sensitive to brain damage individually, have never been tested as a battery for validity in relating to type, location or process of cerebral pathology, and are subject to a permissive clinical interpretation with few (if any) published standards available for reference or comparison purposes.

Clearly, a "flexible" battery would be preferred by those clinicians who feel a need to impose their own imprint on their clinical evaluations and want to avoid achieving the level of clinical competence required by a system of clinical evaluation that demands knowledge of extensive research findings and adherence to a body of knowledge that represents competent clinical assessment. The question comes down to whether we favor a personal and impressionistic approach or a scientific approach in clinical neuropsychology — do we want to base our discipline on science or art?

Ralph M. Reitan
Deborah Wolfson

Acknowledgements

We are grateful to those who helped us with the production of this volume. Jacquelyn Tarpy was involved in all aspects of editing, proofreading, and organizing. Keith Kasnot's original medical illustrations made the difficult and complex concepts more understandable. Frank Wallis and Sharon Flesher gave us invaluable technical advice and suggestions. Kathleen Wilson typed the many drafts of the manuscript.

CONTENTS

I

TRAUMATIC DAMAGE AND MECHANISMS OF REPAIR OF BRAIN TISSUE

Description of Damage and Pathological Changes Following Traumatic Brain injury

Most of the knowledge concerning structural changes of the brain following head injury has been based upon gross and microscopic studies of brains at post-mortem examinations. Since there is no doubt that similar types of damage often occur in the brains of persons who have experienced less severe non-fatal injuries, autopsy examinations have contributed a great deal of information regarding the nature of pathological changes associated with both focal and diffuse effects of head blows.

Most persons who sustain a fatal head injury die within the first 24 hours post-injury. Therefore, much of the information derived from post-mortem examinations has been based upon study of the relatively immediate effects of brain trauma. In more recent years, however, intensive medical care has led to longer survival periods for head trauma victims and the consequences of initial damage have become more understood. These consequences have reflected particularly evidence of ischemic damage and damage to axons. Such information has in turn led to the realization that a severe head injury invariably has diffuse effects in addition to whatever focal lesions may have been caused by the trauma. Obviously, this diffuse involvement is a significant factor in determining a patient's eventual outcome. Such pathological changes, which would be expressed as long-term consequences of head injury, cannot be explained on the basis of information gained from autopsy studies. However, Oppenheimer (1968) has published studies of patients who had sustained a head injury and later died of unrelated causes. His results suggest that even relatively mild closed head injuries may result in long-term pathological evidence of brain damage.

The major categories of traumatic brain injury and the primary and secondary effects that have been observed in post-mortem studies will be reviewed in this section.

Types of Head Injury

Most investigators differentiate between closed head injury (sometimes called blunt injury) and penetrating head injury (often referred to as missile injury). A closed head injury, which may injure the scalp and deform the skull, may also be accompanied by a fracture of the skull bone (Fig. 1-1).

Adams' (1975) classification of missile injuries

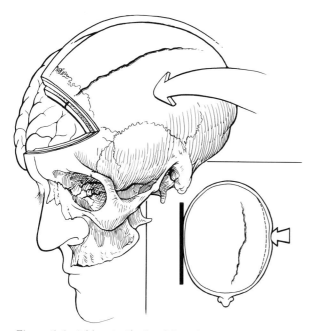

Figure 1-1. A blow to the head (INSET) may result in skull deformation and linear fracture. Patients with a skull fracture may have no other evidence of central nervous system injury.

includes depressed skull fractures, penetrating wounds, and perforating injuries. Depressed skull fractures are injuries in which the force of the blow has caused a relatively focal fracture of the skull with depression of the bone below the normal level of the skull-table (Fig. 1-2). *Depressed skull fractures* show a considerable degree of variation. In some cases the depression may be so minimal that the injury can barely be classified as depressed; in other instances the depression of the skull bone is severe enough to establish a direct route to the brain through soft tissue. Whether contusion or laceration of underlying cerebral tissue accompanies a depressed skull fracture depends upon the degree of the depression and the extent to which the fractured bone is driven into the brain tissue.

Adams describes *penetrating injuries* as those in which an object penetrates through the scalp and skull directly into the brain but does not pass through the brain. Such wounds may be caused by a variety of objects, ranging from knife blades and nails to bullets and shrapnel.

The final classification, *perforating injuries,*

are those in which an object penetrates the skull with sufficient force to pass completely through the brain and leave an entrance and an exit wound. Perforating brain wounds are usually caused by penetration by a bullet (Fig. 1-3).

In penetrating and perforating brain wounds the pathology is represented by laceration of brain tissue at the point of impact, hemorrhage in the regions of the brain that are damaged and destroyed by penetration of the object, and the resultant swelling and edema (particularly in the areas of principal damage). In addition to focal damage along the path of penetration, contusions may also occur in areas remote from the point of injury. This is particularly common in cases of high velocity missile penetration. These remote contusions seem to be essentially similar to those

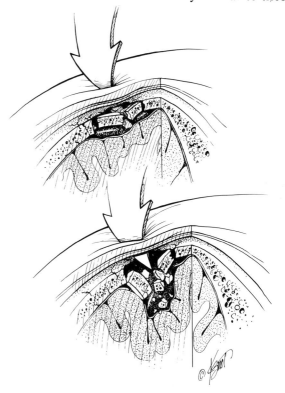

Figure 1-2. A depressed skull fracture occurs when a strong force makes contact with the skull over a small area. In a closed (simple) depressed skull fracture (TOP) there is no laceration of the scalp overlying the injured area. In an open (compound) fracture (BOTTOM), the scalp is lacerated above the area of injury, thus establishing a direct route for infection to occur.

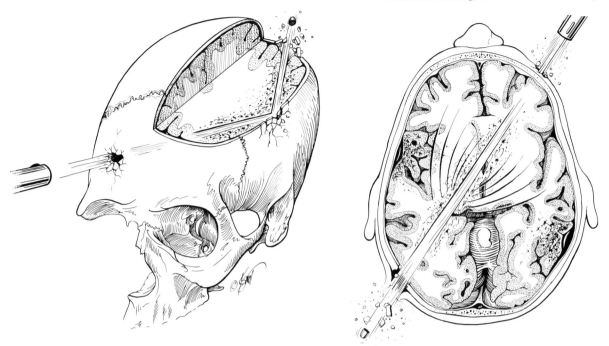

Figure 1-3. Missile wounds to the head often cause extensive damage to the scalp and brain. Hemorrhage and contusion may occur in areas distant to the missile tract, due to the displacement of the brain by the sudden pressure wave.

observed in cases of closed head injury. The forces which displace the brain within the cranial vault and cause the brain to impact against the skull are most probably the cause of the remote contusions.

Secondary changes, associated particularly with bleeding and edema, occur with penetrating wounds as well as with closed head injuries. There is usually only one path of penetration in this type of wound, but objects such as bullets may ricochet within the cranial vault and cause multiple tracts of damage. Obviously, the extent of cerebral damage in penetrating and perforating brain wounds varies tremendously, but the damage is generally widespread and extends beyond the area of penetration and the missile track.

Primary Mechanisms of Head Injury

In instances of closed head injury primary damage falls into two categories: (1) macroscopic lesions, represented by contusions, and (2) microscopic lesions, demonstrated by direct damage to nerve fibers. Although a contusion does not occur in every instance of closed head injury,

it appears that axonal damage is frequently present. Adams, Mitchell, Graham, and Doyle (1977) studied head-injured patients and found that every person with a primary brainstem lesion also demonstrated damage in the cerebral hemispheres.

The principal manifestation of diffuse damage following closed head injuries is represented by shearing of axons (Fig. 1-4). In the early stages following a head injury pathological evidence of axonal damage is demonstrated by the appearance of retraction balls (beads of axoplasm at the end of each axon, formed from torn and damaged axons) and microglial stars (small clusters of hypertrophied microglial cells). Wallerian degeneration of the distal portions of severed axons is a slower process that may take six to eight weeks to occur. Breakdown products resulting from this process may be subject to identification for two or more years following the injury.

As pointed out by Adams (1975), the neuropathological changes are quite characteristic in patients who survive severe closed head injury for more than six to eight weeks. There may be contusions of the cerebral cortex (particularly involving the orbital frontal surface and the frontal and temporal poles) with generalized enlargement of the ventricular system (reflecting atrophy of the white matter). This atrophy undoubtedly is a result of degeneration of axons due to shearing forces and axonal damage. Adams (1975) notes that this evidence of reduction of the amount of white matter increases in accordance with the duration of survival and that after a severe closed head injury the brainstem is usually smaller than normal because of degeneration of fiber tracts. In fact, degenerating fiber tracts may be recognized macroscopically by their abnormally white appearance.

Characteristic lesions of the corpus callosum adjacent to the superior cerebellar peduncles are also often present. Lesions of the white matter (shown by breakdown of myelin) can be demonstrated by certain staining techniques, and it appears likely that damage to the myelin sheaths of axons is a direct result of tearing of nerve fibers by the pressure forces generated within the cranial vault by the head blow. In addition, vascular and anoxic damage may also play a significant role in

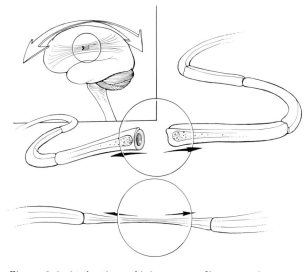

Figure 1-4. At the time of injury nerve fibers are often stretched and torn, resulting in axonal damage. Diffuse injury to axons is only visible microscopically.

white matter degeneration.

Secondary Mechanisms of Head Injury

Edema. Secondary damage may also occur in addition to the primary damage caused by contusions and direct damage to nerve fibers. Secondary damage is a result of bleeding or edema. Bleeding may be manifested by specific lesions (such as epidural, subdural, or intracerebral hematomas), but almost certainly is also represented by small hemorrhages that may occur on a widespread basis. In many instances cerebral edema, which results from the accumulation of excess fluid in the brain, is demonstrated by focal swelling around contusions and hematomas. The most probable etiology is that damaged cerebral vessels leak fluid into the lesion and the fluid subsequently spreads into the surrounding white matter by passing between the myelin sheaths (Fig. 1-5) (Klatzo, 1967).

Factors contributing to cerebral edema include vascular dilatation, decreased cerebral perfusion, and increased vascular permeability resulting from shear strains on small blood vessels. Even in the absence of focal lesions one or both cerebral hemispheres may be edematous. Postmortem examination of edematous brains often reveals small, compressed, or obliterated ventricles, pallor or grayness of the white matter, and early reactive gliosis.

Ischemia. Besides sustaining vascular lesions representing secondary effects of head injury (which can usually be identified through standard diagnostic techniques such as computed tomography), the patient with a significant head injury may also suffer widespread ischemic brain damage. Death of cells due to ischemia results when the cerebral blood flow is reduced below a critical level. Ischemic damage of the brain is particularly common in persons who have experienced a severe episode of total circulatory arrest or status epilepticus.

Adams (1975) noted that a high proportion of

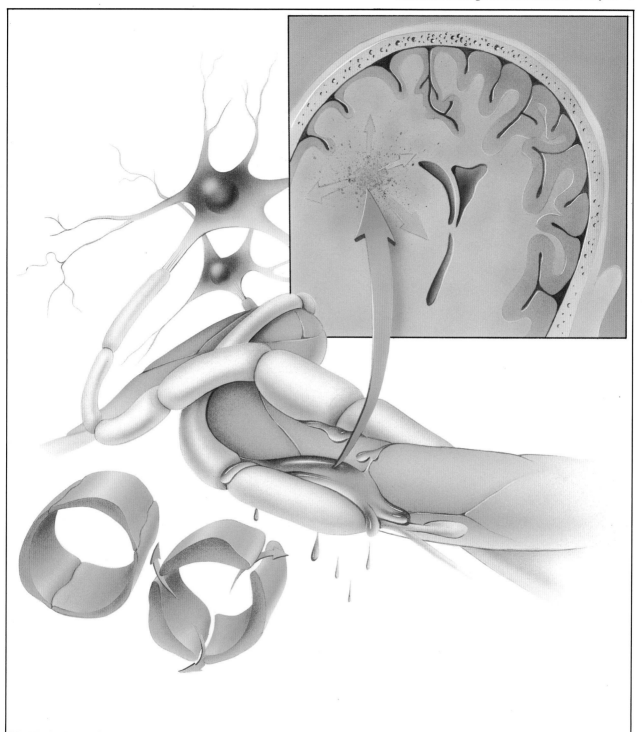

Figure 1-5. Cerebral edema, a specialized form of swelling in which the brain substance expands because of an increase in tissue fluid, frequently develops adjacent to areas of cerebral contusion. Increased permeability of cerebral vessels allows fluid (plasma filtrate) to escape into the surrounding tissue, causing the volume within the cranial vault to increase and intracranial pressure to rise. Computed tomography (CT) is the technique used most frequently to identify cerebral edema. In a healthy vessel, normal CNS homeostasis requires intact endothelial cells and tight junctions (LEFT). In edema, plasma escapes into the extracellular space when the tight junction of the endothelial cell is destroyed (RIGHT).

patients with head injuries demonstrate neuronal necrosis and infarction throughout the brain, even when the condition is not recognized macroscopically. After excluding patients with cardiac arrest, status epilepticus, infarction associated with contusions as well as other infarcts, and necrosis due to fat emboli, Adams found an incidence of 26% of ischemic neocortical damage in the arterial boundary zones between the major cerebral arteries (Fig. 1-6). Of these cases, 11% had lesions restricted to the occipital lobes. In the remaining 89% the lesions involved in the frontal, temporal, and parietal regions. In most cases the ischemic damage was bilateral. In slightly more than 50% of the cases there was evidence of cortical infarction and in about 30% of the cases there was evidence of multiple foci of ischemic brain damage scattered throughout the cortex. Ischemic damage was also frequently found in the basal ganglia. These findings indicate that ischemic brain damage is a significant factor in head injury and probably has distinct significance in producing neuropsychological deficit in the patients who survive.

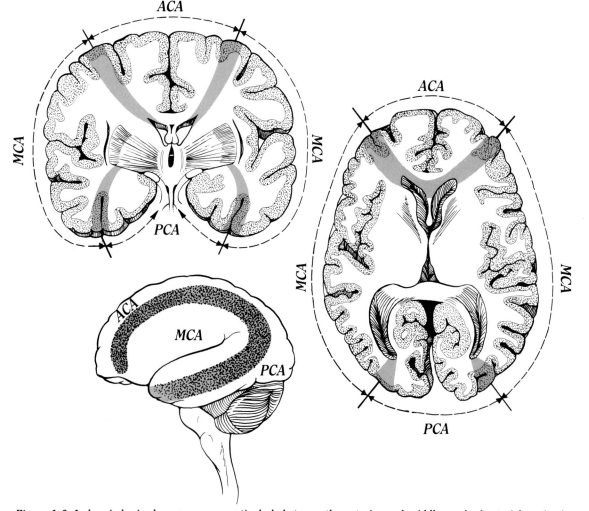

Figure 1-6. Ischemic brain damage occurs particularly between the anterior and middle cerebral arterial territories. This type of damage is significantly more common in patients who have sustained an episode of increased intracranial pressure or an episode of hypoxia (a systolic blood pressure of <80 mm Hg for at least 15 min). Ischemic brain damage is frequently found in head-injured patients who remain in a vegetative or severely disabled state. *ACA,* anterior cerebral artery; *MCA,* middle cerebral artery; *PCA,* posterior cerebral artery.

Contusion and Axonal Shearing

As noted in the preceding section, besides damage due to penetration, contusions and direct damage to nerve fibers constitute the significant aspects of primary brain damage (see Reitan & Wolfson, 1986b).

Contusions are caused by damage to the blood vessels and represent areas of bleeding into the surrounding tissue. These lesions can be identified using computed tomography. The second class of lesions, involving direct damage to nerve fibers, can be evaluated only through microscopic examination. Although nerve fiber damage may lead to cerebral atrophy (and therefore be visualized by computed tomography), the immediate effects of nerve damage are usually not subject to assessment with imaging techniques.

The mechanisms of cerebral damage have also been previously reviewed (Reitan & Wolfson, 1986b). It should be noted that both contusions and damage of nerve fibers result from either acceleration or deceleration injuries, distortion of the skull, linear and rotational shearing of brain tissue, and tearing against bony protuberances on the inner surface of the skull.

Diffuse cerebral damage, which is believed to occur in most (if not all) instances of significant head blows, is highly variable between subjects. However, diffuse damage may be of great clinical significance to the individual patient. With minor diffuse damage the patient is likely to have little disturbance of consciousness, although delayed effects may result in eventual deterioration. In cases of severe diffuse damage to the nerve fibers the patient may never regain consciousness, deteriorate clinically, and remain in a persistent vegetative state until death occurs.

Nerve fiber damage concerns injury to axons and the resulting consequences. Typical changes, referred to as *chromatolysis,* occur within the cell body soon after injury and consist of swelling, dissolution of Nissl bodies, and displacement of the nucleus to the peripheral part of the cell (Fig. 1-7).

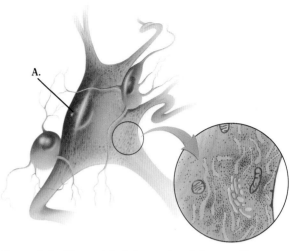

Figure 1-7. *Chromatolysis* is a series of degenerative changes which occur in the neuronal body whose axon is injured. The cell body swells and becomes distended, the nucleus (*A*) is displaced toward the periphery of the cell, and the Nissl bodies undergo dissolution (INSET).

This process may progress to death and dissolution of the cell or, in cases of less severe injury, it may be arrested and gradually reversed over a period of months. Depending upon the degree of cellular damage and the facilitation of recovery by the internal environment, it appears that a critical point of injury may exist. If the cell is damaged beyond this critical point the metabolic repair processes are insufficient to effect recovery. Of course, many other damaged cells may not have reached this critical point and for them recovery is possible. An effect of this type leads logically to the presumption that some cells may continue to live but their recovery may not be complete.

In addition to direct damage of neurons, it must also be recognized that head trauma can cause significant disruption of both the anatomical status and function of blood vessels of the brain. While most large hemorrhages are easily identified, in many cases it is also possible to visualize microscopic hemorrhages (Fig. 1-8). Damage to blood vessels can alter blood flow, causing changes in arterial blood pressure which may in turn limit cerebral perfusion. Arterial hypertension may contribute to brain swelling, extracellular edema, and an increase of fluids in the damaged areas. Exper-

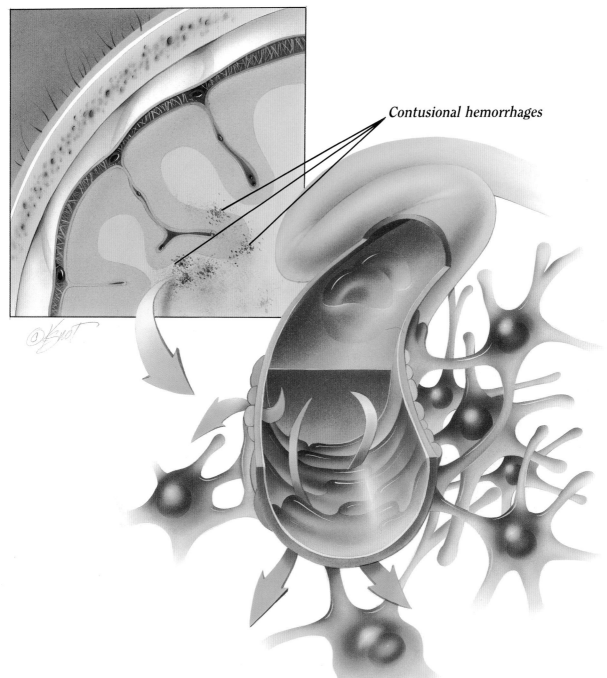

Figure 1-8. *Contusional or petechial hemorrhages* are discrete small hemorrhages in the gray or white matter that result from injury to small blood vessels (capillaries). The injured vessels allow blood to escape into the surrounding tissue. The lesions range in size from 3–4 mm to 1–2 cm. In severe trauma many such areas of hemorrhage may exist.

imental studies have suggested that responses of this kind may occur within the first few minutes following the injury. It appears likely that structural damage to neurons and blood vessels, together with alterations of physiological functions, may also lead to disorders of the neurotransmitter system and cause neurochemical dysfunction of the neuron.

Effects of Damage at the Cellular Level

There are two types of cells in the nervous system: neurons and glia. The function of glial cells within the central nervous system is similar to the role of connective tissue cells in other parts of the body. In other words, glial cells serve as supporting cells. In addition, glial cells separate groups of neurons from each other and may also have some role in nutritive functions and production of myelin. Glial cells are divided into five major classes: astrocytes, oligodendrocytes, microglia, ependymal cells, and Schwann cells (Fig. 1-9). It is estimated that there are probably about nine times as many glial cells as nerve cells.

Astrocytes are divided into two types: (1) fibrous astrocytes (located extensively in the white matter) and (2) protoplasmic astrocytes, (found primarily in the gray matter and associated with cell bodies, dendrites, and synapses of neurons). Oligodendrocytes occur in conjunction with myelinated central axons, wrapping themselves around the axon in a tight spiral. Microglia are small cells that react particularly to injury, acting as phagocytes. The ependymal cells line the inner surface of the brain.

Before discussing impaired function resulting from brain injury, it may be advantageous to provide a brief statement of additional aspects of the cellular composition of the nervous system. Neurons perform the signaling function of the nervous system and communicate between cells over junctions called *synapses.* The human brain is estimated to be composed of more than ten billion neurons and each neuron is estimated to have about one thousand synaptic connections.

Although neurons can be classified into many different types, they have certain common characteristics. Neurons consist of a cell body, dendrites, axon, and pre-synaptic terminals of the axon through which communication with dendrites of other neurons is achieved at the synapse (Fig. 1-10). The cell body is involved in the synthesis of macromolecules and contains the nu-

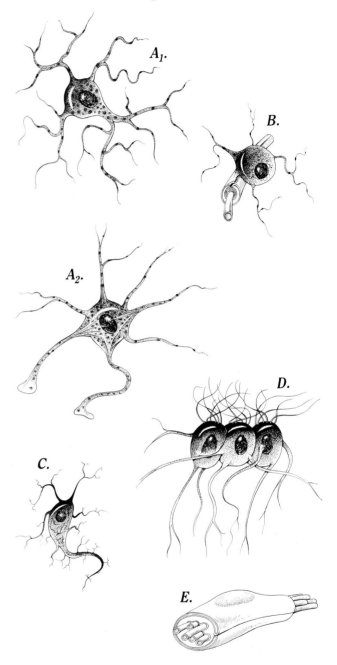

Figure 1-9. The five types of glial cells. *A (1, 2)*, astrocytes react to injury of the CNS by swelling or hypertrophy. The tips of the astrocytic processes are called *end feet* and attach to blood vessels. *B,* oligodendrocytes wrap around axons in the CNS to produce a myelin sheath. *C,* microglia proliferate in size and number during inflammatory or degenerative processes and become macrophages. *D,* ependymal cells, which have important secretory and absorptive functions, line the ventricular cavities. *E,* Schwann cells are located in the peripheral nervous system and produce myelin to encase axons.

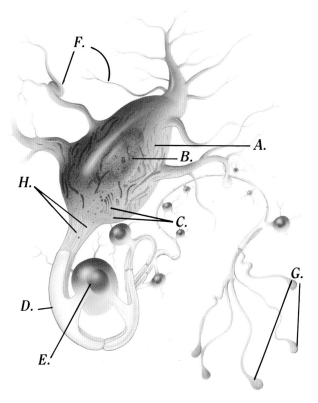

Figure 1-10. A typical neuron. *A*, cell body; *B*, nucleus, *C*, Nissl bodies; *D*, axon; *E*, oligodendrocyte; *F*, dendrites; *G*, boutons; *H*, neurofibrils.

cleus, ribosomes, rough endoplasmic reticulum, and Golgi apparatus. Macromolecules are organized into organelles within the cell body and these are transported to other regions of the neuron.

In general, the dendrites receive communicational information which proceeds to the cell body and then to the axon before being transferred at the synapse to another neuron. Thus, the cell body has multiple extensions (known as *dendrites*) and the axon, which is a tubular process, may extend over a considerable distance. Large axons are sheathed by a fatty insulative material called *myelin* which facilitates high-speed conduction. Axons divide into many fine branches near their terminal point, called the *presynaptic terminal.* This terminal makes contact with the receptive surfaces of other cells (principally dendrites but sometimes the cell body) and, through both electrical and chemical processes, communicates with

either other cells or with effector cells (muscles and glands).

Cellular damage, particularly involving shearing or cutting of axons, results in interference and interruption of transport of axons, and interference and interruption of transport of materials within the cell (Fig. 1-11). Cellular damage may have a number of adverse effects: (1) degeneration of presynaptic terminals resulting in a reduction of synapses, (2) degeneration of the distal segment of the axon (Wallerian degeneration), and (3) a dual response of microglial cells consisting of (a) removal of the residual of degenerating tissues (phagocytic action), and (b) proliferation within the central nervous system which impairs the prospect of functional reconnection of neurons.

The biochemical processes underlying synaptic transmission relate to the secretory function of nerve cells. Within the cell body proteins and lipids are synthesized and incorporated into membranes within the endoplasmic reticulum and Golgi apparatus of the cell body. Organelles are formed from these components and transported from the cell body into the axon and conducted toward the presynaptic terminal (Fig. 1-12). Some of the material is deposited along the axon but the rest of this substance reaches the terminals and appears to be involved in the release of neurotransmitter substances. The membranes of the synaptic vesicles become partially degraded by lysosomes and are returned to the cell body. Thus, the degraded membrane is partially recycled.

Two mechanisms of transport of materials within the cell have been identified (Fig. 1-13). The first mechanism, upon which synaptic transmission depends, is referred to as *rapid transport* and is estimated to have a rate of about 400 mm/day. In addition to carrying materials from the cell body toward the presynaptic terminals (anterograde transport), the rapid transport mechanism also carries presumably worn out material back to the cell body (retrograde transport), either for degradation or for reconstitution and reuse.

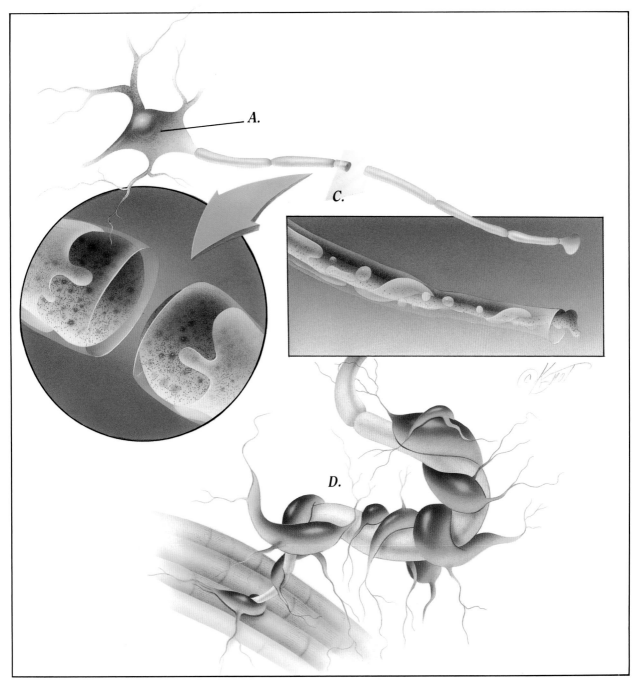

Figure 1-11. Reactions to axonal transection may include *A, chromatolysis*, a process during which the cell body swells and becomes distended and the nucleus is displaced toward the periphery; *B*, the formation of *retraction balls*, an accumulation of the cellular material which cannot pass the site of damage; *C, Wallerian degeneration*, in which the axon distal to the transection disintegrates and the myelin degenerates; *D*, regrowth and formation of a *traumatic neuroma*, consisting of Schwann cells, connective tissue cells and fibers, macrophages, and an abundance of tangled aberrant nerve fibers which may disrupt normal reconnection of neurons and be the source of severe pain.

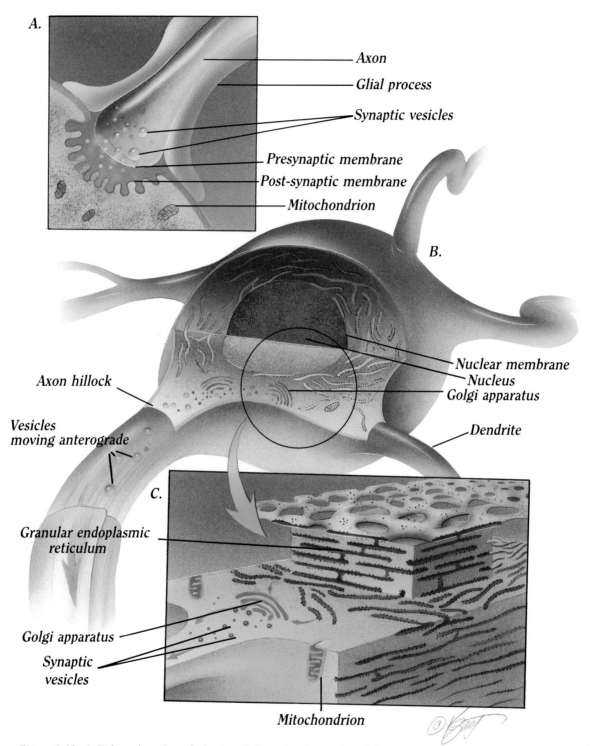

A.
Axon
Glial process
Synaptic vesicles
Presynaptic membrane
Post-synaptic membrane
Mitochondrion

B.
Nuclear membrane
Nucleus
Golgi apparatus
Dendrite

Axon hillock

Vesicles
moving anterograde

C.

Granular endoplasmic
reticulum

Golgi apparatus

Synaptic
vesicles

Mitochondrion

Figure 1-12. *A*, Enlarged section of a bouton. Information is transferred from one neuron to another (or between neurons and receptor or effector cells) at *synapses*, specialized regions of cellular contact. Boutons contain synaptic vesicles, unique cellular organelles. These vesicles in turn contain chemical transmitter substances which produce excitation or inhibition of the postsynaptic neuron. *B*, The neuronal cell body showing the major components as seen in an electron micrograph. *C*, Enlarged section of the cell body, illustrating the major organelles.

A second type of transport of materials within the cell is referred to *axoplasmic flow.* This process occurs in the anterograde direction only and is estimated to proceed at a rate of only 0.5–3 mm/day. Considering the fact that some axons extend for over a meter in length, it appears that the mechanisms of intracellular distribution of material is a significant factor in maintenance and nurturance of the extensive structure of the neuron. Thus, when damage occurs to the axon, there may well be consequences in both directions because of the anterograde and retrograde transport of materials. If the materials synthesized in the cell bodies are not available for distribution within the cell, the axon and synaptic terminals cannot receive their normal metabolic support and degeneration results. Because of impairment of retrograde supply to the cell body there are also

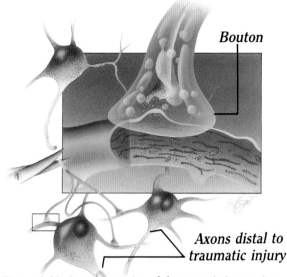

Figure 1-14. A representation of the synaptic interactions between neurons. The enlargement (INSET) shows the initial stages of degeneration in a synapse distal to the injury of an axon.

changes in the cell body itself.

The next step in this process involves atrophy, shrinkage, or degeneration of synaptic terminals (Fig. 1-14). Besides the electrical signals which pass between cells at the synapse there are also nutritive or trophic interactions between neurons. When axons are sheared or severed as a result of traumatic injury, degenerative changes occur not only in the neurons that are damaged, but also in subsequent neurons that receive synapses from the damaged neurons. In fact, involvement of the dendrites of the subsequent neuron may lead to impairment of these presynaptic tissues and result in transsynaptic or transneuronal impairment. Transneuronal deficits are the basis for distance effects that extend well beyond the site of the lesion.

The final step in this general description concerns the actions of glial cells in response to injury. Microglia play a role in phagocytosis, absorbing the debris resulting from injury to neurons as well as the products of degeneration (Fig. 1-15). However, the proliferation of microglia also interferes with any effective restoration of severed synaptic connections within the central nervous system.

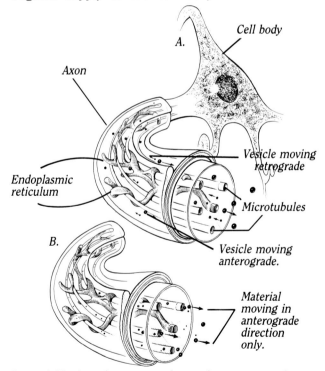

Figure 1-13. *Axonal transport* refers to the movement of proteins and other substances along the axon. Diagram *A* shows that the movement occurs in both directions: *anterograde,* from cell body toward the axon terminal, and *retrograde,* from the axon terminal toward the cell body. *Axoplasmic flow* (*B*) occurs in the anterograde direction only.

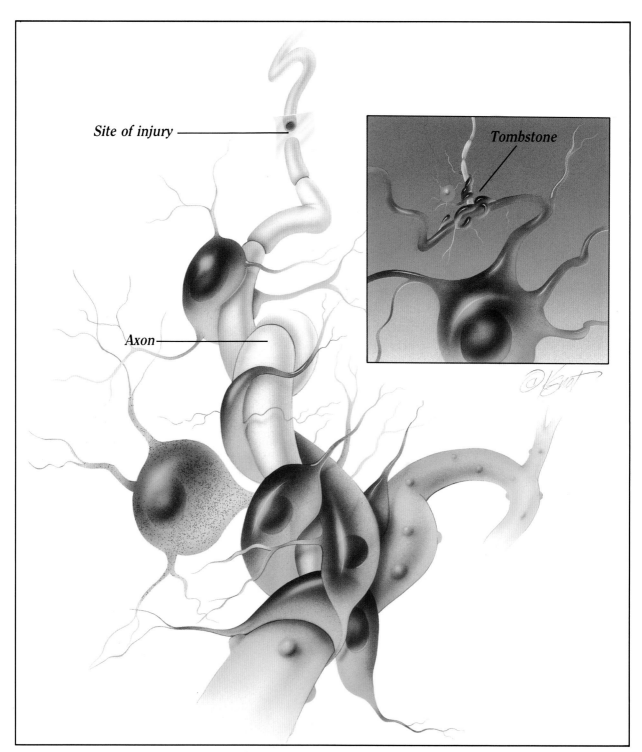

Site of injury

Axon

Tombstone

Figure 1-15. Microglial cells surrounding an axon after traumatic injury. Although microglial cells appear inactive in normal adult brain tissue, they become activated during inflammatory or degenerative processes. These cells are able to undergo rapid proliferation and migrate quickly toward the site of injury to act as macrophages. The nodule (INSET) of microglial cells found where a neuron once lay is called a *tombstone* (traumatic neuroma).

Direct Consequences of Sectioning Axons

When an axon is sectioned by the shearing forces that may accompany either acceleration or deceleration head injuries, the ends of the axon retract from each other and begin to swell. These swollen bulbs are known as *retraction balls* and consist principally of the substances that are ordinarily moved within the cell by axonal transport (Fig. 1-11). The sealed ends of the severed axon prevent the substances from escaping and thus the retraction balls are formed. Both parts of the severed axon swell because the system of rapid transport within the axon occurs in both anterograde and retrograde directions.

With axonal shearing (Fig. 1-16) there is also usually some damage of blood vessels, and in the area of specific damage the axon and the myelin sheath rapidly deteriorate. Macrophages from the general circulation may enter the injured area and remove damaged and degenerating tissue. Glial cells (including both astrocytes and mi-croglia) also act as phagocytes. However, proliferation of fibrous astrocytes also occurs and leads to the formation of a glial scar which, as noted above, may prevent re-establishment of connections within the central nervous system.

The axon degenerates both proximally and distally from the point of sectioning (Fig. 1-17), but the proximal degeneration extends back only for a short distance. Within a few days the effect of the axonal sectioning is seen in the cell body and, if the entire cell dies, degeneration appears at the axon hillock and progresses through the rest of the proximal segment. Degeneration of the distal segment of the axon (called Wallerian degeneration) appears about twenty-four hours after the initial insult, but within two weeks may progress to the axon terminal and thus eliminate synapses with adjoining cells. Wallerian degeneration may continue for two to three months. As this procedure continues degeneration across neurons may occur.

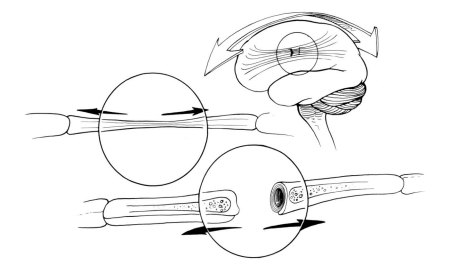

Figure 1-16. Axonal shearing may occur in acceleration as well as deceleration injuries. The nerve fiber may be stretched or completely severed, producing the manifestations of diffuse head injury.

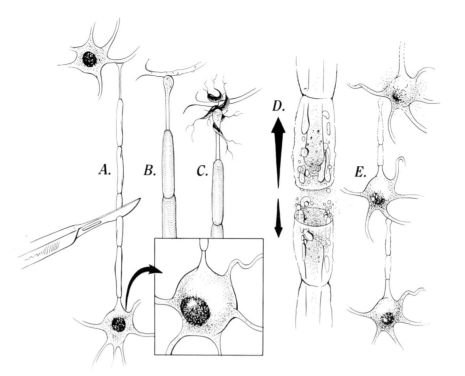

Figure 1-17. This illustration shows the changes which occur in a neuron in response to an injury. When a neuron is severed *(A)*, a series of degenerative processes occur. The neuronal body whose axon is injured shows marked changes (INSET). The cell body swells and becomes distended, the nucleus is displaced toward the periphery, and the Nissl bodies undergo dissolution. Nissl body breakdown begins in the center of the cell and spreads outward *(central chromatolysis)*. A lesion of the axon near the cell body produces a greater central effect than a more distant lesion. In the distal portion of the neuron *(B)*, the axon and myelin sheath completely disintegrate. The process is known as *secondary* or *Wallerian degeneration*. Microglial cells proliferate and migrate to the site of injury *(C)*, frequently interfering with normal regeneration of nerve fibers. At the site of resection *(D)*, the formation of *retraction balls* occurs, probably due to the accumulation of cellular material in the microtubules. Because nutritive material cannot reach cells distal to the injury, these cells may also degenerate *(E)*.

The axon terminal responds very quickly to interference or interruption of transport of materials from the cell body. When the axon is sectioned, the terminal begins to swell and show other changes within twenty-four hours. Within six to seven days proliferating glial cells separate the terminal from adjoining neurons with which synaptic connections had existed.

The next step in this sequence of Wallerian degeneration involves the entire distal portion of the axon and occurs about one week after the appearance of initial degenerative changes in the axon terminal. First, the myelin sheath surrounding the axon draws away and begins to disintegrate. Then the axon swells and becomes beaded, and

structures called *neurofibrils* begin to fill the axon. Glial cells absorb the necrotic material and transport it away from the injured area.

Damage of axons within the central nervous system permits little (if any) functional reconnection because of the interference of the glial cells. However, in peripheral nerve injuries the axon may begin to regenerate if the cell survives and may grow along the connective tissue sheath through which the nerve originally ran. This process may continue to the point that previous synaptic connections are re-established.

Typical changes in the cell body after sectioning of the axon were described briefly above. The first reaction of the cell body is represented by swelling, which may be quite substantial. The nucleus of the cell moves away from a central position, usually opposite to the position of the axon hillock, and may also show evidence of swelling. The rough endoplasmic reticulum in the cell body breaks apart and moves to the periphery of the swollen cell. When the endoplasmic reticulum is stained it appears as Nissl substance.

When axons have been severed, the Nissl substance of the cell body dissolves — a process known as *chromatolysis.* This process may continue for one to three weeks following sectioning of the axon and various biochemical changes occur within the cell body (especially protein synthesis, which may be involved in regenerating the severed parts of the axon). As noted, regeneration may occur in peripheral nerves and appropriate connections may be re-established. In these cases chromatolysis within the cell body discontinues and the cell body regains its usual appearance. However, if the appropriate synaptic connections are not eventually restored, the cell may atrophy and degenerate entirely.

Cells in different locations show various reactions to axonal injury and in some instances do not undergo chromatolysis. For example, Purkinje cells of the cerebellum do not undergo these changes after axonal damage (Fig. 1-18). In addition, animal studies have demonstrated that chromatolysis is more pronounced in younger animals and axonal interruption usually leads to complete degeneration of the cell. In adult animals there is a greater tendency for regeneration of neurons and restitution of the normal condition. Chromatolysis is also more pronounced when the axonal lesion is close to the cell body. For example, peripheral nerves that are sectioned close to the cell body within the central nervous system are more likely to show prolonged chromatolysis and a diminished potential for recovery.

It has been noted that axonal lesions within the central and peripheral nervous systems react somewhat differently. Lesions of neurons within the central nervous system demonstrate chromatolysis after axonal injury, but proliferation of glial cells (resulting in glial scars) inhibit regrowth and restoration of synaptic connections. These circumstances cause severe atrophy and, for neurons within the brain that have sustained axonal damage, result in limited recovery. The role of glial cells following injury of neurons is not fully understood, but it is clear that they function as phagocytes to remove debris and necrotic material.

Glial cells are much more common than neurons. Astrocytes are predominant in the grey matter and oligodendrocytes predominate in the white matter. Oligodendrocytes normally appear to be involved in the formation of myelin in the central nervous system. One oligodendrocyte may contribute to the myelin sheath of as many as twenty axons. After the process of chromatolysis has begun following an injury, glial cells proliferate around chromatolytic neurons.

Besides their phagocytic action, glial cells also appear to intervene between pre-synaptic and post-synaptic elements of the synapse, apparently interrupting the pre-synaptic and post-synaptic connections.

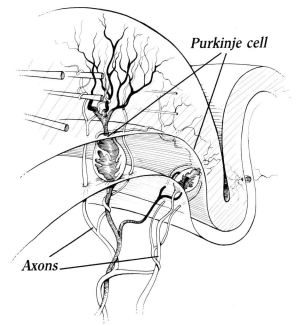

Figure 1-18. A typical Purkinje cell in the cerebellum, showing the ways in which axon collaterals loop from one Purkinje cell to another.

This mechanism leads to a reduction in the number of synapses established by the neuron and in turn is responsible for a reduction in amplitude of evoked response potential in damaged neurons. However, even with reduced synaptic input, chromatolytic neurons can still be activated through activation of remote synapses that previously had not been functionally involved. In addition, new areas of sensitivity develop on the cell body and along the axon. Thus, in some instances, a damaged cell may be able to maintain relatively normal function even when the action of glial cells has reduced the total number of synapses. Compensating mechanisms seem to be important in maintenance of function when axonal damage has led to certain changes which cause initial dysfunction.

Transneuronal Degeneration and Distance Effects

When an axon is severed, trophic (nutritive) effects may have a profound influence on either the organs (muscle and glands) which are innervated by the neuron or on additional neurons in a system which forms synaptic junctions with the terminals of the damaged axon. There is a loss of tone and contractibility when a muscle is deprived of innervation due to destruction of the neuron serving it (Fig. 1-19). The affected muscle fibers lose their functional capability and within a few weeks the affected muscle may demonstrate loss of tissue substance or bulk. The affected muscles may show a striking degree of atrophy, apparently representing severe impairment of normal muscle metabolism. Thus, there is no doubt that normal innervation has a significant effect on the function of effector organs.

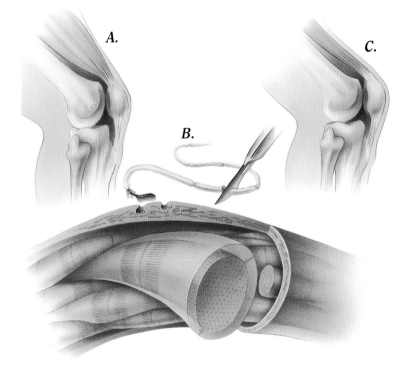

Figure 1-19. An illustration of *secondary* or *Wallerian degeneration.* When a nerve is severed, degenerative changes occur in the proximal as well as the distal portions of the axons. Because nutrients can no longer reach the muscle innervated by the severed fiber, the muscle begins to atrophy. *A,* a healthy thigh muscle before injury; *B,* severance of a neuron, causing degenerative changes in the axon and resulting secondary degeneration in the muscle fiber; *C,* atrophied thigh muscle, which may occur days or weeks after the injury.

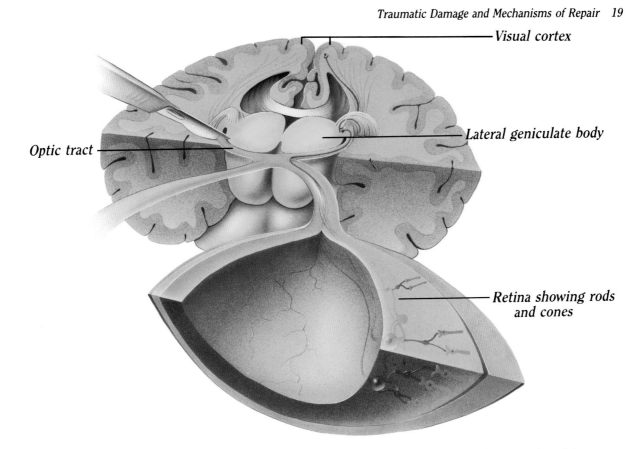

Figure 1-20. Post-synaptic neurons in the lateral geniculate body undergo severe atrophy after sectioning of the optic tract.

Similar distance effects may be noted in neurons organized into a sensory system. In the visual system, for example, two neurons represent the pathway from the retina to the striate cortex. The first of these neurons has receptor organs (rods or cones) in the retina and the axons of these cells join at the optic disc to form the optic nerve. These axons lead to the lateral geniculate body of the thalamus where synapses are formed with the neurons that constitute the geniculostriate tract. These neurons in turn extend from the lateral geniculate body via their axons to the striate cortex of the occipital lobe.

After sectioning of the axons of the optic nerve the terminals of the neurons that originate in the retina show evidence of rapid degeneration in the lateral geniculate body (Fig. 1-20). Several months after sectioning the optic nerve the postsynaptic neurons in the lateral geniculate body undergo severe atrophy. These findings suggest that the neurons which form the geniculostriate tract depend upon stimulation from the neurons that originate in the retina to maintain their normal condition. However, in other systems within the brain this degree of transneuronal degeneration is not prominent.

There is considerable speculation about whether transneuronal degeneration results from elimination of the electrical activity or from trophic influences (which may be necessary for survival of postsynaptic neurons). It is possible that some kind of biochemical substance is released by synaptic terminals which has an effect on the structure and function of the postsynaptic cell. It may be that electrical stimulation as well as trophic influences affect transneuronal degeneration.

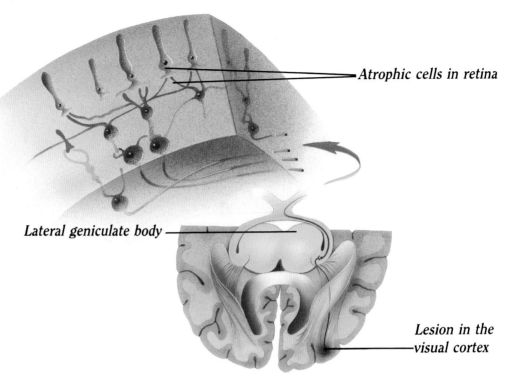

Atrophic cells in retina

Lateral geniculate body

Lesion in the visual cortex

Figure 1-21. Transneuronal degeneration can occur in a retrograde as well as an anterograde direction. A lesion in the visual cortex of the occipital lobe may cause neurons in the lateral geniculate body and the retina to undergo atrophic changes (compare to Figure 1-20).

There are two additional points which should be emphasized. First, transneuronal degeneration may cross more than one synapse and therefore have considerable distance effects. For example, sectioning of the optic nerve within the visual system not only causes degeneration of neurons that originate within the lateral geniculate body, but also has an adverse effect on neurons within the visual cortex, resulting in some degree of degeneration of the visual cortex.

The second point to be established is that transneuronal degeneration can also progress in a retrograde direction. Lesions in the visual cortex cause loss of neurons in the lateral geniculate body and after a few months these losses may be reflected by atrophy of the cells that originate in the retina (Fig. 1-21). It is apparent that damage in one location may have widespread deleterious effects on neuronal function in distant locations.

At this point a brief statement of the short-term consequences of injuries to axons may be given: (1) Axonal damage precipitates adverse structural responses within the cell body; (2) Wallerian degeneration occurs and leads to deterioration of the distal segment of the axon; (3) Impairment of the cell body leads in turn to diminution of synapses; (4) Glial cells respond to the deteriorating and necrotic substance resulting from neuronal injury; and (5) Functional deterioration or death of the neuron leads to transneuronal degeneration, often crossing more than one synapse, and thus having distance effects. Neurons within the central nervous system of the adult are not capable of reproduction or cell division; as a result, damage or death of nerve cells brings about permanent structural limitations.

Mechanisms of Impairment and Mechanisms of Recovery

Although there is no doubt that recovery of brain functions does occur following a cerebral insult or injury, the mechanisms (particularly those concerned with long-term recovery) are very poorly understood. However, some information is available about the mechanisms of impairment or the factors that produce deficit. For example, it has long been observed that sudden insults to the brain result in greater and more profound deficits than comparable damage which occurs as a result of a slower process of destruction. A sudden insult appears to cause more abrupt functional disruption of the brain, does not provide an opportunity for adaptational processes to be employed, and produces more severe losses.

Admittedly, it is difficult to compare immediate damage with slowly progressive damage because of the association between secondary effects and sudden insult. In other words, sudden insults may result in secondary damage, particularly in the form of bleeding and edema, which in turn may make the lesion considerably more extensive and impairing than if the same area of destruction had been a result of a slower process. Nevertheless, acute disruption of function in a normal brain, for whatever reasons, causes much more significant deficit than a slowly progressive process of destruction.

In addition to clinical observations in support of this point, the principle seems to extend to neuropsychological impairment as well as clinical neurological deficit. Hom and Reitan (1984) evaluated neuropsychological correlates of both rapidly growing and slowly growing intrinsic cerebral neoplasms of the left and right cerebral hemispheres. Within the groups there were basically similar degrees of deficit in somatosensory functions depending upon the hemisphere involved. However, the deficits were significantly more profound in persons with rapidly growing intrinsic neoplasms than in persons with slowly growing tumors.

Secondary effects are undoubtedly significant in producing neuropsychological deficits in persons with brain tumors. Such secondary effects can include intracranial hypertension, compression of tissue, metabolic changes and edema, infarction or hemorrhage, and venous obstruction. Rapidly growing and slowly growing tumors may also vary in their degree of necrosis and cystic degeneration. Thus, there is a host of factors that may produce the observed differences, but the generalization still exists. In terms of recovery as well as initial impairment, the full extent of primary and secondary involvement may play a significant role.

Research with animals has also contributed to the understanding of the ways in which the mechanisms of impairment interact with the mechanisms of recovery. Many investigations of cerebral lesions have been done with animals, including production of a single lesion, production of a larger lesion in stages, or production of lesions in various locations according to a time-separated sequence. In general, of course, a principle of mass action is in effect and the principle of equipotentiality of function of cerebral tissue in various locations diminishes in significance as one progresses along the phylogenetic scale, giving way to a principle of regional localization. However, in terms of initial damage, several general principles can be stated: (1) A small lesion produces less deficit than a larger lesion in the same area; (2) A larger lesion, produced suddenly and totally, causes more deficit than a lesion of the same size that is incurred by a step-wise production of the lesion distributed over time. Thus, a lesion produced in stages appears to cause less deficit than a total lesion produced at one time; and (3) Lesions produced in different areas in a time-separated sequence appear to cause less profound impairment than lesions which are effected concurrently.

These observations and experimental results imply that the process of recovery or restitution of function begins almost immediately after the initial insult to the brain. With a slower process of destruction (as contrasted with a sudden insult), the less severe deficits with the slower process imply that recovery mechanisms begin to operate even while the destructive process is continuing. The fact that two-stage operations cause lesser effects than extirpation done in a single stage also implies that the second stage effects are ameliorated by the recovery effects of the first stage. In fact, the basic principle that seems to be operative is that if the insult is distributed in time the overall deficits are less, suggesting that the recovery process has had an opportunity to become initiated at an earlier point. Undoubtedly, the interaction of mechanisms of impairment and recovery are more complicated than implied above, but there does seem to be significant interaction.

Many hypothetical and theoretical explanations for recovery of brain function following insult have been proposed. Wall (1980), who has presented a concise review of these ideas, feels that it is extremely unlikely that mechanisms of mitotic cell duplication or sprouting of destroyed or severed axons, in a manner similar to peripheral nerve regrowth, are significant. Tissue of the liver, kidney, or skin is relatively undifferentiated in its cellular composition and when damage occurs the process of mitotic duplication of cells represents the mechanism of repair. As cells divide through the process of mitosis the new cells migrate and differentiate into functioning cells. However, in the central nervous system there is no evidence of mitotic division of neurons as a response to injury. Sprouting or growth of axons within the central nervous system also seems to be an unlikely explanation.

As noted above, when an axon is sectioned the portion distal to the cell body degenerates. In time the severed end of the proximal portion of the axon emits sprouts which tend to grow and, in the peripheral nervous system, apparently are guided by Schwann cells. This growth continues and may eventually reach the original effector organ with reinstitution of the original function. However, this same mechanism does not occur within the central nervous system. Even though sprouts are emitted from severed axons, glial cells interfere with functional growth necessary to re-establish

the original connections. Thus, in the peripheral nervous system there is a considerable difference between the repair process and regeneration of nerve tissue. Even though the sprouting of injured central axons may establish some connections, the organization of neurons is incorrect, the original input is lost, and meaningful reconnections are minimal. Wall concludes that there is little (if any) evidence for successful regeneration of severed axons in the brain or spinal cord insofar as meaningful reorganization of neuronal contacts are concerned.

However, these considerations do not rule out the possibility that temporary impairment of functional nerve transmission within the central nervous system may be followed by partial or complete recovery. Such a condition is clearly demonstrated by the temporary interference with nerve impulse conduction caused by a local anesthetic agent. Wall also points out that demyelination of the axon may significantly impair transmission of nerve impulses even though some degree of function may remain. Partially demyelinated axons may also be readily subject to adverse influences in other respects and show significant variation in adequacy of nerve transmission (as in patients with multiple sclerosis). In addition, remyelination of axons may also occur, resulting in more adequate function and at least partial recovery. In summary, mitotic cell duplication, which occurs in a number of organs, does not appear to be a viable explanation of recovery of function following injury to the central nervous system. The mechanism of sprouting from the ends of severed axons, which occurs in peripheral nerve regrowth, also seems entirely unlikely as a basis for functional recovery following brain injury.

Wall (1980) points out that "explanations" of recovery following brain injury also suffer from two additional afflictions: (1) A tendency to use technical terminology to name a condition without realizing that naming is not explanation, and (2) A tendency to use technical words that are essentially mystical in character because they refer to conditions which have not been demonstrated and have neuropathological mechanisms which are not understood. As an example of this tendency Wall cites the concept of "post-traumatic amnesia" as an explanation of the failure of head-injured subjects to remember the circumstances of injury. Obviously, any such "explanation" is entirely circular because by definition "post-traumatic amnesia" coincides with inability to remember circumstances of the head injury.

Wall feels that terms such as "shock," "diaschisis," and "disorganization of neural functioning" are terms that fall essentially in this category. Neural shock is used to describe temporary disruption or cessation of nervous system functioning, but the nature of "shock" and its mechanisms are poorly understood. Therefore, use of the term does little to explain the condition in question.

Diaschisis is a term coined by von Monakow (1905) to indicate a condition in which injury to the brain causes a loss of functional continuity between various centers of the brain or neuronal tracts, thus representing distance effects of the primary injury. While edema has been proposed as the pathological change responsible for diaschisis (Kertesz, 1979; Russell, 1981), the mechanisms are so poorly understood that Wall views the term as being mystical. Nevertheless, von Monakow's original conception has been adopted and elaborated upon by some authors (Seron, 1979; Smith, 1979) who differentiate between deficits associated with the initial location of brain damage and deficits resulting from impaired functional continuity with more distant brain centers. The primary deficits caused by the injury are relatively discrete in nature and functionally part of the same configuration of the primary deficit, as contrasted with generalized depression of cerebral activity presumably due to a loss of continuity between centers. Since initial impairment clearly improves in many cases following brain insult, some theory apparently was necessary to "explain" the transient nature of the impairment, and the concept of diaschisis seems to have filled this void.

Some authors (Gazzaniga, 1974; Laurence & Stein, 1978) have postulated that diaschisis is the mechanism of impairment with initial depression of functions which then recover spontaneously. Other authors (e.g., Smith, 1981) postulate that diaschisis, because of its disruption of neural networks (distance effects), may result in permanent changes in functions that are not directly associated with the location of the initial lesion. Obviously, these details of "explanation" suffer in terms of credibility when the condition itself is hypothetical (if not, as described by Wall, mystical).

Wall (1980) also takes exception to explanations of recovery following brain injury that involve the concept of redundancy of neural tissue. He points out that the notion of redundancy, in terms of central nervous system functioning, generally implies the existence of alternate systems or circuits in the brain which can "take over" functions that were impaired in the original system or circuitry. A second notion of redundancy may possibly relate to compensatory systems or mechanisms which may be initiated following damage to the substrate, but such a concept of redundancy does not change the fact that the original deficit is still present. In this latter concept redundancy merely refers to a method or manner of adapting to the original deficit by using, for example, muscle groups for performance of an activity (even though in an impaired fashion) that were originally subserved by the damaged system.

The concept of redundancy of brain tissue is widely known and referred to frequently. There have been numerous claims that only a small fraction of the large number of neurons in the brain are actually used. The redundancy concept presumes that there is a substantial number of neurons essentially "in reserve," ready to become active when the original system of neurons is damaged or destroyed. There is, in fact, evidence indicating that such a system, which implies a significant degree of plasticity or interchangeability of functions for neurons in various parts of the brain, may exist in the developmental process of the immature organism. Thus, children with a totally atrophic or amputated cerebral hemisphere may still develop some of the cognitive functions that would normally be subserved by the absent cerebral hemisphere. In other words, the neuropsychological effects of a damaged or limited immature brain may be quite different from the effects of a lesion imposed on a mature or adult brain. In addition, the process of developing cognitive abilities with a damaged or limited brain is quite different from the process of developing such abilities with a normal brain (Reitan, 1985b).

Wall (1980) argues against the concept of redundancy to explain recovery principally on the basis that alternative systems or circuits in the brain, which can be activated when the initial system fails, have not been documented in terms of basic neuroanatomy or neurophysiology. However, it should be noted that there is some evidence to support the hypothesis that regions within a cerebral hemisphere which perform related functions may permit substantially better recovery when the entire region is not destroyed than when destruction is total (Penfield & Roberts, 1959; Reitan & Wolfson, 1985b).

Wall feels that the redundancy theory is entirely inadequate to explain the loss of previously acquired abilities. He points out, for example, that in the slow destruction of peripheral nerve tissue in leprosy the process of destruction must extend to over 50% of the neurons before clinical manifestations appear. He feels that such evidence is weak because the clinical tests used to measure performance fail to test the limits of the underlying neural system and, as a result, very possibly fail to demonstrate deficits that could have been demonstrated with more sensitive procedures.

Exactly the same kind of objection to the "redundancy" explanations of recovery following brain injury apply with respect to neuropsychological testing. In years past certain areas of the cerebral cortex have been identified as being "silent" (or at most representing "association tissue" with the nature of the "associations" being unspecified). The fact that these areas have not been shown to have specified and recognized functions does not serve as a basis for concluding that they have no identifiable functions. It must be remembered that

"absence of evidence is not evidence of absence." Because evidence for the function of these association areas has not been produced does not mean that such evidence will never be discovered. More specifically, it would be advantageous for scientific theory to develop with a greater degree of cognitive sophistication than that represented by the child who complains that he has no socks because he is not able to find them.

The development of neuropsychological evaluation of brain functions bears out the fact that there are both general and more specific types of function subserved by the cerebral cortex (Reitan & Wolfson, 1985a; Reitan & Wolfson, 1986b), and the problem in the past has been that an adequately comprehensive examination of brain-behavior relationships has not been available. Such techniques have now been developed, represented particularly by the Halstead-Reitan Neuropsychological Test Battery, and even small lesions located in the so-called "association" areas reflect significant evidence of neuropsychological impairment. In fact, examinations of thousands of patients with careful neurological and neurosurgical evaluation of the brain include few instances in which persons with identified cerebral cortical lesions fail to show evidence of neuropsychological deficits. Thus, except for a greater degree of equipotentiality of cerebral tissue in immature brains during the developmental period, the possibility of redundancy of brain tissue as an explanation for recovery following neuropsychological deficit does not seem to be plausible.

Wall (1980) points out that there is a category of explanation for recovery of functions, *partial secondary solutions,* which does not demonstrate relevance to the long-term recovery process. The principal consideration in this regard refers to temporary impairment of brain tissue resulting from pathological influences in which eventual full recovery of function ensues.

Impairment can be caused by many types of pathology, and even though brain tissue may be totally destroyed in certain areas, there are boundary areas in which the damage and impairment is at least partially reversible. It is not reasonable to propose, for example, that every brain lesion causes either irreversible death of nerve cells or no impairment whatsoever. In any lesion of the brain many nerve cells must certainly occupy an intermediate position of damage which may result in death of the cells or in partial or complete recovery.

In the case of a cerebral thrombosis, for example, the area of the brain which is principally involved will sustain irreversible ischemic damage and necrosis. However, the cells surrounding this area will be involved to a differential degree (as far as morphological damage is concerned) and will continue to have a degree of supporting function, particularly relating to blood supply. These cells may recover as new capillaries gradually form and establish collateral blood supply, and the involved tissue may return to relatively normal function. Beyond this area of tissue that is impaired but not totally destroyed the nerve cells can be expected to be unaffected and totally normal.

Most kinds of brain lesions are probably similar in terms of having an area of principal destruction and pathology and an area of damaged but not totally destroyed tissue which eventually extends into normal tissue. This is almost certainly true, despite the definite distance effects which occur on a transneuronal basis or, with many lesions, on a secondary basis. Even conditions which are not represented by focal lesions must be considered to have the potential for impairment of nerve tissue with eventual return of function.

In toxic encephalopathy, for example, nerve tissue may be impaired or totally destroyed in its function. However, as the toxin is reduced one would necessarily expect some recovery of function. Viral encephalitis represents a similar kind of situation. In the case of brain trauma it is extremely likely that the injury may cause temporary impairment of some tissue with eventual recovery of function, even when other areas of the brain are totally and permanently destroyed.

Problems exist, however, with the concept of temporary and reversible impairment of brain tissue following disease or damage. The first of these concerns is that the repair processes which are currently known relate particularly to vascular and metabolic changes. In turn, these changes involve short-term repair and recovery processes which are probably essentially complete within weeks of sustaining the initial damage. Therefore, the long-term improvement shown by many individuals (including persons who have sustained permanent and irreversible cerebral damage) is not explained.

The basic unexplained problem concerns the continuing long-term recovery that is routinely seen after an insult to the brain. Any explanation for the long-term recovery process can hardly appeal to the vascular and metabolic changes that represent the immediate repair process following a brain insult. In fact, at present there are only vague hypotheses about the biological bases of the long-term recovery process. Obviously, the short-term changes cannot be used to explain the spontaneous recovery that may extend over a period of many months.

Possible Mechanisms of Long-term Recovery of Functions

As mentioned above, collateral sprouting within the central nervous system has been proposed as a mechanism for long-term recovery of functions (Raisman & Field, 1973). In brief, when axons within the central nervous system are severed, the terminal synaptic regions are disconnected from the neuron and do not have input (Fig. 1-14). However, nearby intact axons seem to be able to respond in some manner to the presence of these evacuated synaptic regions and send out sprouts which occupy them (Fig. 1-22). Thus, the synaptic regions, which have been separated from their previous axonal connections, are again activated. This mechanism is distinctly advantageous in the peripheral nervous system because of the common function, concerned with muscular contraction, that is served.

Within the central nervous system, however, the situation is much more complex and the tasks subserved by axons which are close to each other

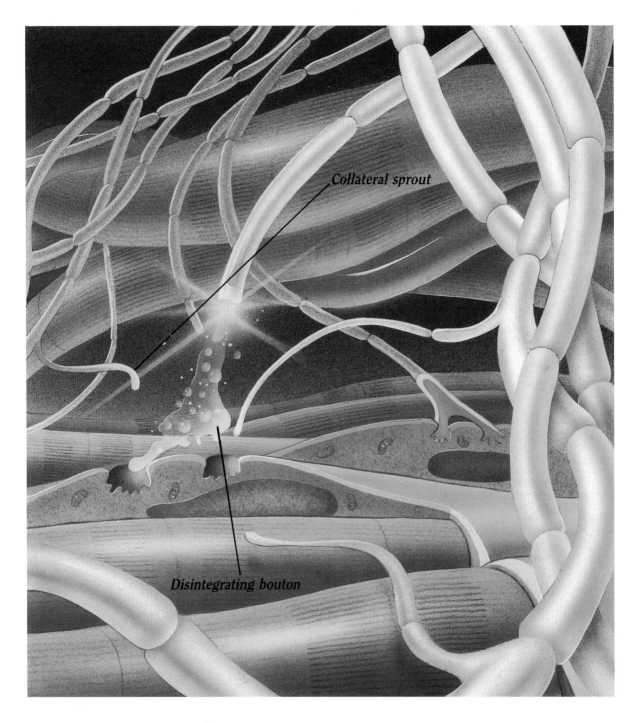

Figure 1-22. When an axon is severed, degeneration occurs proximal and distal to the injury. In this illustration the distal end of the axon is shown disintegrating, leaving the synaptic regions served by that axon available to be occupied by sprouts of nearby axons.

may be quite different. Therefore, a different function may be produced if sprouting from a nearby axon reactivates an empty synaptic region. There is a question of whether formation of nerve sprouts contribute to restoration of initial function or introduce deviant or even disadvantageous functions. Nevertheless, the evidence indicates that nearby axons may produce sprouts to occupy evacuated terminal synaptic regions and must be considered a possible structural basis for recovery of function.

There are additional questions regarding adaption to damage which may be relevant to long-term recovery of function. Wall and his colleagues have found evidence that circumstances which decrease input activity may result in a compensatory increase of excitability. In other words, it may be possible that synapses which have not been destroyed by a lesion can be brought to a state of increased action through mechanisms which are not fully understood.

It appears that there is some type of homeostatic mechanism whereby a partial loss of input produces a compensatory reaction which permits the diminished input to have an increased synaptic effectiveness. Regardless of whether this increase is brought about by morphological change, a change of substances transported along the axon, or other physiological mechanisms, an increased excitability within the central nervous system, stemming from a decrease of input activity, would represent an adjustment that could be of considerable significance concerning the recovery process.

In a series of experiments Wall and his colleagues created situations in cats in which afferent input to a region of the brain was partially destroyed or reduced. Their studies indicated that in every instance the cerebral cells which had lost their input began to respond to afferent systems which had not been impaired. Apparently the connection to the denervated zone had initially been inhibited in these intact afferent systems, but as soon as the major (normal) input was removed the inhibition was also removed and a new excitatory

pathway was created (Fig. 1-23). In some instances the response to intact afferent systems was almost immediate; in other instances days or weeks were necessary for the new receptive field to reach a full state of excitability.

The process by which normally ineffective input becomes effective is difficult to answer. Induced neuronal sprouting may play some role in longer-term reactions, but it seems perhaps more likely that unknown processes of reduction of inhibitory mechanisms come into play and permit the emergence of existing contacts. However, normally ineffective afferent input does appear to become operational and there seems to be a trans-synaptic diminution of inhibitory mechanisms which permits the function of a new excitatory pathway to emerge.

Wall and his colleagues (Dostrovosky, Millar, & Wall, 1976) have also studied the effects of cutting peripheral nerve fibers on the function of cells within the spinal cord. Clusters of cells within the spinal cord were identified with receptive fields in the leg of the cat. Within days or weeks after sectioning of the peripheral nerve, the cell cluster within the spinal cord began to respond to input from other areas of the leg. Under these circumstances, with input from the periphery diminished, one would hardly postulate axonal sprouting as a mechanism for establishing these new connections. The diminution of impulses resulting from the section of peripheral nerve may have led to the change in receptiveness, or there may have been some influence caused by transport mechanisms into the spinal cord via dorsal routes.

Nevertheless, the adaptability of function within the central nervous system following reduction of peripheral input demonstrated the remarkable capacity of the central nervous system to adapt to peripheral injury. As a response or adaptation to injury, it appears that the central nervous system undergoes very subtle changes in function that may underlie the process by which function returns.

In summary, Wall points out that nerve cells show a type of homeostatic response which permits

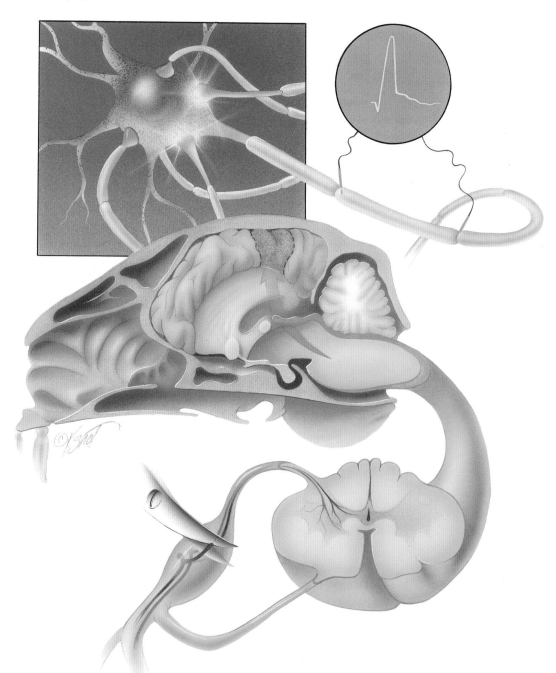

Figure 1-23. In the Wall et al. experiments the afferent input pathway to a region in a cat's brain was partially destroyed. The damaged cerebral cells (which had lost their input) began to respond to unimpaired afferent systems, establishing a new excitatory pathway.

them to adjust their excitability or augment excitatory effects when input is reduced. Sprouting may occur when nerve fibers have been damaged and have left terminal synaptic regions vacant. Nerve connections which are not normally operative may become active if the usual afferent input is diminished or destroyed. Both sprouting and unmasking of ineffective connections, as a response to injury, may constitute mechanisms whereby long-term recovery of functions is possible following injury.

Recapitulation of the Effects and Reactions to Traumatic Brain Injury

The types of damage a brain may sustain as a result of trauma are well documented. Primary or direct damage to brain tissue occurs as a result of the initial impact and is represented by injury to neurons, supporting cells, and blood vessels. Significant blows to the head routinely result in generalized and widespread cerebral damage as well as focal damage. Primary damage may result from penetration, pressure gradients, and rotational and shearing forces (especially involving areas where the brain is compressed within the skull or where the brain has been torn over rough surfaces on the inner surface of the skull) (Fig. 1-24).

Secondary effects of primary damage may also occur and result in further serious and significant damage. Secondary damage is caused by bleeding and edema. Bleeding may be focal, as in hemorrhages and contusions, or may be in the form of widespread petechial hemorrhages. Brain edema may be relatively focal and clearly involve one cerebral hemisphere more than the other, but often the swelling is rather widespread in nature. Because the skull is an inflexible structure, swelling of cerebral tissue in one area displaces tissue in some other area and may result in permanent and even fatal consequences. Tearing of brain tissue over the tentorium as a result of brain edema, compression of tissues, and even displacement of brain tissues through the foramen magnum all represent important mechanisms of secondary damage (Fig. 1-25).

In addition to the primary and secondary pathological effects of brain trauma, adverse influences on cellular mechanisms may also occur. As described above, these involve particularly the interruption of axonal transport and axoplasmic flow within the neuron. This impairment of normal metabolic functions causes changes within the cell body and degeneration of axons and dendrites. These metabolic changes may be sufficiently severe to cause death of the neuron. Impairment of function or death of the neuron affects synaptic interactions by limiting mediation of both electrical signals and nutritive (trophic) interactions between neurons. Thus, damage to the neuron as well as impairment of its synaptic interactions may result in atrophy and degenerative changes in other neurons that receive synapses from the damaged neurons. As researchers have demonstrated (particularly in the sequence of neurons that constitute the visual system), these transneuronal changes have adverse effects at distant sites.

Supporting cells, which consist mainly of glial cells (oligodendrocytes, astrocytes, ependymal cells, and microglia) proliferate following injury and are involved in absorbing the cellular debris and toxic products of degeneration and necrosis. These cells function as phagocytes and in this sense have the positive effect of removing damaged and necrotic tissue. However, the proliferation of these supporting cells also creates a problem. Within the central nervous system as well as the peripheral nervous system there is a tendency for neurons to regenerate and attempt to re-establish connections that were disrupted by the injury. Within the central nervous system the proliferation of glial cells tends to block effective restoration of synaptic connections. In other words, the rapid proliferation of glial cells interferes with the ability of damaged neurons to re-establish their prior connections. This fact has led to the often stated conclusion that functional regeneration within the central nervous system is not possible. Nevertheless, there definitely are short-term recovery functions represented by biological repair (especially in the form of redevelopment of vascularization and diminution of swelling) that may lead to a restoration of physiologic processes. Restored vascularization particularly may result in improved cerebral oxygenation and recovery of tissue that has been damaged but not destroyed.

Thus, the short-term biological recovery and repair processes definitely can serve as a basis for improvement of function of the damaged brain tissue. However, these processes are essentially completed in a relatively short time, usually within

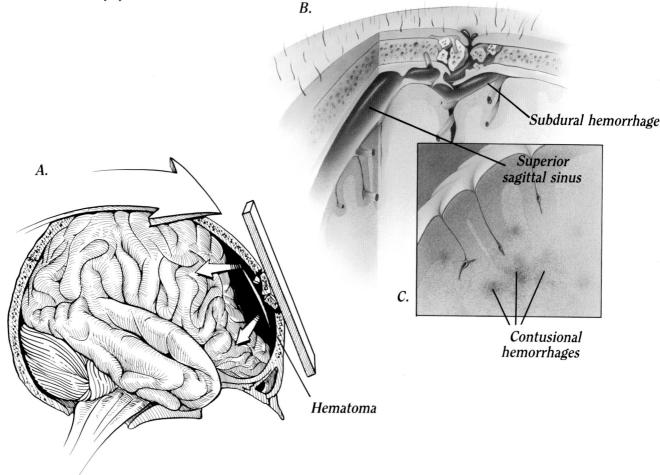

Figure 1-24. *A,* A blow to the head may cause inward deformation or fracture of the skull at the site of the blow, and the force of the blow may be directed to the underlying cortex. If the fracture causes laceration of an artery, blood will collect and form a convex mass (hematoma) that indents the brain. The cranial vault can accommodate up to 75 cc of extra volume without showing any clinical symptoms. Beyond this volume, symptoms occur abruptly and may result in a catastrophic outcome. *B, Subdural hemorrhage* occurs in 5% of the patients who sustain a head injury. In most cases the bridging veins that extend from the cerebrum to the dura are torn where they enter the superior sagittal sinus. The volume of subdural hematomas varies. The rapidity with which the volume increases is more important than the absolute volume. *C, Contusional hemorrhages* are discrete hemorrhages in the gray or white matter. They range in size from 3-4 mm to 1-2 cm. Hemorrhages result from shearing or tearing of the blood vessels.

one month or less. In fact, in many persons who have sustained a brain injury these processes are probably essentially complete either by the time the patient is ready for discharge from the hospital or soon afterwards. Nevertheless, as experienced clinicians have observed, the recovery of functions and general improvement of intellectual and cognitive abilities continues for a much longer period of time. This latter process of improvement may be referred to as *long-term recovery,* and relatively little is known about its biological basis.

Long-term Recovery

Theories abound whenever there is a paucity of facts. There is ample evidence that recovery from the impairment associated with brain damage actually does occur over an extended period of time. It is difficult to dissociate spontaneous or unassisted recovery (which presumably occurs on a biological basis) from facilitated recovery (which can result from either a specifically designed and structured brain retraining program or the influences of the general environment).

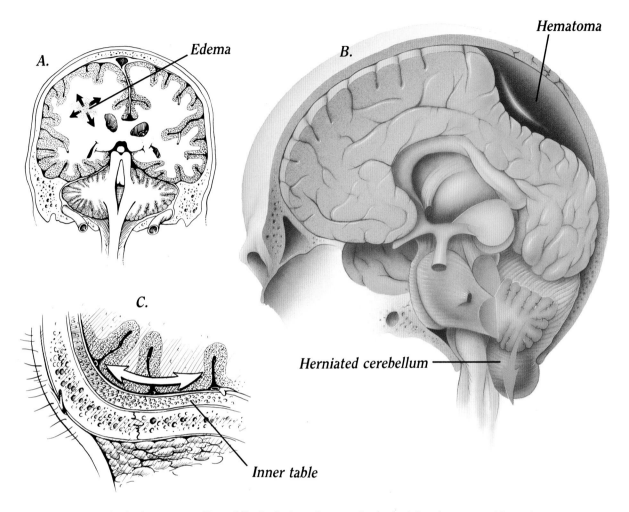

Figure 1-25. *A, Cerebral edema,* or *swelling of the brain,* is an increase in the brain's volume caused by an increase in the brain's fluid content. As the edema increases the gyri become flattened, the sulci narrow, and the ventricles narrow and are displaced to the opposite side. *B,* Herniation of the cerebellar tonsils into the foramen magnum (*tonsillar herniation*) may result from a hematoma. An acute increase of 150 cc or more is almost invariably associated with herniation. In this type of herniation the tonsils of the cerebellum are forcibly compressed around the medulla. Vital functions are lost as the medulla is pushed ventrally against the clivus and the edge of the foramen magnum. *C,* Edema may displace the cerebral spinal fluid and cause the gyral crests to be abraded by the rough inner table of the skull.

Although animal studies provide some data suggesting that axonal sprouting and restoration of synapses may occur to some degree, it is very doubtful that these mechanisms can be fully responsible for the degree of recovery that often occurs in individual cases. This recovery gradient has generally been considered to be progressive in nature, with the major recovery occurring during the first several months following the cerebral insult or injury and a gradual progression of the recovery curve to an asymptotic level.

In this volume (Chapter III) evidence is presented for the first time that this recovery curve is not continuously progressive. Instead, it appears to be biphasic in nature, at least for persons who sustain primary or secondary tissue damage as a result of the injury. The biological basis for this deterioration of abilities, which tends to occur in the same behavioral areas as the initial deficit and the initial spontaneous recovery, is presently unknown. It is probable that some type of gliotic reaction occurs in the long-term recovery period (more than one year after the injury) and is responsible for this reversal of the recovery curve. Further pathological studies will be necessary in order to identify the biological changes that are responsible for the long-term regression of abilities.

Theories of long-term recovery (as opposed to mechanisms such as neuronal sprouting and augmented neuronal excitability due to reduced input) center around two principal postulates: (1) Neuropsychological recovery depends upon and makes use of the remaining brain tissue which has not been fully destroyed and still subserves the general cognitive ability that has been impaired, and (2) Recovery depends upon redundant brain tissue, which presumably has not been fully utilized, and therefore is available to subsume the function that was impaired by the injury. The first of these postulates can be referred to as the *alternative brain tissue hypothesis;* the second represents the *redundant brain tissue hypothesis.*

The *alternative brain tissue hypothesis* presumes that cognitive functions originally subserved by the destroyed cerebral tissue may be gradually acquired by uninjured adjacent tissue which was involved in functions similar to the functions of the destroyed area (Fig. 1-26, A). For example, Penfield and Roberts (1959) have observed in adults that a relatively large area of the cerebral cortex of the left cerebral hemisphere is specifically involved in language functions. When only part of this "language" area of the cerebral cortex has been destroyed, the remaining tissue involved in language functions is available to subsume the impaired functions and thus provide a biological basis for the recovery that occurs.

Roberts (1958) has presented some evidence suggesting that the potential for recovery of language functions in an adult is greatly reduced if the entire language area is destroyed. Only those persons who have remaining functional tissue in the language area are good candidates for significant recovery of language functions, apparently regardless of the biological status of remaining tissue in the left cerebral hemisphere or the bio-

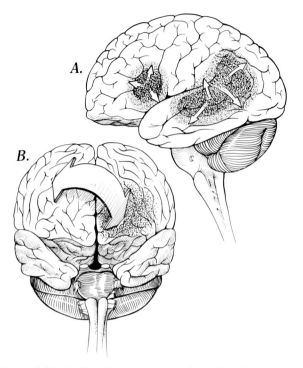

Figure 1-26. *A, The alternative brain tissue hypothesis* assumes that undamaged tissue surrounding an area of injury will eventually take over the functions of the injured area. *B, The redundant brain tissue hypothesis* postulates that tissue even in the non-damaged hemisphere will be able to assume the functions of the injured tissue.

logical condition of the right cerebral hemisphere.

The *alternative brain tissue hypothesis* rather obviously does not include a specific role for tissue of the other cerebral hemisphere in the recovery process, and in this respect observes the specialization of right and left cerebral functions. However, for those intellectual and cognitive functions that are diffusely distributed throughout the cerebral cortex, one would presume that this theory would permit all of the remaining cerebral cortex to be involved in the recovery process. If the remaining cortex were unimpaired biologically, one would further postulate that all of this remaining tissue would increase the prospect of recovery of the diffusely distributed abilities in comparison with those abilities that are dependent upon more focal (limited) areas of cerebral cortex. Although some investigators have hypothesized that certain cognitive abilities recover more rapidly than others, no research has been done comparing the recovery rate between focal and diffusely distributed neuropsychological functions. We would postulate that no clear difference would emerge if such a study were conducted.

The *redundant brain tissue hypothesis* postulates a potential for a much more general reorganization of brain functions following a head injury. According to this hypothesis distant brain tissue (even in the non-damaged hemisphere) will assume some or all of the lost or impaired functions as the recovery process progresses (Fig. 1-26, B). There is substantial evidence that in children the unaffected cerebral hemisphere can assume a significant role in cognitive development, even including abilities that would normally be the function of the damaged or impaired cerebral hemisphere. In adults, however, it appears that the organization of brain-behavior relationships is much more firmly established (crystalized), and the potential for involvement of distant brain tissue in recovery of a specific function is less likely or perhaps even impossible.

It is interesting to note that these two theories of recovery of functions following brain damage are closely related to theoretical conceptualizations of brain-behavior relationships. The history of theorizing in this area has ranged from extreme positions of equipotentiality to postulates of localization of functions represented by a patchwork mapping of each function within its delimited cortical area (see Reitan & Wolfson, 1985b for a more complete review and critical evaluation of these various theories of brain-behavior relationships).

Many investigators have adopted an intermediate theoretical position, postulating that certain abilities have a regionally localized substrate and other abilities are generally distributed throughout the cerebral cortex. Motor and sensory-perceptual functions are probably the most strictly localized abilities with language and verbal skills representing the next degree of localization.

A number of investigators have described language abilities and visual-spatial and manipulatory skills as being differentially represented in the left and right cerebral hemispheres (Reitan, 1955b; Wheeler & Reitan, 1962). These studies suggest that visual-spatial skills are most heavily depen-

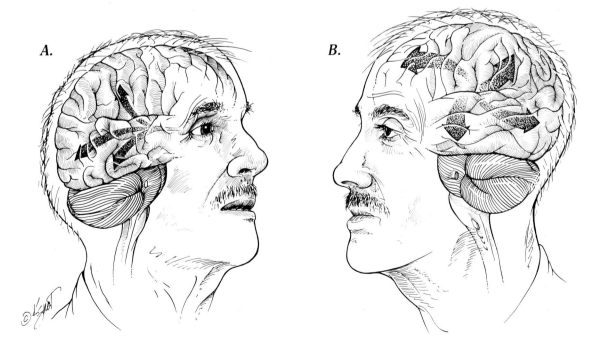

Figure 1-27. *A*, Visual-spatial skills appear to be most dependent on the posterior cortex of the right cerebral hemisphere. *B*, Research studies have indicated that concept formation, reasoning and logical analysis skills are diffusely represented throughout the cerebral cortex.

dent upon the posterior cortex (parietal, occipital, and posterior temporal areas) of the right cerebral hemisphere. Although considerable emphasis has been given to localizing abstraction, reasoning, and logical analysis skills in the anterior parts of both frontal lobes, our investigations indicate that these abilities are diffusely represented throughout the cerebral cortex (Reitan & Wolfson, 1985a; Reitan & Wolfson, 1986b) (Fig. 1-27).

Considering the differential and specialized functions of the two cerebral hemispheres, the redundant brain tissue hypothesis appears to be somewhat less likely than the alternative brain tissue hypothesis concerning recovery of function after a brain insult. The former theory is more closely related to a equipotentiality concept of brain-behavior relationships and the latter is more closely aligned with a regional-localization hypothesis. As noted above, a considerable amount of evidence suggests that the equipotentiality notion is probably much more relevant in development of brain-behavior relationships through the childhood years and that a regional-localization hypothesis is more reflective of the status of the adult brain. The theory of Reitan and Wolfson invokes both of these concepts for different categories of neuropsychological functioning in the adult (Reitan & Wolfson, 1986b).

Finally, the redundant brain tissue hypothesis has had basic support from the presumption that many neurons in the brain have no particular function but in effect represent unused tissue. Most persons have heard the contention that a large proportion of nerve cells in the brain have no specific function largely because of failure to develop ("exercise") the brain through environmental experiences. It is entirely possible that this notion developed largely because investigators were unable to determine the function of certain areas of the brain and labeled these areas "association" areas without specification of the "associations" that they served.

As neuropsychological investigative work has developed, researchers have gradually learned more about the particular functions of these "association" areas and determined that they subserve significant abilities that are quite different from those subserved by other areas. Using the Halstead-Reitan Battery to study thousands of persons with unequivocal evidence of brain lesions (including very small lesions in some instances), we have found that essentially all of these persons show some degree of impairment, either in general or specific neuropsychological functions, regardless of the particular location of the lesion. In other words, now that we know how to identify and measure the functions that are represented by the brain generally and specifically, we rarely (if ever) find persons with definitely identified brain lesions who do not show significant neuropsychological deficits, regardless of how small the lesion may be. It appears, then, that cerebral cortical tissue is functionally occupied in a neuropsychological sense regardless of its location and that the redundant brain tissue hypothesis is not likely to be generally tenable. A considerable amount of evidence is available, for example, to demonstrate that when a child has sustained an extensive lesion of one cerebral hemisphere early in life that the child's developing abilities are generally compromised, since the remaining cerebral hemisphere by itself is not sufficient to subserve the entire ability structure.

Obviously these comments do not provide a comprehensive explanation of recovery of functions following insult, damage, and destruction of brain tissue. As we noted at the beginning of this section, the biological bases of long-term recovery are poorly understood and will require much research before all aspects of this phenomenon are completely appreciated.

II

PROGNOSIS AND OUTCOME FOLLOWING BRAIN INJURY

When to Assess Outcome

Jennett and Teasdale (1981) have raised the question of when outcome should be assessed in the individual patient and have correctly recognized that the answer to this question depends upon two factors: (1) How detailed a categorization of outcome is required, and (2) The nature and duration of spontaneous recovery. An additional factor, of course, relates to the influence of brain-training programs on eventual recovery and outcome. Obviously, if outcome is to be assessed after the entire recovery process is completed, there will be a great deal of variation from one patient to another. This is particularly true if outcome is assessed in detail concerning eventual neuropsychological status as well as social and vocational recovery.

Jennett & Teasdale (1981) indicate the importance of the outcome categories that are considered. In some studies the question has only been one of death versus survival. By the time the patient is ready for discharge from intensive care it is usually possible to determine confidently whether he/she will survive long term, although some patients may remain in a persistent vegetative state for a considerable period of time before they expire.

There may be no definitive method to predict the eventual outcome and quality of life of the head injury victim, but some studies have related the period of time following the injury to results obtained with the Glasgow Outcome Scale (see pp. 60–62). Jennett, Teasdale, Galbraith, et al. (1977) reported on a sample of 534 head-injured persons who had survived 3 months after the injury and were then evaluated at 6 and 12 months post injury. Between the third month and the twelfth month the results indicated gradual progression from categories of *Vegetative State, Severe Disability,* and *Moderate Disability* to the category of *Good Recovery.* While 7% of this sample had been classified in the *Vegetative State* 3 months after the injury, the percentage had dropped to 5% at the time of the 6-month evaluation and declined to 3% by the 12-month examination. Subjects with a classification of *Severe Disability* at 3 months post-injury showed a rather striking reduction at 6 months (from 29% to 19%), with only a mild additional reduction (from 19% to 16%) at 12 months. Persons with *Moderate Disability* represented 33% of the sample at 3 months, 34% at 6 months, and 31% at 12 months post-injury.

The failure to achieve a reduction in the percentage of subjects in the *Moderate Disability* group at the 6-month and 12-month intervals reflected the improvement of patients who initially were more severely disabled. However, the *Good Recovery* category, limited by the end of the scale, showed substantial increments at each later evaluation, rising from 31% at 3 months to 42% at 6 months and 50% at 12 months.

In terms of the Glasgow Outcome Scale, a total of 64% of the head-injured subjects had achieved *Moderate Disability* or *Good Recovery* 3 months after the injury. This percentage had risen to 76% at 6 months and to 81% at 12 months. These authors noted that of the patients who had achieved a classification of *Good Recovery* or *Moderate Disability* by 12 months, two-thirds had already reached this level within 3 months of the injury and 90% had done so within 6 months.

Jennett, Snoek, Bond, and Brooks (1981) found that 10% of their sample (150 patients) who were classified in the categories *Severe Disability* or *Moderate Disability* at 6 months improved to the category of *Moderate Disability* or *Good Recovery* within 12 months. Eighty-two of these patients were followed for more than 18 months and only 5% were able to be reclassified into a category better than the one in which they were placed at 12 months. However, these authors recognize that these three categories of disability are broad in nature and that a degree of improvement may continue to occur even though the patient does not meet the criteria for a change of category. In fact, when a six-category scale was used instead of a three-category scale, between the 6-month and 12-month examinations nearly twice as many patients showed improvement significant enough to be reclassified. Thus, it is clear that gradual and progressive recovery may occur which can be revealed only by more refined assessment than that customarily provided by the Glasgow Outcome Scale.

Jennett and Teasdale (1981) conclude that (1) Most of the recovery that will be achieved by an individual patient will occur within the first 6 months following the injury, (2) It is usually possible to maintain contact with the majority of patients over this period of time for purposes of standardized assessment of outcome, and (3) Six months after the injury has occurred is an appropriate time for outcome assessment. They also cite the study by Roberts (1980) in which persons who had sustained severe head injuries were followed for 20 years. Roberts found that almost all subjects who had made good recoveries had done so within the first 6 months post-injury.

In contrast to these studies, our findings suggest that recovery of higher-level neuropsychological functions continues for a much longer period (although at a decreasing rate), and that there may well be a difference between recovery criteria oriented toward neurological findings and criteria oriented toward neuropsychological capabilities. In fact, Jennett, Snoek, Bond, and Brooks (1981) indicate that at 6 months post-injury they found no neurological abnormalities in 25% of persons who had sustained a severe head injury. In cases of severe head injury it is unusual to see full recovery (no impairment) of neuropsychological functions within this time period.

It can be seen, then, that the question of when to assess outcome may vary with the type of examination. An assessment 6 months post-injury may be appropriate to determine the physical neurological condition and the results of the Glasgow Outcome Scale. However, if questions regarding outcome are oriented toward neuropsychological, social, and vocational recovery, a considerably longer period of time may be more appropriate.

Dikmen, Reitan, and Temkin (1983) used measures from the Halstead-Reitan Neuropsychological Test Battery to study 27 patients with a head injury (2 subjects with penetrating injuries, 11 with brain contusion, and 14 with concussion). The patients were usually examined within one month following the head injury and re-examined at 12-month and 18-month intervals. Of the 12 neuropsychological measures that were used, 9 showed no differential recovery rate between the first year and the 12-month and the 18-month interval; however, those subjects who initially demonstrated more severe impairment showed a greater absolute degree of recovery than the persons who had initially demonstrated lesser impairment.

The results of this investigation, which showed little evidence for a decreasing rate of recovery over time, would raise questions about the many reports in the literature that claim that the greatest degree of recovery occurs during the first 6 months or, at most, during the first year post-injury. Admittedly, however, it is difficult to answer this question on the basis of statistical analyses of differences in the slope of the recovery curve at different time periods following head injury, especially since some degree of variability must be expected and all the changes are essentially in the direction of improvement.

Ideally, to assess recovery following a serious head injury, repeated evaluations should be made over a minimum of 18 months. Using neuropsychological tests for this purpose has been complicated by the occurrence of practice-effects with repeated testings, but this problem may be attenuated if the Halstead-Reitan Battery is used and the test scores are converted to Neuropsychological Deficit Scale scores (see Chapter III).

The Medical Orientation Toward Outcome

In terms of a medical approach, evaluation of outcome following traumatic head injury is probably best represented by the criteria used in the Glasgow Outcome Scale. As noted previously, the categories of the Glasgow Outcome Scale include *Death, Vegetative State, Severe Disability, Moderate Disability,* and *Good Recovery.* Even though the category of *Good Recovery* specifies that the subject has not necessarily returned to normal in all functions and that there may be persisting sequelae (such as bilateral anosmia or mild impairment on some psychological tests), the patient

must be able to participate in normal social life activities and have the ability to return to work. It should be recognized that the categories of *Good Recovery* and *Moderate Disability* include many patients with significant neuropsychological deficits that may be of critical significance concerning the patient's potential for achieving his/her pre-injury quality of life.

Becker, Miller, and Greenberg (1982) state a concerned but limited conceptualization of outcome. They feel that it is important to identify categories of outcome (as the Glasgow Outcome Scale does), and that such categories should cover the full range of outcome in head-injured patients; however, the categories should still be general enough to provide "sufficiently large numbers in each group to provide accurate statistical analysis."

From the above criterion it is apparent that for these authors the orientation concerning outcome is to provide a basis for grouping which will permit statistical evaluation of data. It is noteworthy that this aim neglects entirely any requirement that procedures for assessing outcome reflect the unique aspects of recovery, as well as remaining deficits, for the individual subject. Becker et al. go on to point out, "Firm predictions of outcome become less feasible when outcome categories are established that make fine distinctions between levels of intellectual, behavioral, and socioeconomic disability. Currently, prognosis in head injury falls far short of such subtle predictions. This in no way diminishes the importance or desirability of such information: the present limit of knowledge on the subject must, however, be recognized."

Although this may be a reasonable and straightforward recommendation for evaluating outcome in the medical area, neuropsychological assessment goes well beyond the broad categories of outcome and permits an assessment that does make relatively fine distinctions between levels of intellectual and behavioral disability. Neuropsychological evaluation extends beyond the medically recognized limitations of predictions (Dikmen & Reitan, 1976). Using the Halstead-Reitan Battery, neuropsychological evaluation has the advantage of considering both interindividual and intraindividual comparative data in the initial evaluation following head injury and can be used as a basis for predicting later status (Dikmen & Reitan, 1976). More specifically, neuropsychological evaluation has not been satisfied with merely identifying a range of predictor variables and a range of outcome variables, based on large numbers of subjects, in which the relationship of the two sets of variables is largely lost for the individual case.

It must be recognized that in science the customary methodological approach is to analyze data based on large numbers of subjects using statistical procedures that represent an abstraction of the group characteristics. Although this method does serve as a basis for generalization of the obtained results, by its very nature it neglects the critical need to derive information applicable to the individual person. In terms of clinical values, the individual subject is the unit of interest and concern.

A commitment to establish outcome categories that are sufficiently broad to produce large numbers of subjects in each group for statistical analysis has some value in producing known distribution characteristics, but this approach can be stifling in terms of developing methods for individual clinical predictions. Unfortunately, methodological advances in developing scientific procedures for analysis relevant to the individual case have not been the hallmark of statistical procedures, despite the fact that medicine and surgery continually focus on the individual subject. The methods of clinical neuropsychology permit not only generation of objective data for inferential statistical analyses of intergroup differences, but also provide detailed information based on the same data for clinical evaluation of the individual subject.

When using the Halstead-Reitan Battery, identical rigor exists in the collection of data for individual clinical evaluation as for generation of research data used for group comparisons. Standardization of assessment and evaluation procedures, as provided in clinical neuropsychological evaluation, has a tremendous advantage in integrating clinical and research methodology.

Factors That Influence or are Related to Outcome

Except for age and brain damage sustained prior to the injury in question, most of the medical and surgical studies involved with predicting outcome are concerned with the primary and secondary effects of the injury itself. Thus, as we have noted elsewhere in this volume, studies concerned with prognosis essentially must be viewed as being concerned with the predictive significance of any early post-injury manifestations. Even the early outcome factors (the primary and secondary effects of head injury, which are often identified as prognostic indicators), are still outcome factors. It is helpful conceptually to view the predictive model as being concerned with early outcome vs. later outcome following head injury.

Although there are many reasons for wanting to use early outcome indicators as a reliable basis for predicting eventual long-term outcome, it should be recognized that the primary and secondary effects of the lesion are tremendously variable between subjects and usually are not fully understood even in the individual patient. On the other hand, a complete neuropsychological evaluation provides a consistent and standardized assessment of brain functions which permits a comparison of the individual patient with control subjects and other experimental groups and therefore may provide a better basis for predicting eventual outcome.

In most cases it is possible to administer the Halstead-Reitan Battery within 30 days after the head injury. (Of course, in some instances orthopedic injuries may prevent a patient from being

GLASGOW OUTCOME SCALE

POORER PROGNOSIS	BETTER PROGNOSIS
GLASGOW COMA SCALE SCORE <**7**	GLASGOW COMA SCALE SCORE >**7**

Old Age	
	Youth

Pupillary light reflex	Pupillary light reflex
Pupils are dilated and do not react to light	Pupils constrict in response to light

Caloric test with ice water Eyes do not deviate	Caloric test with ice water Eyes deviate to irrigated side

Motor response to noxious stimulus results in decerbrate rigidity	Motor response to noxious stimulus results in a defensive gesture (localization)

MRI scan showing subdural hematoma	Normal MRI scan

Brainstem Auditory Evoked Response is deficient	Brainstem Auditory Evoked Response is normal

tested). Because of the differences in orientation between the medical and the neuropsychological approaches toward identification of prognostic factors as well as assessment of outcome, this section will review some of the conventional medical studies concerned with outcome. The neuropsychological studies, particularly those involving the Neuropsychological Deficit Scale, are considered in Chapter III.

Factors that have Relatively Little Influence on Outcome

Jennett and Teasdale (1981) have presented a brief summary of factors related to brain injury that shows little difference among persons who, according to the Glasgow Outcome Scale, are classified in the categories of *Dead* or *Vegetative State*. The data presented were based upon persons with severe head injuries (Jennett, Teasdale, Braakman, et al., 1979). These investigators found that among these variables the circumstances under which the injury had occurred had relatively little significance for the patient's eventual outcome.

Fifty-four percent of the subjects were classified in the *Dead* or *Vegetative State* categories, regardless of whether the injury had been sustained in a road accident, an alcoholic fall, a work-related incident, or in an assault. With such a high percentage of the subjects classified in either the *Dead* or *Vegetative State* categories, it is apparent that the victims in this group had sustained a very severe brain injury. In this sample, the proportion of persons classified as *Dead* or *Vegetative State* was only slightly greater for persons who had sustained skull fracture (54%) compared with persons who did not have evidence of a skull fracture (43%).

Impairment of motor functions (specifically, hemiparesis or hemiplegia) was present in nearly half the group, and these subjects were compared with head-injured subjects who had normal motor functions. The proportion of subjects classified in

the *Dead* or *Vegetative State* categories decreased to approximately 30%, but showed little difference in these two groups. Patients with right and left hemisphere damage were also compared, and these groups had nearly identical proportions in the *Dead* or *Vegetative State* category as compared with the *Moderate Disability* or *Good Recovery* categories.

Jennett et al. also identified a separate group of subjects who had sustained a major chest injury in addition to brain trauma. While these subjects had a slightly greater representation in the *Dead* and *Vegetative State* categories than persons without such injuries, the difference was not very striking.

Finally, a group of persons with extracranial injuries in addition to a head injury was compared with a group of subjects who had only a head injury. No differences were present using the gross categories of outcome in the Glasgow Outcome Scale. It must be recognized that these results relate to only the very general categories that are provided by the Glasgow Outcome Scale and do not purport to answer all questions regarding neuropsychological, social, and vocational aspects of outcome. For example, when damage particularly involves the right cerebral hemisphere as compared with the left side of the brain, there may be distinct patterns of neuropsychological deficit which, in turn, will have a differential effect on intellectual, cognitive, and probably vocational outcome for the individual.

The Influence of Chronological Age

The natural tendency of trying to identify the differential significance of *individual* factors on outcome following head injury and then comparing their significance raises many procedural difficulties. It is often impossible to determine the influence of each contributing factor in isolation because the unit of interest is the individual patient, in whom many separate factors may coexist. In this section we will follow the traditional procedure of attempting to assess separate factors and their influence on outcome, but it always must be recognized that every patient represents an individual person and the factors themselves show variability in their significance between patients.

It could readily be argued that any attempt to consider a factor in isolation represents a methodologically inadequate approach. Instead, the prognostic indicator of outcome should be a more global type of measure which reflects the full interaction, for the individual subject, of the many variables that represent brain impairment. Some of these variables may obviously have existed before the brain injury was sustained (factors such as chronological age and previous brain damage); other factors represent the primary and secondary effects of the head injury itself. Although an attempt may be made to consider these factors individually (such as age, pre-existing brain damage, the presence of an intracranial mass lesion, duration of coma, post-traumatic amnesia, intracranial hypertension, measures of cerebral circulation and metabolism, etc.), a global measure, which more accurately represents the overall condition of the brain for the individual subject, may be more useful as a basis for prognosis. We believe that the Neuropsychological Deficit Scale, based on the Halstead-Reitan Battery, may be such a measure (see Chapter III).

Among investigators who elect to consider single factors individually, chronological age has been claimed to be the most important single determinant of outcome from severe head injury. Becker, Miller, and Greenberg (1982) have summarized a number of studies that support a basis for this generalization (Bruce, Schut, Bruno, Wood, & Sutton, 1978; Fell, Fitzgerald, Moiel, & Carem, 1975; Harris, 1971; Hieskanen & Sipponen, 1970; Jamieson & Yelland, 1972; Jennett, Teasdale, Braakman, Minderhoud, & Knill-Jones, 1976; Jennett, Teasdale, Galbraith, Pickard, Grant, Braakman, Avezaat, Maas, Minderhoud, Vecht, Heiden, Small, Caton, & Kurze, 1977; Overgaard,

Christensen, Hvid Jansen, Haase, Land, Pederson, & Tweed, 1973; Pagni, 1973; Pazzaglia, Frank, Frank, & Gaist, 1975; Robertson & Pollard, 1955; Rossanda, Selenati, Villa, & Beduschi, 1973).

Jennett and Teasdale (1981) also state that age is probably the most widely acknowledge influence on outcome. In a study based upon 668 cases of severe head injury, represented in age categories from 5 years to more than 75 years, these investigators found a steadily progessive age relationship among subjects who were classified in the categories of *Dead* or *Vegetative State.* Conversely, when chronological age was plotted for subjects in the categories of *Moderate Disability* or *Good Recovery,* the reverse relationship was demonstrated; nearly 60% of the youngest age groups were in these categories and essentially no person over the age of 70 was in either of these two categories.

In addition to observing the potent influence of chronological age on outcome, these authors further state that this influence is independent of the state of coma, eye movements, and pupillary reactions. However, in patients with an extremely severe head injury, the head injury itself, rather than the patient's age, is the overruling factor. Thus, the severity of the brain damage, when sufficiently pronounced, certainly can determine the outcome for the individual patient regardless of his/her age.

More detailed evaluations have suggested that other variables may be of special significance, and Becker, Miller, and Greenberg (1982) have cautioned against interpreting the age-related outcome data as having a direct causal relationship. In a series of 496 patients with a severe head injury, Carlsson, von Essen, and Lofgren (1968) noted that the cause of death was related to medical factors to which the elderly were more susceptible.

Becker, Miller, Ward, Greenberg, Young, and Sakalis (1977) confirmed these findings in their study of 160 patients with a severe head injury. When considering death due to cerebral causes, they found essentially a constant death rate across the age range (subdivided into 20-year categories from 0–80 years). However, there was a steady progression in proportion of deaths due to systemic causes, ranging in the four age categories from 9% to 19%, 23%, and 43% in the oldest subgroup. Systemic factors include the conditions that produce hypoxemia, arterial hypotension, and anemia. Thus, it would not appear that the direct effects of brain trauma are necessarily more severe in older persons than younger persons, but that older persons do not tolerate the insult as well as younger persons.

Some types of lesions (such as intracranial hematomas) have been reported to be more frequently encountered in older patients. In addition, however, older brains in general have very probably experienced more previous trauma and biological change represented by cerebral vascular deterioration and primary neuronal degenerative changes. In one sense, it is possible to postulate that the brains of older persons tolerate traumatic insult less well than the brains of younger persons because of previous damage due either to prior injury or biological deterioration (see Reitan & Wolfson, 1985b for a more detailed discussion of the normal and pathological changes associated with aging).

The Influence of Pre-existing Brain Damage

A common observation among neurologists and neurosurgeons is that a pre-existing head injury makes the brain more vulnerable to damage resulting from a second brain injury. Becker, Miller, and Greenberg (1982) note that many neurosurgeons have observed a patient's excellent recovery from a head injury only to see "the same patient devastated by a second head injury that seemed initially to be much milder than the first." Reitan (1979) has generalized this observation to apply to facilitated neuropsychological recovery (brain-retraining), noting that either a subsequent

brain injury, a developing illness with systemic effects that may secondarily influence the brain, or significant emotional stress all represent factors that have a disproportionately impairing effect on the recovery and retraining of brain-injured patients. Thus, it would appear that even though recovery may seem to have occurred, a previous injury renders the brain somewhat more susceptible to impairing stresses.

As Becker, Miller, and Greenberg (1982) point out, the pre-existing brain damage does not need to be traumatic in nature. They note that hydrocephalic patients who have regained function after cerebrospinal fluid shunting or patients who have recovered from a stroke may later be rendered significantly disabled by an apparently minor head trauma. Reitan and Wolfson (1986b) have presented similar case results, illustrating the adverse effects of head injuries in alcoholics, polydrug abusers, and persons who had previously developed cerebrovascular disease.

The same principle, relating to the cumulative effects of brain damage, have been cited in studies of the progressive deterioration sometimes shown by boxers (Corsellis, Bruton, & Freeman-Browne, 1973; Roberts, 1969). Autopsy examinations of the brains of boxers indicate the presence of small areas of pathology, probably initially represented by petechial hemorrhages, which appear to have not only cumulative significance with additional head blows, but eventually become progressive in nature even after the cessation of further blows to the head.

Because of the difficulty in fully describing and quantifying the severity of the initial insult and the subsequent injuries that follow, there are relatively few carefully controlled studies of the effects of pre-existing brain damage. However, clinical experience certainly suggests that when persons who have previously sustained brain damage experience a subsequent head injury, the resulting deficits are often much more severe than would have been expected.

The Influence of Type and Severity of Damage to the Brain

Although the severity of brain damage is related to the force of the blow to the head, there are many more specific factors, involving acceleration/deceleration injuries and rotational and shearing effects, that may reflect the damage sustained. However, direct evidence of the force of the blow is rarely available, and, in cases of blunt injury, even the point of impact is often difficult to discern precisely. Thus, inferences regarding the force are usually drawn from the observed consequences. These effects may include duration of coma and post-traumatic amnesia (factors often presumed to involve axonal shearing and brainstem involvement), tissue damage in instances of penetrating wounds (which often can be estimated at surgery), intracranial mass lesions resulting from focal bleeding, intracranial hypertension associated with edema, and alterations in cerebral circulation and metabolism. Therefore, many factors, most of which are based upon clinical observation or special diagnostic studies following the injury, are involved in estimating the force of the blow and the type and severity of the resulting brain damage.

The Influence of Blunt vs. Penetrating Injury

With respect to outcome there are distinct differences between a blunt injury of the head and a penetrating injury. In the latter type of insult, the skull and brain are penetrated (usually in a rather localized area) and the underlying damage to the brain — while it may be quite extensive in many cases — involves an area of focal as well as diffuse damage. Low velocity penetrating injuries (such as stab wounds) may cause essentially only focal damage in the vicinity of penetration. High velocity penetrating injuries, frequently associated with bullet wounds, cause more extensive brain damage.

In either type of penetrating injury there may be entry of foreign objects (such as bone frag-ments, skin, and hair) into the wound, and complications may include infection, intracranial hemorrhage, bleeding from dural venous sinuses, problems related to distant distribution of bone or missile fragments, and distant hemorrhages. It should be noted that many patients with a penetrating head injury do not immediately lose consciousness; impaired consciousness may occur later as a result of the secondary effects of the injury.

In cases of blunt (closed) head injury the force of the blow may be applied to the brain much more generally. Shock waves may travel through the brain, causing compression effects of brain tissue and tearing of brain tissue and blood vessels over rough protuberances on the inner surface of the skull. These factors result in extensive shearing of axons and focal areas of cerebral bleeding that involve the anterior frontal and anterior temporal areas more frequently than other locations.

More than half of all severe head injuries occur in traffic accidents. In motor vehicle accidents approximately 80% of the victims are operators or occupants of the the vehicle and 20% are pedestrians. Falls or other blows to the head account for an estimated 20% of severe head injuries (Eisenberg, 1985). The force of the blow to the head is generally much greater in motor vehicle accidents than in other types of injuries and cause much more generalized and diffuse damage. When the injury is sustained through a fall, older persons are more frequently the victims and there is a higher proportion of resulting hematomas (Becker, Miller, & Greenberg, 1982; Bowers & Marshall, 1980; Jennett, Teasdale, Braakman, et al., 1979). Mortality is particularly high in instances of penetrating gunshot wounds: among 424 such cases studied by Kaufman, Loyola, Makela et al. (1983), 60% of the victims died at the scene of the accident, 8% were dead by the time they reached the emergency room (or died in the emergency room), 17% died during their hospitalization, and only 15% survived.

The Influence of Focal Lesions Resulting from Brain Injury

Focal areas of brain damage are particularly prevalent in cases of penetrating injury or depressed fractures. Areas of bleeding may occur in the epidural space, the subdural space, or within the brain tissue. Adverse effects, including death, occur frequently among persons who experience such lesions. These conditions can be treated surgically when identified, and failure to identify and treat the lesions has been viewed as a highly significant factor in causing death that might have been avoided (Rose, Valtonen, & Jennett, 1977).

Becker, Miller, Ward, et al. (1977) found that the outcome of head-injured patients with an intracranial mass lesion was significantly worse than among head-injured patients who sustained only diffuse brain damage. In a series of 160 patients, 62 had intracranial mass lesions which were treated by surgical decompression. Fifty-six percent of these subjects had evidence of abnormal motor responses; 49% of the patients with diffuse brain injury had similar impairment. Impairment of reflex eye movements and bilateral absence of pupillary light response was also significantly greater in the group with mass lesions of the brain. The mortality rate in this group was 40% (compared with 23% in the group with diffuse injury). When evaluated in terms of long-term outcome, 29% of the patients with a mass lesion were classified in the category of *Good Recovery.* Forty percent of the patients with diffuse brain injury were classified in this category.

The type of mass lesion also has a differential effect. Patients who have sustained an epidural hematoma generally fare the best; persons with an acute subdural hematoma fall in an intermediate position; and patients with an intracerebral mass lesion have the poorest outcome.

Even though epidural hematomas are associated with better outcome than other types of mass lesions, they frequently occur in head injuries eventually resulting in either death or a poor outcome. Of course, variable degrees of damage to the rest of the brain occurs among patients with an epidural hematoma, and these conditions may not be comparable from one case to another. Therefore, the significance of a hematoma alone is difficult to evaluate; however, if a diagnosis and surgical treatment are effected promptly, several authors estimate that the mortality rate with such lesions should be under 20%, and probably within the range of 5%–10% (Becker, Miller, & Greenberg, 1982; Hooper, 1959; Jamieson & Yelland, 1968).

Becker, Miller, and Greenberg (1982) have studied differential factors related to the clinical state of patients with an epidural hematoma and have identified certain conditions that have adverse effects on outcome. For example, they found that patients who were in a coma at the time of surgical treatment had a mortality rate 3 times as high as patients who were only drowsy and able to converse at the time they were taken to surgery. If a patient in a coma had never had a lucid interval since the time of the injury, the frequency of death was twice as great as in the patient who had experienced a lucid interval.

Patients who had bloody cerebrospinal fluid had a mortality rate twice as high as patients who had clear cerebrospinal fluid (Gallagher & Browder, 1968). Patients who had bilateral dilatation of the pupils or bilateral decerebrate rigidity at the time of surgical intervention rarely made a good recovery.

Becker, Miller, and Greenberg (1982) estimate that if patients with an acute subdural hematoma receive prompt diagnosis and surgical intervention, it should be possible to hold the number of deaths below 50%. However, in various studies the mortality rate has ranged from 50%–95%. There are many factors besides the presence of an acute subdural hematoma that relate to severity of brain injury in individual patients, and these additional factors contribute to the variance in mortality rates. A number of circumstances lead to higher mortality rates, including the presence of bilateral hematomas and evidence of severe damage of the brain besides the hematoma itself.

Evacuation of the hematoma through burr holes rather than a craniotomy has also been associated with a higher mortality rate. Decerebrate rigidity appears to be associated with a higher mortality rate, particularly among patients who do not receive prompt and effective surgical treatment. Finally, older persons beyond 60 years of age tend to do poorly; age does not seem to be a significant variable in persons under 60 years old (Cooper, Rovit, & Ransohoff, 1976; Fell, Fitzgerald, Moiel, & Carem, 1975; Harris, 1971; Jamieson & Yelland, 1972; Ransohoff, Vallo, Gage, & Epstein, 1971; Richards & Hoff, 1974; Tallala & Morin, 1971).

Jennett, Teasdale, Braakman, et al. (1979) report that in persons with a severe head injury the incidence of hematomas increases progressively in accordance with chronological age: below 20 years of age there is a 30% frequency; between 20 and 40 years there is a 45% frequency; between 40 and 60 years there is a 65% frequency; and beyond 60 years of age the incidence is 71%. However, in interpreting this data, Jennett and Teasdale (1981) indicate that the association between the presence of a hematoma and the patient's age spuriously tends to implicate age. With or without an intracranial hematoma, age has a significant effect on outcome. When the data are adjusted for increased frequency with advancing age, increased mortality occurred only among those persons under 20 years who tended to have a poorer outcome when a hematoma was present.

The outlook is relatively poor in cases of intracerebral hematomas. Surgeons differ in their preference for treatment procedures. Internal decompression by amputation of the frontal or temporal poles has often been used, but intracranial hypertension following surgery remains in about 70% of the cases. In their series, Becker, Miller, and Greenberg (1982) found that 58% of the patients who had intracerebral hematomas died, 21%

were categorized as *Vegetative State* or *Severe Disability,* and only 21% eventually achieved a classification of *Moderate Disability* or *Good Recovery* according to the Glasgow Outcome Scale.

The Influence of Adverse Factors Occurring Shortly After Brain Injury

Respiratory problems can occur very shortly after a head injury and influence outcome and complicate recovery. A brief period of apnea frequently occurs after the head blow. Although respiration resumes spontaneously in most cases, the period during which the patient was not breathing may clearly have an adverse effect. In addition, gag reflexes may be depressed and aspiration of blood or emisus may occur. Chest injuries as well as facial injuries may also cause respiratory difficulties.

In some instances of head injury reduced blood pressure and resulting shock may be a significant factor. While this is often due to internal or external hemorrhage, systemic hypotension may occur in patients who are confined to an upright position following a significant head injury.

Although epileptic seizures do not occur often in the very early phases following a head injury, when they do occur it is a warning that intracranial focal bleeding may be present. Seizures may be associated with more general effects on the brain such as hypoxia, cerebral vasodilation, and intracranial hypertension. These factors, in turn, may represent significant manifestations of secondary brain damage and result in a poorer outcome. In addition, the occurrence of seizures soon after the injury has been associated with the development of post-traumatic epilepsy as a long-term effect of the brain injury (Jennett, 1975; Jennett & Lewin, 1960).

Additional factors which result in poor outcome may be observed after the patient is hospitalized. Abundant evidence is present to demonstrate that patients who sustain a severe head injury have impaired oxygenation. Froman (1968) estimated that hypoxemia might involve up to 85% of unconscious patients with a head injury. Arterial hypotension and anemia are additional adverse factors that occur principally in persons with multiple injuries (rather than injuries involving only the head). Although there are excellent mechanisms within the brain to maintain oxygen delivery, a head injury may disrupt these mechanisms. Miller, Sweet, Narayan and Becker (1978) did not find that adverse systemic effects of this kind had a significant effect on outcome in patients who had a mass lesion. On the other hand, when diffuse brain injury was present, patients who also had hypoxia and hypotension or anemia tended to be classified in the categories of *Dead, Vegetative State,* or *Severe Disability.*

The Influence of Autonomic Nervous System Dysfunction

Additional abnormal circumstances have been associated with autonomic nervous system dysfunction and have an adverse association with outcome. These factors, which are probably indicators of brainstem dysfunction, include abnormalities of respiration, aspects of cardiovascular function, and regulation of body temperature. Respiratory abnormalities and systolic hypertension have also been related to poor prognosis. However, Jennett and Teasdale (1981) note that these abnormalities occur in only a minority of severely head-injured patients and, when they did occur, injuries and complications involving other parts of the body and systemic functions were also present. In fact, North and Jennett (1974) found that abnormal breathing patterns seemed to be much less significant with respect to outcome than had previously been reported.

Nevertheless, Jennett, Teasdale, Braakman, et al. (1979) did find that autonomic nervous system abnormalities were more commonly associated with an outcome of *Death* or *Vegetative State* than *Moderate Disability* or *Good Recovery.* When pa-

tients showed periodic respiration (i.e., rhythmic or patterned variations of breathing intensity which occur in repetitive cycles) in the first week following a severe head injury, the percentage of patients categorized as *Dead* or *Vegetative State* was 62%. Forty-seven percent of the patients who did not demonstrate periodic respiration were in these categories. Only 30% of the patients with periodic respiration were classified in the category of *Moderate Disability* or *Good Recovery* (compared with 45% who did not show evidence of periodic respiration).

Compared to subjects who were not tachypneic, 65% of the head-injured persons who showed respiration rates greater than 30 per minute were classified as *Dead* or *Vegetative State* and 28% were categorized as *Moderate Disability* or *Good Recovery.* Of the subjects who were not tachypneic, 44% were classified in the *Dead* or *Vegetative State* category and 46% were in the *Moderate Disability* or *Good Recovery* categories.

Among patients whose pulse rates were greater than 120 during the first week after head injury, 60% were classified in the *Dead* or *Vegetative State* categories and 31% were in the *Moderate Disability* or *Good Recovery* categories. Of the head-injured patients who were not tachycardic, 47% were categorized in the *Dead* or *Vegetative State* categories and 31% were in the *Moderate Disability* or *Good Recovery* categories.

Persons with elevated blood pressure following head injury also tended to do more poorly than head-injured persons who were not hypertensive. Fifty-eight percent of the hypertensive subjects were classified in the *Dead* or *Vegetative State* category and 31% were in the *Moderate Disability* or *Good Recovery* categories. Of the normotensive subjects, 50% were classified in the *Dead* or *Vegetative State* and 40% were in the *Moderate Disability* or *Good Recovery* categories.

Finally, head-injured subjects with elevated body temperature were classified more frequently in the *Dead* and *Vegetative State* categories (59%)

and less frequently in the *Moderate Disability* and *Good Recovery* categories (29%). Forty-eight percent of the normothermic subjects were classified in the *Dead* or *Vegetative State* categories and 45% were in the *Moderate Disability* or *Good Recovery* categories. It is certainly true that head-injured subjects with autonomic abnormalities also tend to have more severe brain damage, but insofar as the autonomic abnormalities represent overall severity of injury, they appear to have some significance with respect to eventual outcome.

The Prognostic Significance of Deficits Shown on the Neurological Examination

In addition to impairment of consciousness, hemiparesis or hemiplegia and abnormal brainstem signs (especially involving eye movement and pupillary responses) have been evaluated as prognostic indicators. Jennett, Teasdale, Braakman, et al. (1979) found that lateralized motor impairment of the extremities had little significance in patients classified in the Dead or *Vegetative State* categories.

In contrast, abnormalities of brainstem reflexes are definitely related to outcome as well as to mortality rates (Braakman, Gelpke, Habbema, et al., 1980; Jennett, Teasdale, Braakman, et al., 1976; Jennett, Teasdale, Braakman, et al., 1979; Levati, Farina, Vecchi, et al., 1982; Narayan, Greenberg, Miller, et al., 1981). Bilateral impairment of pupillary reflexes was particularly serious, and was associated with an 85%-90% mortality rate. Absent or impaired eye movement, considered generally, was associated with a mortality rate ranging between 70% and 90%.

The Influence of Elevated Intracranial Pressure

Elevated intracranial pressure following head injury is associated with increased mortality (Fig. 2-1). Miller, Becker, Ward, et al. (1977) found that patients with normal intracranial pressure had a 14% mortality rate and patients who had an elevation of 20 mm/Hg had a 55% mortality rate. Narayan, Greenberg, Miller, et al. (1981) found that 44% of their head-injured sample had evidence of intracranial pressure above 20 mm/Hg and a mortality rate of 51%. In the remaining 56% of the sample, in whom intracranial pressure did not reach the specified level, the mortality rate was only 16%. Intracranial hypertension is related to the score on the Glasgow Coma Scale, but Eisenberg, Cayard, Papanicalaou, et al. (1983) have shown that elevated intracranial pressure has predictive significance with respect to mortality that goes beyond the variance accounted for by the Glasgow Coma Scale score.

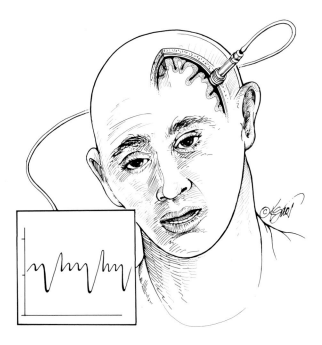

Figure 2-1. A subarachnoid screw may be inserted to monitor the patient's intracranial pressure. When intracranial hypertension exists, the pressure of the CSF rises above 15 Torr (200 mm of water). Since the normal pressure within the cranium is less than 15 Torr, an increase in pressure above this level will decrease the blood flow, reduce the CSF, and shift neural parts from one intracranial compartment to another. This shifting is known as *herniation*.

The Influence of Cerebral Blood Flow and Metabolism

A relationship exists between the severity of head injury and cerebral blood flow or level of cerebral oxygen consumption for each hemisphere. When these levels fall below a critical level, a poor outcome or death is probable (Fig. 2-2). In some instances there is a dissociation between cerebral blood flow and oxygen metabolism; blood flow may increase beyond the normal range, and this condition also is adversely associated with outcome. Studies of regional cerebral blood flow have shown both abnormally low levels and abnormally high levels in the frontal and temporal lobes, the areas that are usually most significantly damaged in head injury (Bruce, Langfitt, Miller, et al., 1973; Enevoldsen, Cold, Jensen, & Malmros, 1976; Overgaard & Tweed, 1974). The relationship between ischemia or hyperemia and the clinical condition of the head-injured patient to variables such as

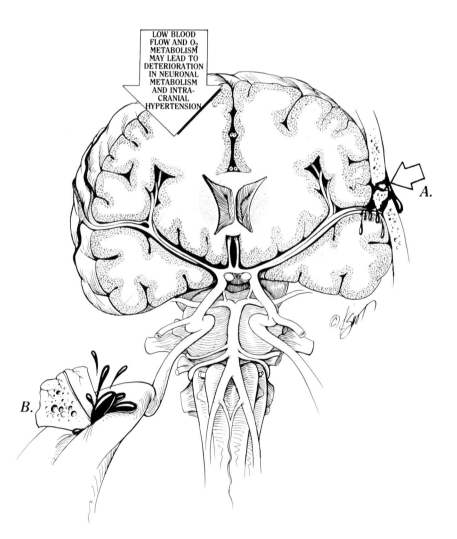

LOW BLOOD FLOW AND O₂ METABOLISM MAY LEAD TO DETERIORATION IN NEURONAL METABOLISM AND INTRA-CRANIAL HYPERTENSION

A.

B.

Figure 2-2. A skull fracture which causes a hematoma (A) may cause increased intracranial pressure and eventually lead to uncal herniation. An impaired blood supply to the brain due to an arterial injury (B) can cause hypoperfusion and necrosis of brain tissue.

evoked potentials, intracranial pressure, or eventual outcome is uncertain (Muizelaar & Obrist, 1985).

In addition, responsiveness of the cerebral circulation to vasoactive stimuli has been studied in relation to regional cerebral blood flow. Although results have been related closely to the areas of the brain that most frequently sustain surface damage, the significance of the findings has not been closely correlated to outcome. Sequential measures of cerebral blood flow in the same patients have also been studied, allowing investigators to determine that an abnormal finding initially might become normal within days. Studies of this kind have yielded results which appear to relate more validly to eventual outcome than instances of only a single measurement (Obrist, Langfitt, terWeeme, O'Connor, et al., 1977).

Finally, various techniques have been developed to measure cerebral vascular transit time which, in turn, appears to be related to cerebral blood flow. However, there is a considerable degree of variability among normal subjects, and the usefulness of such measurements has not yet been clearly demonstrated.

Thus, relating cerebral blood flow measurements to severity of head injury and outcome has been relatively confusing. Part of the difficulty with these measurements may very well relate to intraindividual changes in the status of the cerebral vasculature, especially shortly after the injury, and investigations which reflect these changes over time for the individual subject promise to be of greater value. In fact, Muizelaar and Obrist (1985) have shown significant relationships between hemispheric cerebral blood flow and motor deficits which represent degrees of severity of involvement of the contralateral hemisphere as well as a striking relationship between cerebral metabolic rate and the Glasgow Coma Scale score. Patients with a Glasgow Coma Scale score of 8 or less showed evidence of distinct depression of cerebral metabolic rate; their scores fell below half of the normal mean value.

The Electroencephalogram and Outcome

Electroencephalographic tracings do not appear to relate very closely to the patient's clinical condition or his eventual outcome. This is particularly true when only one EEG is obtained following a head injury. In fact, a single, relatively normal EEG may suggest that brain damage is minimal, and changes in the patient's condition (for example, the development of an intracranial hemorrhage) may not occur for several hours or even days post-injury. However, research has indicated that the information obtained even with serial EEG's has limited prognostic value.

A major problem is that many patients with unequivocal clinical evidence of cerebral damage have normal EEG's. Walker and Jablon (1959) found that approximately 50% of patients with hemiplegia or hemiparesis following brain injury had normal EEG's in follow-up studies. Only 40% of patients who had sustained a penetrating head injury had abnormal EEG's. In many of these instances when abnormal EEG's were found, the results suggested diffuse rather than focal EEG abnormalities, even when lateralized cerebral contusions were present together with permanent hemiplegia. However, some studies have suggested that diffuse EEG abnormalities persist only for about 6 months in patients with focal lesions, but that focal EEG deficits may continue for longer periods of time in a significant number of patients.

In general, EEG findings are correlated with the severity of brain damage and the patient's clinical course. Nevertheless, in many instances EEG tracings may initially be abnormal following a mild head injury but return to normal within a very short period of time (Dow, Ulett, & Raaf, 1943). In other instances persons who have sustained a head injury may have an abnormal EEG in spite of the fact that they show no clinical evidence of significant impairment of brain functions (Bickford & Klass, 1966; Poole, 1970). Such findings may be related to the fact that to a degree, abnormalities are present in a proportion of the general population, and the EEG abnormalities therefore may have been present before the head injury. Other investigators have also documented examples of normal EEG tracings among patients with severe brain impairment (Chatrian, White, & Shaw, 1964).

Although EEG changes may occur immediately after a brain insult, they often appear only after the patient has shown clinical evidence of either improvement or deterioration (Dawson, Webster, & Gurdjian, 1951; Rodin, 1967). Rodin, Whelan, Taylor, et al. (1965) compared EEG tracings of persons who suffered an acute fatal head injury which resulted in death within 48 hours with another group of subjects who survived a severe head injury. The two groups showed no particular differences, except that those who died from the head injury had a tendency to demonstrate lower EEG amplitudes.

In terms of focal slow-wave activity, Williams (1941) found some instances in which focal discharges correlated with clinical symptomatology, but he also observed many cases in which focal EEG patterns were present without focal clinical symptoms.

The reliability of slow-wave (delta) foci are also subject to question. Dawson, Webster, and Gurdjian (1951) as well as Rodin, Whelan, Taylor, et al. (1965) found that following head injury these foci changed location both within and between the cerebral hemispheres. These investigators concluded that delta foci were of little clinical significance in cases of head injury.

Electroencephalographic tracings are not dependable as a predictor of post-traumatic epilepsy, although a change in EEG pattern from slow-wave to focal spike activity is seen in some persons who eventually develop epilepsy. Nevertheless, Jennett and van der Sande (1975) were not able to demonstrate any differences in diffuse as compared with focal EEG abnormalities among patients who eventually developed post-traumatic epilepsy.

Some patients who became epileptic following a head injury had normal EEG tracings that became abnormal only after the onset of seizures. Many other patients with persisting EEG abnormalities, even including focal spiked activity, did not develop seizures. Thus, the consensus appears to be that the EEG is not of value in predicting the development of post-traumatic epilepsy in patients who sustain a head injury.

Nevertheless, it should be noted that EEG abnormalities do show some relationship to the extent and severity of brain damage as manifested by correlations with the duration of post-traumatic amnesia, the presence of dural tearing, depressed skull fractures, intracerebral hematoma, and penetrating head injuries. In each of these instances the incidence of EEG abnormalities is increased (Walker & Jablon, 1959; Williams, 1941).

Sensory Evoked Potentials and Their Relation to Outcome Following Head Injury

With the development of computer averaging techniques it has become possible to evaluate the integrity of sensory systems that extend from the receptor organ to the cerebral cortex (Fig. 2-3). The sensory modalities most commonly tested are vision, hearing, and touch. An appropriate sensory stimulus can be administered to the end organ which will elicit time-related evoked potentials, averaging out the signal from the random ongoing cerebral activity that is also recorded. In practice, a flash of light might be delivered to the retina (visual stimulation), a tone pip may be the stimulus to the cochlea (auditory stimulation), or any procedure which causes peripheral nerve depolarization (tactile stimulation) can be administered to the skin.

When the sensory stimulus arouses a peripheral receptor, a depolarization wave travels toward the central nervous system at velocities that are determined by the diameter of the nerve fiber. The time interval from the point of stimulation to ar-

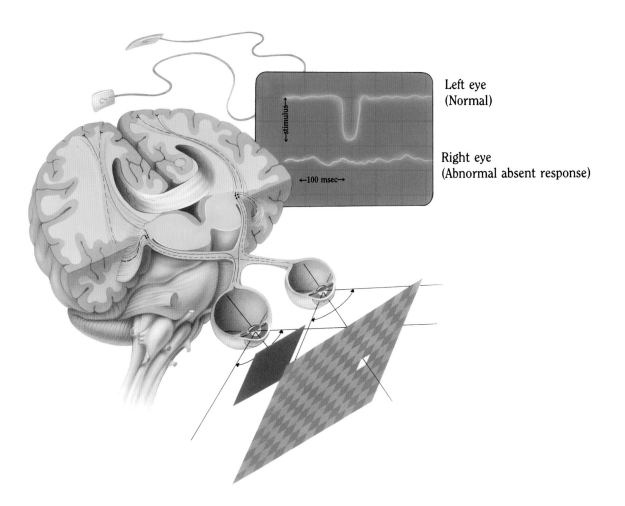

Figure 2-3. *Visual Evoked Responses.* For this test the patient wears a patch over one eye and views a reversing checkerboard pattern on a screen. Electrodes are placed midline in the parietal and occipital regions. In a normal response a major positive wave, which originates in the receptive visual cortex, occurs approximately 100 msec after the stimulus is presented. A unilateral abnormality suggests a prechiasmatic lesion; bilateral delays are much less specific. Prolonged latencies may occur in up to 66% of patients, many of whom have no clinical evidence of neuritis. In more severe cases, no response is elicited.

rival of the nerve impulse at the primary sensory cortical receiving area is related to the distance traveled, the presence or absence of neuronal abnormality, the conduction velocity of the axons, and the number of synapses involved in the sensory system. Arrival of the nerve impulses at the cerebral cortex generates potentials that may be recorded for seconds after stimulation. In practice,

however, evoked potentials are generally recorded for 100-1000 milliseconds.

The evoked potential wave is analyzed for latency, amplitude, duration, and morphology. The latency of each wave is the most commonly used clinical variable. Parietal lobe lesions can often be accurately localized on the basis of somatosensory evoked potentials, although abnormalities in these potentials may also be caused by lesions in the pre-rolandic area of the frontal lobe.

Localizing a lesion to the temporal lobe (Fig. 2-4, A) customarily requires both auditory and visual evoked potentials. Both potentials would be depressed by a lesion that involves the concurrent involvement of the auditory and visual pathways in the temporal lobe.

Lesions in the posterior part of the hemisphere, especially involving the occipital lobe, correlate well with visual evoked potentials (Fig. 2-4, B). However, in such cases, it is advisable to obtain electroretinograms concurrently in order to identify any receptor dysfunction in the retina.

Brainstem dysfunction can also be differentiated from involvement at the level of the cerebral hemispheres by using visual, auditory, and somatosensory evoked potentials (Fig. 2-4, C). This is possible because somatosensory and auditory pathways traverse regions of the lower part of the brain (medulla, pons, midbrain, and the lower part of the diencephalon) but the lateral geniculate body is the most caudal area of the visual system between the retina and the striate cortex.

In individual cases it is possible to demonstrate relative abnormality of areas involved in the visual system and demonstrate impairment in the brainstem by using somatosensory and auditory evoked potentials. Conversely, a deviation from normality using visual evoked potentials may well indicate damage of the more rostral portions of the diencephalon or areas of the brain within or adjacent to the geniculostriate tracts. Although sensory evoked responses may be useful in identifying areas of major structural damage within the brain, frontal lesions are difficult to identify because no specific sensory stimulus leads directly to the frontal cortex (Fig. 2-4, D).

Evoked potential recordings done during the first few days after a head injury have been studied with relation to the neurological condition of the patient at later times following the head injury (Greenberg, Becker, Miller, & Mayer, 1977). Initial

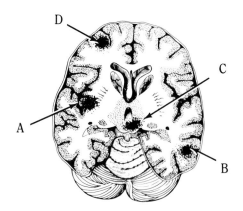

Figure 2-4. Typical sites of cerebral lesions. Lesions in the temporal lobe (*A*) are best localized by using both visual and auditory evoked potentials. Lesions in the posterior area (*B*) generally correlate well with visual evoked potentials. Visual, auditory, and somatosensory evoked potentials are frequently used to differentiate a brainstem lesion (*C*) from a cerebral lesion. Frontal lesions (*D*) pose a particularly difficult problem in identification because the frontal cortex receives no specific sensory stimuli.

readings which demonstrated severe evoked potential abnormalities implied that residual or permanent neuronal dysfunction would later be present; mild evoked potential abnormalities were associated with a good prospect for functional recovery (Greenberg, Mayer, & Becker, 1976). Severely abnormal evoked potentials have been used to predict persisting blindness, deafness, and hemiplegia, apparently because profound alteration occurs only when the neuronal substrate has been irreversibly damaged.

The duration of coma has also been related to visual, auditory, and somatosensory evoked potentials. These potentials, obtained during the first week after injury, identified 80% of patients who were comatose at the time of the evaluation but would become responsive within 30 days of the injury (Greenberg, Mayer, Becker, & Miller, 1977). The identification of the patients who would recover consciousness was based on the fact that their multi-sensory evoked potentials were only mildly abnormal. The remaining 20% of the patients who did not regain consciousness within 30 days were among the older members of the population. In addition, the evoked potentials data suggested that the duration of the coma following a head injury was a result of bilateral involvement of the cerebral hemispheres rather than a brainstem dysfunction. This finding corresponds with a number of other studies that have suggested that brainstem damage plays a limited role in the production of unconsciousness (see Reitan & Wolfson, 1986b).

Additional studies have related evoked potentials to eventual outcome after a head injury. Greenberg, Becker, Miller and Mayer (1977) obtained multi-sensory evoked potentials on patients within a week after they had sustained a head injury and repeated the examination about 14 days following the injury. These investigators then correlated the results with eventual outcome as assessed by the Glasgow Outcome Scale.

The patients in this study were divided into two groups: (1) *Persistent Vegetative State* and *Death,* and (2) *Good Recovery, Moderate Disability,* and *Severe Disability.* Evoked potentials recorded an average of 3 days after the injury were not definitive for visual and auditory avenues, but the somatosensory evoked potential was significantly related to outcome. Auditory brainstem and somatosensory evoked potentials taken an average of 14 days post-injury were predictive of a poor outcome. When the somatosensory evoked potentials recorded during the first week following the head injury were only mildly abnormal, 90% of the patients were eventually classified in the *Moderate Disability* or *Good Recovery* categories.

Although these findings are encouraging, it is important to recall the comments made by Jennett and Teasdale (1981), noting that it is of relatively little help to the clinician to know that a patient under his care has one or more features known to be associated with a good or poor outcome. They point out that it is of limited value to know that a certain proportion of patients with certain characteristics will die or will recover. Data which associate a particular circumstance with a particular outcome rarely have a sufficient degree of accuracy to permit any reliable statements about the indi-

vidual patient who has recently sustained a severe head injury.

The Significance of Routine Diagnostic Findings on Outcome

Routine diagnostic studies frequently include plain skull x-rays, computed tomography, cerebral angiography, evaluation of intracranial pressure, monitoring respiration, studies of cerebral circulation and metabolism, the electroencephalogram, multi-sensory evoked potential recordings, cerebrospinal fluid studies, and occasionally, ventriculography. As we have noted previously, plain x-rays of the head and neck have relatively little significance to the eventual outcome unless the x-ray demonstrates the presence of intracranial air or gas and foreign bodies. Such findings could imply the potential development of intracranial infection and this, in turn, might have an adverse prognosis.

We have previously discussed the significance of intracranial mass lesions and the increased mortality associated with them. In fact, general observation indicates that death following head injury is considerably more frequent in the first 3 days post-injury than during the ensuing period. These early deaths often result from secondary bleeding in the form of hematomas. Brain visualization techniques (computed tomography, angiography, and air studies) are useful in identifying intracranial mass lesions and, in this sense, contribute information that is relevant to outcome.

Neurological surgeons recognize the importance of identifying intracranial bleeding in the early phases after a head injury, since an intracranial hematoma is the most common cause of death in patients who lose consciousness following an initial lucid interval. Computed tomography often differentiates between epidural, subdural, and intracerebral hematomas, and such findings are significant for predicting eventual outcome.

In addition, it is sometimes possible to differentiate between edema and infarction and between hemorrhage and contusion. Diffuse or generalized edema of the brain is demonstrated by inability to identify the Sylvian fissure and compression of the lateral ventricles, sometimes to the point of being unable to visualize the ventricles at all. Evidence suggests that diffuse or generalized edema is not a particularly ominous indicator with respect to outcome; however, signs of increased density, associated with hemorrhage and contusion, are correlated with an increased mortality and poor recovery, especially when the lesions are bilateral (Sweet, Miller, Lipper, Kishore, & Becker, 1978). In many such cases death is attributable to severe intracranial hypertension.

Cerebral angiography has two major values: (1) It gives an estimate of the speed of cerebral circulation, and (2) It demonstrates any spasms of major cerebral arteries which may result in ischemic damage to the brain (Scialfa & Christi, 1973). Cerebral vasospasm is also associated with impaired cerebral circulation (Macpherson & Graham, 1974).

Ventriculography may provide information that aids in describing the nature of the brain damage and permits measurement of intraventricular pressure at the time of the procedure. Such data may be useful in predicting the eventual outcome.

Intracranial Pressure and Outcome

It is generally agreed that intracranial pressure equivalent to 10 mm/Hg or less is normal and that a sustained pressure beyond 20 mm/Hg is abnormal. In about half of the patients who expire following a severe head injury, the apparent cause of death is intracranial hypertension (Miller, Becker, Ward, et al., 1977). The prognosis is very poor when the intracranial pressure is sustained at 40mm/Hg or greater (Johnston, Johnston, & Jennett, 1970).

Miller, Becker, Ward, et al. (1977) found that head-injured patients with normal intracranial pressure had a 14% mortality rate; subjects who had elevations above 20 mm/Hg had a 55% mortality rate. As mentioned earlier, Narayan, Greenberg, Miller, et al. (1981) found intracranial pressures of 20 mm/Hg or greater in 44% of their sample, and 51% of these patients died. Of the remaining 56% of the sample, in whom intracranial pressures were less than 20 mm/Hg, only 16% expired. In summary, there appears to be little doubt that elevated intracranial pressure has a very significant relationship to poor outcome, particularly in the early period following a severe head injury.

Respiration as Related to Outcome

We have previously noted that abnormal breathing patterns are related to eventual outcome. Breathing patterns are also significant with regard to severity and location of brain damage following a head injury. Abnormal respiratory patterns are common in patients with definite evidence of lesions of the medulla, cerebellum, and pons. In lesions confined to the cerebellum, however, there appears to be no significant pattern of abnormal breathing (North & Jennett, 1974). In general, abnormal respiratory patterns following head injury are associated with a significantly higher mortality rate, regardless of the particular type of respiratory abnormality.

Apnea lasting more than 5 seconds after a period of hyperventilation has also been suggested as a correlate of brain damage. Jennett, Ashbridge and North (1974) found that apnea lasting for 5 seconds occurred rarely among normal subjects but was not uncommon when brain damage and lethargy were present in combination. In addition, a number of investigators have studied the influence of hypoxemia and mortality rate (Brackett, 1971). These studies consistently indicate an increased mortality rate among patients with hypoxemia.

Cerebrospinal fluid measurements also have some predictive significance with respect to outcome in persons with severe head injury, primarily because of changes that may be related to respiration or reduced cerebral blood flow. The carbon dioxide content in cerebrovenous blood and cerebrospinal fluid is generally similar, but when the carbon dioxide content increases in the cerebral drainage system the results may suggest a reduced cerebral blood flow and in turn be associated with a poor outcome. Direct changes in the cerebrospinal fluid may also be caused by respiratory changes resulting from head injury.

Post-traumatic Amnesia and Outcome

The importance attributed to post-traumatic amnesia (PTA), defined as the interval between the occurrence of the injury and the time the patient has regained continuous memory of on-going events, can readily be established by a brief reference to comments of authorities in the field. Jennett and Teasdale (1981) refer to an editorial in the journal *Lancet* (1961) that agreed with Brock (1960) in concluding that PTA is the best measurement for assessing the severity of a head injury.

Becker, Miller, and Greenberg (1982) state that, "The duration of amnesia after injury probably is the best simple yardstick for determining the severity of diffuse head injury and the total toll of brain dysfunction." At a later point in the same article, these authors state that "... post-traumatic amnesia is at present one of the most important correlates with the extent and severity of psychological as well as physical deficits following injury." They go on to say, "There is a close association between the duration of post-traumatic amnesia and many aspects of the sequelae of head injuries, such as the incidence of post-traumatic epilepsy and psychological sequelae, and the length of time before the patient returns to work."

Jennett and Teasdale (1981) state that PTA "appears to be a reliable guide to the severity of diffuse brain damage, which has been reflected in the acute stage by the depth and duration of coma."

Finally, these same authors point out that "... outcome is closely correlated with the duration of PTA, although there are some patients who make a satisfactory recovery even after a month or more of PTA."

Considering these conclusions, there can hardly be serious questions about why PTA is so often used as a criterion of severity of brain damage in cases of closed head injury. It should also be noted that other instruments, such as the Glasgow Coma Scale, are also used extensively in this respect. In fact, Levin (1985) recognized the importance of the Glasgow Coma Scale as an indicator of severity of brain damage in his comment, "Prior to the induction of the Glasgow Coma Scale in 1974, the duration of PTA was probably the most widely used index of severity of brain injury."

Jennett and Teasdale (1981) have presented a scale, originally proposed by Russell, that explicitly relates duration of PTA to severity of brain injury. The *Very Mild Injury* category correlates with PTA of less than 5 minutes; *Mild Injury* relates to PTA of 5–60 minutes; *Moderate Injury* corresponds with 1–24 hours of PTA; *Severe Damage* relates to PTA of 1–7 days; *Very Severe Damage* was presumed when PTA lasted from 1–4 weeks, and *Extremely Severe Damage* corresponded with a period of PTA lasting more than 4 weeks.

Using the Glasgow Outcome Scale Jennett and Teasdale (1981) present data showing the relationship between the duration of PTA and outcome at 6 months following head injury. When PTA was less than 14 days, none of a sample of 101 patients was classified as *Severely Disabled.* Seventeen percent were categorized as *Moderate Disability,* and 83% were classified as having *Good Recovery.* Among 96 patients whose period of PTA extended from 15 to 28 days, 3% were *Severely Disabled,* 31% were *Moderately Disabled,* and 66% had *Good Recovery.* In this study 289 patients had PTA of more than 28 days, and these patients fared considerably less well than those with shorter duration of PTA. Of these 289 patients, 30% were *Severely*

Disabled, 43% were *Moderately Disabled,* and 27% made a *Good Recovery.*

Duration of PTA is not an absolute determinant of eventual outcome, but there can be no doubt that there is a strong relationship between the two variables. Nevertheless, PTA has been used in many studies as if it were a definitive indicator of severity of brain damage and has been used to assess the validity of other indications of eventual impairment. Although it may be the "best yardstick," it is apparent that there is a considerable degree of variability in outcome of persons with comparable PTA and many patients (even with extended PTA) appear to eventually be placed in the category of *Good Recovery.* However, Jennett and Teasdale (1981) state, "In patients whose PTA has exceeded three weeks it is almost always possible to detect impairment of performance on some tests of cognitive function, even six months after injury, and some degree of measurable deficit is often permanent."

These same authors also have studied the risk of late epilepsy in association with duration of PTA. They estimate that 1% of patients will develop late epilepsy when PTA has lasted less than 24 hours; however, the estimate increases to 4% when PTA has lasted more than 24 hours. These investigators also subdivided their cases in accordance with the occurrence of early epilepsy. Early epilepsy is associated with a substantial increase in the rate of occurrence of late epilepsy, but the relationship with PTA continues to show a difference. Among these cases of early epilepsy, PTA of less than 24 hours was associated with a 22% occurrence of late epilepsy; PTA of more than 24 hours corresponded with late epilepsy in 30% of the cases.

While these values indicate the association between duration of PTA and aspects of outcome, it must again be emphasized that statistics have limited value for predicting the eventual outcome for an individual patient; a head-injured subject may be classified in any outcome category almost regardless of the duration of PTA.

As noted in *Traumatic Brain Injury Volume I* (Reitan & Wolfson, 1986b), PTA has been used extensively as a criterion of severity of brain injury against which the validity of psychological test results have been assessed. There are distinct difficulties in determining the duration of PTA in many cases and definite scientific weaknesses implicit in establishing a variable which is dependent upon the patient's own assessment and determination of the point in time that he left a state of confusion and memory impairment and regained continuous memory and appreciation of events in his environment. There probably is no other instance in which a "scientific" variable is determined by the judgement of a confused and bewildered person who has just recovered from a state of impaired consciousness and memory. Thus, it is not surprising that disparities have been shown between retrospective estimates of PTA by patients and direct inquiry and measurement while the patient was under continuous observation in the hospital (Gronwall & Wrightson, 1980).

In an attempt to standardize procedures for evaluating PTA and retrograde amnesia, Levin, O'Donnell and Grossman (1979) developed the Galveston Orientation and Amnesia Test (GOAT). This test consists of eight questions concerned with orientation to person, place, and time, the day of hospital admission, and events before and after the injury. This test can be administered on a repeated basis, providing information on which to base an estimate of duration of PTA. These investigators found that PTA duration was longer in patients with severe diffuse closed head injuries or bilateral mass lesions than in patients with unilateral mass lesions (Levin, O'Donnell, & Grossman, 1979). They also found that PTA lasting more than 14 days was associated with residual disability at 6 months following the head injury as determined by the results of the Glasgow Outcome Scale. However, results of the Galveston Orientation and Amnesia Test were not found to be very closely related to duration of coma as evaluated by the Glasgow

Coma Scale, even though the relationship was significant (Levin, Papanicolaou, & Eisenberg, 1985) and the conclusion was that the duration of coma does not accurately predict the duration of PTA.

Aphasic Deficits and Outcome

Earlier studies of outcome involving patients who had become aphasic following a head injury centered on war casualties (Russell & Espir, 1961) and there are extensive studies still in progress of persons who sustained a penetrating head injury in Vietnam (Mohr, Weiss, Caveness, et al., 1980). This latter study, which evaluated 1030 head-injured veterans, found that 24% had been aphasic after sustaining the head injury. As might be expected, a high proportion (79%) of these aphasic subjects had lesions principally involving the left cerebral hemisphere and a lower percentage (18%) sustained injuries principally of the right cerebral hemisphere. Fluent aphasia was more commonly associated with left temporal-parietal injuries; nonfluent or motor aphasia was more common in patients with left frontal lesions. Mohr and his associates found that patients with motor aphasia recovered fully within 6 years of the injury, and recovery was most likely in those subjects who did not initially suffer from right hemiparesis. Patients with fluent aphasia showed a considerably greater tendency to have persisting deficits.

A number of studies have been performed among aphasic patients who have suffered a closed head injury, but the incidence of aphasia is considerably less in this category (except among patients who develop a space-occupying lesion, such as a hematoma, in the language area of the left cerebral hemisphere). As with patients who had sustained a penetrating head injury, the most rapid improvement occurs during the first months following the injury. Full recovery (or only mild, selective residual deficits) may be the end result, but Levin, Grossman, Sarwar, and Meyers (1981) estimate that significant residual impairment occurs

in more than half of the closed head injury patients who develop aphasia following the injury.

After sustaining a head injury some degree of recovery is a general phenomenon. The time course relating to recovery of ability in eye opening, obeying commands, and spontaneous speech following injury among aphasia subjects has been plotted by Bricolo, Turazzi, and Feriotti (1980). Najenson, Sazbon, Fiselzon, et al. (1978) have also plotted recovery curves relating to comprehension of gestures, oral language, oral expression, reading, writing, and articulation. Investigators have typically found that some degree of aphasic deficit persists even when some recovery occurs (Thomsen, 1975). The permanence of the deficits relates generally to indications of more severe lesions in the language area of the left cerebral hemisphere.

Prognostic Significance of Glasgow Coma Scale Scores

The Glasgow Coma Scale has been studied in some detail with respect to its prognostic significance, using results of the Glasgow Outcome Scale to assess the patient's eventual status following head injury. We have given a description of the Glasgow Coma Scale previously (Reitan & Wolfson, 1986b) and will briefly review it here for interested readers. The *Glasgow Coma Scale* is a 15-point scale based on the patient's ability to obey verbal commands (a 5-point scale ranging from a total absence of verbalization under any circumstances to normal verbal responsiveness and conversation); the stimulus required to induce eye opening (a 4-point scale ranging from failure to open the eyes under any circumstances to spontaneous eye opening); and motor responsiveness (a 6-point scale ranging from no motor response whatsoever to appropriate motor responses).

The *Glasgow Outcome Scale,* which has been used to evaluate the prognostic significance of the Glasgow Coma Scale, includes five categories: (1) *Good Recovery,* (2) *Moderate Disability,*

GLASGOW COMA SCALE

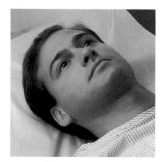
Spontaneous

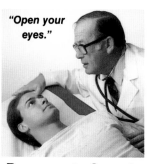
Response to Speech

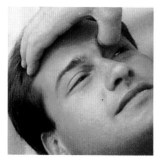
Response to Pain

EYE OPENING (E)

Spontaneous 4
To Speech 3
To Pain 2
No Response 1

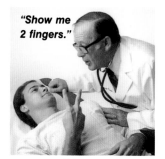
Obeys

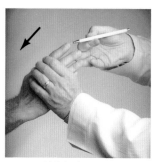
Localizes

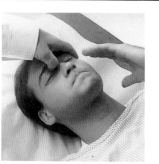
Withdraws

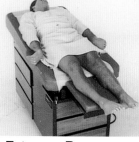
Extensor Response

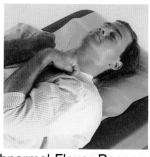
Abnormal Flexor Response

MOTOR RESPONSE (M)

Obeys 6
Localizes 5
Withdraws 4
Abnormal
Flexion. 2
Extensor
Response. 2
No Response 1

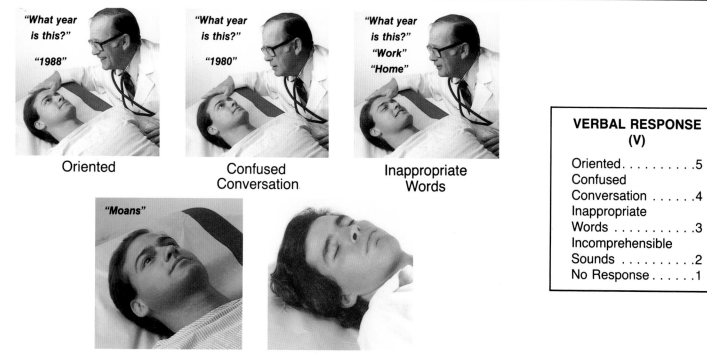
Oriented

Confused Conversation

Inappropriate Words

Incomprehensible Sounds

No Response

VERBAL RESPONSE (V)

Oriented. 5
Confused
Conversation 4
Inappropriate
Words 3
Incomprehensible
Sounds 2
No Response 1

(3) *Severe Disability*, (4) *Persistent Vegetative State*, and (5) *Death.*

It is obvious that neither of these Scales requires a detailed examination. In fact, they are deliberately quite simple and are based upon limited observations in order to achieve reliability in rating. It is possible, therefore, to train any careful observer to use these Scales and excellent reliability, or agreement among raters, has been demonstrated (particularly for the Glasgow Coma Scale) (Teasdale & Jennett, 1976).

The first investigation of the relationship between these Scales was reported by Jennett, Teasdale, Braakman, Minderhoud, and Knill-Jones (1976). These investigators used results obtained with the Glasgow Coma Scale 24 hours post-injury. Subdividing scores into intervals (11–15 representing relatively good scores and categories of 8–10, 5–7, and 3–4 representing degrees of impairment). In many studies coma has been operationally defined as a total score of 8 points or less. The results of this study indicated that the following proportions of patients, using the four categories of the Glasgow Coma Scale given above, fell in the *Good Recovery* or *Moderate Disability* categories, as indicated by the Glasgow Outcome Scale 6 months after injury as follows: 91%, 59%, 28% and 13%, respectively. Conversely, the number falling in the *Vegetative State* or *Dead* categories, in accordance with Glasgow Coma Scale scores were: 6%, 27%, 54% and 80%. These data indicate that the status of the patient on the Glasgow Coma Scale, 24 hours after injury is significantly related to general categories of outcome six months after injury.

Among the three areas of function (Verbal, Motor, Eye Opening) of the Glasgow Coma Scale, the patient's best Motor response correlated most closely with his/her eventual outcome. Eisenberg (1985) states that among more severely injured patients (those whose Glasgow Coma Scale score was 8 or less), the motor examination during the first 3 post-injury days yields only slightly less predictive power than the total Glasgow Coma Scale score. However, Becker, Miller, Ward, Greenberg, Young, & Sakalas (1977) note that abnormal motor responses carry a significant adverse prognosis for outcome only for patients who have diffuse brain injury. Patients with mass lesions who had been evaluated prior to operative decompression did not show a significant relationship between abnormal responses and adverse outcome.

Becker, Miller, and Greenberg (1982) also note that failure to open the eyes on command or with painful stimulation has significance for outcome only during the first 72 hours after injury. After 72 hours eye opening may occur among patients who remain in a persistent vegetative state.

It should also be noted that although verbal responsiveness is used as part of the operational definition of recovery from coma, the fact that a patient is responding verbally does not mean that he/she has regained continuous consciousness and memory. Often patients will verbalize during the period of post-traumatic amnesia, but later have no memory of doing so. Considering the relatively restricted data and general categories included in the Glasgow Coma Scale and the Glasgow Outcome Scale, qualifications of this nature are to be expected.

Since the initial study of the prognostic significance of the Glasgow Coma Scale in 1976, large scale investigations have been instituted and a great deal of additional data is available. Eisenberg (1985) has summarized the results of eight studies, each of which includes more than 100 patients and is consistent with respect to a Glasgow Coma Scale score of 8 or less obtained 6 or more hours after injury (Bowers & Marshall, 1980; Braakman, Gelpke, Habbema, et al., 1980; Gennarelli, Spielman, Langfitt, et al., 1982; Jennett, Teasdale, Braakman, et al. 1979; Langfitt & Gennarelli, 1982; Levati, Farina, Vecchi, et al., 1982; Miller, Sweet, Narayan, & Becker, 1978; Saul & Ducker, 1982). These investigators studied patients in various centers including Glasgow, the Netherlands,

Los Angeles, Milan, Philadelphia, Richmond, San Diego, Maryland, and the Seven Seas Center U.S.A. study (which included 1107 patients).

Mortality rates varied among the studies by as much as 17%. In these eight studies patients classified in the category of *Good Recovery* according to the Glasgow Outcome Scale ranged from 12% to 48%; patients in the *Moderate Disability* category ranged from 6% to 19%; subjects in the *Severe Disability* comprised from 4% to 14%; patients in the category of *Persistent Vegetative State* ranged from 1% to 6%; and the category of *Death* included from 33% to 50% of the patients. Studies of the mortality rate of head-injured subjects with Glasgow Coma Scale scores ranging from 3 to 8 show a progressive decline in various studies; a score of 3 had the highest mortality rate and a score of 8 had the lowest. Nevertheless, there were striking differences in the mortality rates reported in accordance with Glasgow Coma Scale scores from the various centers. Eisenberg (1985) attributes these differences more to the mixture and variability of patients at each entry Coma Scale score than to the therapeutic competence of the individual centers.

While the Glasgow Coma Scale score has been shown to relate significantly to outcome in terms of statistical analyses, the unit of value continues to be the individual head-injured subject. Much additional investigation is needed, in terms of initial assessment procedures as well as evaluation of the eventual quality of life, to improve the meaningfulness of such predictions for individual patients.

Evaluation of Outcome
Using the Glasgow Outcome Scale

The Glasgow Outcome Scale was developed by Jennett and Bond (1975) to assess outcome following head injury (Jennett, Teasdale, Galbraith, et al., 1977) and non-traumatic coma (Bates, Caronna, Cartlidge, et al., 1977). The Scale is in-

tended to reflect the overall social capability or dependence of the patient, based on evaluation of specific mental and neurological deficits.

Evidence suggests that the Glasgow Outcome Scale can be used reliably by different raters. In one investigation, 150 persons who had survived severe head injury were classified independently by a neurologist and a neurosurgeon. There was over 90% agreement in categorization, both at 6 months and 12 months following the head injury (Jennett, Snoek, Bond, & Brooks, 1981). As noted earlier, the four categories of classification based on the Glasgow Outcome Scale are *Vegetative State, Severe Disability, Moderate Disability,* and *Good Recovery.* Of course, for many persons who sustain a head injury, death is a fifth category.

Definition of Categories of Outcome

It should be recognized initially that the category of *Death* should be further subdivided according to the cause of death. Some patients die from the primary damage resulting from direct impact to the head and brain; other patients succumb to the effects of secondary brain damage, usually resulting from edema and severe intracranial hypertension or bleeding after the patient has recovered from unconsciousness. In addition, death may be caused by problems resulting secondarily from the head injury, including factors such as pneumonia associated with prolonged coma, pulmonary embolism, and renal failure.

The Vegetative State. Jennett and Plum (1972) identified the vegetative state as a category of outcome following head injury in which there is no behavioral evidence of cerebral cortical functioning. Nevertheless, there may be quite a number of responses, which include eye opening (and even the occasional ability to track movement with the eyes), postural reflexes with the limbs, and a grasp reflex of the hands. Observers sometimes interpret these responses as signs of early recovery of consciousness. However, experience indicates that many patients who show such signs never regain the ability to speak or perform other tasks, and these reflex types of behavior apparently reflect brain stem functions.

The vegetative state, of course, can be caused by conditions other than head injury. For example, diffuse cerebral hypoxia, a condition which sometimes occurs in patients who have been resuscitated after cardiac arrest, may also result in vegetative state. In cases of head injury, however, the vegetative state probably results from severe axonal shearing caused by the force of the blow. Patients may persist in the vegetative state for considerable periods of time extending over weeks, months, or even years.

The course and duration of the vegetative state has been studied to some extent, but such questions are complicated by the dismal prognosis and its effect on use of heroic measures to maintain life. Jennett and Teasdale (1981) conclude that the "vegetative state is regarded as death temporarily postponed." In addition, there may be some difficulty in classification depending upon the clinician's evaluation of responses as being due only to brainstem activity (as compared with a cerebral component). Some clinicians have been inclined to classify patients as being in a persistent vegetative state even though occasional words may be said, although Jennett and Teasdale (1981) disagree with this practice and emphasize that the classification should be used only for patients who show no psychologically meaningful responses.

Among patients who were confidently categorized by Jennett and Teasdale (1981) as being in the vegetative state, 7% eventually became capable of independent, although impaired living. No patient who was classified in the *Vegetative State* category 3 months after the injury ever gained independent status, although 10% of these patients did regain consciousness but remained totally dependent.

It would appear that anyone who remains in the vegetative state three months after head trauma has little if any chance for regaining an independent existence. Jennett and Teasdale (1981) state that the longest survivor known to them, in a continuous vegetative state, died 18 years after sustaining a head injury. More commonly, however, duration of life is considerably less. Jennett and Teasdale (1981) indicated that of 94 patients judged to be in a vegetative state one month after the injury, 50% had died within a year. When the classification was still present at 3 months post injury, 60% were dead within one year.

A number of conditions have been described which should be differentiated from the persistent vegetative state. The *locked-in syndrome,* described by Plum and Posner (1980), leaves the patient paralyzed and unable to speak, but nevertheless responsive and apparently aware of his environment. The patient with locked-in syndrome may be able to communicate by blinking or making movements with his jaw or eyes. In fact, ingenious methods of facilitating communication using computer displays have been developed for such persons. This condition results from interruption of motor pathways in the ventral part of the pons.

Akinetic mutism, a condition described by Cairns, Oldfield, Pennybacker, et al. (1941), results from cystic or neoplastic lesions in the vicinity of the anterior diencephalon. These patients may show some movement at times and even occasionally say words. In addition, they may appear to be aware of their surroundings. Some patients who have recovered from akinetic mutism state that they are able to recall events that occurred while they were mute.

The patient with *global aphasia* should also be differentiated from the patient in a persistent vegetative state, but these patients are usually able to engage in many activities that indicate the presence of remaining cerebral cortical functioning.

Finally, in some instances, the persistent vegetative state may resemble aspects of some psychiatric disorders, including catatonic schizophrenia and possibly hysterical coma. In general, however, it is not difficult to differentiate these conditions from the absence of cerebral cortical functioning following head injury.

Severe Disability. Jennett and Bond (1975) identify patients in this category as persons who are dependent on some other person for at least some activities during every 24-hour period. The disability may relate to physical impairment (such as spastic paralysis of the limbs), pronounced dysphasia which limits communication both expressively and receptively, or severe impairment of higher-level brain functions that requires permanent supervision, often in a mental hospital. In some instances these higher-level deficits may be manifested as disinhibited, irresponsible, and even psychopathic behavior. Jennett and Bond (1975) described the least impaired of persons included in this category as patients with definite impairment of cognitive and memory functions who are dependent upon others during every 24-hour period for activities such as dressing, feeding, or cooking of meals. Therefore, any person who suffers impairment following a head injury who is not totally independent for at least daily periods is classified in the *Severe Disability* category.

Moderate Disability. Persons who are impaired by head injury but still able to care for themselves, travel by public transportation, and are capable of some work are classified in the category of *Moderate Disability.* Within this classification a great deal depends upon the particular nature of the patient's deficit and the type of work that might be appropriate. For example, a person with severe dysphasia may be able to carry out certain occupational tasks that do not require facility in verbal communication. In other instances, as pointed out by Jennett and Teasdale (1981), the brain-injured person is actually not able to carry out the job to which he is assigned but is either assisted in his duties or excused for not carrying them out by other persons in his environment. In other words, the person is not capable of performing his work but is permitted to continue in his occupation through the assistance or indulgence of others.

These authors do not feel, therefore, that return to work, in its own right, should be a final criterion in determining the degree of disability. Many patients who have moderate disability, in terms of the Glasgow Outcome Scale, may have physical or mental difficulties, including hemiparesis, ataxia, cranial nerve deficits, post-traumatic epilepsy, or intellectual, cognitive, and personality deficits. Those persons who are able to attend to their personal needs only and are able to engage in occupational activities to some degree would be classified in the *Severely Disabled* category rather than only in the *Moderately Disabled* category.

Good Recovery. This final category characterizes head-injured patients who are able to participate in a normal social life and return to work. In many instances the patient has not returned to work for various reasons, but classification in this category requires a judgement that the patient possesses the basic abilities necessary to return to work. Thus, there may be some residual deficits on neuropsychological measures or persisting losses of a physical nature, but these should not prevent the patient from functioning relatively normally.

As a critique of the categories of classification representing the Glasgow Outcome Scale, it must be recognized that neuropsychological evaluation identifies many patients who would fall in the *Good Recovery* category who, nevertheless, show significant deficits in various areas of higher-level neuropsychological functioning which severely restrict returning to pre-morbid activities. In fact, subjects who have sustained a head injury and find it impossible to return to the demanding activities of professional tasks are totally neglected by these classifications of outcome. They are identified as having achieved a good recovery although they are not able to carry out their pre-morbid activities. Many such subjects, when evaluated in centers for rehabilitation, are considered to be normal, to have no significant difficulties, and therefore be inappropriate subjects for rehabilitation.

Basically, the question concerns what should be rehabilitated when the subject shows no evidence of disability? In these instances it is extremely important that detailed neuropsychological evaluation be performed, examining both the strengths and weaknesses of brain-related abilities, so that a proper neuropsychological diagnosis of disability may be made (as contrasted with the frequent impression, based upon casual observation, that no disability exists). Cases of this kind were illustrated in Volume I of *Traumatic Brain Injury* (Reitan & Wolfson, 1986b).

Jennett and Teasdale (1981) recognize the possibility of a more refined subdivision of the four categories representing survivors of head trauma. Initially the subjects may be divided into patients who die and patients who survive. Survivors may be subdivided according to those who are in a persistent vegetative state and those who are conscious. Conscious subjects, in turn, may be severely disabled or may be relatively independent, and degrees of disability may be classified within the four categories described above or be divided into a better and worse subclassification for each category.

The situation still exists, however, in which many persons who have sustained a relatively mild brain injury have significant impairment which is not recognized by clinical observation and examination and requires neuropsychological testing in order to define the nature and degree of the deficit. In many individual cases, these latter deficits may have great significance for adaptation to everyday living, particularly for technical and professional occupations, and to the overall quality of living.

Validation of Outcome Assessments

It is difficult to validate the Glasgow Outcome Scale because it is based upon predetermined categories of outcome rather than upon primary data concerned with evaluation of deficits. A possible approach might be to consider prognostic indicators following head injury and their relationship to classifications obtained in using the Glasgow Outcome Scale. However, even this approach would have significant difficulties because the validity of the prognostic indicators can be determined only in terms of the outcome classifications, and thus the procedure is based on interdependent variables rather than upon independent and dependent variables. In other words, one cannot validate prognostic indicators in terms of concordance with outcome indicators or outcome indicators in concordance with prognostic indicators unless the validity of one or the other is known initially.

Of course, the Glasgow Outcome Scale is presumed to be valid for the criteria used to classify the patient into an outcome category. However, as noted earlier in this chapter, prognostic indicators must be viewed in most cases only as early outcome indicators rather than later outcome indicators. Prognostic indicators that predate the head injury are generally unknown in the individual case and the only relevant data, in terms of the effects of brain trauma, are available only after injury has been sustained. A definite need exists, though, for determining the significance of early results of head injury for eventual outcome classifications.

Some studies have been done in which the nature of the disability has been related to categories of recovery as shown by the Glasgow Outcome Scale. Jennett, Snoek, Bond, and Brooks (1981) have studied the significance of psychological vs. physical disabilities with relation to the proportion of persons falling in various outcome categories. The physical disability was more limiting than the psychological impairment in only about 25% of their sample of 150 head-injured survivors. In more than half of these subjects, the psychological deficit was a more significant disability than the physical impairment. The psychological and physical deficits were considered to be about equally significant in just less than 20% of the subjects.

In terms of total assessment, the psychological deficits were equal or equivalent to the physical deficits for determining disability in 72% of the cases. There was no particular differential relationship of psychological and physical bases for disability depending upon the outcome category. Among patients classified in the category of *Severe Disability,* nearly two-thirds had more significant psychological disorders and the ratio was only slightly less among persons in the categories of *Moderate Disability* and *Good Recovery.*

Bond (1976) studied 56 patients and attempted to differentially relate social handicaps and behavior to psychological and physical deficits. He found that psychological impairment was of greater significance. Physical deficits did contribute to social handicap as a whole and also, significantly in a statistical sense, to work capability. However, psychological deficits also contributed a social handicap, as a whole, to work capability, leisure activities, and cohesion of family relationships. Impairment of sexual activity and adjustment was not found to be significant with respect to either physical or psychological deficits.

Bond also found that the severity of disability was related to residual manifestations of both physical and psychological impairment. Patients who were classified in the category of *Good Recovery* were described principally as only having mild changes in personality. (We must note that careful and detailed neuropsychological evaluation of such patients often identifies significant intellectual and cognitive impairment that, without the advantage of neuropsychological evaluation, is described as mild changes in personality.) In patients with moderate disability, psychological and physical deficits were found in about equal proportions. The physical deficits were usually represented by a mild degree of hemiparesis, cranial nerve palsies, or occasional instances of post-traumatic epilepsy.

Studies of reaction time demonstrated that impairment is present in persons who have sustained traumatic brain injury and that reaction time improves during the course of recovery (see Reitan & Wolfson, 1986b for a more detailed review of psychological deficits following traumatic brain injury). Von Zomeren and Deelman (1978) have shown that head-injured subjects who had experienced longer periods of coma (as compared to patients who had experienced shorter periods of coma) demonstrated initially more severe deficits in reaction time. The group with initially more severe deficits also showed greater improvement in reaction time over a 24-month period following the injury but, nevertheless, did not reach the level of performance shown by the group with a shorter period of coma.

The above finding suggests that the degree of initial impairment is related to the absolute degree of recovery over time following head injury. Dikmen, Reitan, and Temkin (1983) showed that rather than being specific to reaction time, this effect is general in nature, as demonstrated by recovery curves on an extensive battery of neuropsychological tests. Although persons with more serious brain damage suffer more significant initial impairment than subjects with less severe damage, the more severely damaged subjects also achieve a greater absolute degree of recovery than subjects who are less seriously impaired initially. Nevertheless, the group with more significant initial damage still shows more residual deficit at an eventual outcome point in the recovery process.

In terms of intellectual ability (principally as measured by the Wechsler Adult Intelligence Scale), studies generally reveal some degree of impairment following traumatic brain injury with the potential for at least a degree of recovery in time. Mandleberg and Brooks (1975) found evidence of impairment on the WAIS following head injury but, in follow-up studies of these patients, reported that Verbal IQ appeared to reach an asymptotic level approximately 5 months after the injury; Performance IQ reached an asymptotic level 13 months after the injury. In a final examination performed 3 years after the injury, these investigators felt that WAIS results had returned to normal levels regardless of the duration of post-traumatic amnesia (which was used to infer the severity of the injury).

Levin (1985) points out that this conclusion is at variance with the findings of many other investigators who have studied the eventual outcome of Verbal IQ and Performance IQ following severe head injury. Other investigators (Levin, Grossman, Rose, & Teasdale, 1979; Norrman & Svahn, 1961; Roberts, 1980) have demonstrated that persons who have sustained a severe head injury show definite and permanent impairment on the WAIS. Obviously, this conclusion should not imply that the permanent deficits of intelligence, as measured by the WAIS, represent the complete evaluation of intellectual and cognitive functioning. In fact, many neuropsychological tests are generally more sensitive to such impairment than Verbal IQ and Performance IQ measurements (see cases presented in *Traumatic Brain Injury Volume I* and in this volume).

Levin, Grossman, Rose, and Teasdale (1979) studied the degree of recovery on the WAIS approximately one year post-injury and found a correlation between recovery and the average range of intellectual functioning only in patients who had achieved a good overall recovery. The category of *Moderate Disability* related to variable IQ values and the patients in the *Severely Disabled* category were consistently intellectually impaired. These researchers also found that duration of coma and the presence of oculovestibular deficits, which they used as an indicator of severity of brain damage, were correlated with the degree of later cognitive and intellectual deficit. Verbal IQ was less closely related to the duration of coma (as shown by the Glasgow Coma Scale) than Performance IQ, a finding that has previously been reported by Kløve and Cleeland (1972).

Somatosensory and Motor Skills

Levin (1985) comments that in studies of the effects of traumatic brain injury, "perceptual and motor skills have generally been accorded a minor role as compared to memory and information processing." This has been true only for those neuropsychologists who have elected to study memory and information processing rather exclusively. The significant impairment of perceptual and motor skills resulting from traumatic brain injury, as well as many other types of neuropsychological deficits, have long been recognized by those who have investigated problems in this area (Reitan & Wolfson, 1986b).

Investigation of the adequacy of visual perception has shown that patients with closed head injuries have significant impairment in recognition of photographs of faces (Levin, Grossman, & Kelly, 1977), even though a severe deficit of this type is rare. Brain injury also may cause impairment in recognition of letters of the alphabet tachistoscopically presented in the peripheral aspects of the visual field. This finding occurred even though identification of similar letters in the area of macular vision was intact (Hannay, Levin, & Kay, 1982). As might well be expected, more deficient performances were shown by patients who had a Glasgow Coma Scale score of 8 or less, indicating that the deficit was more pronounced among persons with severe head injuries.

Auditory perceptual functions have also been studied. Bergman, Hirsch, and Najenson (1977) found that auditory perceptual skill of the ear contralateral to a unilateral temporal lobe lesion showed evidence of impaired perception of competing sentences presented to the two ears simultaneously. The intactness of the auditory pathways from the cochlea to the brain cortex have also been investigated extensively by recording of auditory evoked potentials (see pp. 50–53, this volume).

Tasks dependent upon tactile perception as the primary sensory input (even though the overall task may be considerably more complex) have also been investigated. Hom and Reitan (1982) have compared performances with the right hand compared with the left hand on the Tactual Performance Test in patients with right and left cerebral neoplastic, vascular, and traumatic injuries. The results indicated that lateralized vascular lesions cause the most consistent and striking contralateral deficits. Neoplastic lesions occupied an intermediate position, and traumatic head injury, as might be expected because of the generalized effects of a severe blow from the external environment to the head, showed a lesser lateralized effect.

Dikmen, Reitan and Temkin (1983) found evidence indicating that impairment on the Tactual Performance Test was quite severe after initial damage, probably because of the complexity of the task (as contrasted with the rather isolated element of tactile input). In fact, recovery of skill on the Tactual Performance Test was relatively slow over an 18-month period, again probably due to the complexity of the task. Many research findings have suggested that rather simple tasks can be performed satisfactorily by persons with cerebral damage, whereas impairment of performance becomes much more obvious, in comparison with normal controls, on tasks that involve unexpected, complex, or higher-level aspects of brain functions.

Tasks involving visual-motor performances have also been studied in relation to traumatic brain injury. Probably the principal example in this regard involves the Trail Making Test. Prior research (Reitan, 1958) has indicated that in adults Part B of this test is more sensitive to cerebral damage than Part A; Part B requires integration of numerical and alphabetical sequences, whereas Part A requires only connection of individual numbers in sequence. However, the test appears to be quite complicated in terms of its overall requirements, necessitating functional integrity of both the left and right cerebral hemispheres (Reitan & Tarshes, 1959). It is likely that the poor performances of brain trauma subjects on this test, even though they show improvement over an 18-month period (Dikmen, Reitan, & Temkin (1983), probably relate to the simultaneous requirements of the task.

Rather than attempt to isolate the factors which contribute to impairment, as suggested by Levin (1985), it is important to recognize that clinical measurement of brain-related deficits also requires the use of tasks that involve input and integration of several related neuropsychological elements in the performance of the task at hand. Most problem-solving functions in everyday life do not depend exclusively on the use of factorially pure abilities, but require the integrated and organized use of various skills.

Emotional Disturbances and Outcome

Emotional difficulties of adjustment are common among persons with traumatic brain injury. In some instances the emotional problems are reactive, stemming from significant intellectual and cognitive impairment and the distressing effects of these deficits when they impair adaptation to prior living activities and patterns. Over and beyond such reactive difficulties, however, it is likely that brain injury itself, in a primary sense, causes some degree of emotional problems. A number of studies have been performed to evaluate the emotional status of patients following significant head injury, and these were described in *Traumatic Brain Injury Volume I* (Reitan & Wolfson, 1986b, pp. 90–92).

Because outcome studies require a longitudinal design, evaluation of outcome following the development of emotional difficulties has not been studied in detail. However, Dikmen and Reitan (1977b) used the Minnesota Multiphasic Personality Inventory (MMPI) to evaluate head-injured patients shortly after their injury (usually within one month), 12 months after the initial examination, and again 18 months later. Trend analyses of the three evaluations indicated significant improvement, especially on the Hypochondriasis, Depression, Hysteria, Psychasthenia, and Schizophrenia scales. The findings suggested that patients with a head injury have relatively numerous complaints indicating depression, anxiety, somatic problems, and strange experiences shortly after the injury, but that these complaints tend to decrease in time.

This same study considered the relationships between results on the Halstead-Reitan Battery, in terms of severity of impairment, and resulting indications of emotional distress as demonstrated by results on the MMPI. The findings indicated that patients with more serious neuropsychological deficits also showed evidence of greater emotional difficulties than subjects who were only mildly impaired. Those patients who were more seriously impaired in intellectual and cognitive functions also were more likely to demonstrate continued abnormalities on the MMPI 12 months post-injury.

Currently available evidence suggests that there is an interaction between severity of damage and resulting emotional problems of adjustment, even though spontaneous improvement in emotional status occurs in time following head injuries. Additional studies are needed that are specifically designed to identify variables which will permit prediction of the adequacy of emotional outcome.

Outcome Studies Regarding Social Aspects of Behavior

General observations have indicated that subjects who sustain brain trauma often suffer significant changes in their social behavior. Oddy, Humphrey, and Uttley (1978) evaluated 50 young adults 6 months after closed head injury using interviews with relatives, the Katz Adjustment Scale, and determination of subjective complaints of the patients. These researchers concluded that there was deterioration in social functioning, characterized by a decreased number of close friends, diminished frequency of social outings, and a rise in feelings of loneliness.

Thomsen (1974) interviewed 50 patients 2 years after they had sustained a severe closed head injury and found that the principal complaint was loneliness. As might be expected, social contact was particularly diminished for subjects who had residual aphasia. While the evidence makes it clear that social adjustments may be impaired by traumatic brain injury, additional studies are needed to determine the types of deficits that lead to a poor social outcome in order to gain insight into the mechanisms involved and intervention strategies or procedures that might be helpful.

Post Head Injury Employment as an Indicator of Outcome

Various studies have reported quite variable results concerning the proportion of head-injured subjects who are able to return to an employment level that is essentially similar to their pre-injury employment status. Dresser, Meirowsky, Weiss, et al. (1973) found that approximately 75% of head-injured veterans of the Korean war were gainfully employed 15 years after their injury. These were cases primarily of penetrating head injuries. The factors that characterized the veterans who had returned to work were higher premorbid scores on the Armed Forces Qualification Test, the depth of missile injury, the presence and severity of motor deficit, and the duration of coma. These latter variables would appear to be reflections of the severity of brain damage, suggesting that those persons with less severe damage had a greater potential for post-head injury employment.

Oddy, Humphrey, and Uttley (1978) found that 71% of subjects with a period of post-traumatic amnesia from 1 to 7 days returned to work; only 27% returned to work when PTA was longer (more than 7 days). Variables related to severity of injury, particularly if physical disability was a residual, were also significant in this respect. In general, the severity of brain injury appears to be a major determinant, but other factors, including age among older persons, pre-existing personality problems or a psychiatric condition, alcoholism, etc. may all be significant variables.

There is no doubt that occupational outcome after head injury is determined by many factors. The severity of brain injury, the nature and type of neuropsychological deficit, emotional difficulties following head injury (which may be exacerbated in patients with prior psychiatric difficulties, see Aita & Reitan, 1948) all represent significant factors.

Final Comments

It is important to note that nearly all of the studies reviewed above have been oriented toward outcome through measurement of initial deficits and evaluation of recovery. As would be expected, these studies indicate that following a head injury most patients show a degree of improvement in time. Of course, details regarding the initial damage and deficit constitute early prognostic indicators that improve prediction of the degree of recovery that might be expected for individual persons. Nevertheless, we must again emphasize Jennett and Teasdale's (1981) comment: "It is seldom realized how little help it is to the clinician to know that an individual patient under his care has one or more features known to be associated with a bad or a good outcome. Only when the brain damage is at one extreme or the other of severity, in a category in which all patients will die or all will recover, does the clinician have a useful guide; but only a small minority of patients have such distinctive characteristics. For the rest it is of limited value in decision-making to know that a given fraction of patients with certain characteristics will die (or recover). For the care of individuals the doctor needs to know for a given patient what the probabilities of alternative outcomes are." (Pp. 327–328.)

The fundamental purpose of outcome studies is to generate information that will be useful in predicting outcome for the individual head-injured subject, and group statistics are of limited value in this regard. Because the critical question concerns outcome for the individual head-injured subject, compilation of statistics regarding recovery of memory, language functions, or results on selected psychological tests appears to be of more academic interest than clinical significance. This area clearly needs studies that focus on variables, or combinations of variables, that will permit prediction of recovery for the individual person.

Dikmen and Reitan (1976) conducted a study during which neuropsychological function was systematically monitored over an 18-month period together with detailed clinical neurological examination and EEG reports. These findings permitted establishment of an initial baseline for type and severity of impairment. A number of data-sets were composed from findings shortly after the head injury to be used as predictor variables for eventual outcome. Eventual outcome was based upon clinical evaluation of neuropsychological test results obtained 18 months after the injury with each subject classified either into a category that showed definite and significant residual impairment or a category that showed relatively normal performances or only mild impairment.

The first data-set used for predictive purposes was derived from neurological evaluation shortly following the injury. Nine variables were available for each subject, and using discriminant analyses, these variables correctly classified 76% of the subjects to their appropriate groups.

A second discriminant analysis utilized 10 variables derived from the full complement of information that included the initial neurological evaluation, neurological evaluation 3 months following the injury, initial and 3-month EEG recordings, and neuropsychological evaluation shortly after the injury. This data-set resulted in a 94% correct prediction rate, a finding that appears to be highly promising with respect to the potential for eventually devising a method for making accurate predictions.

The final data-set that was based on 15 variables derived entirely from neuropsychological tests. This data-set permitted a 91% correct prediction rate.

These findings would suggest that neuropsychological data, obtained usually within one month post-injury, provides information that is quite relevant to eventual outcome and degree of recovery. Obviously, a longitudinal study was needed to obtain this information and cross-validation is necessary, particularly because the study was based only upon 34 subjects. It appears from these findings, however, that it would be possible to develop a data-set which, with appropriate weighting of individual variables, could be used as an accurate basis for predicting eventual neuropsychological status of head-injured persons.

Figure 2-5. Responses to cerebral trauma at a cellular level.

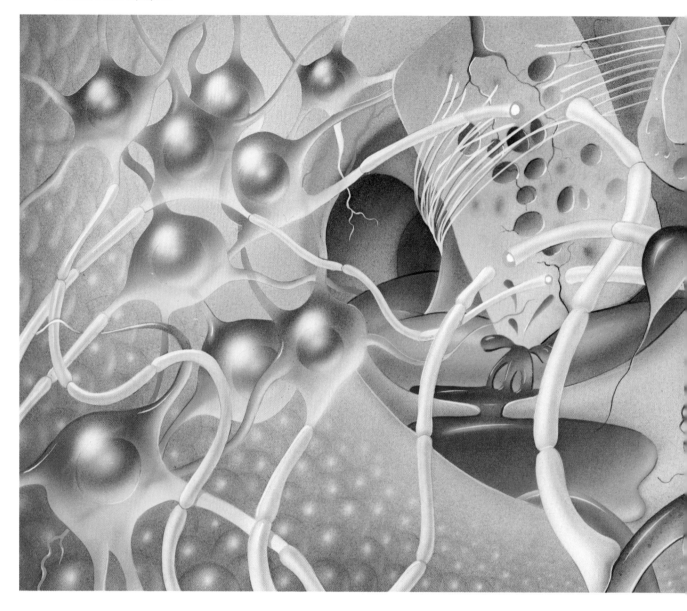

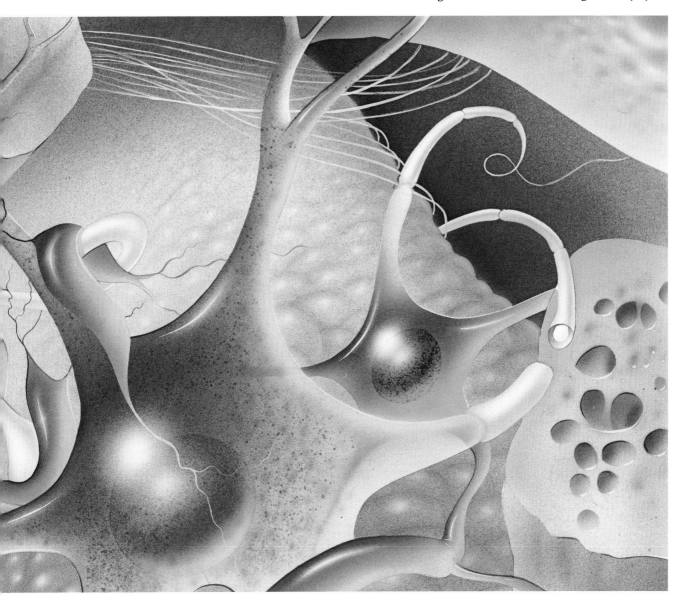

III

DEVELOPMENT, SCORING, AND VALIDATION OF THE GENERAL, LEFT, AND RIGHT NEUROPSYCHOLOGICAL DEFICIT SCALES

Various measures and procedures have been used to evaluate the severity of brain injury, and in turn these measures have been used to predict eventual outcome of cognitive abilities. Sometimes a global neurological evaluation — including the clinical neurological examination, specialized diagnostic methods (such as computed tomography), observations at surgery, duration of unconsciousness and post-traumatic amnesia, and other available information — has been used to classify head injuries as severe, moderate or mild (Aita, Reitan, & Ruth, 1947). However, this method is inescapably impressionistic and reflects the judgement and prejudices of the person who reviews the records for each patient.

A main criticism of this method is that the sources and types of information vary from one patient to another and are combined in a subjective manner to reach a final conclusion. Under such circumstances it may be difficult to replicate the evaluation exactly and the resulting classification of the severity of the head injury may reflect the bias of the individual who decides upon the classification. Therefore, although use of the full range

of pertinent information might be thought to be the most valid procedure, efforts have been made to identify more explicit variables or conditions for categorizing head injury cases according to severity of impairment.

In 1932 Russell proposed using the duration of time required to fully recover consciousness as a valid index of the severity of brain damage. By "full consciousness" Russell particularly emphasized the return of continuous, on-going memory of events that occurred in the patient's environment; Russell believed that the recovery of consciousness was finally established only when normal memory of events had returned.

There is a problem, however, with defining the "return of normal memory." Jennett and Teasdale (1981) indicate that the patient's own account of the time at which memory was regained is the criterion to be used. For these researchers, then, the interval between the time the injury occurred and the point at which the subject says that his memory has returned constitutes the period of post-traumatic amnesia. In fact, Jennett and Teasdale believe that the advantage of this definition of post-traumatic amnesia is that one can obtain the information directly from the patient even if months or years have passed since the time of the injury; the criterion will not be affected even if original notes, hospital records, or other supporting information has been lost or misplaced or is unavailable.

In the past many procedures have been adopted in which patients are asked to assess and evaluate their own cognitive condition. For example, Luria interviewed his patients to learn their own assessment of their neuropsychological deficits after brain disease or injury in order to determine what psychological tests he would administer. Basically, this same procedure is used and recommended by some modern neuropsychologists (Lezak, 1983).

It may be of interest to the neuropsychologist to learn what patients think to be the time at which they recovered consciousness and their opinions of their neuropsychological deficits; however, on the face of the situation, it would seem that an impaired patient is hardly the best source or judge of such information. In fact, it seems almost ludicrous to base a supposedly scientific variable — a criterion used to evaluate the severity of a brain injury and predict the patient's eventual cognitive outcome — upon that patient's own report of when he/she recovered from post-traumatic amnesia. Even though some patients are quite specific in identifying the first thing that they remembered after the accident or the event occurring at the time their memory returned, such reports can hardly be considered reliable indicators of the time that full return of memory functions occurred.

A majority of the studies of alertness, memory, and learning referred to earlier (Reitan & Wolfson, 1986b) demonstrated that most persons still had significant impairment of memory and learning abilities even after the period of post-traumatic amnesia (using the criteria described above). Anyone who has ever observed patients closely after they have sustained a significant head injury severe enough to cause loss of consciousness realizes that

it is very difficult to define the point in time at which complete and continuous memory functions have returned. In fact, recovery of consciousness and memory is a gradual process that is probably not basically distinguishable from the longer-term recovery that has been reported to occur over months and even years following a head injury.

Duration of unconsciousness and post-traumatic amnesia are not necessarily closely related to the severity of damage or the neuropsychological impairment. It is well known that some persons who have sustained a penetrating head injury with severe damage to their brain tissue may not lose consciousness. Even in cases of closed head injury the period of unconsciousness may continue for months, and when the patient finally recovers he/she may show no more significant neuropsychological impairment than a patient with a closed head injury who had a much shorter period of post-traumatic amnesia (Reitan & Wolfson, 1986b).

Jennett and Teasdale (1981) implicitly recognized that the duration of post-traumatic amnesia (PTA) often cannot be accurately estimated, but they point out that it is almost always possible to estimate whether it lasted for minutes, hours, days, or weeks, and that even these gross judgments are a satisfactory index of the severity of a head injury. These authors propose the following scale for evaluating severity of head injury based on duration of unconsciousness: less than 5 minutes, *Very Mild;* 5–60 minutes, *Mild;* 1–24 hours, *Moderate;* 1–7 days, *Severe;* 1–4 weeks, *Very Severe;* more than 4 weeks, *Extremely Severe.* Jennett and Teasdale emphasize that many studies have established the "close relationship between the duration of PTA and various sequelae of head injury"; in fact, they state explicitly that the best way to describe a series of patients is either by (1) noting the minimum duration of PTA, or (2) charting the distribution of PTA durations.

Recommendations such as those made by Jennett and Teasdale have tended to establish the duration of post-traumatic amnesia as an important measure and probably the most widely-used procedure for evaluating the severity of closed head injury and assessing the validity and degree of impairment shown on various psychological measures and testing procedures. It must be recognized, however, that duration of post-traumatic amnesia is a very crude and approximate index, determined exclusively by someone who is possibly the least capable of an accurate appraisal of the situation: the brain-injured, psychologically impaired person who has recently sustained head trauma and is just barely recovering consciousness and memory functions.

Another measure that has been widely used to assess severity of brain injury and predict eventual outcome is the Glasgow Coma Scale. There is no doubt that the scores obtained on this Scale have a significant relationship to various measures of eventual outcome, and it has been proven to be a very useful instrument. Scores are based on the patient's responses to well defined and explicit stimuli. This procedure promotes reliability in assessment and scoring among personnel with various degrees of training. In addition, the Scale can be repeated at any interval, allowing the examiner to plot the patient's course of recovery.

Despite the advantages of the Glasgow Coma Scale, its value is limited by the simplified nature of the procedures on which it is based. As described previously (Reitan & Wolfson, 1986b), the Scale is based upon three types of behavior: (1) *Eye Opening* (with responses ranging from no opening of the eyes to spontaneous eye opening), (2) *Motor Response* (with responses ranging from no motor response to extensor response, abnormal flexion, withdrawal, localization of the stimulus, or spontaneous compliance); and (3) *Verbal Response* (with responses ranging from no verbal response to incomprehensible sounds, inappropriate words, confused conversation, and normal verbal communication).

Although the Glasgow Coma Scale was originally devised to be used with patients in various stages of coma, it is nevertheless based upon behavioral responses. One can hardly expect to do a very meaningful or complete neuropsychological (behavioral) examination on a partially comatose patient. Therefore, the purpose for which the Scale was developed requires that the content of the examination be quite limited (and even primitive) as a behavioral assessment of brain functions. As noted above, the Glasgow Coma Scale can be used when more complete neuropsychological assessment is obviously impossible and, in addition, the results have been shown to have definite predictive value. Because of its nature, however, the Scale cannot be a substitute for a complete neuropsychological evaluation and must be viewed as a limited and relatively gross evaluation of responsiveness.

The above comments are not intended to demean the value either of estimates of the duration of post-traumatic amnesia or the Glasgow Coma Scale. It is clear, though, that these rather simplistic procedures overlap very little with the complete neuropsychological examination in describing behavioral correlates of traumatic brain injury. Complete neuropsychological evaluation is necessary in order to comprehensively assess residual deficits of cerebral trauma along the many relevant dimensions of behavior that relate to brain function.

Our recommendation is that the patient receive a complete neuropsychological evaluation at approximately the time he/she is medically stable enough for discharge from the hospital (at least as far as the head injury is concerned; orthopedic injuries or other problems may require extended hospitalization). This point in time is hardly a precise criterion in terms of its meaning, but in clinical practice it does relate to recovery of a certain degree of stability of both biological and behavioral functions. Of course, it is highly advantageous to repeat the neuropsychological examination later at specified dates and compare the results in order to assess recovery or deterioration of cognitive functions.

The complexity of a complete neuropsychological examination, the many areas of function involved, and even the necessary use of various strategies of measurement create a problem concerning standardization, objectivity, and quantitative assessment of the results (Reitan & Wolfson, 1986b). There is, of course, no substitute for a complete neuropsychological evaluation to validly assess a patient's relevant cognitive functions; however, it is also useful to have a quantitative score which reflects the overall adequacy of neuropsychological functioning.

Two very similar indexes which have been proposed for this purpose are the Halstead Impairment Index (Halstead, 1947a) and the Average Impairment Rating (Russell, Neuringer, & Goldstein, 1970). Each of these measures was based on a number of variables and has been shown to achieve an impressive degree of reliability in differentiating between groups of subjects with and without cerebral damage. The reliability of each of these two indexes generally exceeds the reliability achieved with individual measures.

Unfortunately, neither of these composite indexes is based upon a complete set of neuropsychological tests which had been devised to reflect neuropsychological aspects of brain functions generally, and neither assesses the patient's degree of deficit regarding the principal neuropsychological methods of inference (level of performance, patterns and relationships among test results, specific deficits characteristic of brain injury, and comparisons of functional efficiency on the two sides of the body using the same tasks).

The General Neuropsychological Deficit Scale (G-NDS) was devised to provide a comprehensive summarical evaluation of brain-behavior relationships for individual subjects. Normative and validational data for the G-NDS are presented below. Fortunately, it also appears that the G-NDS is not significantly affected by positive practice-effects on readministration of the Halstead-Reitan Battery. This apparently occurs because the G-NDS was devised to reflect changes of clinical significance rather than variations of normal performances. Sensitivity to severity of impairment, coupled with freedom from practice-effects, promises to make the General Neuropsychological Deficit Scale a highly useful measure for evaluating clinically significant changes in neuropsychological status in individual or group evaluations, clinical or research needs, and assessment of improvement or deterioration.

THE GENERAL NEUROPSYCHOLOGICAL DEFICIT SCALE

The General Neuropsychological Deficit Scale (G-NDS) was devised to evaluate adult subjects (15 years of age and older) and represents a subject's performances on 42 variables derived from the Halstead-Reitan Battery for Adults. The 42 variables were divided into four groups to reflect deficits in accordance with each of the methods of neuropsychological inference: (1) *Level of Performance* (variables 1–19); (2) *Pathognomonic Signs* (variables 20–31); (3) *Patterns and Relationships Among Test Results* (variables 32 and 33); and (4) *Right-Left Differences* (variables 34–42). A score is obtained for each of these categories as well as a total score for all 42 variables.

Each variable (except for pathognomonic signs, described below) is scored on a scale ranging from 0 to 3 points. A score of *0* corresponds with a perfectly normal performance. A score of *1* is still within the normal range, but represents a performance that was not quite as good as might be ideally expected.

A significant dividing point occurs between scores of *1* and *2;* scores of *0* and *1* represent the normal range and scores of *2* and *3* depict impaired performances. A score of *2* represents mild to moderate neuropsychological impairment and a score of *3* represents severe impairment. Transformation of raw scores into scaled scores of *0, 1, 2,* or *3* can be done quite straightforwardly by using the information provided in Table 3-1.

Table 3-1. Rules for computing the General Neuropsychological Deficit Scale score.

Level of Performance

Variable	0	1	2	3
1. Verbal IQ	90+	82–89	73–81	≤72
2. Performance IQ	90+	82–89	73–81	≤72
3. Impairment Index	0–.2	.3–.4	.5–.7	.8–1.0
4. Category Test	0–25	26–45	46–64	65+
5. TPT — Total Time	0′–9.0′	9.1′–15.0′	15.1′–25.0′	25.1′+
6. TPT — Memory	8–10	7	4–6	0–3
7. TPT — Localization	7–10	6	3–5	0–2
8. Seashore Rhythm Test (# correct)	28–30	25–27	20–24	0–19
9. Speech-sounds Perception Test (errors)	0–6	7–10	11–15	16+
10. Finger Tapping — Dominant Hand	55+	50–54	41–49	0–40
11. Finger Tapping — Non-dominant Hand	49+	45–48	37–44	0–36
12. Trail Making Test — Part A	0″–26″	27″–39″	40″–51″	52″+
13. Trail Making Test — Part B	0″–65″	66″–85″	86″–120″	121″+
14. Tactile Form Recognition — Total Time	0″–16″	17″–23″	24″–33″	34″+
15. Bilateral Tactile Stimulation — Total errors	0	1	2–3	4+
16. Bilateral Auditory Stimulation — Total errors	0	1	2	3+
17. Bilateral Visual Stimulation — Total errors	0	1	2–3	4+
18. Tactile Finger Recognition — Both hands (errors)	0–2	3–4	5–8	9+
19. Finger-tip Number Writing — Both hands (errors)	0–3	4–6	7–11	12+

Pathognomonic Signs

Variable	Score
20. Dysnomia	3
21. Auditory verbal dysgnosia	3
22. Visual number dysgnosia	3
23. Visual letter dysgnosia	3
24. Body dysgnosia	3
25. Dyscalculia	2
26. Dysgraphia	2
27. Dyslexia	2
28. Constructional dyspraxia	2
29. Central dysarthria	1
30. Spelling dyspraxia	1
31. Right-Left confusion	1

Table 3-1. (continued)

Patterns

Variable	0	1	2	3
32. Verbal IQ/Performance IQ Difference	0–5	6–10	11–19	20+
33. If Impairment Index 0.0–.4, score is 0. If Impairment Index .5–1.0, then derive score from Full Scale IQ. If FS IQ:	<90	90–95	96–100	101+

Right-Left Differences

Variable	0	1	2	3
For Variables 34, 35, and 36: Divide non-dominant hand by dominant hand and subtract from 1.0				
34. Finger tapping	.08–.12	.13–.16 .07–.05	.17–.21 .04–(−.03)	.22 or more (−.04 or less)
35. TPT	.38–.26	.25–.15 .39–.42	.14–.05 .43–.50	.04 or less .51 or more
36. Grip strength	.08–.12	.13–.17 .07–.06	.18–.20 .05–.00	.21 or more (−.01 or less)
37. Tactile Form Recognition	0–1″	2″–3″	4″–5″	6″+
The score is the difference in seconds between the two hands				
For Variables 38, 39, and 40: The score is the difference in errors between the right and left side				
38. Bilateral Tactile Stimulation	0	1	2	3+
39. Bilateral Auditory Stimulation	0	1	2	3+
40. Bilateral Visual Stimulation	0	1	2	3+

For Variables 41 and 42: (1) Determine the percentage of errors by the hand with the greater number of errors; (2) Enter the table in the row with the total errors made; (3) Determine the score

41. Tactile Finger Recognition
42. Finger-tip Number Writing
Table for Variables 41 and 42:

Total Errors	0	1	2	3
21 or more	50–54	55–57	58–60	61+
18–20	50–54	55–57	58–62	63+
15–17	50–54	55–58	59–63	64+
12–14	50–55	56–58	59–63	64+
9–11	50–56	57–59	60–63	64+
6–8	50–56	57–63	64–70	71+
3–5	50–59	60–67	68–79	80+
0–2	50	1 error	100	—

(% applies to columns 0–3)

Pathognomonic signs (variables 20–31), derived from the Reitan-Indiana Aphasia Screening Test, are scored differently than the other variables because each of these signs is presumed to represent brain dysfunction (rather than a range of performances that extends from normal to impaired). In order to score the pathognomonic sign variables it is necessary to have experience and clinical competence with the Aphasia Screening Test. In order to facilitate the development of these clinical skills among neuropsychologists, Reitan (1984) has provided many illustrations of interpretation of results for individual patients and reviewed the area of aphasia and related disorders.

Each of the pathognomonic sign variables was assigned a score ranging from *1* to *3*. These scores were derived from data that reflected the extent to which each of the types of deficit was intercorrelated with other deficits (Reitan, 1984). Therefore, if the patient demonstrates dysnomia, a score of *3* is assigned because dysnomia appears to have more pervasive significance (and more serious neuropsychological consequences) than some of the other pathognomonic signs.

In practice, it is necessary to review the results of the Aphasia Screening Test for the individual subject, determine if any deficits are present, and assign the indicated score for each pathognomonic sign that is present. The next step is to add the scores in each of the four sections of the G-NDS and finally, to add these four resulting scores in order to obtain a total G-NDS score for the subject.

Table 3-2 presents mean scores for each of the four sections and the average total General Neuropsychological Deficit Scale score for a number of groups of subjects. For purposes of preliminary validation, a non-brain-damaged control group as well as groups with generalized cerebral damage, left cerebral damage, and right cerebral damage were taken from a previously published study that explored another question (Reitan, 1985a). As noted in Table 3-2, the control group (No Cerebral Damage) was composed of 41 subjects; the groups

with generalized, left, and right cerebral damage were composed of 23, 25, and 31 subjects respectively. All groups were comparable in distributions of chronological age, years of formal education, and gender.

The control group (subjects who had no evidence of brain damage) had a mean G-NDS score of 17.20 points for the total of all 42 variables. Performances on the 19 variables in the Level of Performance section were the principal contributors to this total, but the two variables reflecting Patterns and Relationships had approximately the same average weight as the Level of Performance variables. Pathognomonic signs occurred rarely among the control subjects and (as will be noted by comparisons with the mean points for the total of 42 items), Right-Left Differences had an intermediate weighting.

These results indicate that each variable had a mean between *0* and *1* points (normal scores), averaging 0.41 points per item. These data confirm that the control subjects did indeed generally fall within the range of normal performances.

Before inspecting the results for the groups with generalized, left, and right cerebral damage, we will consider the combined results for these groups (listed as Heterogeneous Brain-Damaged in Table 3-2). This group of 79 subjects had a mean total G-NDS score of 51.34 points, with each of the 42 variables contributing an average of 1.22 points. (Obviously, subjects with brain damage are not impaired on every item and their overall average performance reflects a combination of these normal and impaired performances.) The Level of Performance items contributed more per item to the total than the other categories, with Patterns and Relationships and Right-Left Differences falling at an intermediate position.

Pathognomonic signs contributed the least number of points, reflecting the previous finding that specifically abnormal performances are seen relatively infrequently, even if the subject has a cerebral lesion (Reitan, 1984). The particular path-

Table 3-2. Mean scores on sub-sections and total General Neuropsychological Deficit Scale scores for various groups with cerebral lesions and a non-brain-damaged group.

	N	$\overline{X}$ Level of Perf. Nos. 1–19	$\overline{X}$ Signs Nos. 20–31	$\overline{X}$ Patterns Nos. 32–33	$\overline{X}$ Rt/Lt Diff. Nos. 34–42	Total 1–42
No Cerebral Damage	41	11.95	.54	1.34	3.37	17.20
Mean Points Per Item		0.63	.04	0.67	0.37	0.41
Generalized Cerebral Damage	23	31.57	6.35	2.65	10.65	51.22
Left Cerebral Damage	25	32.20	7.08	2.72	12.44	54.48
Right Cerebral Damage	31	32.84	1.16	2.32	12.52	48.90
Total Heterogeneous BD	79	32.27	4.54	2.54	11.95	51.34
Mean Points Per Item		1.70	0.38	1.27	1.33	1.22
Generalized CVD	15	34.53	7.60	2.27	11.67	56.07
Left CVD	15	36.53	11.80	2.07	13.80	64.33
Right CVD	15	38.67	3.73	3.07	18.00	63.47
Total CVD	45	36.58	7.71	2.47	14.49	61.29
Mean Points Per Item		1.93	0.64	1.24	1.61	1.46
Diffuse Head Injury	15	31.33	7.60	2.60	10.27	52.20
Left Head Injury	15	29.07	8.40	2.20	9.80	49.47
Right Head Injury	15	27.27	5.93	1.80	8.73	43.73
Total Head Injury	45	29.22	7.31	2.20	9.60	48.47
Mean Points Per Item		1.54	0.61	1.10	1.07	1.15
Total Brain Damage	169	32.60	6.12	2.43	12.00	53.22
Mean Points Per Item		1.72	0.51	1.22	1.33	1.27

ognomonic signs included for evaluation in the Halstead-Reitan Battery were derived entirely from the Aphasia Screening Test.

The Aphasia Screening Test includes many items concerned with receptive and expressive aspects of language impairment which tend to occur with damage of the left cerebral hemisphere and contains fewer specific signs associated with right cerebral damage. Therefore, patients with left cerebral lesions show many more pathognomonic signs than patients with right cerebral lesions. The group with generalized cerebral damage, involving both cerebral hemispheres, had a substantially greater incidence of pathognomonic signs than the group with right cerebral damage. These results suggest that a patient's left cerebral hemisphere has to be significantly impaired in order to obtain a clearly defective score on the Pathognomonic Sign section of the G-NDS.

The mean values for the groups with generalized, left, and right cerebral damage were approximately equivalent in all other instances; in fact, the total score for each of these groups failed to show statistically significant differences. This finding indicates that the General Neuropsychological Deficit Scale generates an equivalent degree of impairment for brain-damaged subjects regardless of whether neurological information classifies the patient as having generalized, left, or right cerebral damage.

Comparisons of the Heterogeneous Brain-Damaged Group with the control group (No Cerebral Damage) reflect highly significant differences for each of the four sections as well as for the total score on the G-NDS. The total score for the brain-damaged subjects (a mean of 51.34) was almost exactly three times as large as the mean for control subjects without cerebral damage (a mean of 17.20). Each of the sections contributed significantly to the overall difference between the groups with and without cerebral damage. Even the Pathognomonic Signs section was of definite value in this regard because of the limited number of

defective performances demonstrated by control subjects. This finding supports the observation previously reported by Wheeler and Reitan (1962) that when pathognomonic signs do occur they have definitive significance for cerebral damage.

Table 3-2 also reports the results of the four sections of the General Neuropsychological Deficit Scale in groups of patients with generalized, left, and right cerebrovascular disease and groups of patients with diffuse (generalized), left, and right cerebral lesions resulting from craniocerebral trauma. Within each category of lesion type, the groups had equivalent age, education, and gender distribution.

The patients with vascular disease were consistently slightly more impaired on the total score than the groups with heterogeneous generalized, left, and right cerebral damage. This finding is consistent with data previously reported by Hom and Reitan (1982), in which patients with lateralized cerebrovascular lesions had somewhat more striking deficits than patients with lateralized intrinsic brain tumors or patients with left or right cerebral damage from a head injury.

This prior finding of Hom and Reitan (1982) was also reflected by the evidence that patients with cerebrovascular lesions (strokes) demonstrated greater impairment on the left side of the body than the right side. The patients with left cerebrovascular lesions had the greatest incidence of left pathognomonic signs, as would be expected from the contribution of items from the Aphasia Screening Test. The patients with generalized cerebrovascular brain damage (which obviously includes left as well as right cerebral lesions) occurred next in frequency, followed by the subjects with right cerebrovascular disease.

At this point we should note that the G-NDS was devised as a procedure for evaluating the general adequacy of brain functions, and was *not* designed as a measure to differentiate between left and right cerebral lesions. In fact, the sections on Patterns and Relationships and Right-Left Differences deliberately do not specify the direction of the differences involved. Determining the presence of lateralized cerebral damage requires a second step which logically follows the initial determination of whether cerebral damage of any kind is present. The Right and Left Neuropsychological Deficit Scales, which address this problem, will be presented later in this chapter.

Patients with brain damage due to head injury were essentially comparable in total scores on the G-NDS regardless of the category of traumatic brain damage (diffuse, left, or right). (It should be noted, though, that the group with right cerebral damage tended to perform somewhat better than the other groups.) The scores for the head-injured subjects were also approximately comparable to the level of deficit shown by the groups with heterogeneous brain damage. Among the head-injured subjects who had right cerebral damage, the incidence of pathognomonic signs was somewhat higher than in the previous groups considered. This finding reflects the fact that head injury, even though lateralized according to neurological and neurosurgical information, almost invariably has widespread effects within the cerebral hemispheres (Reitan & Wolfson, 1986b).

Mean values for the total of 169 brain-damaged subjects are given at the bottom of Table 3-2. It is apparent that Level of Performance variables contribute most per item toward the total score, with Patterns and Relationships and Right-Left Differences at an intermediate position.

Pathognomonic signs contribute least, although as noted above, when pathognomonic signs are present they are particularly significant because they rarely occur among control subjects. Therefore, although pathognomonic signs cannot be expected to occur in every brain-damaged subject, they are almost a certain indication of cerebral damage when they are present. (Note the essential absence of pathognomonic signs in the group without cerebral damage.)

The mean scores for the total of 169 subjects

approximate rather closely the mean scores for the 79 heterogeneous brain-damaged subjects, although it must be recognized that this latter group constitutes more than half of the patients that were used to obtain the total means.

The data presented in Table 3-2 were reorganized for presentation in Table 3-3 in order to provide a direct comparison of patients with generalized, left, and right cerebral lesions across categories of heterogeneous, cerebrovascular, and craniocerebral trauma. The results indicate that the total G-NDS score was quite similar regardless of whether the damage was generalized or involved the left or right cerebral hemisphere (mean values of 52.87, 55.80, and 51.21, respectively). In fact, the means were generally similar to those presented in Table 3-2 where the data was organized according to heterogeneous cerebral damage, cerebrovascular disease, and head injury.

The contributions from each of the four sections were also rather closely comparable, except that the Pathognomonic Signs section score contributed less toward the total score for the group with right cerebral lesions than for the groups with left or generalized cerebral damage. However, as intended in developing an overall indication of severity of neuropsychological deficit, the scores in total were generally quite comparable regardless of whether the brain lesion was generalized or involved the left or right cerebral hemisphere. It is obvious that the mean for every category was nearly 50 points or higher, compared with a mean of only 17.20 points for the non-brain-damaged control group.

Table 3-4 presents statistical comparisons of groups that recapitulate the results presented above. Matrix A indicates that no differences approached statistical significance in groups with lateralized (left or right) or generalized cerebral lesions. However, Matrix B makes it clear that patients with cerebral vascular lesions were more seriously impaired than groups with heterogeneous (mixed) or traumatic cerebral lesions.

Table 3-3. Comparative performances on the General Neuropsychological Deficit Scale of groups with generalized, left and right cerebral lesions.

	N	Level of Performance	Signs	Patterns	Rt/Lt Diff.	Total
Heterogeneous Generalized	23	726	146	61	245	1178
Generalized CVD	15	518	114	34	175	841
Generalized HI	15	470	114	39	154	783
Total (Generalized)	53	1714	374	134	574	2802
Mean		32.34	7.06	2.53	10.83	52.87
Left Heterogeneous	25	805	177	68	311	1362
Left CVD	15	548	177	31	207	965
Left HI	15	436	126	33	147	742
Total (Left)	55	1789	480	132	665	3069
Mean		32.53	8.73	2.40	12.09	55.80
Right Heterogeneous	31	1018	36	72	388	1516
Right CVD	15	580	56	46	270	952
Right HI	15	409	89	27	131	656
Total (Right)	61	2007	181	145	789	3124
Mean		32.90	2.97	2.38	12.93	51.21

Table 3-4. t-ratios comparing groups of subjects on the General Neuropsychological Deficit Scale according to areas of cerebral damage and types of cerebral lesions (Matrices A, B, and C), and controls vs. brain-damaged (Matrix D).

Matrix A	1	2
1. Heterogeneous generalized		
2. Heterogeneous left	$t = .70; p < .489$	
3. Heterogeneous right	$t = .52; p < .605$	$t = 1.18; p < .242$
Matrix B	1	2
1. Total heterogeneous		
2. Total CVD	$t = 3.17; p < .002$	
3. Total HI	$t = 1.08; p < .284$	$t = 3.42; p < 001$
Matrix C	1	2
1. Total generalized		
2. Total left	$t = -1.11; p < .271$	
3. Total right	$t = .20; p < .840$	$t = 1.28; p < .204$
Matrix D	1	
1. Controls		
2. Total brain-damaged	$t = 19.79; p < .0001$	

Note: Because of the clear-cut nature of the findings, the authors decided not to encumber either the text or the reader with the results of multivariate statistical analyses customarily performed before doing comparisons of paired groups.

Matrix C was based on all of the brain-damaged subjects reported above, and again showed no evidence of differential G-NDS scores in accordance with lateralized or generalized cerebral damage. Finally, Matrix D reports the comparison between the control group and the total brain-damaged group and the results are striking. It is apparent that the G-NDS is a remarkably sensitive variable.

Table 3-5 presents distributions of the scores on the G-NDS for 41 control subjects and 169 brain-damaged subjects. These scores are organized according to corresponding percentile ranks. Thus, the lowest total score for the control patients was 7 points (corresponding with a percentile rank of 5) and the highest score was 35 points (corresponding with a percentile rank of 100).

The brain-damaged subjects had quite a different scale, with a score of 22 points corresponding with the 5th percentile, a score of 51 points corresponding with the 50th percentile (note the consistency with which mean and median scores for the various groups centered around 50 or slightly higher), and a score of 113 points corresponding with the 100th percentile. This table indicates that none of the control subjects scored above 35 total points on the G-NDS, but 85% of the brain-damaged subjects had scores higher than 34 points and 80% had scores higher than 38 points.

Although there was some overlap in the distribution of control subjects and brain-damaged subjects (as would be expected from the likelihood that some control subjects would perform relatively poorly in terms of brain-related measures and some brain-damaged subjects with mild injuries and high pre-morbid cognitive levels would perform relatively well), the overall differentiation between the groups was striking. The results shown in Table 3-5 make it quite clear that the total score for the G-NDS permits identification of a very effective cut-off score for differentiation between patients with and without cerebral damage.

Table 3-5. Distributions of scores on the General Neuropsychological Deficit Scale for control and brain-damaged groups.

%ile	G-NDS Scores	
	N = 41 Controls	N = 169 Total Brain-Damaged
100	35	113
95	32	84
90	25	79
85	24	75
80	22	70
75	21	67
70	20	62
65	19	59
60	18	57
55	17	55
50	16	51
45	15	49
40	14	47
35	13	45
30	12	42
25	11	40
20	10	38
15	9	34
10	8	30
5	7	22

Using various cut-off scores for the General Neuropsychological Deficit Scale, Table 3-6 presents information regarding false-positives and false-negatives among both control and brain-damaged groups. If one were to use a cut-off score between 12 and 13, none of the brain-damaged subjects would be incorrectly classified, but 68% of the control subjects would fall in the "brain-damaged" range. Obviously, this error-rate in correct classification of the control subjects would not be acceptable. The results indicate that a cut-off score between 25 and 26 would result in the least error of classification in both groups. Using this as the cut-off score, 10% of the control subjects would fall in the brain-damaged range and 8% of the brain-damaged subjects would fall in the control range.

Table 3-6 presents additional information for use by clinicians who have reasons, based on external data, to suspect that the subject may have performed poorly (due to initially low general intelligence or other factors) even though still a non-brain-damaged subject, or that the individual may have performed well (due to a high level of premorbid abilities) and still have sustained some brain damage. In our data distribution, however, no control subject had a score of 35 or more points; however, 85% of the brain-damaged subjects fell in this range.

Finally, a review of the data suggests that using the G-NDS we can present preliminary classification scores that best characterize normal, mildly impaired, moderately impaired, and severely impaired neuropsychological abilities (Table 3-7). As noted previously, 10% of the control subjects had total scores of 26 or more and appear to represent controls who were relatively less able than the rest of their group. Eight percent of the brain-damaged subjects had scores of 25 or less and represented those persons with very mild brain damage that left them relatively unimpaired. As illustrated in Table 3-7, persons with scores of 25 points or less would be classified in the *Normal* range in terms

Table 3-6. Accuracy of classification of control and brain-damaged subjects at various cut-off scores for the General Neuropsychological Deficit Scale.

Cut-Off Score	Controls	Total Brain-Damaged
35 +	0%	85%
34 −	100%	15%
33 +	5%	87%
32 −	95%	13%
26 +	10%	92%
25 −	90%	8%
25 +	15%	93%
24 −	85%	7%
13 +	68%	100%
12 −	32%	0%

of the adequacy of their neuropsychological functions.

Scores of 26 to 40 represent the category of *Mild Impairment.* No control subject had a score above 34; however, 17% of the brain-damaged subjects had scores between 26 and 40. Obviously, the total of brain-damaged subjects with scores of less than 40 points (25%) represents a conservative figure with respect to classification of mild impairment.

Moderate Impairment corresponds with total General Neuropsychological Deficit Scale scores between 41 and 67. No control subjects fell in this

Table 3-7. Tentative categories of deficit corresponding to score ranges on the General Neuropsychological Deficit Scale (based on 169 brain-damaged subjects and 41 control subjects).

G-NDS Score

68 or more	Severe Impairment	(No controls fell in this range) (25% of brain-damaged subjects had NDS scores of 68 or more)
41–67	Moderate Impairment	(No controls fell in this range) (50% of brain-damaged subjects had NDS scores of 41–67)
26–40	Mild Impairment	(No controls had NDS scores above 34) (17% of brain-damaged subjects had NDS scores of 26–40)
0–25	Normal Range	(10% of controls have scores of 26+ and are impaired controls) (8% of brain-damaged subjects have scores of 25 or less and are unimpaired brain-damaged subjects)

range, but 50% of the brain-damaged subjects had scores in this range. Thus, moderate impairment is represented by the point that includes a total of 75% of the brain-damaged subjects.

The category of *Severe Impairment*, represented by NDS scores of 68 points or more, extends far beyond the distribution of control subjects and represents the 25% of brain-damaged subjects who performed most poorly on the General Neuropsychological Deficit Scale.

The above information relevant to classification of subjects according to the degree of neuropsychological impairment obviously is based upon the statistical spread of G-NDS scores. The classification would certainly have relevance for practical assessments of impairment in everyday living,

but research of this nature has not yet been done.

Although the G-NDS differentiates strikingly between control and brain-damaged subjects and serves as an excellent general indicator of neuropsychological impairment without being strikingly influenced by generalized, left, or right cerebral damage (and is even quite sensitive in groups of head-injured subjects where chronological age is generally considerably lower), we must still emphasize the need for careful and competent clinical interpretation of the test results for the individual subject. There is a striking degree of variability among brain-damaged subjects, both in terms of their degree of cognitive impairment and the specific nature of their deficits. Each of these factors has great significance for clinical evaluation and recommending programs for remediation and management. There is no substitute for competent clinical evaluation to describe the individuality of impaired brain-behavior relationships, a condition that must be recognized in terms of respect for the subject as a person.

Effect of Repeated Testings on the General Neuropsychological Deficit Scale (G-NDS)

Repeated testing of head-injured patients and other brain-damaged subjects is often required for clinical assessment of possible improvement or deterioration as well as for research evaluations. However, differentiating between the effects of spontaneous biological recovery, facilitated recovery through brain retraining, and positive practice-effects has posed a formidable problem.

There have been many attempts to solve this problem in various ways. The most common solution is to identify the amount of "improvement" expected on the basis of positive practice effect, to subtract that amount from the scores obtained, and to consider any resulting change to be a reflection of improvement or deterioration. The procedure used to accomplish this aim has been to employ a control group that has not been head-injured or trained in the interval between testings. The neuropsychological tests are then administered on the same schedule to this control group and the head-injured group. The "improvement" obtained by the control group is considered to be an estimate of the practice effect. Scores for individuals or groups on the second testing are then statistically adjusted. The amount of practice effect shown by the control subjects is subtracted and any remaining improvement or deterioration of performance is considered to be either spontaneous or facilitated recovery or deterioration.

As the reader is probably aware, such procedures are far from satisfactory. There is no way to know that the amount of practice-effect (improvement on successive testings) of a control group would be perfectly equivalent to the practice-effect expected from brain-injured subjects. It is entirely possible that subjects with a brain injury would not be able to profit as much or learn as much from previous exposure to the tests as control subjects. Variations might even be expected to occur differentially among brain-damaged subjects, with more impaired persons being able to profit from earlier testing experiences less well.

Finally, the procedure is grossly inadequate in providing an adjustment of the scores for individual subjects. A process in which the subject's raw score is adjusted on the basis of group results loses the uniqueness that characterizes the performance of the individual.

Rather than use adjustments based on test-retest results of control subjects, we felt that we might have found a solution to this problem of evaluating practice effect through the scoring system used for the G-NDS. The scores assigned for the 42 variables taken from the Halstead-Reitan Neuropsychological Test Battery for Adults reflect categories of performances extending from perfectly normal to severely impaired. The score assigned to the variable corresponds with a range of performances, and our postulate was that these four categories of scores (*0, 1, 2,* and *3*) represented differences, at least to a degree, in the clinical significance of the test results. In other words, minor changes or variations should have no consistent effect on the test results.

If a person was initially perfectly normal on a particular measure, he/she might still continue to be perfectly normal on a subsequent examination, even though the absolute difference in scores reflected a degree of positive practice-effect. Our postulate was that practice-effect did not represent a clinically significant change, and therefore would not be reflected by a transformation of the raw data to a scoring framework that was oriented toward clinically significant changes in performance.

In order to test this hypothesis, we administered the Halstead-Reitan Battery for Adults to 25 normal subjects. We deliberately selected persons who might be comparable in age to groups of head-injured patients, but also selected the 25 subjects to reflect excellent educational backgrounds and high levels of intelligence. Our purpose in selecting very bright subjects was to be certain that they had the ability to comprehend all of the testing procedures and, when retested, to be able to take full advantage of the initial testing experience. It has been observed that seriously impaired persons typically gain little insight or understanding of a test based on the first administration and, as a result, demonstrate little positive practice-effect.

We therefore composed a group of 25 men with a mean age of 41.64 years (SD, 8.75) and a mean educational level of 16.76 years (SD, 2.07). These were all persons who had professional or management-level occupations. They all were in good health and functioning normally. Their mean Verbal IQ was 128.44 (SD, 8.28); mean Performance IQ was 125.80 (SD, 8.02); and mean Full Scale IQ was 129.26 (SD, 7.06). Six of these 25 men had doctoral degrees, 11 had master's degrees, 3 had completed college, 4 had completed two or three years of college, and one had completed only high school. Each subjects was tested initially and retested with the complete Battery 12 months later.

The results of these subjects on the G-NDS for the initial and 12-month testings are shown in Table 3-8.

On the initial testing the mean G-NDS score was 12.48 and on the second testing the mean score was 10.92. Both scores were well within the normal range but showed no significant difference between each other. A question might be raised regarding whether these very bright subjects may have performed so well on the first examination that a "ceiling effect" precluded achievement of a better score on the second examination. Inspection of raw-score distributions argued against this hypothesis.

The mean scores for each of the four sections of the G-NDS are also shown in Table 3-8. The pattern of comparative contribution is essentially similar to the pattern reported for control subjects (see Table 3-2). The means for the initial and 12-month testings showed no significant differences for any of the four sections. It is possible that these subjects performed slightly better on the 12-month testing than they had initially, but none of the differences was statistically significant and from these data we therefore have no reason to believe that practice-effects over a 12-month period have any substantial influence on the General Neuropsychological Deficit Scale. Further evaluation is necessary, but these preliminary findings suggest that the G-NDS may prove to be very useful in assessing clinically significant changes (either improvement or deterioration) in individual as well as group evaluations.

Results on the General Neuropsychological Deficit Scale for Head-Injured Subjects Tested Initially and Re-examined at 12 and 18 Months

With support from the National Institute of Neurological and Communicative Disorders and Stroke (NINCDS), we had an opportunity at the University of Washington to administer the Halstead-Reitan Battery to head-injured subjects three times: when the patients were ready for discharge from the hospital, 12 months later, and again 18 months following the initial testing. These patients were studied very systematically and completely, not only neuropsychologically, but also medically by neurosurgeons, electroencephalographers, and neuro-otologists. This is the group of patients from which we selected illustrative examples for neuropsychological interpretation in the latter part of this volume.

This group of patients has been described in detail elsewhere (Dikmen & Reitan, 1976; Dikmen, Reitan & Temkin, 1983). These subjects were primarily from a university community. They were very bright and appeared to be highly motivated during the neuropsychological testing. As a group,

Table 3-8. Results on the General Neuropsychological Deficit Scale for initial and 12-month testings of 25 bright normal controls.

	Level of Performance	Pathognomonic Signs	Patterns	Rt/Lt Diff.	Total NDS Score
Initial testing	6.72	0.52	0.84	4.40	12.48
12-month testing	5.92	0.60	0.52	3.88	10.92
t	1.57	0.62	1.07	0.77	1.59
p <	.20	.60	.30	.50	.20

Table 3-9. Mean scores on the General Neuropsychological Deficit Scale for groups of head-injured subjects with evidence of cerebral tissue damage (Group 1) and cerebral concussion (Group 2) on three examinations (initial, 12-months, and 18-months).

CEREBRAL TISSUE DAMAGE GROUP		Level of Performance	Pathognomonic Signs	Patterns	Right/Left Differences	Total
Initial Exam	Mean	31.44	6.83	2.72	12.06	53.06
	SD					18.33
12-month Exam	Mean	19.61	4.06	2.06	8.33	34.06
	SD					17.05
18-month Exam	Mean	20.11	3.94	2.72	9.72	36.50
	SD					18.14
CEREBRAL CONCUSSION GROUP						
Initial Exam	Mean	14.18	0.54	2.09	8.55	25.36
	SD					11.45
12-month Exam	Mean	9.64	0.45	1.64	6.64	18.36
	SD					7.86
18-month Exam	Mean	9.09	0.91	1.27	7.55	18.82
	SD					6.95

they were considerably more intelligent than the average (as reflected by scores on the Wechsler Scale). Therefore, they might be expected to perform better than the average of the general population.

Table 3-9 presents mean G-NDS scores for one group of subjects whose available neurological evidence unequivocally indicated the presence of cerebral tissue damage (Group 1) and another group of subjects whose head injury apparently resulted only in cerebral concussion (Group 2). The first group earned a mean total G-NDS of 53.06 and on the initial examination performed much worse than the group with cerebral concussion. For the patients who had a cerebral concussion and no definitive evidence of cerebral tissue damage, the mean was only 25.36. As shown in Table 3-10, these means were significantly different (p <.001).

Both groups showed substantial improvement on the 12-month testing, but the larger absolute improvement occurred in Group 1, where the greatest deficit was initially present. On the 18-month testing neither group demonstrated any further improvement, although the group with cerebral tissue damage continued to have significantly worse G-NDS mean scores.

Figure 3-1 presents details of statistical evaluation of the significance of changes on successive testings for both Groups 1 and 2. In addition, the data are graphed for each of the four sections as well as the total General Neuropsychological Deficit Scale. As shown, the group with evidence of cerebral tissue damage consistently performed worse than the group with cerebral concussion. We did not feel that further statistical testing of these differences was necessary because the results would only have shown them to be highly significant. Our focus in statistical evaluation was based upon change (or difference) between scores on the three examinations, presuming that positive practice-effect was essentially inoperative (see results reported above on normal subjects tested initially and at 12 months).

Table 3-10. Statistical comparisons of results on the General Neuropsychological Deficit Scale for a group with cerebral tissue damage and a group with concussion.

	Total	
	t	p <
Initial Testing	4.35	.001
12-month Testing	2.77	.01
18-month Testing	2.99	.01

Considering the results for the group with cerebral tissue damage, each of the four sections showed evidence of significant improvement between the initial and the 12-month examination. This improvement stands in contrast to the lack of any such change in normal subjects, and would certainly seem to represent spontaneous recovery. (None of these subjects had been enrolled in any formal rehabilitational program.) The consistency of these changes resulted in a highly significant difference for the total G-NDS scores, with a substantial degree of improvement being manifested.

Similar results were obtained for the group with cerebral concussion, except for variables concerned with the pathognomonic signs and patterns and relationships between test results. Only two variables contributed to the Patterns score, thereby limiting the prospect of finding a significant difference. A definite degree of improvement occurred on the total G-NDS, even though the absolute degree of improvement was not as great as for the subjects with cerebral tissue damage.

There was no further improvement in any of the comparisons between the 12-month and the 18-month examinations. For the sections, the changes usually were not statistically significant but in two instances the group with cerebral tissue damage showed significantly poorer scores (Patterns and Relationships and Right-Left Differences).

Figure 3-1. Proportion-of-maximal-deficit score, according to inferential method, for head-injured groups with cerebral tissue damage and cerebral concussion tested initially and at 12 and 18 months.

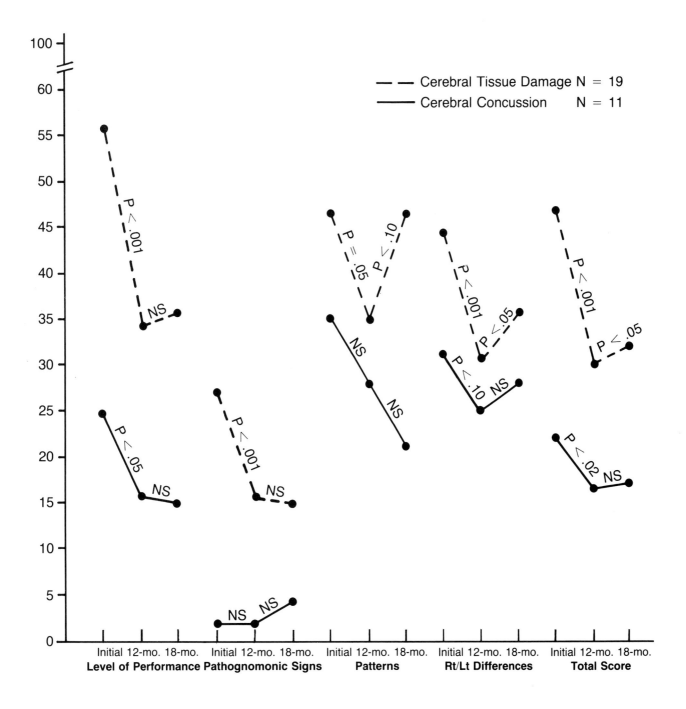

The overall changes for the group with cerebral tissue damage showed a highly surprising result, with significantly poorer performance (p <.05) on the 18-month examination as compared with the 12-month examination. The evidence suggests that instead of demonstrating continued improvement during the 12th to 18th months post-injury, patients with actual cerebral tissue damage in fact show at least a mild degree of deterioration. Thus, our data indicate that improvement is not merely a leveling-off process that gradually ceases, but actually is a biphasic phenomenon.

Many patients with a head injury and evidence of cerebral tissue damage eventually show deterioration of neuropsychological functions that previously had been spontaneously recovered. The neuropathological bases for such changes are presently unknown, but these findings indicate the need for further biological studies during what has been presumed to be the late recovery period but actually appears to represent a period of late spontaneous deterioration. The necessary studies must be oriented toward revealing the biological changes experienced by damaged cerebral tissue over a much more extended time period than has presently been investigated. Obviously, the short-term biological changes (see Chapter 1 on Damage and Repair of Brain Tissue) are not relevant to this long-term result. Some type of adverse long-term effect (e.g., microgliosis) will probably be found to occur during the 12th to 18th month period following cerebral tissue damage.

Finally, we must note that our longitudinal study of head-injured subjects was scheduled and funded for follow-up for only 18 months. No information at all is available regarding the course of any further spontaneous changes that may occur later than 18 months following the injury, and such studies should be conducted. Obviously, such investigations, as well as the findings reported above, would require cross-validation. A review of the individual cases included in our current report strongly suggest that mild but definite deterioration occurs in the 12th to 18th month post-injury period, and the consistency among individual cases served as the basis for producing a statistically significant result even though the mean difference score was relatively small.

The finding of a long-term deterioration of previously recovered abilities during the 12-month to 18-month period following traumatic cerebral tissue damage also has implications for rehabilitation. The presumption has generally been that the spontaneous recovery process is monotonic with the absolute degree of improvement gradually decreasing with the passage of time.

Jennett and Teasdale (1981) studied 500 survivors of a head injury and found that of those who made a good or moderate recovery, two-thirds had done so within 3 months and 90% within 6 months of the injury. Among the remaining 10%, only 5% of those who were followed for 18 months or more showed significant clinical improvement compared to their status 12 months after injury. These investigators suggest not only that a gradually progressive recovery curve occurs, but that most head-injured persons have achieved the degree of spontaneous recovery of which they are capable within 6 months following the injury.

Although our investigation was not designed to determine whether recovery was completed in less than 12 months, for many persons it appears that spontaneous improvement, as measured by neuropsychological tests, continues to occur beyond the 6-month period. However, the finding that deterioration of previous improved abilities regularly occurs in persons with cerebral tissue damage during the 12th to 18th month post-injury period must necessarily influence expected outcomes of facilitated (brain retraining) programs. It would appear that basic biological changes, as yet not known, will eventually operate against spontaneous recovery, and probably also against improvement brought about by brain retraining.

Reitan (1982) has commented on the excellent potential for retraining of impaired abilities in brain-injured persons, but has also emphasized the tenuous and insecure nature of these regained abilities over the course of time. These comments were based on clinical observations of individual patients, and led to the conclusion that abilities regained through a combination of spontaneous and facilitated recovery were much more susceptible to deterioration under the pressure of either emotional or pathophysiological stress than abilities which had never been impaired. Either emotional stresses, or the influence of pathophysiological conditions such as systemic disease states, may have such adverse effects, and we must now add an additional factor of long-term spontaneous deterioration that undoubtedly interacts with other variables and, in fact, may lay the groundwork for adverse effects of other types of negative influences.

The full contingent of significant factors, both positive and negative, must be considered in developing, applying, and evaluating the progress of rehabilitation for individual subjects, but possible spontaneous neuropsychological deterioration and the need for continued brain-retraining should be assessed in the long-term period following injury. Considering the statistically significant improvement (which was not found among control subjects) between the initial and 12-month testings, it is unequivocally clear that despite the fact that their G-NDS scores were in the normal range, the group with cerebral concussion sustained a degree of impairment from their mild head injury.

It is interesting to note, however, that the results of initial neuropsychological testing for this group produced a mean G-NDS score of 25.36 that was nearly within the normal range. We should also reiterate that the subjects were mainly from a university community and more intelligent than average. A review of their initial test results, in terms of clinical interpretation, often yielded a basis for suspecting some impairment in spite of good levels of performance, but it frequently was not possible to be certain that any impairment was

present. Nevertheless, the change shown on the 12-month examination was unquestionably significant statistically (p <.02), with the mean G-NDS score being 18.36. As the reader will recall (Table 3-8), control subjects who were tested initially and retested 12 months later showed no significant improvement on the G-NDS.

It appears, therefore, that despite their relatively good scores, a mild degree of neuropsychological deficit was actually present in these subjects at the time of the initial testing. This conclusion could not be inferred with complete confidence without follow-up testing and the use of a procedure such as the G-NDS. The approach illustrated above may represent a research approach to resolve the dilemma surrounding the question of brain impairment in mild head injury and relieve the "confusion" surrounding this issue that is so frequently cited (Alves & Jane, 1985; Rosenthal & Berrol, 1986).

Age and Gender Effects

An additional investigation was conducted to determine whether there were any significant differences between females and males and between older and younger persons on the General Neuropsychological Deficit Scale. Using control subjects and persons with left and right cerebral damage, Herring (1983) performed a careful study of the effects of cerebral damage in men and women. He found that there were no consistent sex differences and concluded that, "Sex is not a major determinant of neuropsychological ability structure." These same groups of subjects were used to investigate the General Neuropsychological Deficit Scale.

There has recently been a number of reports of the differences between men and women regarding the differential effects of lateralized cerebral lesions on the Verbal and Performance scores of the Wechsler Scale. Although a number of these reports have concluded that lateralized specialization of verbal and performance skills is greater among men than women, other investigations have been essentially negative. Herring and Reitan (1986) studied this question and found that both males and females with lateralized cerebral lesions had essentially similar patterns of Verbal IQ-Performance IQ scores, although the differences were somewhat smaller for women than men.

A reasonable approach to gender differences in neuropsychological functions and cerebral organization would be to perform a comprehensive comparison of neuropsychological functions, including many more measures than just the Wechsler Scale, so that any differences could be viewed in a proper general context. Herring (1983) is the only investigator so far to have adopted such an approach. He had sufficient case material available from Reitan's files to be able to use an extensive range of neuropsychological test data and to use controls comparable in age, education, type of lesion, location of lesion, etc. Herring found certain small and relatively minor differences in his extensive investigation, including results indicating that women perform slightly better than men on the Digit Symbol subtest and men perform better than women in finger tapping speed with the dominant hand.

Reitan and Wolfson (1986a) have reviewed the literature regarding aging effects on the Halstead-Reitan Battery. The results show that older persons demonstrate significant deficits, especially on tests that have been found to be especially sensitive to impairment of cerebral functions.

Gender and Age Effects on the General Neuropsychological Deficit Scale

Investigation of the General Neuropsychological Deficit Scale utilized control subjects (N = 56) and groups with unequivocal evidence of left cerebral damage (N = 48) and right cerebral damage (N = 48). In this study we deliberately avoided including subjects with craniocerebral trauma because of the evidence of generalized as well as focal damage among these patients. All subjects with lateralized cerebral lesions had either neoplastic or vascular disease, conditions of pathology arising from within the brain rather than from an adverse external influence, such as a blow to the head.

The 56 control subjects were subdivided according to sex into groups of 28 younger and 28 older subjects. The younger females had a mean age of 23.07 years and the older females had a mean age of 46.43 years. Comparable age means for the younger and older male controls were 25.14 years and 45.50 years. Age differences between the two younger control groups and the two older control groups were not significant but, obviously, the older groups were significantly different in age from the younger groups.

The 48 subjects with right cerebral lesions and the 48 subjects with left cerebral lesions were subdivided into groups of 24 males and 24 females. These four groups of brain-damaged subjects had mean ages that ranged from 43.96 to 47.88 years. They were not significantly different either from each other or from the older controls. Mean grades of education among the various groups ranged from 10.88 to 12.29 years and no overall differences were present on this variable. Therefore, distributions of age and education were essentially similar in all groups.

A major feature of the design of this study related to establishing comparability of brain lesions in each of the four groups so that controlled comparisons of males and females could be accomplished. Not only was laterality of the lesion considered, but careful attention was paid to comparability of groups with respect to specific lesion site, lesion type (neoplastic or vascular), lesion etiology (fast or slow-growing intrinsic tumors vs. extrinsic tumors; cerebral vascular accidents vs. arteriovenous malformations), and chronicity and severity of the condition. Control of these many aspects of brain damage, as well as age and educational levels, increased the probability that any differences between females and males could be attributed specifically to the variable of gender.

Table 3-11. Mean values on the General Neuropsychological Deficit Scale for control groups and groups with left or right cerebral lesions.

Group	Level of Performance	Pathognomonic Signs	Patterns	Rt/Lt Diff.	Neuropsychological Deficit Scale Score
Younger Female Controls	10.50	0.50	0.71	6.36	18.07
Younger Male Controls	7.64	0.29	1.29	4.57	13.74
Older Female Controls	15.00	0.46	1.71	8.14	25.64
Older Male Controls	15.29	0.36	2.21	6.00	24.00
Left Cerebral Damage (Females)	32.46	5.58	2.54	13.58	55.58
Left Cerebral Damage (Males)	33.17	8.00	2.46	12.62	55.83
Right Cerebral Damage (Females)	36.13	3.29	2.20	14.96	56.58
Right Cerebral Damage (Males)	35.96	3.21	3.17	18.50	60.84

Table 3-11 presents the mean General Neuropsychological Deficit Scale scores for the eight groups. It is apparent immediately that the control groups, regardless of whether they were composed of older or younger subjects, performed much better than any of the brain-damaged groups. Mean G-NDS scores were very similar for the older males and older females, but they performed significantly worse than the younger male and younger female control subjects. Although the mean score for the younger male control subjects was somewhat better than for the younger female control subjects, this difference was not statistically significant.

It is apparent from these results that chronological age has an influence on the G-NDS and further studies must be done to examine this variable. It is not surprising that chronological age is a significant variable; this finding confirms results that have consistently been reported earlier (Reitan, 1955d, 1967; Reitan & Wolfson, 1986a). The

G-NDS cut-off score between 25 and 26, as derived from the studies reported above, must be used cautiously with older persons.

On the G-NDS all brain-damaged groups performed much more poorly than the control subjects, with mean values ranging from about 55 to 60. The design of this study permitted comparisons of lateralization effects as well as age and gender influences. As noted earlier, the G-NDS was not designed to reflect differences in left and right cerebral functions. Instead, it was designed to reflect the severity of neuropsychological deficit generally considered.

Confirming the results reported above, the present findings reflected no significant differences in either women or men with respect to lateralization of cerebral damage. In addition, comparisons of the scores of women and men yielded very similar mean values for the G-NDS regardless of the cerebral hemisphere involved.

These findings supported several conclusions: (1) On the General Neuropsychological Deficit Scale, older control subjects (both male and female), scored worse (at statistically significant levels) than younger control subjects. (2) Male and female control subjects of comparable age distributions (older *or* younger groups) did not differ significantly on the G-NDS, although younger males tended to perform somewhat better than the other groups (p <.10). (3) All brain-damaged groups performed much more poorly than any of the control groups, with differences being highly significant statistically. (4) No brain-damaged groups were significantly different from each other, regardless of whether this damage was generalized or lateralized to the left or right cerebral hemispheres. (5) Males and females of comparable age and cerebral lesion showed no significant differences in G-NDS scores. Tables 3-12, 3-13 and 3-14 present t-ratios and probability levels.

Finally, brief comments will be offered concerning the means for each of the sections (Level of Performance, Pathognomonic Signs, Patterns and Relationships, and Right-Left Differences) of the General Neuropsychological Deficit Scale. Table 3-11 indicates that pathognomonic signs make a negligible contribution for either older or younger control subjects. Essentially, control subjects can perform these tasks from the Aphasia Screening Test without difficulty.

The groups with left cerebral damage had higher scores on the pathognomonic signs section than either males or females with right cerebral damage. Obviously, this finding is to be expected because of the heavy contribution to the section on pathognomonic signs of organic language deficits (dysphasia).

In other respects, the scores for men and women with left or right cerebral damage were essentially equivalent, leading to total General Neuropsychological Deficit Scale scores that were quite similar among groups. This finding, based upon carefully controlled and closely comparable groups of subjects with left and right cerebral lesions, emphasizes the equivalent importance of each cerebral hemisphere in overall neuropsychological functioning.

Although it seems that many psychologists have tended to value the left cerebral hemisphere more than the right (apparently because of prejudgments concerning the significance of language functions), the present results, based upon a set of measures — the Halstead-Reitan Battery — that was designed and tested to reflect impairment regardless of lateralization, localization, and type of cerebral damage, underscore the equivalent significance of the right and left cerebral hemispheres.

Left and Right Neuropsychological Deficit Scales (L-NDS and R-NDS)

Goodglass and Kaplan (1979) have emphasized the complementary importance of tests that are (1) generally sensitive to cerebral functions, and (2) selectively sensitive to lateralized or regionally localized functions. It is necessary to have individual tests in each of these categories in order to obtain a complete evaluation of brain functions for the individual subject.

The process by which the Halstead-Reitan Neuropsychological Test Battery evolved necessarily required the development and selection of tests in each of these two categories. The Battery was developed not only through formal research investigations but also through the study of thousands of individual subjects. Each subject constituted a separate experiment in which the general question being asked was whether the neuropsychological test results permitted accurate and detailed inferences regarding the brain pathology involved. Obviously, some patients have diffuse or generalized cerebral damage, and others have damage that principally involves one area or another. In many instances both diffuse and focal damage is present; therefore, an adequate neuropsychological test battery must include tests to reflect these various conditions.

Table 3-12. Comparisons of younger and older female and male control groups on the General Neuropsychological Deficit Scale.

	1	2	3
1. Younger Female Controls			
2. Older Female Controls	t = 2.54 ; p < .02		
3. Younger Male Controls	t = 1.76 ; p < .10	t = 3.88 ; p < .001	
4. Older Male Controls	t = 1.83 ; p < .079	t = .37 ; p < .718	t = 3.13 ; p < .005

Total Younger Controls vs. Total Older Controls   t = 3.95 ; p < .0001

Table 3-13. Comparisons of control subjects and groups with left or right cerebral lesions.

	1	2
1. Older Controls		
2. Left Cerebral Damage	t = 9.72 ; p < .0001	
3. Right Cerebral Damage	t = 8.31 ; p < .0001	t = 1.28 ; p < .204

Table 3-14. Means, standard deviations, and t-ratios for groups of 28 male and female control subjects on age, education, and the General NDS and its component parts.

		Control Variables		NEUROPSYCHOLOGICAL DEFICIT SCALE				
		Age	Educ.	Level	Signs	Patterns	Rt vs Lt	Total NDS
Females	Mean	34.75	13.32	12.75	0.64	1.21	7.25	21.86
	SD	13.13	3.04	5.61	1.26	1.18	2.90	8.54
Males	Mean	35.36	13.18	11.54	0.32	1.75	5.29	18.89
	SD	11.89	2.99	6.85	0.66	1.33	3.59	9.84
	t ratio	0.17	0.15	0.71	1.19	1.59	2.20	1.18
	p <	.90	.90	.50	.25	.20	.05	.25

As we have emphasized elsewhere, it is also important to view the neuropsychological data in accordance with the four major methods of inference regarding brain-behavior relationships in order to understand the brain of the individual subject. These methods use both interindividual and intraindividual approaches in assessing the test results (Reitan, 1966a; 1974).

Finally, it is important that the content of an adequate neuropsychological test battery cover completely the neuropsychological functions subserved by the brain. Thoroughly studying Halstead-Reitan Battery test results of thousands of patients gradually revealed the range of neuropsychological functions that may be impaired by cerebral damage and, as these areas of deficit were revealed, the Halstead-Reitan Battery was expanded to include tests which would provide neuropsychological findings that correlated with the pathological results determined by the complete neurological evaluation (in many cases including surgery and autopsy). Within this framework it is apparent that Neuropsychological Deficit Scales for the two cerebral hemispheres would augment and complement the significance of the General Neuropsychological Deficit Scale that was previously described.

Interest in the specialized functions of the two cerebral hemispheres has a long history, especially in the area of aphasia (Reitan, 1984). Other areas of neuropsychological functioning have also been investigated in considerable detail, including differential sensory-perceptual and motor skills of the two sides of the body (Hom & Reitan, 1982, 1984) and their relationships with higher-level aspects of neuropsychological functioning (Reitan, 1970); evaluation of differential higher-level neuropsychological functions of the left and right cerebral hemispheres in such areas as verbal vs. performance intelligence (Reitan, 1955b); auditory perceptual skills (Milner, 1962); basic language vs. visual-spatial constructional skills (Reitan, 1964; Wheeler & Reitan, 1962); and the extensive number of studies of persons with commissurotomies (Sperry, Gazzaniga, & Bogen, 1969).

In fact, the interest in the unique functions of each cerebral hemisphere has been so intense that a serious scientific question has arisen concerning why we have two brains (Mountcastle, 1962). It is apparent that an adequate procedure in neuropsychological assessment must be directed toward elucidation of the differential functions of the two cerebral hemispheres and, in addition, provide a basis for comparing the adequacy of each hemisphere for the individual subject.

The development, content, and methodological organization of the Halstead-Reitan Battery has been shown to permit accurate classification of (1) persons with and without cerebral damage (Reitan, 1955a; Wheeler, Burke, & Reitan, 1963); (2) persons with damage to the left or right cerebral hemisphere (Reitan, 1964; Wheeler, Burke, & Reitan, 1963; Wheeler & Reitan, 1962); and (3) persons with various types of cerebral lesions (Reitan, 1964).

Differentiations of this type have been possible not only using multivariate statistical methods, but also have been shown to be quite accurate in individual clinical evaluation. However, development of skill in clinical evaluation has been heavily dependent upon acquisition of extensive experience. Development of the G-NDS, the L-NDS, and the R-NDS should be useful to the less experienced clinician, although scoring procedures of this kind can never be expected to replace clinical insight and understanding. Therefore, the purpose of developing the L-NDS and the R-NDS was to provide a set of rules, based on results obtained with the Halstead-Reitan Battery, for differentiating between left and right cerebral lesions, to have a method for directly comparing the adequacy of cerebral functioning for the individual subject, and to provide a preliminary test of the validity of the procedure.

The General Neuropsychological Deficit Scale (G-NDS) was developed to reflect the extent to which an individual's performances deviated from a normal standard (thus showing severity of impairment). The G-NDS deliberately did not provide for comparative assessment of the two cerebral hemispheres. In fact, the validational studies reported earlier in this chapter showed that although the G-NDS was highly sensitive to cerebral damage, it did not differentiate between left, right, and generalized cerebral damage using separate categories of cerebrovascular, traumatic and heterogeneous brain lesions. The G-NDS, in accordance with its design, proved to be a very sensitive general indicator of neuropsychological status. Although this section is concerned specifically with the L-NDS and the R-NDS, the reader is urged to use the lateralizing scales in conjunction with the G-NDS in clinical evaluation and interpretation.

Rules for Scoring the L-NDS and the R-NDS

The L-NDS is based on 21 measures and the R-NDS is based on 13 measures drawn from the Halstead-Reitan Battery. Because of the differing number of contributing variables to each of these NDS scores, it would be possible to compute a mean L-NDS or R-NDS score for each subject. Data to be presented below suggest that this is a refinement which is not of critical importance. It should be noted, however, that both the L-NDS and the R-NDS utilize patterns or relationships among higher-level neuropsychological functions, comparisons of performances on the two sides of the body, and the presence of specific or pathognomonic deficits.

Table 3-15 lists the 21 variables that determine the L-NDS and Table 3-16 presents similar information for the R-NDS. Each table provides information for converting raw data to scores of *0, 1, 2* and *3*. These converted scores were designed to reflect the extent of differences in left or right cerebral functions.

The first category, *0,* represents a perfectly normal performance. The converted score of *1* is still within the normal range, but reflects a possible very mild deviation toward differential functions of the two cerebral hemispheres. The score of *2* represents a mild to moderate degree of de-

viation between left or right cerebral dysfunction. Finally, scores that fall in the highest category, *3,* reflect definite and significant lateralized differences.

Since many of the variables contributing to the L-NDS and the R-NDS constitute manifestations of impaired cerebral functions, these Scales should be viewed as representing procedures for identifying dysfunction of one cerebral hemisphere or the other in addition to providing an intraindividual comparison. In fact, because of their composition, the L-NDS and R-NDS are probably not adequately designed for routine comparisons of differential functions of the two cerebral hemispheres among normal (non-brain-damaged) individuals.

Finger Tapping, Grip Strength, and the Tactual Performance Test are scored according to the same procedure that is used for scoring the G-NDS, but the conversion ranges reflect differences in left or right-sided performances. Variables 11 through 21 of the L-NDS (which are manifestations of dysphasia and related left-hemisphere deficits) and variable 11 from the R-NDS (constructional dyspraxia) are viewed as pathognomonic signs, and are scored in exactly the same manner as they are scored in the G-NDS. If one of these deficits is judged to be present, a converted score (*1, 2,* or *3*) is assigned to reflect the significance of the deficit. For example, if a patient demonstrates dysnomia, it would contribute 3 points to the L-NDS total score, regardless of the severity or pervasiveness of the naming deficit. Correspondingly, the presence of constructional dyspraxia would contribute 2 points to the R-NDS, regardless of the severity of the deficit. Scoring of these particular variables depends upon clinical evaluation of the subject's performances on the Reitan-Indiana Aphasia Screening Test and it is necessary for the neuropsychologist to have sufficient clinical competence to be able to make the judgements that are required. (*Aphasia and Sensory-perceptual Deficits in Adults* [Reitan, 1984] was written specifically to assist the clinician in developing this type of clinical competence.)

Table 3-15. Variables that contribute to the Left-Neuropsychological Deficit Scale and rules for scoring each variable from perfectly normal results (0) to serious deviations (3) (see text).

	0	1	2	3
1. **VIQ/PIQ Difference**	0–5	6–10	11–19	20+
2. **TPT** (RH S's) RH vs LH Divide non-dominant hand by dominant hand and subtract from 1.0 Score 0 if unable to perform with either hand	.38 or Less	.39–.49	.50–.59	.60 or More
3. **Tapping** (RH S's) RH vs LH Divide non-dominant hand by dominant hand and subtract from 1.0	.07 or More	.06–.04	.03 to –.02	–.03 or Less
4. **Grip Strength** Divide non-dominant hand by dominant hand and subtract from 1.0	.07 or More	.06–.04	.03 to –.02	–.03 or Less
5. **Tactile Form Recognition-Time** RH minus LH If any error occurs with RH except for □ & △, score 3.	1″ or More	–2″ or –3″	–4″ or –5″	–6″ or More
6. **Bilateral Tactile Stimulation** Right side minus Left side (12 trials)	– or 0	1	2	3 or More
7. **Bilateral Auditory Stimulation** Right side minus Left side (4 trials)	– or 0	1–2	3	4
8. **Bilateral Visual Stimulation** Right side minus Left side (12 trials)	– or 0	1	2	3 or More
9. **Tactile Finger Recognition** Score 0 when LH has more errors than RH. If RH has more errors than LH, use table on next page to determine score.				
10. **Finger-tip Number Writing** Score 0 when LH has more errors than RH. If RH has more errors than LH, use table on next page to determine score.				

Table 3-15. Continued

For Variables 9 and 10: (1) Determine the percentage of errors by the RH; (2) Enter the table in the row with the total errors made; (3) Determine the score.

Table for Variables 9 and 10:

Total Errors		**0**	**1**	**2**	**3**
21 or more		50–54	55–57	58–60	61 +
18–20		50–54	55–57	58–62	63 +
15–17		50–54	55–58	59–63	64 +
12–14	%	50–55	56–58	59–63	64 +
9–11		50–56	57–59	60–63	64 +
6–8		50–56	57–63	64–70	71 +
3–5		50–59	60–67	68–79	80 +
0–2		50	1 error	100	—

	Score
11. Dysnomia	3
12. Auditory verbal dysgnosia	3
13. Visual number dysgnosia	3
14. Visual letter dysgnosia	3
15. Body dysgnosia	3
16. Dyscalculia	2
17. Dysgraphia	2
18. Dyslexia	2
19. Central dysarthria	1
20. Spelling dyspraxia	1
21. Right-left confusion	1

Table 3-16. Variables that contribute to the Right-Neuropsychological Deficit Scale and rules for scoring each variable from perfectly normal results (0) to serious deviations (3) (see text).

	0	1	2	3
1. **VIQ/PIQ Difference**	0–7	8–12	13–21	22 or More
2. **TPT** (RH S's) RH vs LH Divide non-dominant hand by dominant hand and subtract from 1.0 Score 0 if unable to perform with either hand	.29 or More	.28–.24	.23–.11	.10 or Less
3. **Tapping** Dom vs non-dom hand Divide non-dominant hand by dominant hand and subtract from 1.0	.12 or Less	.13–.18	.19–.26	.27 or More
4. **Grip Strength** Divide non-dominant hand by dominant hand and subtract from 1.0	.12 or Less	.13–.18	.19–.26	.27 or More
5. **Tactile Form Recognition-Time** RH minus LH If any error occurs with LH except for □ & △, score 3.	1″ or Less	2″ to 3″	4″ to 5″	6″ or More
6. **Bilateral Tactile Stimulation** Right side minus Left side (12 trials)	+ or 0	−1	−2	−3 or Less
7. **Bilateral Auditory Stimulation** Right side minus Left side (4 trials)	+ or 0	−1 to −2	−3	−4
8. **Bilateral Visual Stimulation** Right side minus Left side (12 trials)	+ or 0	−1	−2	−3 or Less
9. **Tactile Finger Recognition** Score 0 when RH has more errors than LH. If LH has more errors than RH, use table on next page to determine score.				
10. **Finger-tip Number Writing** Score 0 when RH has more errors than LH. If LH has more errors than RH, use table on next page to determine score.				
11. **Constructional dyspraxia** Score 2 points				
12. **Inf + Voc/2 minus PA**	Minus values to 2.5	3–3.5	4–5.5	6 or More
13. **Inf + Voc/2 minus BD**	Minus values to 2.5	3–3.5	4–5.5	6 or More

Table 3-16. (cont.)
For Variables 9 and 10: (1) Determine the percentage of errors by the LH; (2) Enter the table in the row with the total errors made; (3) Determine the score.

Table for Variables 9 and 10:

Total Errors		0	1	2	3
21 or more		50–54	55–57	58–60	61+
18–20		50–54	55–57	58–62	63+
15–17		50–54	55–58	59–63	64+
12–14	%	50–55	56–58	59–63	64+
9–11		50–56	57–59	60–63	64+
6–8		50–56	57–63	64–70	71+
3–5		50–59	60–67	68–79	80+
0–2		50	1 error	100	—

After the individual items are scored in the L-NDS and the R-NDS, the converted scores are added to provide a total L-NDS and R-NDS for each subject.

Validational Studies of the L-NDS and R-NDS

Several preliminary studies were done to determine the validity of the L-NDS and R-NDS. We used the same groups of subjects that had been evaluated with the G-NDS (reported earlier in this chapter). These groups consisted of samples used in a previous investigation (Reitan, 1985a) and were composed of 41 subjects who had no past or present evidence of cerebral damage, and three groups of brain-damaged subjects who were heterogeneous in their etiology but categorized on the basis of independent neurological evidence into categories of generalized cerebral damage (N = 23), left cerebral lesions (N = 25), and right cerebral lesions (N = 31). These groups therefore provided a total of 79 brain-damaged persons, classified into groups with generalized, left, and right cerebral damage, to be compared with a control group. The demographic characteristics of these groups were previously reported (Reitan, 1985a); the groups were comparable for chronological age, education, and gender distributions.

We also studied the L-NDS and R-NDS in groups within the same etiological categories, again classified as generalized, left, and right cerebral damage (Table 3-17). The etiologies investigated were cerebrovascular disease (N = 45) and traumatic brain injury (N = 45). The group with generalized diffuse cerebrovascular disease had a mean age of 52.33 years (SD, 7.0) and and mean education of 10.27 years (SD, 3.02). The subjects with left cerebrovascular disease had a mean age of 52.00 years (SD, 10.14) and a mean education of 10.60 (SD, 2.68). The group with right cerebrovascular disease had a mean age of 50.47 (SD, 8.55) and a mean education of 9.80 (SD, 2.07).

The subjects with generalized (diffuse) traumatic brain injury had a mean age of 37.13 (SD, 10.68) and a mean education of 10.73 (SD, 3.04). The group with left traumatic brain injury had a mean age of 37.13 (SD, 10.10) and a mean education of 10.73 (SD, 3.73). The subjects with right traumatic brain injury had a mean age of 36.93 (SD, 10.74) and a mean education of 11.60 (3.20).

Obviously, the subjects with cerebrovascular disease were, as expected, older than the subjects with traumatic brain injury; however, within etiologies there were no intergroup differences of statistical significance in age or education between any pairs of groups. Specific diagnoses within the

Table 3-17. Means, standard deviations and probability levels for various groups with and without evidence of cerebral damage on the Left and Right Neuropsychological Deficit Scales.

	N		Left NDS	Right NDS	Difference: L-NDS Minus R-NDS	t ratio: L-NDS vs. R-NDS
No Cerebral Damage	41	Mean	2.59	2.39	0.20	.32
		SD	2.54	2.53	3.98	p<.70
Generalized Cerebral Damage	23	Mean	10.96	7.87	3.09	1.23
		SD	8.11	5.64	11.82	p<.20
Left Cerebral Damage	25	Mean	18.80	3.48	15.32	5.70
		SD	10.71	4.08	13.18	p<.001
Right Cerebral Damage	31	Mean	2.61	17.00	−14.39	7.03
		SD	3.75	8.54	11.15	p<.001
Total Heterogeneous BD	79	Mean	10.16	10.06		
		SD	10.35	8.78		
Generalized CVD	15	Mean	13.00	9.67	3.33	1.36
		SD	6.56	6.45	9.13	p<.10
Left CVD	15	Mean	26.47	3.60	22.87	6.34
		SD	11.12	3.16	13.51	p<.001
Right CVD	15	Mean	3.73	20.47	−16.74	9.48
		SD	2.24	6.23	6.54	p<.001
Total CVD	45	Mean	14.40	11.25		
		SD	12.00	8.87		
Diffuse HI	15	Mean	11.00	7.80	3.20	1.09
		SD	8.24	6.67	11.02	p<.25
Left HI	15	Mean	16.40	5.73	10.67	4.17
		SD	10.44	3.09	9.60	p<.001
Right HI	15	Mean	6.67	11.13	−4.46	2.87
		SD	6.24	6.67	5.82	p<.02
Total Head Injury	45	Mean	11.36	8.22		
		SD	9.30	6.15		
Total Generalized Brain Damage	53	Mean	11.55	8.36	3.19	2.11
		SD	7.79	6.23		p<.05
Total Left Brain Damage	55	Mean	20.24	4.13	16.11	8.95
		SD	11.49	3.72		p<.001
Total Right Brain Damage	61	Mean	3.89	16.41	−12.52	9.56
		SD	4.47	8.28		p<.001
Total Brain Damage	169	Mean	11.61	9.89		
		SD	10.70	8.27		

groups with cerebrovascular disease and traumatic brain injury were also generally comparable.

The subjects with left cerebrovascular lesions (N = 15) had diagnoses of middle cerebral artery thrombosis (5), middle cerebral artery aneurysm (1), middle and posterior cerebral artery thrombosis (1), anterior cerebral artery thrombosis (2), internal carotid artery thrombosis (4), and arteriovenous malformation (2).

The subjects comprising the group with right cerebrovascular lesions (N = 15) had diagnoses of middle cerebral artery thrombosis (5), posterior cerebral artery thrombosis (1), and internal carotid artery thrombosis (9).

The subjects with generalized cerebrovascular disease (N = 15) had diagnoses of hypertensive encephalopathy (4), cerebral arteriosclerosis (10), and bilateral partial carotid artery occlusion (1).

Among the subjects with generalized traumatic brain injury (N = 15), 10 subjects had sustained a closed head injury, 2 had evidence of a depressed skull fracture, and 3 had sustained an open penetrating wound.

Subjects with left cerebral traumatic lesions (N = 15) had suffered closed head injuries (6), depressed skull fractures (5), and penetrating head wounds (4).

The group with right traumatic injuries (N = 15) included 9 subjects with a closed head injury, 3 with a depressed skull fracture, and 3 with a penetrating head injury.

As might well be expected, evidence of cerebral contusions as well as epidural, subdural, and intracerebral hematomas were present in some patients. A number of subjects had developed post-traumatic epilepsy, and many of the subjects, particularly those who demonstrated evidence of lateralized damage, showed positive findings on the physical neurological examination. Nevertheless, within the general groups of cerebrovascular disease and traumatic brain injury, the three groups seemed to be relatively comparable, except for generalized or lateralized cerebral damage. Thus, it does not seem likely that any emerging differences

in scores on the L-NDS as compared with the R-NDS would be attributable to age, education, or a specific type of injury of damage (although, as we have noted, the group with cerebrovascular disease was clearly older than the group with traumatic injuries).

In terms of procedure, the Halstead-Reitan Battery for Adults had been administered to each subject individually by a carefully trained technician who had no knowledge of the diagnoses or the purposes of the present study. In addition, neuropsychological testing was done without prior knowledge of the neurological findings for each subject. The neurological examinations were performed by neurologists and neurological surgeons; their diagnostic conclusions were based upon conventional clinical procedures and were not influenced by psychological test results. Only subjects in whom the neurological diagnoses were definitive were considered for inclusion in the study.

Statistical analyses of the L-NDS and R-NDS distributions involved computations of means, standard deviations, and t-ratios. Because of the striking intergroup differences in the NDS distributions, and the relatively small number of intergroup comparisons, alpha slippage was not considered to be a problem and a multivariate analysis of variance was deemed unnecessary prior to computation of the t-ratios comparing pairs of groups.

Mean G-NDS scores are listed for each group in Table 3-2 and the reader may wish to refer to these scores in conjunction with a review of the information in Table 3-17. Our attention will be directed principally to the L-NDS and R-NDS scores.

The group without evidence of cerebral damage had a mean L-NDS score of 2.59 and a R-NDS mean of 2.39, yielding a mean difference of 0.20 between these values. This difference did not approach statistical significance. As will be noted in comparison of comparable mean values for the groups with cerebral damage, the non-brain-damaged group had quite low means. Although the L-NDS and R-NDS could conceivably be used as indicators of the presence or absence of cerebral damage generally considered, the G-NDS is the more appropriate instrument for this purpose.

The groups with a heterogeneous etiology of brain damage, although categorized according to generalized, left, or right cerebral involvement, showed striking differences depending upon the cerebral hemisphere involved. The group with left cerebral damage had a mean L-NDS score of 18.80; this group had a mean R-NDS score of only 3.48. Conversely, the group with right cerebral damage had a mean R-NDS score of 17.00 and a mean L-NDS score of 2.61. As will be noted in Table 3-17, the differences between these mean values were highly significant, indicating that the L-NDS and R-NDS corresponded closely with the hemisphere involved.

The group with generalized cerebral damage did not show a significant difference between the L-NDS and the R-NDS scores, even though the L-NDS was composed of 21 variables and the R-NDS was based on only 13 variables. (Nevertheless, as will be noted below, the L-NDS generally tended to have a higher mean value across groups than the R-NDS, and this result probably is a function at least in part of the difference in the number of variables contributing to each value.)

The results for the groups with cerebrovascular disease suggest initially that the absolute values for the L-NDS and R-NDS were somewhat higher than for the groups with heterogeneous etiology. This is not surprising, in consideration of prior findings (Hom & Reitan, 1982) indicating that persons with cerebrovascular disease are rather generally impaired on neuropsychological measures. However, the disparities between the L-NDS and R-NDS, in accordance with lateralization of cerebral damage, were even more striking than for the groups with heterogeneous damage. Again, the group with generalized cerebrovascular disease did not show a significant difference between the L-NDS and R-NDS.

Finally, the results on the groups with traumatic brain injury followed the same general pattern, although the scores were somewhat better than in the groups with cerebrovascular disease. As would be expected, subjects with generalized cerebral damage resulting from a head injury failed to show a significant difference between the L-NDS and the R-NDS. However, both groups with lateralized cerebral damage showed significant differences, with the elevated value corresponding with neurological evidence of the hemisphere involved.

It must be noted, though, that in the head-injured group the differences between the L-NDS and the R-NDS were not as pronounced as in the comparisons involving patients with cerebrovascular disease. This finding is entirely to be expected in consideration of the abundant evidence (Reitan & Wolfson, 1986b) of widespread cerebral damage in cases of traumatic injury, particularly in the form of axonal shearing, even when available clinical neurological and neurosurgical findings implicate only a single cerebral hemisphere.

In cases of traumatic brain injury the comparative values of the L-NDS and R-NDS strongly suggest a greater degree of neuropsychological impairment in the hemisphere that supposedly was not involved (as compared with the involved hemisphere). This finding also confirms the clinical observation made many years ago (Reitan, 1964) that in cases of traumatic brain injury, one should expect to see evidence on the Halstead-Reitan Battery of involvement of both cerebral hemispheres, even though one hemisphere might be principally involved. Nevertheless, the findings in Table 3-17 still indicate that statistically significant differences between mean values on the L-NDS and R-NDS are present in accordance with the neurological and neurosurgical classification of lateralized damage.

Finally, Table 3-17 presents results for combined groups. Although the group with generalized brain damage had mean L-NDS and R-NDS scores that were not much different than in the individual samples, the difference just reached statistical significance at the 0.5 level because of the increased number of subjects. The combined groups with left cerebral damage and right cerebral damage showed highly significant differences between the L-NDS and R-NDS in the expected direction.

Table 3-18 presents information about the level of L-NDS or R-NDS scores that appear to have clinical significance for differential involvement of the two cerebral hemispheres. In our sample of subjects without cerebral damage (N = 41), none had an intraindividual difference as large as 10 points between the two Scales. However, one subject (2%) had a difference in favor of the L-NDS of 9 points and another subject had a difference this large in favor of the R-NDS. Subjects with generalized cerebral damage showed substantial differences between the L-NDS and R-NDS rather consistently, suggesting that one cerebral hemisphere was more impaired than the other, despite the fact that neurological information led to a diagnosis of generalized cerebral involvement.

The group with generalized cerebrovascular disease tended to show a greater degree of equivalence between the two cerebral hemispheres than either the group with traumatic cerebral damage

or heterogeneous cerebral damage, but the general conclusion should be that when damage is generalized in nature, it is entirely possible that one cerebral hemisphere may be considerably more involved than the other.

Among the groups with left or right cerebral damage, a rather striking differentiation was possible on the basis of intraindividual differences between the L-NDS and the R-NDS. For example, none of these subjects was misclassified when the difference between the two lateralizing NDS scales was 9 or more points. (As noted above, however, 5% of the control subjects had differences this large.) With a difference of 10 or more points in either direction, no control subjects were included and a large percentage (87%) of patients with cerebrovascular disease and approximately 70% of patients with heterogeneous etiologies were correctly classified. Among subjects with traumatic cerebral damage, however, the incidence of correct classification was much lower, ranging between 20% and 33%, even though every subject who had a difference this large was correctly classified.

Table 3-18. Percentages of subjects with no cerebral damage (controls) or generalized, left, or right cerebral damage with L-NDS and R-NDS differences of varying magnitudes.

	L-NDS Minus R-NDS:→	7 or More			8 or More			9 or More			10 or More		
	N	L>R	R>L	Total	L>R	R>L	Total	L>R	R>L	Total	L>R	R>L	Total
No Cerebral Damage	41	7%	7%	15%	5%	5%	10%	2%	2%	5%	0%	0%	0%
Heterogeneous Cerebral Damage	79												
Generalized	23	43%	17%	61%	39%	17%	56%	39%	13%	52%	30%	13%	43%
Left	25	0%	72%	72%	0%	72%	72%	0%	72%	72%	0%	72%	72%
Right	31	71%	3%	74%	71%	3%	74%	71%	0%	71%	68%	0%	68%
Cerebral Vascular Damage	45												
Generalized	15	27%	7%	33%	20%	7%	27%	20%	7%	27%	20%	7%	27%
Left	15	0%	87%	87%	0%	87%	87%	0%	87%	87%	0%	87%	87%
Right	15	87%	0%	87%	87%	0%	87%	87%	0%	87%	87%	0%	87%
Traumatic Cerebral Damage	45												
Generalized (Diffuse)	15	33%	27%	60%	33%	27%	60%	27%	20%	47%	20%	13%	33%
Left	15	0%	67%	67%	0%	53%	53%	0%	40%	40%	0%	33%	33%
Right	15	27%	0%	27%	27%	0%	27%	20%	0%	20%	20%	0%	20%
Total Cerebral Damage	169												
Generalized	53	36%	17%	53%	32%	17%	49%	30%	13%	43%	25%	11%	36%
Left	55	0%	75%	75%	0%	71%	71%	0%	67%	67%	0%	65%	65%
Right	61	64%	2%	66%	64%	2%	66%	62%	0%	62%	61%	0%	61%

The lateralizing power of the L-NDS and R-NDS scores was clearly indicated by the finding that scarcely any subjects in the groups with left or right cerebral damage were misclassified when the difference between the Scales was 7 points or more. Thus, the results suggest that a difference of 7 or more points between the two Scales (regardless of the direction involved) is sufficient to raise a question of differential functioning of one of the hemispheres. It must be noted, though, that 15% of our control group showed a difference of 7 to 9 points between the two Scales (even though these subjects did not have any independent evidence of cerebral damage).

The L-NDS and R-NDS scores described in this chapter appear to have definite validity for neuropsychological dysfunction of the left and right cerebral hemispheres. Differences between the L-NDS and R-NDS scores were substantially larger in subjects with lateralized cerebral lesions than in groups with generalized involvement or subjects without cerebral damage. It would appear that these lateralizing Scales may also be applied validly to subjects with generalized cerebral damage when a question exists about the impairment emanating from differential involvement of the left and right cerebral hemispheres.

The results suggest that the L-NDS and R-NDS are not subject to direct application in persons without independent neurological evidence of cerebral damage, even though some subjects in this group may show fairly substantial differences in the neuropsychological adequacy of the two cerebral hemispheres. The NDS scales, as currently proposed, are oriented toward deficits in performance (including variables that should be positive only in cases of cerebral damage, such as aphasic manifestations) rather than to achievement scores. It appears, however, that it would be possible to develop a G-NDS as well as L-NDS and R-NDS scales, based on achievement scores, for evaluating differential functioning of the left and right cerebral hemispheres among non-brain-damaged subjects.

IV

THEORIES OF BRAIN-BEHAVIOR RELATIONSHIPS

Introductory Comments

Theories are conceptual formulations that become necessary because of a paucity of facts. Individual theories, however, take advantage of documented information to provide a basic structure for postulating a more complete explanation than the one available from the facts themselves. Therefore, development of a theory depends upon some prior knowledge about the situation in question, but the theory attempts to organize this prior knowledge in a way that leads to a fuller and more complete understanding.

Since theory development is dependent upon prior knowledge, the emerging theory may suffer from errors in the available "facts" that are used: (1) The information selected to provide the basic structure is sometimes composed of only partially-true facts; (2) Facts are often selected by a theorist because they support his/her pre-existing biases or interests and therefore do not represent a complete or impartial representation of all available facts; and (3) The elaboration of the basic factual structure (insofar as it is complete or accurate) is developed according to the biases or prejudices of the theorists. It is clear from these observations that given the same facts, two theorists may develop similar, or perhaps quite different, theories.

The accuracy of the "facts" available, their selection and/or omission, and their organization are all relevant to the emerging theory.

In addition to these considerations, some theories are developed to provide a reasonable and logical assessment and evaluation of the subject matter in a particular area. Such theories depend upon an extrapolation (invoked essentially gratuitously, although perhaps reasonably), to explain known circumstances.

As a simple example, we might cite the well known fact that results from the arithmetic portion of the Reitan-Indiana Aphasia Screening Test and the Wechsler Arithmetic subtest are both more sensitive to brain damage than the results of the Information and Vocabulary subtests of the Wechsler Scale. On theoretical grounds, one might wonder why the results of certain tests are more sensitive than the results of other tests to the biological condition of the brain. A simple theoretical formulation to explain this situation might be that immediate problem-solving abilities are required when doing arithmetic problems, whereas only stored (previously accumulated) information is necessary to perform well on the Information and Vocabulary subtests. Of course, this theoretical formulation requires the postulate that immediate problem-solving tasks place more of a stress upon brain functions than tests dependent upon stored information.

Other theories may be formulated to explain more detailed aspects of the subject matter. An explanation, in this sense, refers to organizing known facts in a meaningful framework with relation to other known or partially-known facts. An example of a simple theoretical formulation in this regard might also refer to facts previously developed using the arithmetic aspects of the Aphasia Screening Test and the Wechsler Arithmetic subtest. The facts indicate that the results on these two arithmetic tests do not relate to the left cerebral hemisphere in the same way. The arithmetic performances on the Aphasia Screening Test seem to be much more dependent upon the status of the left cerebral hemisphere than the right cerebral hemisphere (Wheeler & Reitan, 1962), whereas the Wechsler Arithmetic subtest is generally related to adequacy of brain functions without lateralization significance.

What theoretical explanation could be postulated to account for arithmetic being closely dependent upon the left cerebral hemisphere in one instance and in another instance having no lateralization effect, even in the same subjects? Obviously, a theoretical construct in this regard would necessarily refer to differences in the nature of the arithmetical operations used by the two tests. It appears that the Aphasia Screening Test requires the ability to perform simple, discrete arithmetical computations (left hemisphere) and the Arithmetic subtest of the Wechsler Scale requires verbal comprehension of arithmetical data, an evolution of quantitative relationships, and ability in arithmetical and numerical analysis (general brain functions).

These simple examples make it clear that theoretical constructs may be quite different, even when relating to apparently similar content. Rather than concluding that there is little value or validity in forming theoretical constructs (because the attractiveness and plausibility of any

theory is principally a function of the creative imagination of its author), it is apparent that a theoretical construct has value insofar as it generates a hypothesis that can be tested experimentally. Although this type of heuristic value is important, the theory or theoretical construct, even though apparently well-founded on available facts, cannot be considered.to be established until it can be used to accurately predict future outcomes that can be independently verified.

Historical Perspectives

Historical reviews of the ways in which the brain relates to behavior have been published by a number of persons (Boring, 1929; Riese, 1959). These theories have followed a general organizational plan in which sensory input represents the first element, central processing the second element, and motor responsiveness the third element. Sensory input is related to the identified primary receptor areas of the cerebral cortex and these areas, which serve to receive incoming information, are related in turn to secondary sensory areas. The secondary sensory areas are customarily assigned a task involved in additional processing or integration of incoming information.

The motor areas of the cerebral cortex constitute the anatomical basis for responses imposed upon the environment which presumably represent the completion of the response cycle. Again, it has been customary to assign the fundamental aspects of motor response to the primary motor areas, and to recognize that the secondary motor areas provide some type of modulation, co-ordination, or integration of motor responses.

The aspect of brain function which is presumed to intervene between sensory (incoming) and motor (outgoing) functions has been identified as higher-level brain functioning, with a distinction made between this aspect of brain-behavior relationships and the lower-level aspects (sensorimotor performances). The principal differences among theories of brain-behavior relationships have concerned higher-level brain functions.

Halstead (1947a) classified theories of brain-behavior relationships into three categories: (1) Holistic Theory, (2) Aggregation Theory, and (3) Regional Localization Theory. *Holistic theory* contended that all parts of the cerebral cortex served essentially a similar role in central processing and there was no significant localization of functions. However, holistic theory did recognize that the severity of a deficit was related to the quantity of cerebral tissue removed.

Aggregation theory emphasized the localization of primary sensory input areas within the cerebral cortex which were interconnected by an extensive network of intracortical fibers. It was believed that these sensory areas provided a basis for integrated comprehension of sensory stimuli coming from the external environment, which in turn provided a basis for insightful and intelligent responses. The aggregation theorists who emphasized the network of sensory areas essentially conceptualized intelligence as knowledge or awareness of the external environment. However, other aggregation theorists felt that equivalent emphasis should be given to the motor components of intelligent behavior, arguing that it was necessary to integrate the sensory systems of the cerebral cortex with the motor response systems.

It should be noted that neither the holistic nor the aggregation theories were very explicit in identifying the components of higher-level central processing, which involves skills such as language, concept formation, judgement, and reasoning. This omission may well have stemmed largely from the fact that early investigators based their studies and drew their conclusions from observing the effects of cerebral extirpation in lower animals. Studies of the effects of brain lesions in human beings, however, made it quite clear that language functions were heavily dependent on the status of the left cerebral hemisphere, and the observations of aphasic manifestations, initially associated with right hemiparesis and hemiplegia, led to characterization of the left side of the brain as the dominant hemisphere.

When an area of significance — such as the dependence of verbal and language functions on the left cerebral hemisphere — has been established, one can nearly count with certainty on the fact that future investigations will attempt to explore the details. In other words, the "more about less" approach in scientific investigation will come into play. Although there were debates about whether aphasic manifestations were a result of general intellectual impairment (Marie, 1906) or highly specific deficits represented by losses of the "instrumentalities of speech" (Goldstein, 1939), it was essentially inevitable that some investigators would proceed to a position of relatively extreme localization, with different behavioral functions (such as reading, writing, arithmetic, etc.) each being assigned to a small specific compartment of the cerebral cortex.

Such theories of extreme localization of specific abilities have gradually lost their popularity, particularly because the abilities themselves were recognized as being complex and composed of many functions and the fact that brain lesions in human subjects are rarely so exactly specified that they permit verification and validation of the localization claims. Nevertheless, many studies have contributed to a regional-localization theory which postulates that various areas within the cerebral cortex are committed to different types of psychological functions. The so-called "association areas" of the cerebral cortex have been particularly vulnerable to being assigned higher-level cognitive functions (because the primary and secondary sensory and motor areas already had their assigned tasks).

The frontal agranular cortex serves as a particularly striking example. Considering its location with relation to the sensory and motor areas, the association cortex in the posterior parts of the cerebral hemispheres might well be assigned tasks of integration of sensory input with motor functions. The frontal agranular cortex, however, being relatively isolated in the frontal poles, appeared a very likely candidate for some type of special higher-level function. In addition, gross observation of the brains of human beings (compared with subhuman animals) suggests that the frontal lobes are greatly developed in humans. These factors have had at least a partial role in the attribution of abilities such as reasoning, judgement, executive functions, and concept formation to this area. One investigator of the effects of sectioning fibers to the anterior frontal areas went so far as to refer to such operations as "removals of the soul" (Rylander, 1939).

Holistic Theories

The *Holistic Theory* of brain-behavior relationships can be traced back to investigations performed in the 19th century (Flourens, 1843), in which areas of the cerebral hemispheres in dogs were extirpated and post-operative observations were made. Goltz (1881) noted that removal of larger areas of cerebral cortex produced greater defects, but concluded that extirpation of cerebral tissue, regardless of localization, was represented essentially as a manifestation of generalized dullness or impairment of attention.

Ferrier (1886) performed similar experiments on dogs and monkeys and again failed to observe any differential behavioral effects associated with the areas of damage. Nevertheless, he felt that the frontal lobes might serve to integrate sensory and motor functions and, in this way, have a special relationship to the more complex performances related to intelligence. Loeb (1902) felt that extensive destruction of cerebral cortex in *both* hemispheres was necessary to produce clear evidence of deficit in dogs, and he believed that even bilateral frontal resection had little effect.

The earlier investigators based their conclusions essentially on gross observations of their experimental animals. By the time Lashley performed his experiments on rats (1929), scientific

methods of observation had developed within the field of psychology in terms of learning experiments. Lashley not only varied the size and location of lesions in the brains of rats, but he was also able to study the effects quite systematically by recording the rat's ability to learn a maze. Using this procedure, he was even able to study differential effects of relatively simple and complex mazes. This additional sophistication of experimental technique lent considerable emphasis to his findings.

Lashley's results supported the principals of equipotentiality and mass action. *Equipotentiality* referred to the finding that each lesion of the cerebral cortex, regardless of its location, had equivalent effects. The *principle of mass action* was based on the observation that the degree of deficit in maze-learning ability was correlated with the amount of cerebral cortex destroyed. In addition, the results indicated that any particular lesion was more clearly manifested behaviorally by more difficult mazes than mazes that were simple in nature.

Aggregation Theories

The earlier aggregation theories (Munk, 1890) emphasized the importance of the primary sensory areas of the cerebral cortex, their relationship to other areas through extensive intracortical connections, and their influence in mobilizing the functions of the brain in understanding the external environment. Intelligence therefore stemmed from incoming information to the brain and depended upon a complex network of neuronal connections.

Von Monakow (1905) insisted that the motor components of intelligence also be considered within this framework. He suggested that an interaction between sensory and motor areas of the cerebral cortex and their complex relationships represented the essence of intelligence. Aggregation theories agreed with holistic theories insofar as larger areas of damage would cause more significant and pervasive impairment. In addition, von Monakow proposed the term *diaschisis* to represent acute or transitory manifestations of cerebral disturbance (as contrasted with more permanent deficits). In fact, diaschisis represented a temporary interference or interruption between various sensory or motor centers of the cerebral cortex and a resulting loss of functional continuity.

More modern theories of brain-behavior relationships have also emphasized the importance of sensory reception and motor function. For example, Halstead (1947a) included in one of his four factors of "biological intelligence" the Directional Factor, which served to deliver information to the cerebral cortex and to carry responses to the external environment. Luria (1970) placed considerable emphasis on the primary, secondary, and tertiary sensory receptive areas and their importance in comprehending environmental stimuli as well as their integrative functions involved in the transition from lower-level (sensory and motor) to higher-level brain functions.

From this brief summarization it can be seen that the aggregation theories, in a historical sense, emphasized the lower-level aspects of brain functions, with less emphasis on higher-level functions (including speech, concept formation, reasoning, visual-spatial problem solving, and abstraction).

Regional-Localization Theories

Regional-Localization theories have attempted to integrate knowledge of the differential functions served by various areas within the cerebral cortex with the theories more heavily oriented toward input and output. As early as 1836 Dax recognized impairment of language functions, right hemiparesis or hemiplegia, and left cerebral damage as associated phenomena (Benton, 1964). Broca's observations (1861) of patients with sudden losses of verbal communicational skills and damage in the left frontal-temporal area had long been recognized but not explicitly integrated in certain of the earlier theories. While the right cerebral hemisphere has been shown to have some primitive abilities concerned with language functions (although this evidence has been derived primarily from persons with cerebral lesions dating back into childhood), there is no doubt that an area within the left cerebral hemisphere — which includes the posterior inferior frontal lobe, the temporal lobe, and the adjacent lower parts of the parietal lobe — is intimately involved in expressive and receptive aspects of language and verbal functioning (Penfield & Roberts, 1959).

Halstead believed that he had localized "biological intelligence" in the anterior frontal lobes of both cerebral hemispheres, and investigators in the area of behavioral neurology have recently again placed strong emphasis on this area (Benson, 1979).

The pronounced effect of lesions in the posterior part of the right cerebral hemisphere on visual-spatial skills (Hécaen & Albert, 1978) contribute further support for the significance of various regions within the cerebral cortex regarding different types of deficits and corresponding abilities. There is no doubt that a regional-localization set of hypotheses must be considered in developing a concept of brain-behavior relationships, with current evidence centering most strongly on differentiation of the specialized functions of the left and right cerebral hemispheres.

Although it is appealing to identify differential and specialized functions that are related principally to various regions of the cerebral cortex, the existence of higher-level brain functions that are diffusely distributed throughout the cerebral cortex must also be considered. In most theories general neuropsychological functions are postulated to be interactions of identified centers and integration between centers, thus effecting an overall network that is diffusely spread throughout the cerebral cortex. Because stimulus precedes response, such theories often describe these networks of general cortical function as originating in sensory-reception areas and extending their influence through various regions or zones to involve the cerebral cortex generally.

Another example would be Luria's postulate of the widespread influence of the anterior frontal lobes in terms of executive functions (which he believed were involved in every complex behavioral process). Our research, however, has suggested that basic abilities (as contrasted with content-related abilities) in the area of abstraction, reasoning, and logical analysis are diffusely distributed throughout the cerebral cortex and that there is *no* particular center or region which is principally responsible for such skills.

Many theories have proposed that the degree of cortical damage is related to the resulting overall impairment. For example, Goltz (1881) concluded that the extent of cerebral damage was represented by increasing degrees of generalized dullness or defect in attention. Several theories have emphasized the importance of alertness and attention in registration of incoming information (e.g., Block 1 in Luria's theory), but with the discovery of the activating effect of the ascending reticular activating system on the cerebral cortex, there has been a tendency to relate attention, concentration, and alertness to this system. This system, in turn, with its activating effect on the sensory receptive centers, would place a greater emphasis on the areas where these centers are located, namely the non-frontal parts of the cerebral cortex.

Our data, however, have indicated that attention, alertness, and concentration can be significantly impaired with major lesions in any location of the cerebral hemispheres, and this factor seems to follow a "mass action" principle. It is apparent that a neuropsychological theory of brain-behavior relationships must consider input and output functions, specialized abilities that relate to regional areas within the cerebral cortex, higher-level functions that are diffusely distributed, and the mechanisms that permit immensely complex functional integrations between all of these elements.

Molecular Theories

Many theories have been proposed relating the behavioral and biological aspects of brain functions (Finger & Almli, 1984; Gazzaniga, 1985; Geschwind & Galaburda, 1984; Levy, 1985; Pribram, 1971; Shaywitz, Shaywitz, Cohen, & Young, 1983). In these individual contributions it is difficult to discern the extent to which a formal theory is presented versus a marshalling of evidence in support of a particular view of brain-behavior relationships. Nevertheless, many of these statements present evidence that is without question of great significance regarding the biological bases of behavior.

For example, Scheibel (1977) has summarized his extensive studies relating dendritic tissue and function and behavioral changes associated with aging. Although his purpose is to identify biological aspects of brain functions that underlie deterioration of higher-level neuropsychological functions in the aged, his conclusions about the importance of dendritic function and its relationship to behavior has much more general significance.

Scheibel notes that dendrites constitute 70%–90% of the total membrane area of the neuron. If one considers neuronal function to have significance for behavior (as one inevitably must), this fact alone indicates that dendrites must play a very significant role in the information processing capabilities of the individual person. Scheibel has found evidence of a definite reduction in the spine systems and dendritic arborization among the aged, especially in persons with clinical indications of dementia. Therefore, a principle of brain-behavior relationships that may be of very definite significance relates to dendritic function.

Many such important statements have been presented in the literature, and it is beyond the scope of the current presentation to summarize all of these findings. Woodruff and Baisden (1986) have reviewed some of the basic biological principles that underlie molecular theories of brain-behavior relationships, and at present we will restrict our comments to a brief review of some of these principles.

Woodruff and Baisden identify three principles of organization of brain-behavior relationships which they feel are fundamental to theory development. These include (1) the hierarchichal (caudal to rostral) organization of brain function, (2) the separation of sensory and motor systems in an anatomical and functional sense and the implications of the separation of these systems for behavior, and (3) the laterality of cerebral function and possibly localization of function. These authors offer a fourth principle, which they consider to be tentative in nature, to the effect that the brain functions as a cluster of "unit modules" that join and interact with each other as linked distributed systems (Mountcastle, 1979).

An understanding of the hierarchical organization of the central nervous system has developed mainly from studies of lesions placed in animals at various levels. For example, if the spinal cord is isolated from the brain, a number of reflex-responses may still be elicited, including withdrawal from an aversive stimulus, a scratching response when cutaneous irritation is present, muscle-stretch reflexes that provide the basic aspects of postural support, and the flexion-crossed extension reflex, with reciprocal inhibition, that permits co-ordinated movements of all four limbs. However, spontaneous or volitional behavior of the limbs is not demonstrated.

When the medulla, pons, and cerebellum are added to the isolated spinal cord (a condition of low decerebration), the previous responses can still be elicited and in addition the animal is capable of swallowing food or water when it is placed in the mouth. Besides withdrawing from aversive stimuli, the animal may also demonstrate growling, hissing, and biting. Co-ordination of limb movement increases to the point that the animal

may engage in rudimentary aspects of locomotion, but precision of response is poor. The low decerebrate animal cannot walk or even right itself completely. If the midbrain is preserved, however, motor functions tend to recover in a fairly brief period of time, and the animal can right itself and locomote spontaneously.

In cases of high decerebration, just caudal to the posterior limb of the mammillary bodies, the animal can demonstrate walking, running, and even climbing ability. Preservation of the diencephalon permits the animal to demonstrate emotional responses and allows basic autonomic functions. Although movement of the limbs may be co-ordinated and patterns of movement may appear nearly normal, the animal does not relate accurately or appropriately to specific stimuli in the environment. Such an animal demonstrates the capability for sensorimotor integration and movements become organized into behavioral sequences. Although emotional responses may occur, these have been called examples of "sham" rage because of the lack of specific direction or a focused target for the response.

The evidence of hierarchical organization of central nervous system functioning clearly demonstrates an additive principle inasmuch as each level adds additional behavioral capabilities. Other points of information, such as the release phenomenon (demonstrated perhaps most strikingly in instances of decerebrate rigidity), also illustrate the interaction of higher and lower levels of the central nervous system. However, it must be recognized that this information is very fundamental and basic; it is derived particularly from experimental study of animals and adds relatively little to the understanding of higher-level neuropsychological deficits or to the organization of intellectual and cognitive functions as they relate to the brain.

The next major principle of organization of brain function cited by Woodruff and Baisden concerns the differentiation of sensory and motor systems within the spinal cord and brain. Although further research investigating these systems continues at a rapid rate, it has a long history, dating back to the discovery by Johannes Müeller in 1836 of the "specific energies" of nerves. Müeller observed that the nerve pathways for different senses were separately organized and, when stimulated, subserved the specific sense to which the system was devoted.

As reviewed by Reitan and Wolfson (1985b), Fritsch and Hitzig (1870) discovered the motor areas of the cerebral cortex and, through electrical stimulation, demonstrated their potential for eliciting contraction of muscles in various parts of the body. Thus, the sensory-motor dichotomy within the central nervous system has long been understood.

Woodruff and Baisden point out that the division between sensory and motor areas occurs very early during embryogenesis. It is manifested in the dorsal (sensory) and ventral (motor) organization of columns of the spinal cord, maintains this organization in the brainstem, and continues to be manifested in the sensory and motor areas of the cerebral cortex. These investigators further relate the differentiation of sensory and motor functions within the central nervous system to language disorders, which clearly can, in general, be differentiated into receptive and expressive aspects. At this level of function, however, the individual subject with dysphasia nearly always shows evidence of both receptive and expressive disorders (Reitan, 1984).

Considering the length of time that the sensory and motor differentiation has been known and the pervasiveness of this principle within the central nervous system, it is not surprising that many theories of brain-behavior relationships have used the concept. In their review of the historical conceptualizations of nervous system functioning, Reitan and Wolfson (1985b) have noted that Munk (1890) postulated that the aggregate functioning of various sensory areas in the cerebral cortex produces an integration of comprehension of stimuli from

the outside environment that results in intelligent behavior.

Von Monakow (1905) agreed with the theoretical conceptualization proposed by Munk, but also insisted on the importance of motor areas in the cerebral cortex and their role in integrating responses stemming from the brain. Essentially every theory of brain-behavior relationships either explicitly or implicitly provides for sensory (input) and motor (output) functions; without a mechanism for perceiving the external environment, and without a provision for the brain to exert its influence through responses on the external environment, there could be no behavior.

As will be noted later, Luria especially emphasized the reception of information in primary sensory zones within the cerebral cortex and further analysis and integration of this information through secondary and tertiary sensory areas. These sensory areas are then integrated with the motor response systems of the brain and nervous system with modulation imposed by the anterior frontal areas.

Woodruff and Baisden cite these aspects of Luria's neuropsychological theory, but criticize the theory because it does not state in specific detail the cellular basis for behavior. Specifically, they say, "As a general theory of brain function it falls short in that it does not lead from the molar level of analysis to the more cellular." Our review of these so-called molar theories, later in this volume, will show clearly that such theories are the *only* ones, in fact, that have any specific meaning with relation to higher-level aspects of brain functions. Theories that attempt to relate cellular (especially neuronal) functions to cognitive activity and behavior fall far short of doing any kind of justice to the complexity of the behavior aspect of brain functions.

The final principle cited by Woodruff and Baisden concerns laterality of function in the human brain, which is presumed to be related to asymmetry of structure. Although these authors note that in most activities the functions of the two cerebral hemispheres are generally coordinated, they fail to recognize that certain higher-level abilities are diffusely distributed throughout the cerebral cortex. Instead, their explanation relates only to functions that are principally lateralized and subserved individually by each cerebral hemisphere, with some type of integration produced by commissural connections of the two cerebral hemispheres to produce integrated behavior.

Woodruff and Baisden also state (p. 49) that there is "nothing special" about lateralization and that it represents only a special case of localization of functions. They say, "As language developed it was simply parceled into one hemisphere, rather than being segregated from other functions along the anterior-posterior axis. A general corollary to this position would be that the more discrete and specialized a function becomes, the more localized it is likely to be."

This latter statement appears to be in direct conflict with the observation that the highest aspect of brain functioning, relating to abstraction, reasoning, and concept formation, is generally distributed throughout the cerebral cortex rather than being localized. In one sense, this highest level of brain function might be thought to be quite specialized, even though it is not discrete in nature.

Theories based on the anatomical, physiological, and chemical substrates of brain function appear at this point in our knowledge to contribute little in their own right to understanding of behavior subserved by the brain. The connection between the cellular and chemical functions of the brain and behavior are still too widely separated to postulate any explicit and meaningful integration. In fact, even in reviews of biologically based theories of brain functioning (such as the review of Woodruff and Baisden), the only considerations of behavioral aspects of brain functions as such are essentially drawn from clinical and behavioral observations rather than from structural, physiological, or chemical knowledge.

In spite of criticisms that behavioral theories of brain functions do not lead from the molar level of analysis to the more cellular level, the molar theories have the advantage of including behavior in the brain-behavior equation. We must also note, however, that the behavioral theories risk neglect of the "brain" aspect of the equation. It is imperative, therefore, that molar or behavioral theories be derived directly from observations or data that actually reflect the biological condition of the brain rather than only to provide a statement of psychological functions. If the theory neglects or ignores the brain it becomes a psychological theory rather than a neuropsychological theory. A psychological theory may be useful in understanding behavior, but it does not aid in understanding brain-behavior relationships.

Developmental Theories

Developmental theories of brain-behavior relationships have been preoccupied with the specialized functions of the left and right cerebral hemispheres and the ways in which these different abilities, subserved by each hemisphere, have evolved.

Kolb and Whishaw Theory. Kolb and Whishaw (1980) have proposed a theory which is based on the premise that abilities, early in the course of development, are relatively simple in nature and become more complex in a cognitive sense as the individual develops. The essential feature of this theory is concerned with the organization of the brain as it subserves simple and more complex cognitive functions.

The authors postulate that simple cognitive functions are initially represented bilaterally, but particular abilities develop an increased dependence on one of the cerebral hemispheres as the neuropsychological functions of the individual develop and become more complex.

Simple cognitive functions presumably are not lateralized but are generally distributed throughout the brain; more complex cognitive abilities (such as language and visual-spatial skills) are differentially lateralized. As determined by the eventual outcome, Kolb and Whishaw's theory proposes that language functions become increasingly represented in the left cerebral hemisphere during the course of neuropsychological maturation and spatial and manipulatory abilities relate more closely to the right cerebral hemisphere. Recognizing that the "association" areas of the cerebral cortex are not already committed to primary or secondary sensory and motor functions, Kolb and Whishaw's theory postulates that these association areas are especially involved in complex cognitive functions and serve as the principal location of higher-level brain functions.

The developmental context in which this theory is based would, then, presume that young children have a general representation of their relatively simple abilities throughout the cerebral cortex, and the specialized functions of the left and right cerebral hemispheres develop as the child grows older and cognitive skills become more complex. A considerable amount of evidence is available to support the contention that brain functions in the young child are not well localized. A focal lesion does not necessarily give rise to highly specific neuropsychological deficits. Secondly, lateralized cerebral damage in a young child does not totally preclude development of abilities that would normally be associated with the damaged area. For example, children who have sustained lateralized cerebral lesions early in life and have undergone hemispherectomy are not totally devoid of language functions, even when the left cerebral hemisphere has been removed.

Available evidence suggests that the potential of cerebral cortical tissue to subserve particular abilities is much greater (regardless of the location or lateralization of the tissue) early in life than after physical maturation. It would seem likely, in accordance with the theory of Kolb and Whishaw, that there may be a progression from diffuse to more specific representation of particular abilities.

It is certainly apparent that intellectual and cognitive abilities develop in complexity as the child grows into adulthood. There appear to be some features of the Kolb and Whishaw theory that relate to known events in the developmental sequence.

It is possible to examine the postulates of this theory in more detail, particularly with relation to simple cognitive functions. According to the theory, simple cognitive tasks presumably are not well localized in the cerebral cortex. However, even a cursory review of the literature indicates that some of the most simple types of cognitive tasks are very closely dependent upon one of the cerebral hemispheres.

It has long been known, for example, that relatively simple tactile cognitive functions, such as finger localization and object identification (stereognosis), are closely dependent upon the intactness of the contralateral parietal area. In tactile finger localization the usual testing procedure involves touching one of the subject's fingers and he/she is required to discern which finger was touched. Quite clearly this is not a complex cognitive task, but a simple cognitive function is involved. On the basis of the Kolb and Whishaw theory one would presume that such a simple cognitive function was diffusely represented in the cerebral cortex.

Research results (Hom & Reitan, 1982) have shown not only that ability in tactile finger recognition is dependent upon the parietal area, but that a distinct lateralization effect is also present. Damage of the left parietal area tends to impair this simple cognitive function for fingers of the right hand; damage of the right parietal area impairs performances on the left hand. In fact, when groups with distinctly lateralized lesions are composed, tactile finger localization abilities on the left and right hands shows a relatively strong inverse coefficient of correlation (Reitan, 1984).

Many other simple cognitive tasks are distinctly lateralized and localized. Aphasic manifestations (such as naming deficits) in right-handed adults who have developed cerebral functions normally are almost invariably associated with damage of the left cerebral hemisphere (Wheeler & Reitan, 1962). Motor deficits of a relatively simple nature have also been shown to have distinct lateralization effects, as demonstrated by evaluation of performances with the Purdue Pegboard (Costa, Vaughn, Levita, & Farber, 1963).

Even in young children these simple types of cognitive performances are distinctly related to the left or right cerebral hemisphere. In fact, the methodological approach in interpreting results from the Halstead-Reitan Battery that serves most effectively to identify children with lateralized cerebral dysfunction is concerned with intraindividual differences on the two sides of the body in a variety of simple cognitive performances. Higher-level neuropsychological abilities may be more diffusely represented in the brains of young children than among adults, but the lower-level neuropsychological functions, which require only simple cognitive abilities, appear to be heavily dependent upon the anatomical organization of pathways within the nervous system and, in turn, have essentially a similar relationship in children and in adults.

A second approach toward testing the theory of Kolb and Whishaw would be to determine whether there were complex cognitive tasks which were diffusely represented in the cerebral cortex and not differentially dependent upon the left or right cerebral hemisphere. The Kolb and Whishaw theory postulates that more complex cognitive abilities, which develop over time, become increasingly specialized in their cerebral lateralization or localization.

One of the most complex higher-level neuropsychological tests is the Halstead Category Test, which measures abilities related to reasoning, abstraction, logical analysis, and concept formation. Prior evidence has indicated that this test is very sensitive to the biological condition of the cerebral cortex (Reitan, 1955a and many ensuing studies).

Results on the Category Test have also been investigated in subjects with lateralized cerebral lesions (Doehring & Reitan, 1962). The findings indicated that performances on the Category Test are quite independent of a lesion's lateralization or localization, despite the Category Test's sensitivity to brain damage. In fact, the pattern of errors on individual subtests was remarkably similar for groups with left or right cerebral lesions as compared with control subjects.

There appear to be quite complex cognitive abilities that are not lateralized or localized in the cerebral cortex but instead are diffusely represented throughout the cerebral cortex. Although language skills become increasingly specialized during the course of development and localize in the left cerebral hemisphere and spatial and manipulatory skills become increasingly dependent upon the right cerebral hemisphere, in developing a theory of brain behavior relationships it is important to recognize that other abilities, including some that are quite complex in nature, are diffusely distributed throughout the cerebral cortex.

In a biological sense, these diffusely distributed abilities, which involve the function of the entire cerebral cortex (including areas that are also devoted to specialized abilities), may be the most important. Nearly every adult with cerebral damage, regardless of whether it is focal or diffuse, shows significant evidence of impairment in abstraction and reasoning abilities, regardless of whether specific deficits (such as aphasic manifestations or constructional dyspraxia) are simultaneously present. As might well be expected from results on the Category Test, persons with cerebral damage much more regularly show generalized deficits than specific deficits which are manifested in measures that are sensitive only to a lesion in either the left or right cerebral hemisphere.

A basic problem with the theory proposed by Kolb and Whishaw concerns not only the fact that simple cognitive functions are often specifically lateralized and localized and that more complex cognitive abilities are sometimes diffusely represented, but that the theory itself is essentially locked in to a concern for explaining the specialized (lateralized) functions of the two cerebral hemispheres. The dramatic differences in functions of the two cerebral hemispheres have been well publicized, but the types of abilities generally dependent upon the entire cerebral cortex, regardless of lateralization or localization, have not received as much attention.

There is a tendency to presume that if an area of the cerebral cortex is clearly related to a specific type of ability (e.g., language and related verbal skills), it does not subserve other neuropsychological functions (such as abstraction and reasoning, even when not in a verbal context). This tendency probably is related to the inclination of some theorists to assign higher-level neuropsychological functions to the "association" areas essentially because of their availability.

In developing a neuropsychological theory of brain-behavior relationships, however, it is important to consider the entire range of abilities critically dependent upon the brain. This criterion cannot be met with regard to human brain-behavior relationships through knowledge derived only from animal studies. A review of the publications cited by Kolb and Whishaw to their own work in their 1980 textbook entitled *Fundamentals of Human Neuropsychology* indicates that their published research has been essentially limited to animal studies.

Goldberg and Costa's Theory. Goldberg and Costa (1981) have also proposed a neuropsychological theory of brain-behavior relationships that emphasizes the individuality of the left and right cerebral hemispheres.

These authors initially review the evidence for neuroanatomical differences between the cerebral hemispheres. Although the two hemispheres appear remarkably similar in gross aspects of structure, and are much more alike than they are different (von Bonin, 1962), many studies have indicated that distinct and fairly consistent anatomical differences between the two cerebral hemispheres exist. These differences, in turn, provide a temptation for the theorist who is motivated to search for an anatomical basis for obvious neuropsychological and behavioral differences in the functions of the two cerebral hemispheres. It must be recognized that it is an extremely difficult task to establish a valid relationship between the anatomical uniqueness of each cerebral hemisphere and corresponding behavioral functions.

As an example of of this problem, scientific studies have reported a decrease in the number of Betz cells in the motor cortex with advancing age among normal subjects, with the decrease becoming particularly apparent after age 55 (Brody, 1955). Independently, Reitan (1967), in measuring finger tapping speed of normal subjects in a cross-sectional evaluation, found no decrements in mean scores until approximately the age of 55, but beyond that age mean values dropped off sharply.

One would be tempted to conclude that the diminution in number of Betz cells was the anatomical basis for the reduction in finger tapping speed. However, it is important to recognize that the evidence relating to a reduced number of Betz cells was derived from persons who, when alive, had finger tapping speeds of unknown frequency. No one has information available on finger tapping speed of individuals with microscopic (histological) evidence of a reduction in the number of Betz cells of the motor cortex.

Before one can draw causal connections between two sets of events, it is necessary at least that those two sets of events be available for the same individuals. It would be hazardous to conclude unequivocally that a decrease in the number of Betz cells was the necessary and sufficient condition to produce a decrement in finger tapping speed, because other changes or circumstances could conceivably be responsible.

This illustration is intended to indicate the difficulty in attributing neuropsychological functions to specific neuroanatomical findings and to temper the (perhaps) natural tendency toward postulating relationships on essentially a permissive and opportunistic basis.

Nevertheless, in their statement of neuropsychological theory, Goldberg and Costa note that fundamental neuroanatomical differences between the hemispheres can lead to a wide range of cognitive consequences and that they have explored one of them which appears to be of considerable importance.

They propose theoretically that the left cerebral hemisphere "... achieves superiority in the utilization of a multiplicity of descriptive systems which are fully formed in an individual's cognitive repertoire and which are relevant to specific classes of materials or tasks." The right hemisphere, conversely, was described as being most crucial in the processing of materials to which none of the descriptive systems pre-existing in a subject's cognitive repertoire is readily applicable, and in assembling new descriptive systems.

This conceptualization describes the left cerebral hemisphere as being more capable of unimodal and motor processing as well as the storage of compact codes, and the right cerebral hemisphere is supposedly more able in performing intermodal integration and in processing novel stimuli. When the individual is involved in the process of acquiring a new descriptive system, the right cerebral hemisphere plays a critical role in the initial stages of acquisition. The left cerebral hemisphere is more able in utilizing codes that are already well-routinized.

These authors become much more specific in attempting to relate the anatomical peculiarities of the left cerebral hemisphere to various aspects of language acquisition. They note that in the left cerebral hemisphere there is a relatively greater representation of the temporal planum, parietal operculum, and pars opercularis of the inferior frontal gyrus, and that these anatomical differences "account for its relatively strong predisposition for elemental phonetic processing." In the right cerebral hemisphere there is a "greater representation of associative zones of intermodal integration," and this presumably "accounts for its relative importance in the formation of the referential basis of semantics."

Syntax may be said to occupy an intermediate position, in that "it is involved in both coordination of the elements of surface structure (for which unimodal learning may be proposed), and also serves a functional role, mastery of which may involve intermodal integration." The necessary requirement of relating unique aspects of anatomical structure and elements of language acquisition *in the same subjects* must again be emphasized, especially since it was totally ignored in the above theoretical statement.

Although Goldberg and Costa identify many studies which support their theory, it is important to note that the results of these studies, even when reaching statistical significance, include a very substantial degree of overlap among groups of subjects. In other words, although independent variables may be exclusively represented among the groups used, the results of dependent variables show a great deal of variability within and between groups even in instances that achieve statistically significant intergroup differences. Therefore, it is an error to treat the conclusions drawn from individual studies as if they were absolute and not subject to a great deal of variability among the subjects on which the principles were established.

Secondly, it is perhaps only natural to select particular points of information from the literature that support one's theoretical position. In one instance, for example, Goldberg and Costa refer to the findings of Semmes (1968) to support their proposed functional differences between the left and right cerebral hemispheres. They state that Semmes proposed that cognitively similar units are represented compactly in the left cerebral hemisphere in contrast to their intermixed representation in the right hemisphere. They use this information with relation to their review of neuroanatomical differences to suggest that these differences "extend to the storage of sets of cognitive elements which may be defined other than on the basis of their sensory modalities."

Specific referral to the results reported by Semmes, however, may be relevant at this point. In her study of tactile functioning of the left hand as compared with the right hand and presumptions concerning responsible cerebral lesions, Semmes used patients with penetrating brain wounds. It is well known that persons with such lesions have extensive and widespread cerebral damage in addition to any evidence of focal involvement (Jennett & Teasdale, 1981). It would be extremely difficult to use findings described as reflecting "compact representation of similar units" vs. "intermixed representation" in the two cerebral hemispheres, with relation to the possible anatomical bases, in this kind of material.

To provide further evidence to support the differential nature of information processing of the two cerebral hemispheres, Goldberg and Costa also use findings derived from the study of patients with commissurotomies as well as persons with congenital absence of the corpus callosum. They make no reference to the fact that the brains of most of the commissurotomized patients had evidence of disease or damage early in life, a factor which in its own right may very well have influenced the organization of behavioral correlates of the two hemispheres.

Also, data from patients with agenesis of the corpus callosum can hardly be thought of as reflecting only an abnormality of the corpus callosum with a presumption that the two cerebral hemispheres are normal in other respects. A review of studies of patients with callosal agenesis (Russell & Reitan, 1955) consistently showed that such persons have failed to develop normally and have evidence of generalized impairment of cerebral functions in addition to having a partial or complete absence of the corpus callosum. Material of this kind scarcely serves to provide evidence pertinent to theories of normal brain functions.

As noted, Goldberg and Costa cite many additional studies in support of their theory. At this point we cannot undertake to review the relevance of each citation and its limitations, but the problem of building a theory on the basis of reports in the literature is filled with many hazards. We should also note that this particular theory, even though presented in a developmental context, presents another example of attempting to explain only the specialized functions of the two cerebral hemispheres and certain aspects of their interrelationships.

Goldberg and Costa note that it is an oversimplification to treat the brain as consisting of two separate processors and that they have a "full appreciation of the fact that interaction of the hemispheres occurs in every on-line process . . ." Nevertheless, they feel that it is necessary to specify the roles of the two cerebral hemispheres before building composite models, and that any concept of interaction would have very little value until "it is clearly established what each element is doing in the ensemble."

It is difficult to resist commenting that a "full appreciation" of the interaction of the two hemispheres, claimed by these authors, may be an overstatement when their concept of the generalized aspects of neuropsychological functioning still refers only to "interaction of the hemispheres" and there is no apparent evidence that any effort has been made to discover the types of neuropsychological functions which are diffusely represented throughout the cerebral cortex regardless of which hemisphere is considered.

Rourke's Theory. Rourke (1982) has also proposed a developmental model of brain-behavior relationships. He acknowledges the theory of Goldberg and Costa (1981) as the principal stimulus for his theoretical position. Reitan (1984) has already reviewed Rourke's theory as follows: "Although Rourke notes that serious students in the area would not contend that an adequate or complete theory of brain-behavior relationships in children is yet possible, he proposes that the right cerebral hemisphere precedes the left cerebral hemisphere in acquisition of abilities." Along with Goldberg and Costa, Rourke believes that the right cerebral hemisphere has a critical role in the initial stages of the acquisition of information and the left cerebral hemisphere deals with the details which he identifies as "utilization of routinized codes that flow from the initial acquisitions."

Rourke's theory is embodied in five postulates: (1) An ontogenetic progression occurs in a developmental context for right cerebral functions, (2) Children's conceptualizations progress from global to specific in accordance with the ontogenetic processing between the hemispheres of the brain, (3) Right hemisphere functions must develop initially for adequate functions, (4) Concept formation also follows this right hemisphere-left hemisphere progression, with the right hemisphere involved in the formation of concepts and the left hemisphere in their articulation, elaboration, and stereotypic application, and (5) Impairment of right cerebral hemisphere functions is of special significance in limiting the development of adaptive abilities.

These are interesting postulates and are supported, in part, by some of Rourke's findings in his study of children with learning disabilities. As noted previously, he and his colleagues have reported findings which postulate two groups of learning-disabled children (Rourke & Finlayson, 1978; Rourke & Strang, 1978, 1983). In addition, Rourke reported results which he believes suggest that children with certain types of disabilities (presumably related to the right cerebral hemisphere but not actually so demonstrated) have special problems with the Category Test (Strang & Rourke, 1983).

Rourke has also found that certain reading, spelling, and arithmetical deficits fall into differential patterns for various groups of children with learning disabilities. Without any biological evidence, Rourke has implied that these patterns of deficits relate to differential impairment of the left and right cerebral hemispheres. These contributions were made during the time he calls "the second phase of neuropsychology," the phase that tended to ignore the "neuro" aspect of the equation.

Concerning the five postulates that serve as the basis of Rourke's developmental neuropsychological theory, it may be that right cerebral functions must be trained before left hemisphere functions become operative in a practical sense. In support of this proposition, one could refer to the historical development of kindergarten training procedures as a forerunner to training in the use of language symbols for communicational purposes. In all probability the brain of the young child is more amenable to training and modification in manipulatory and visual-spatial tasks than training in reading, spelling, writing, and arithmetic. The first point of Rourke's theory seems to be based upon general experience and common sense, even though there is no rigorous scientific evidence to support it.

The second postulate in the theory, concerned with conceptual development from global to specific in association with right to left hemisphere development, is less well supported. As noted previously, Doehring and Reitan (1962) found that in adult subjects (who might represent the ultimate criterion for conceptual development), there were no differences in level or pattern of results on the Category Test in persons with either right or left cerebral lesions. This type of evidence, based on persons with documented brain lesions and emanating from what Rourke describes as the "first phase of neuropsychological theorizing," would seem to be quite important in maintaining contact with the neurological bases of behavior.

The third postulate in Rourke's theory, that development of right hemisphere functions is a prerequisite for adequate development of left hemisphere functions, appears to be a restatement of the first point.

The fourth postulate, that concept formation is basically dependent upon the right cerebral hemisphere and elaboration of the concepts are dependent upon the left cerebral hemisphere, stems principally from Rourke's findings that children with specific arithmetical deficiencies performed more poorly on the Category Test than children who had relatively good arithmetical abilities but were impaired in dealing with language symbols (Rourke, 1982).

It must be noted again that these studies by Rourke and his colleagues were not based upon persons with any documented brain damage or brain lesions whatsoever; they were based upon children with leaning disabilities, and most of these children (although not so reported by Rourke and his colleagues in their studies) have normal neurological findings. Therefore, one must question whether their conclusion has any empirical basis.

We must again state that Doehring and Reitan (1962) found no differences in the effects of actual lesions of the right and left cerebral hemispheres in terms of concept formation. McFie and Piercy (1952), using Weigl's sorting test, found that a significantly larger proportion of patients with left hemisphere lesions than patients with right hemisphere lesions failed the test. Goldstein (1936), using similar abstraction tests, felt that impairment of abstraction ability could result from any cerebral lesion, but that frontal damage had the most adverse effects. Rylander (1939) found no difference in performance of various abstraction tests among persons with left and right cerebral lesions. Halstead (1940) also failed to find any laterality effects when comparing patients in their ability to group heterogeneous objects according to organizing principles. Each of these investigators used subjects with documented brain lesions

to base his conclusions concerning brain-behavior relationships.

Finally, Rourke's fifth postulate is concerned with the significance of limitation of adaptive abilities in persons with right cerebral dysfunction. Rourke is careful to use the term "right-hemisphere systems" rather than right cerebral damage because his data does not refer to persons with documented right cerebral lesions. Therefore, Rourke's inferences are based upon types of impairment or patterns of disability that *he* believes may be related to right cerebral functions. In fact, there is no adequate scientific evidence to support the hypothesis that significant impairment of "adaptive abilities" is specifically related to right cerebral damage, although this certainly is an open question.

In conclusion, one may view Rourke's theory as being of interest, but it is related almost exclusively to the "specialization" concept of cerebral functions. The theory entirely ignores the general characteristics of impaired brain functions. As we previously noted, the abilities of the individual that nature has represented generally in both cerebral hemispheres would appear to be more significant than those that are specialized or limited to either the left or right hemisphere (or areas within each cerebral hemisphere), merely in terms of their more generous anatomical involvement.

As Reitan (1966a) has demonstrated in many studies, certain abilities are generally represented throughout the cerebral cortex and on an *a priori* basis one would think that they would be of special significance for theoretical postulations. In fact, even in terms of clinical evaluation, general as well as specific (or lateralized) measures must always be used in clinical evaluation of the individual patient (Goodglass & Kaplan, 1979). In that sense, a final question must be raised regarding the usefulness of Rourke's theory in clinical application to individual patients.

Theoretical Postulates Regarding Brain-Behavior Relationships in Children with Learning Disabilities

In the last several years many studies have been performed which indicate the differential functions of the two cerebral hemispheres (Gazzaniga & Sperry, 1967; Milner, 1971; Wheeler & Reitan, 1962). The remarkable total scientific effort invested in the study of the functions of the two cerebral hemispheres is revealed in even only a brief review of the literature.

In addition to normals, subjects used in these investigations have included persons with a wide range of various types of developmental and acquired brain lesions and have extended from infants to adults. An extensive range of experimental techniques has been employed, including psychological and neurological examination, dichotic listening, evoked response potentials, reaction time, and many other experimental approaches.

The types of behavioral and psychological functions assessed include many types of simple to complex language performances, including reading proficiency, recognition of letters and words that vary in meaning, and analyses of the grammatical features of language; verbal and performance intelligence; recognition of abstract patterns, famous vs. everyday faces, and many other kinds of spatial configurations; immediate and short-term memory; color-naming ability; flexibility in performances; cognitive processing of geometry; music perception and differentiation of rhythmic beats and tonal patterns; reaction time to various types of stimuli; and shape and texture discrimination as well as other tactile performances.

Considering the appeal that differential functions of the left and right cerebral hemispheres has had to the scientific community in captivating their research efforts, it can hardly be surprising that a number of theories have been proposed, based upon supposed differences in laterality of cerebral functioning, to explain conditions such as learning disabilities. In fact, theorists in this area have recently proposed a range of conceptual formulations (some based upon empirical research evidence), to effect an explanation of differential organization of brain functions between children with learning disabilities and normal children.

As noted by Fisk and Rourke (1983), three approaches have generally been used to obtain relevant data and information: (1) clinical evaluation of individual subjects, (2) use of psychological test results to identify differential (better and poorer) scores to characterize children with learning disabilities, and (3) use of multivariate statistical analyses of test scores to identify clusters that may appear differentially in various subgroups of children.

These investigative approaches have led to conceptualizations, categorizations, and explanations of learning disability which, although not presented as comprehensive theories of brain-behavior relationships, nevertheless imply fundamental principles of brain organization. The great interest in right-left cerebral differences has had a profound effect on the development of these explanations.

Patterns of cognitive deficits or selective relationships among various abilities have been investigated. In turn, these patterns have been related to involvement of the left or right cerebral hemispheres. For example, Boder (1971, 1973a, 1973b), in her study of children with specific reading difficulties, has found that they may be classified as having dysphonetic dyslexia, dyseidetic dyslexia, or show a combination of dysphonetic-dyseidetic dyslexia.

Dysphonetic dyslexics have problems that center in the language or verbal area. These children have auditory-verbal deficits or weaknesses in comprehension skills, and particular difficulties in analyzing words into phonemes. They tend to read words as visual gestalts, neglect phonetics, make semantic substitutions in reading and spelling, and generally fail to analyze words into phonetic units.

The second group of dyslexic children, *dyseidetic dyslexics,* appear to have difficulties in reading because they are impaired in discriminating and analyzing the visual-spatial configuration represented by words. Even though they have adequate ability in phonetic analysis, their difficulties appear in their attempts to sound out words and they have spelling errors that frequently involve reversals and confusion of the proper sequence of letters.

The third group, children with *dysphonetic and dyseidetic dyslexia,* had a combination of the two types of deficits. As one might expect, the dysphonetic dyslexics are presumed to have dysfunction principally of the left cerebral hemisphere; the dyseidetic dyslexics, who had difficulty discriminating and analyzing visual-spatial configurations represented by words, were presumed to have right cerebral dysfunction.

Bakker (1973, 1979, 1982a, 1982b, 1983) has also proposed that ability differences, presumably related to differential impairment of the two cerebral hemispheres, produces two types of dyslexic children. One type depends upon a linguistic-semantic approach to reading and are dyslexic because of difficulties stemming from left cerebral dysfunction. Bakker identifies these children as *L-type dyslexics.* The other group, identified as *P-type dyslexics,* have difficulties in reading principally because of their inability to appreciate the perceptual requirements of words. These visual-form difficulties in perception presumably stem from right cerebral dysfunction.

Pirozzolo (1979) and Pirozzolo and Hess (1976) have also suggested that there are two fundamental types of dyslexia that are differentially related to brain organization of abilities. Persons in one category, identified as *auditory-linguistic dyslexics,* have problems with both receptive and expressive aspects of verbal and language functions and show difficulty with auditory verbal comprehension, in naming common objects, and are slow in carrying out any types of verbal tasks. Other

investigators (Mattis, French, & Rapin, 1975; Denckla & Rudel, 1976) have also reported findings of this type in dyslexic children.

Pirozzolo identifies the second group of dyslexic children as *visual-spatial dyslexics.* The fundamental problem in this group of children relates to difficulties in the area of visual perception and corresponding impairment in learning to recognize letters and words.

Within the framework of differences between right and left cerebral functions, several investigators (as noted in the prior section) have presumed that the cerebral hemispheres develop their organization of abilities at different rates. These differences in development of function presumably have consequences for learning to read.

Carmon, Nachsom, and Starinsky (1976) and Silverberg, Bentin, Gaziel, Obler, and Albert (1979) have studied comparative perception in the left and right visual fields. Their results suggest that younger children depend more upon perception of visual-spatial characteristics of stimulus material (calling principally upon the right cerebral hemisphere) when learning to read and older children rely more on verbal-symbolic characteristics of the stimulus material (relying principally upon the left cerebral hemisphere) when they are reading.

Although it is possible to perform this kind of experiment under laboratory conditions of restricted input to the two sides of the retina, it must be noted that in normal functioning foveal or macular vision must be used to perceive the form discrimination required in reading, and in many cases vision subserved by this part of the retina is bilaterally represented. In addition, in normal reading an individual will move his head and the stimulation of the retina will not be artificially restricted. From a practical point of view, it would be difficult to assess the significance of the differential responsiveness within the visual fields to various types of stimulus material.

It is apparent from the above observations that interest in the differential and specialized functions of the two cerebral hemispheres has had an overwhelming influence, not only in mobilizing research activities but also in various attempts to conceptualize and explain practical kinds of disorders such as reading and learning disability. Again, we must note that theoretical formulations of this condition have consistently appealed only to right vs. left cerebral functions and have failed to even postulate the existence of significant intellectual and cognitive abilities that may be diffusely distributed throughout the cerebral cortex. As the reader will observe, this tendency pervades essentially all aspects of recent theory-building in the area of brain-behavior relationships, thus contributing basically to two-factor theories of cognitive functioning.

These theories might be referred to as representing "lateral specialization" in contrast to the regional-localization approaches previously mentioned. They clearly differ from holistic theories of brain-behavior relationships. Although holistic theories have lost ground almost totally with the current emphasis on right and left cerebral functions, we have noted that evidence derived from study of persons with verified brain lesions indicates that certain higher-level brain functions are diffusely represented throughout the cerebral cortex and other abilities are principally lateralized or even localized in certain regions. This information leads us to point to the value of developing a theoretical framework of brain-behavior relationships that emphasizes both general as well as specialized and specific aspects of neuropsychological functions dependent on brain functions (see the Reitan-Wolfson theory presented later in this chapter).

Luria's Neuropsychological Theory of Brain Functions

Before his death Luria (1970) published a statement of his theory of brain-behavior relationships. In this work, *The Functional Organization of the Brain,* he stated that his theory, which was developed from a new approach to study of brain functions (namely, neuropsychology), was based upon two aims.

The first of these aims was quite practical in nature. He stated (p. 66), "First, by pinpointing the brain lesions responsible for specific behavior disorders we hope to develop a means of early diagnosis and precise localization of brain injuries (including those from tumors or from hemorrhage) so that they can be treated by surgery as soon as possible."

It is clear from this statement that Luria felt that neuropsychological diagnosis of brain lesions in terms of location was an approach in competition with neurological diagnostic methods such as those involving contrast procedures. It must be recognized that computed tomography was already in its early stages at the time this paper was published, and computed tomographic scanning equipment had been installed in many medical centers.

The second aim stated by Luria (p. 66) was as follows: "Second, neuropsychological investigation should provide us with a factor analysis that will lead to a better understanding of the components of complex psychological functions for which the operations of the different parts of the brain are responsible."

Luria was not referring to factor analysis in a technical sense, based upon methods of reducing a correlational matrix into clusters of individual tests. Instead, as he explained later in his paper, he was thinking of a clinical type of factor analysis that involved analysis of results on individual subjects with brain lesions. He felt that it was possible to identify factors, or groups of tests, which showed dysfunction of a particular type in accordance with a lesion in a particular location.

It is apparent from this second aim, as well as other statements made by Luria, that his principal interest was to localize similar or related psychological deficits that corresponded in turn with rather precise areas of the cerebral cortex. In fact, after having discussed briefly the localization of sensory and motor functions in the brain, which he pointed out had been "mapped in precise detail," he noted that probably three-quarters of the cerebral cortex has nothing directly to do with these sensory or motor functions and that the responsibility of neuropsychology was "to proceed further with the mapping of the brain's functions (and) systems responsible for the higher, more complex behavioral processes."

However, Luria's conceptualization of mapping of functions in the cerebral cortex was hardly a simple set of one-to-one relationships. He viewed the basic functions of the brain as being represented by three main blocks.

Block 1, corresponding essentially with the reticular activating system, was responsible for regulating the energy level and tone of the cerebral cortex and for maintaining proper recognition of the significance of incoming stimuli.

Block 2 represented abilities in the analysis, coding and storing of incoming information through the various senses, establishing connections with the third block and effecting integration of incoming information through the various senses.

Block 3 was concerned with executive functions involved in formulation of intentions, plans, and programs for behavior, and thus represented the response or output aspect of brain functions. Although these three blocks compose the major separate aspects of brain functions, integration of these systems constitutes the real key to understanding how the brain mediates complex behavior.

As noted, Block 1, which is located in the lower and upper parts of the brain stem, maintains the energy level and tone of the cerebral cortex. (A brief review of the principal anatomical and functional features of the reticular activating system is presented in Reitan & Wolfson, 1985b). Injury to the ascending reticular activating system (ARAS) may cause the brain to go into a pathological state, characterized by a breakdown of its dynamic processes, deterioration of wakefulness and disorganization of memory traces.

Luria postulated that the breakdown of these "dynamic processes" of the cerebral cortex results in a loss of selectivity of cortical actions and of normal discriminations of stimuli. The ability of the cortex to respond to stimuli appropriately, in terms of their strength or significance, may be impaired with deficits of Block 1 and result in a "weakened cortex." In this case, responses (according to Luria) will be essentially the same to either significant or insignificant stimuli.

As evidence for this contention Luria cites the diffuse and disorganized nature of our thoughts when we become drowsy and the strange and even bizarre associations that the mind may form during dreams or in a state of fatigue. Impairment to Block 1 of the brain, resulting in deficits in normal discrimination of stimuli and the "selectivity of cortical actions" has been observed by Luria to occur in patients with ". . . tumors of the middle parts of the frontal lobes." He notes that others have reported these same deficits in persons with ". . . lesions in the deep parts of the brain." In some respects Luria's Block 1 tends to correspond with the Power Factor of biological intelligence postulated by Halstead.

Block 2 in Luria's neuropsychological theory of brain functions is located behind the central (Rolandic) fissure and is concerned with the analysis, coding, and storage of incoming information, especially through the senses of vision, hearing, touch, and kinesthesis.

Luria postulated that the functions of the second block are much more specific in nature than those of the first block, being distributed in primary receptive areas of various parts of the cerebral cortex depending upon the sensory function involved. Each of these primary receptive zones is responsible for recording and sorting of incoming information. In addition, the incoming information is further organized and analyzed in secondary zones and finally, in tertiary zones. The secondary zones are responsible for coding of sensory input and further organization and understanding of its nature. In the tertiary zones incoming information from the various senses overlap, are combined, and "lay the groundwork for the organization of behavior."

Lesions of each primary zone in Block 2 may cause losses in the appreciation of incoming information that is specific to the particular sense involved, but no marked change in complex behavior occurs. Damage to the secondary zones in Block 2, however, impairs the coding function of the sense involved and leads to disorganization and improper recognition of the incoming information dependent upon the particular sense. However, disturbances in function represented by integration of multi-sensory systems does not occur.

Luria postulated that the differential functions of these areas, in terms of the level of information processing involved, serve as "an important aid for locating the lesion." (It must be noted, however, that in our studies of thousands of persons with cerebral lesions, scarcely any lesions are so highly specific that they fall exclusively in the primary or secondary zones of particular senses. This causes a problem not only in the claim to differential localization of such lesions, but raises a question about the empirical data on which Luria's claim is based.)

Luria states that lesions of the tertiary zones are of greatest interest to neuropsychologists because these zones are responsible for the synthesis of information arriving through various senses into a collection that represents a coherent whole and thus results in complex behavioral disturbances. Since many aspects of human behavior relate to effective understanding and resolution of complex problems, represented by many diverse perceptual experiences, the importance of the tertiary zones can be appreciated. Luria cites visual disorientation in space as a particular example of a deficit resulting from impairment of function in the tertiary zones.

After incoming information from the environment has been registered, coded, stored, organized, and integrated among the various incoming avenues, Block 3 becomes involved in central processing. The third block controls executive functions involved in formulation of intentions, plans, and programs for behavior. Since the third block is responsible for the response element, it is involved in every complex behavioral process.

Luria states that Block 3 is localized in the anterior frontal lobes and performs a final integrative and executive function. Block 3 is involved in no sensory, motor, perceptual, or speech functions and is devoted exclusively to analysis, planning, and organization of programs for behavior. However, Block 3 is very closely related to the functions of Block 1, since both Blocks are concerned with overall efficiency of brain functions.

Block 1 is concerned principally with regulating the tone of the cerebral cortex and mediating attention and concentration. Impairment in Block 1 may result in inadequate registration of response, whereas impairment of Block 3 may result in inadequate expression of response. In one sense both Block 1 and Block 3 may limit the adequacy of cerebral cortical functioning because the limitation may occur either in the incoming (receptive) or outgoing (responsive) functions. In his theory of biological intelligence, Halstead (1947a) incorporated both incoming and outgoing functions into a single factor called the Directional Factor.

The final general aspect of Luria's theory involves the integration of the three Blocks into functional systems. Luria states that every complex form of behavior depends upon the joint operation of several faculties located in different zones of the brain. Disturbances or dysfunction of any one faculty will have an effect upon behavior, but the effect will differ depending upon its relationship with other faculties. Thus, a variety of expressions of brain disorder may be manifested in any one general type of function. Luria offers illustrations of the integration of functional systems by analyzing voluntary movement and by discussing disorders of speech and writing.

Luria points out (p. 68) that, "It was long supposed that voluntary movements are a function of the motor cortex, that is, the large pyramidal cells of the cortex of the anterior convolution of the brain." Although electrical stimulation of the brain identified the motor cortex via corresponding muscular contractions in various parts of the body, the more complex organization of the motor system in the cerebrum has, in fact, long been recognized. Obviously the motor cortex of the precentral gyrus is fundamental in terms of movement. Luria notes that the motor system involves much more than just the motor cortex and includes a system of cortical and subcortical zones, each playing a highly specific role in the functional system of voluntary movement that are necessarily integrated.

Over and beyond the motor strip, Luria identifies the first component as a precisely organized system of afferent input. He notes that it is not possible to regulate voluntary movements adequately only through efferent impulses from the brain to the muscles but that the brain must receive feedback from the muscles and joints as a basis for continual modification of the movement in order to obtain precision.

Therefore, voluntary movement has a sensory or proprioceptive basis which is subserved by the sensory cortex located behind the central sulcus. Damage to the somatosensory cortex can result in significant impairment of voluntary movement.

Next, Luria points out that voluntary movements must be organized with relation to the spatial field and be oriented toward a certain point in space. He feels that spatial regulation of voluntary movements is dependent upon the tertiary parts of the parietal-occipital cortex.

Luria notes that although the primary motor and sensory bases of voluntary movement might still be intact, damage to this area causes the patient to fail in precise spatial organization of the movement. He states specifically (p. 69), "He loses the ability to evaluate spatial relations and confuses left and right. Such a patient may be unable to find his way in a familiar place or may be confused in such matters as evaluating the positions of the hands of a watch or in distinguishing east and west on a map."

This statement, without reference to the differential and specialized functions of the left and right cerebral hemispheres, is vague in its meaning. Confusion of left and right is largely dependent upon the status of the left cerebral hemisphere (Wheeler & Reitan, 1962); confusion in a familiar location or difficulty in evaluating the position of the hands of a watch or distinguishing east and west on a map represent the types of spatial difficulties that are seen much more often in persons with right than left cerebral lesions (Critchley, 1953; Wheeler & Reitan, 1962).

The striking apparent difference between right-left confusion and confusion in dealing with spatial configurations is clearly manifested by a negative correlation between these symptoms in patients with left or right cerebral lesions (Reitan, 1984). As noted at the beginning of this section, the adequacy of theoretical formulations is inescapably directly dependent upon the accuracy of the facts on which the theories are based. If the facts are not accurate, the theory is bound to suffer.

Luria continues in his analysis of voluntary movement to incorporate the function of the premotor cortex. He notes the necessity of constant regulation in voluntary movement, arresting and modulating one of the steps of the movement and making a transition to the next step or phase. When the premotor cortex is damaged, the smooth sequential integration of separate links of motor behavior is impaired and skilled movements disintegrate. Then, even though the subject may still have primary movement capability (motor cortex), sensory feedback (postcentral cortex), and orientation in the spatial field (tertiary parts of the parietal-occipital areas), the smooth sequential flow of skilled movements may still be impaired.

Finally, voluntary movements must be related to the functions of the Third Block of basic brain functions, which is concerned with goal-directed actions and movements that achieve intentional and deliberate purposes. Luria believes (p. 71) that voluntary skilled movements must be regulated by a stable program or stable intention, which is provided by the prefrontal lobes. If this area is destroyed, even though all of the other requirements for skilled voluntary movements are intact, the "goal-linked actions are replaced by meaningless repetitions of already fulfilled movements or impulsive answers to outside stimuli. The whole purposive conduct of the patient is disturbed."

It should be noted that individual patients are encountered who do engage in meaningless repetitions of movements or impulsive responses to outside stimuli, both in terms of specific movements (echopraxia) or verbal communications (echolalia). However, among thousands of brain-damaged patients, such responses are in fact very rarely seen regardless of the specific areas of damage.

Luria presents illustrations done by a patient with a meningioma of the premotor area. The patient did the drawings on the second to fifth day post-operatively. It is apparent that the patient had a marked tendency to draw repetitive lines and that he showed some improvement from the second through the fifth day. However, a meningioma involves the connective tissue covering of the brain and it is highly unusual to see such striking manifestations of cerebral deficit with such lesions. Secondly, even in persons with structural damage of the cerebral tissue, few investigators have observed such perseverative motor deficits, even with anterior frontal lesions.

When citing evidence to support a theory, either in the form of individual case material or other research results, it is important to bear in mind that the test of validity relates to use of the manifestation as a basis for predicting the outcome presumed by the theory. Only in this way can incidentally-associated variables be differentiated from variables that have a direct cause-and-effect relationship.

Luria's Analysis of Speech and Writing According to his Neuropsychological Theory

Luria (1970) presented a detailed analysis of the psychological processes involved in certain aspects of speech and writing and the ways in which these functions relate to the brain. He indicated that the first step in recognition of speech depends upon analysis and differentiation of phonemes (which obviously must be on the basis of prior learning). Many words are quite similar in nature and require subtle distinctions of the sounds involved. These distinctions are made quite readily and even automatically by persons thoroughly familiar with the words and the language, but confusion may occur when such familiarity is not present. Luria notes that in some languages the same word may have quite different meanings depending even upon the pitch of the voice.

In relating the process of differentiating and recognizing phonemes to the brain, it is necessary to determine what part of the brain is responsible for this ability. Luria states that in his investigation of hundreds of patients with brain lesions he has found that "the critical region lies in the secondary zones of the left temporal lobe." The area most frequently associated with such deficits especially involves the posterior part of the superior temporal convolution in the left cerebral hemisphere. Data presented by Luria (1970) indicates, however, that deficiencies of this kind sometimes occur, even though less frequently, in the premotor cortex, the posterior-superior part of the parietal area, and the post-central gyrus.

Luria's reference to highly localized areas of the cerebral cortex must be questioned because his data were based on results obtained from examination of patients with bullet wounds of the left cerebral hemisphere. One could hardly expect the effects of the missile lesions to be localized to such exclusive areas, considering the consistent evidence of widespread damage with such lesions (Reitan & Wolfson, 1986b). Although penetrating brain wounds may cause focal damage, extensive investigation of patients with such lesions indicates that widespread damage, even involving the other cerebral hemisphere, is the rule rather than the exception. In fact, using patients with traumatic brain injuries for the purpose of localizing brain functions is a questionable procedure, considering the primary and secondary effects of such wounds.

Luria continues by stating that articulation has an important relationship to writing. He notes that people frequently pronounce unfamiliar words before attempting to write them. It appears that articulation helps to clarify the word's acoustic structure, which aids in writing the word. Again, in terms of his analysis of the relationship between speech and writing, Luria notes that it is important to have determined the area in the brain responsible for articulation. His studies have indicated that, "A separate area of the brain cortex, in the central (kinesthetic) region of the left hemisphere, controls the articulation of speech sounds."

It should again be emphasized that brain lesions in human beings are very rarely so specifically localized, and it is difficult to have confidence that sufficient material has been available to draw such pinpoint correlations between abilities and localization within the brain. In addition, one must also remember the considerable degree of individual variation that occurs in brain-behavior relationships. However, Luria states that several areas of the cerebral cortex are involved in evaluation of speech sounds and recognition of words.

Using these abilities as a basis, the next step in writing involves coding of the sound units of word (phonemes) into the units of writing (letters). Luria states that this process "calls into play still other parts of the brain cortex, in the visual and spatial zones," without specifying whether he is referring to the left or right cerebral cortex. Although the visual areas are represented in each cerebral hemisphere, a considerable amount of research has indicated that *spatial* functions are

more dependent upon the right cerebral hemisphere than the left.

Nevertheless, Luria goes on to indicate that patients with lesions in the occipital and parietal lobes have a "perfectly normal ability to analyze speech sounds, but they show marked difficulty in recognizing and forming written letters." He emphasizes that visual-spatial limitations are responsible for this difficulty, stating explicitly that persons with occipital and parietal lesions "find it difficult to visualize the required structure of a letter, to grasp the spatial relations among the parts of the letter and to put the parts together to form the whole."

If these observations of spatial difficulties concerning the configuration of letters were, in fact, valid, one would find it necessary to appeal to probable damage of the right cerebral hemisphere as an explanation. In addition, invariant generalizations of this type imply a remarkable specificity of loss of language functions for the individual patient.

On rare occasions one sees instances of a selective and specific deficit with retention of language abilities that one would consider to be closely related, but these cases represent the exceptions. In fact, there is a substantial correlation between aphasic deficits of various types, indicating that if a patient has one type of aphasic loss he is far more likely than not to have other types of aphasic deficits as well (Reitan, 1984). Over and beyond this, it must be acknowledged that the individual person with aphasia often does not show exactly the same deficits, even when attempting the same type of task, on successive occasions.

Head (1926), the noted British aphasiologist, noted long ago that this lack of consistency in demonstrating a specific type of aphasic deficit greatly complicated not only terminology in the area, but especially the potential for developing stable and invariant theories of relationships between particular deficits and areas of brain damage. Although the deficit is often not subject to repeated demonstration (even though similar and related deficits may be present on each examination), one would hardly presume that the brain lesion changes from one location to another between examinations to correspond with the differential results.

Luria continues to pursue the functions required for writing, noting that it is necessary to put the letters in proper sequence in order to form any particular word. He indicates that his "extensive studies" have located the region of the cerebral cortex responsible for this ability, which he refers to as *sequential analysis*. The critical area is in the "anterior region of the left hemisphere." He notes that lesions in the "prefrontal region disturb the ability to carry out rhythmic movements of the body, and they also give patients difficulty in writing letters in the correct order."

Perception of rhythmic sequences, as used in the Seashore Rhythm Test, has recently been shown by Reitan and Wolfson (unpublished study) to have no more relationship to damage in one cerebral hemisphere than the other, even though many American neuropsychologists have attributed such deficits to damage in the right temporal lobe.

Luria proceeds with an even more specific statement, indicating that if the lesion is located deep in the brain and interrupts the connections between the basal ganglia and the cerebral cortex, the patient becomes incapable of writing words at all. Nevertheless, "such a patient, with the higher parts of the cortex undamaged, can recognize phonemes and letters perfectly well."

The Speech-sounds Perception Test obviously requires the subject to recognize and differentiate consonants and consonant combinations. Our experience strongly suggests that any person with a large lesion interrupting connections between the basal ganglia and the cerebral cortex would almost certainly perform poorly on a formal test of this type.

Finally, Luria notes the role of the third block of the brain in providing organization in the expression of thoughts and ideas. He notes that persons with anterior frontal lesions have great difficulty expressing themselves either orally or in writing and have trouble producing a meaningful and progressive statement. These patients tend to repeat themselves over and over, making no progress toward an organized communication, even though they may appear to have great interest in conveying an analysis of the situation involved. We can comment that our studies indicate that generalized involvement of the cerebral cortex, to a severe degree, is a much more common basis for confusion of this type than focal involvement of the anterior frontal areas.

Integration of Neuropsychological Deficits

Luria points out that neuropsychological observations of the type described above are very useful in "dissecting" mental processes as well as in diagnosing the location of brain lesions. He feels that his type of evaluation provides a neuropsychological technique which essentially makes possible a factor analysis of brain-related abilities for the individual subject. Although investigators such as Thurstone and Spearman developed statistical techniques for factor analysis through reducing correlational matrices to their fundamental elements, Luria stated that neuropsychological evaluation can serve essentially the same type of purpose in evaluation of individual brain-behavior relationships.

For example, Luria states that a lesion of the left temporal lobe may cause a person to have "serious difficulty in analyzing speech sounds, in repeating verbal sounds, in naming objects and in writing, but the person retains normal capacities in spatial orientation and in handling simple computations." Objective evaluation of abilities in performing simple computations, with judgments of deficits made without knowledge of the location of lesions, have indicated that left cerebral damage caused such deficits about four times as frequently as right cerebral lesions (Wheeler & Reitan, 1962).

In contrast to his characterization of the effects of a left temporal lesion, Luria goes on to point out that a lesion in the left parietal-occipital area "destroys spatial organization" but "does not affect the patient's fluency of speech or sense of rhythm." Although it is possible to find individual persons who show a great variety of deficits even though certain abilities are retained, the more important conclusion would relate to generalizations across individuals rather than to observations of idiosyncratic individual subjects. If the findings regarding an individual subject are to be given credence, they must be sufficiently firm and pervasive to permit prediction of one circumstance or fact on the basis of knowledge only of the other.

A contention that left parietal-occipital damage destroys spatial organization is true in some cases, but a considerable amount of research has indicated that spatial organization is much more heavily dependent upon the integrity of the corresponding area in the right cerebral hemisphere. Although left parietal-occipital lesions may *not* affect a patient's fluency of speech in some cases (although such impairment is present in many cases with lesions in this area), the contention that such lesions do not effect the sense of rhythm has been clearly contradicted by carefully controlled scientific studies (Reitan & Wolfson, unpublished study). A question must be raised, therefore, about the accuracy of neuropsychological "factor analyses" when they are based upon questionable facts.

Luria points out that many behavioral processes, which may seem to have nothing in common, can be shown to be closely related when one understands how they are subserved by the brain. He asks what there might be in common between capacities for orientation in space, for doing computations, and for dealing with logical complexities in grammar. Luria's research has indicated that all three of these abilities are subserved by the lower part of the left parietal lobe. Because of this, he was prompted to search for an explanation regarding a common factor, and concluded that the

ability to grasp spatial relationships is fundamental to each of the three abilities.

In terms of simple arithmetical processes, Luria cites the problem of subtracting 7 from 31 and notes that this would be performed by first subtracting 7 from 30, obtaining an answer of 23, and then adding 1. He concludes that a spatial factor is represented in this process because "1 is to be *added* by placing it to the right of the 23. A patient with a lesion disturbing his capacity for spatial organization is unable to cope with the problem because he is at a loss whether to place the 1 to the left or the right — in other words, whether to add it or subtract it."

Although the relationship of arithmetical processes to spatial configurations has been cited many times, an empirical approach to this question indicates that deficits in this area occur about four times more frequently with left cerebral lesions than right cerebral lesions (Wheeler & Reitan, 1962).

An equally convincing argument for deficits associated with damage of the left parietal lobe could be offered by citing the pre-eminent role of the left cerebral hemisphere in tasks that require the use of symbols and their relationships. It is likely, in fact, that most persons perform simple arithmetical processes through an understanding of the symbolic relationships of numbers rather than through manipulation of spatial relationships, even though the use of spatial configurations, in the sense of quantities, is often useful in initial instruction. In fact, Luria's explanation faces another difficulty inasmuch as "orientation in space" and "capacity for spatial organization," which he attributes to a left parietal lesion, are much more frequently seen in persons with right cerebral damage. Thus, in terms of a common brain factor, his logical explanation of the common basis for impairment of orientation in space and for doing simple computations appears to be deficient in terms of the basic facts.

However, in developing his theoretical explanation, Luria goes on to include the ability to deal with complex grammatical constructions in the same framework. As an example he cites the ability to grasp the difference between "summer comes after spring" and "spring comes after summer" as requiring a person to make a "clear analysis of the quasi-spatial relations between the elements in each expression."

Again, the basic difficulty with Luria's analysis is that he is willing to attempt to discern a common factor between understanding language symbols and dealing with spatial relationships. The well known relationship of language functioning to the left cerebral hemisphere and spatial relationships to the right cerebral hemisphere confounds the validity of this effort. Luria's examples make it quite clear that the basic facts must be correct if the theoretical formulations or explanations of the "facts" are to have any validity.

Luria also cites a fairly common observation among persons with significant neuropsychological impairment as a basis for presuming that changes in brain function occur when the brain is damaged. He records examples of persons who are unable to engage in specific performances upon request when voluntary organizational effort is required, but who can perform the task when recourse to the analytical process is deliberately avoided.

In our own testing we have observed many instances among persons with left cerebral lesions who, when asked to consider the sentence "He shouted the warning," to explain its meaning, and finally to write the sentence, found that their ability to form the letters correctly deteriorated as they progressed with the writing. Some such patients, in an effort to complete the task, seem deliberately to shut down their voluntary effort and write the whole sentence quickly and on a very automatic basis.

Luria cites this kind of situation as evidence that a "task may invoke a stereotype based on a network of cortical zones quite different from the one that was called on originally when the performance required the help of the analytical apparatus." This kind of theoretical formulation, based upon uncontested observations of specific behavior, does little to explain the brain-related basis of the behavior. Instead, it only represents a presumptive restatement of the observed behavior.

The postulates and theories regarding organization of the brain and its relationship to behavior noted by Luria serve to emphasize the importance of objective initial determination of the facts themselves, a procedure which requires separate and independent evaluation of the biological condition of the brain (independent variables) and the behavioral performances (dependent variables). If both the independent and dependent variables are viewed simultaneously, it is likely that they will be associated permissively in terms of whatever explanatory thoughts occur to the observer.

If the behavioral performances (dependent variables) were analyzed independently of knowledge of the condition of the brain (independent variables) for groups of subjects with lesions in various locations, the next step would be to establish whether a relationship existed between particular kinds of deficits and the location of the lesion. Although such a procedure would be expected in observance even of basic and primary criteria, Luria's approach seems to show little concern for observation of this scientific dictum. As noted earlier by Reitan (1976), the clinical method used by Luria, with intermixture of simultaneous knowledge of independent and dependent variables and use of examining procedures that are not subject to exact replication by others, constitutes a basic disregard for both the conditions and need for cross-validation.

Luria undoubtedly made observations and reached conclusions that have significant value in understanding brain-behavior relationships, but they appear to have been derived in a framework of investigation that was entirely clinically oriented and did not have the safeguards implicit in the use of scientific standards that are routinely expected. Although some of Luria's conclusions agree with findings of other investigators, some of his conclusions disagree with those reached through more carefully controlled scientific investigations. When the initial observations vary in their degree of validity, it becomes quite difficult to formulate a theory concerning the organization of the brain and its relationship to behavior.

Halstead's Theory of "Biological Intelligence"

Although the specific contributions made by Halstead appear in many different sources, his major systematic contribution to clinical neuropsychology is presented in his book, *Brain and Intelligence* (Halstead, 1947a). This monograph is divided into two sections. The first part is a critique of existing concepts of intelligence and a presentation of Halstead's theory of biological intelligence. The second section of his book is concerned with a representation of the various aspects of biological intelligence in the brain.

Halstead was frequently asked to explain what he meant by the term "biological intelligence." In many instances he responded by citing his interpretation of the results of a factor analysis, as will be described below. On other occasions, he related biological intelligence to the adaptive abilities of a healthy brain and nervous system.

Halstead had great respect for human as well as animal adaptive abilities. On one occasion, for example, Halstead and one of the authors (RMR) were discussing some recent findings relating to altered biological functions in rats and corresponding impairment in maze learning abilities. Halstead listened to my (RMR) exposition of these results, considered patiently the "exciting" implications that I felt the results had, and then advised me to go and spend some time with a rat exterminator in order to learn something about the *real* adaptive abilities of rats. Obviously, Halstead felt

that there was much more intelligence implicit in the behavior of rats, as expressed in solution of their own problems, than had been shown in the psychology laboratory.

At other times Halstead talked about the intelligence implicit in the responses and reactions of sheep dogs in tending and herding flocks of sheep. He would cite the selective perception of the sheep dog, the spontaneous ability to discard irrelevant stimuli, the highly appropriate reactions, and the excellent efficiency in achieving the end result that characterized the purposive behavior of these animals. Undoubtedly many aspects of the efficient behavior of sheep dogs was learned, but the important point is that this behavior was learned by a normal brain. It is hardly surprising that Halstead was not much impressed by what he termed "psychometric" intelligence, which he felt was related principally to vocabulary and defined by a criterion of classroom success.

Rylander (1947, p. 65), in discussing a paper presented by Halstead (1947a), said:

> I am sorry to trouble you with the question, Dr. Halstead, but would you be so kind as to give me some sort of definition of your concept of "biological intelligence"? I have been looking through the literature to get a clear idea of that concept and of the theoretical background of your impairment index. While I was at Yale some days ago I asked people there for an explanation of "biological intelligence." They could not tell me and advised to ask you.

In answer, Halstead (1947a, p. 66) responded as follows:

> I am familiar with Dr. Rylander's work on the frontal lobes in which he combines clinical evaluation with measurements by standardized psychological tests. My findings, with, I believe, more exact quantitative methods are in substantial agreement with his. His query as to what I mean by biological intelligence raises a difficult problem in brief communication.
>
> Some years ago Cannon used the title *The Wisdom of the Body* for one of his books. I do

not believe that Cannon intended to omit the nervous system in this concept. In biological intelligence I am trying to direct attention to the "wisdom of a healthy nervous system."

It is my belief that psychometric intelligence, as reflected by the IQ, does not adequately indicate the "wisdom" of the healthy body or of its alteration in the pathological nervous system. We have repeatedly found normal or superior IQ's in neurosurgical patients lacking up to one-fourth of the total cerebrum following frontal lobectomy. Yet our measurements of biological intelligence indicate that these are not normal individuals. Biological intelligence, we believe, with high adaptability, is the normal outcome of the functioning of a healthy nervous system. I shall not try to elaborate the concept further here except to add that biological intelligence seems to have meaningfulness not only in the laboratory but in the psychiatric and in the neurological clinic as well.

It is apparent that there is something appealing in the notion that the healthy nervous system expresses a type of adaptive ability which meets and overcomes problems in many practical aspects of everyday living, both for human beings and animals. Yet, the type of definition offered by Halstead represents merely a conceptual recognition and has little operational value. It is necessary, therefore, to consider the operational definition of the concept, the original evidence for its validity, the extent to which it has been validated by the findings of others, and its clinical applications.

The operational definition of biological intelligence was derived by performing factor analyses based upon a battery of thirteen tests. Halstead (1947a, pp. 38–39) describes the subjects for this study:

> The group finally chosen . . . consisted of fifty healthy adult males, drawn from the head-injury service of the Gardiner Hospital, an Army general hospital in Chicago. All these cases were regarded as medically recovered

from a recent concussive type of head injury. All had experienced an interval of unconsciousness of varying duration up to one hour at the time of the injury. Detailed neurological and psychiatric examinations, including detailed sensory examinations, and complete medical histories were available for each.

More information on these subjects was given in a later section of *Brain and Intelligence* (chapter XV) when Halstead presented a brief statement of the results obtained on patients with closed-head injuries. In this section he pointed out (p. 148) that these patients often did poorly on his tests, which supported his conclusions that "the impairment of biological intelligence in patients convalescing from recent closed-head injuries is similar to that in frontal lobectomies." One cannot be at all sure, then, whether the fifty subjects on whom the factor analyses were based had normal or damaged brains.

The thirteen tests included in the factor analyses included several measures that were later used to determine the Halstead Impairment Index. Tests which contribute to the Halstead Impairment Index are the Category Test, the Tactual Performance Test (Time, Memory, and Localization components), the Speech-sounds Perception Test, and the finger-tapping speed of the preferred hand. Halstead also included the measures based on Flicker-fusion and the Time Sense Test (Memory component), but these tests are routinely omitted by most investigators at the present time because of rather weak validation results (Reitan, 1955a).

The tests that Halstead later used as additional contributors to the Impairment Index, but not included in the factor analysis, were the Flicker-fusion Test (Deviation component) and the Seashore Rhythm Test. Tests which were included in the factor analysis, but which did not contribute to the Halstead Impairment Index, were the Carl Hollow-Square Performance Test for Intelligence, the Henman-Nelson test of Mental Ability, and the Dynamic Visual Field Test (Central Form, Central

Color, and Peripheral components). The intercorrelational matrix for these 13 variables, consisting of 78 coefficients, was analyzed separately by Holzinger and Thurstone. These investigators used somewhat different methods but found similar solutions.

Halstead (1947a) presented the Thurstone solution in terms of four factors. The first factor, as expected in use of the centroid method, produced a general factor which Halstead called the *Central Integrative Field Factor*. The Carl Hollow-Square Test, the Category Test, and the Memory component of the Tactual Performance Test contributed to the second factor, which Halstead called the *Abstraction Factor*. The third factor, called the *Power Factor,* was determined principally by the Flicker-fusion Test, the Memory component of the Tactual Performance Test, and the Central Form component by the Dynamic Visual Field Test. Finally, the fourth factor, the *Directional Factor,* had few significant loadings and was determined by the Time component of the Tactual Performance Test and the Peripheral component of the Dynamic Visual Field Test. The results of this factor analysis, supported by Halstead's interpretation of the factors, served as the basis for the operational definition of the concept of biological intelligence.

Halstead (1947a, p. 142) discussed these four factors in considerable detail in the text of his monograph, and he offered a more concise definition in the last chapter.

A Central Integrative Field Factor (C). This factor represents the organized experience of the individual. It is the ground function of the "familiar" in terms of which the psychologically "new" is tested and incorporated. It is a region of coalescence of learning and adaptive intelligence. Some of its parameters are probably reflected in measurements of psychometric intelligence which yield an intelligence quotient.

A Factor of Abstraction (A). This factor concerns a basic capacity to group to a criterion, as in the elaboration of categories, and involves the comprehension of essential similarities and differences. It is the fundamental growth principle of the ego.

A Power Factor (P). This factor reflects the undistorted power factor of the brain. It operates to counterbalance or regulate the affective forces and thus frees the growth principle of the ego for further ego differentiation.

A Directional Factor (D). This vector constitutes the medium through which the process factors, noted here, are exteriorized at any given moment. On the motor side it specifies the "final common pathway," while on the sensory side it specifies the avenue or modality of experience.

This definition of intelligence, if substantiated, would have represented a very fascinating contribution to knowledge. However, no published replications of the factorial solution have ever appeared, and it is therefore necessary to conclude that there has been no independent cross-validation of the concept of biological intelligence. Considering the fact that the interpretation of Thurstone's factor analysis by Halstead was essentially impressionistic and not subject to the controls of any independently determined criteria, one can only conclude that even to this day the concept of biological intelligence is essentially only an interesting idea.

The second part of *Brain and Intelligence* was concerned with differential representation of abilities which contributed to the concept of biological intelligence in various parts of the cerebral cortex. This question was addressed in terms of results obtained on the Halstead Impairment Index, a summary value which indicates the proportion of tests in which the subject's scores fall in the impaired range. Halstead stated that he found frontal lobe lesions to be associated with evidence of severe impairment, with the mean Impairment Index for patients sustaining frontal lobectomies to be about six times as great as the Impairment Index of normal control subjects and about three times as great as the Impairment Index of subjects with nonfrontal lobectomies (1947a).

Halstead found no differences between patients with excisions from the right or left side of the brain and no relationship between the degree of impairment and the extent of the structural damage. He further stated that impairment of functions, as measured by the Impairment Index, is independent of psychometric intelligence (IQ). Further, impairment was independent of organic language deficits.

Halstead's results, with respect to the differential effects of localized lesions on the Impairment Index, have not been substantiated by the work of other investigators. There may be some prospect of being able to identify left frontal lesions somewhat more readily than right frontal lesions (Meier, 1974; Reitan, 1964), but impairment of language functions with left cerebral lesions is probably the basis for any such achievement.

Chapman and Wolff (1959) have shown that there is a significant association between the extent of tissue involvement and the degree of impairment on Halstead's tests. Everyday observations by many neuropsychologists have borne out this contention inasmuch as small lesions have been associated with lesser impairment and large lesions, involving extensive areas, have been associated with much more serious deficits.

A number of studies (Reitan, 1956; Wheeler, Burke, & Reitan, 1963) have found statistically significant coefficients of correlation of relatively large magnitude between the Impairment Index and IQ measures. It does appear, however, that language dysfunction, *per se,* is not specifically related to results obtained with a number of nonlanguage tests of proved sensitivity to the condition of the cerebral hemispheres (such as the Category Test, for example) or the Impairment Index (Reitan, 1960).

In general, damage of the frontal lobes does not seem to be associated with a more severe level of impairment than damage elsewhere in the cerebral hemispheres, although a great deal of evidence has accrued since the time of Halstead's work to indicate that lesions behind the central sulcus are oftentimes associated with more specific types of losses than the deficits seen with frontal lesions. The current status of knowledge does not substantiate Halstead's finding that the frontal lobes are *especially* involved in subserving higher-level aspects of intellectual and cognitive functions, but they certainly are *significantly* involved.

Halstead (1947a, pp. 148–149) drew certain inferences from his findings, which he viewed as established facts. These were as follows:

Biological intelligence is a basic function of the brain and is essential for many forms of adaptive behavior of the human organism. While it is represented throughout the cerebral cortex, its representation is not equal throughout. It is distributed in a gradient with its maximal representation occurring in the cortex of the frontal lobes.

The nuclear structure of biological intelligence comprises four basic factors which, in unified fashion, enter into all cognitive activities. While these factors make possible the highest reaches of human intellect, their dysfunction, as produced by brain damage, may yield progressively maladaptive forms of behavior, or "biological neurosis."

The frontal lobes, long regarded as silent areas, are the portion of the brain most essential to biological intelligence. They are the organs of civilization — the basis of man's despair and of his hope for the future.

Unfortunately, the concept of biological intelligence has not been adequately documented, either by Halstead or others, despite Halstead's strong belief in such a concept. Further, the heavy representation of fundamental adaptive abilities in the frontal lobes has also failed to be verified. One can still think of the brain as the "organ of civilization — the basis of man's despair and of his hope for the future," but scientific documentation and verification of Halstead's theory of biological intelligence is still lacking.

Halstead's theory of brain-behavior relationships appears to have been misunderstood from the beginning and continues to be misunderstood. Recently, for example, G. Goldstein (1986) has classified Kurt Goldstein's "concept of the abstract attitude and Ward Halstead's theory of biologic intelligence" as perhaps the most well-known examples of neuropsychological deficits defined "along a single dimension of psychologic functioning."

Although K. Goldstein (1939) depicted impairment of the abstract attitude as a single pervasive factor that permeated behavioral impairment of persons with brain lesions (a conclusion which still appears to be true), Halstead's theory was very definitely not a unitary theory composed along a single dimension. In fact, Halstead (1947a, pp. 8–13) explicitly reviewed and discussed unitary or single-unit theories of intelligence and contrasted them with two-factor and multiple-factor theories. Since his theory was composed of four factors, he obviously included his theory among the multiple-factor theories. Complex theoretical formulations may be misunderstood or misapplied, but it is difficult to understand such flagrant misrepresentations of positions which have been clearly and straightforwardly presented in the literature.

Having offered critical comments about the verification of Halstead's theory, it is especially necessary to reiterate a statement of Halstead's contributions to the area of human neuropsychology, because his contributions were substantial. Through his naturalistic observation of patients with brain lesions, Halstead was able to develop a series of standardized experiments (neuropsychological tests) which yield highly significant information about the impairment of adaptive abilities experienced by persons with such lesions. The Halstead Impairment Index, for example, has never failed in any experimental investigation to differentiate between groups of subjects with proved cerebral lesions and subjects with normal cerebral hemispheres. The tests devised by Halstead have provided a valid and systematic basis for further study of human brain-behavior rela-

tionships. The development of such standardized instruments has led to neuropsychological studies which were susceptible to replication and have contributed to increased knowledge of functions subserved by the brain.

It was essential for someone to identify, in a systematic fashion, procedures that would reliably reveal behavioral and psychological deficits associated with brain lesions; Halstead was able to do this. Although Halstead's tests by themselves did not reflect an adequate and complete picture of the behavioral correlates of cerebral functions (Reitan, 1966a), they have served as a core battery to which additional procedures could be added in a systematic fashion (Reitan, 1966a; Reitan & Wolfson, 1985a). Halstead served to stimulate a great deal of investigation and contributed significantly to a renewed interest in the brain as the organ of behavior.

Similarities and Differences in the Theories of Luria and Halstead

Although the theories of brain-behavior relationships of Luria and Halstead are remarkably similar in a number of ways, there are also distinct differences. Both theories stemmed from observations of behavior and psychological performances of persons with brain lesions. Luria based his theory entirely upon such observations, developing a procedure that included many specified tasks for evaluating deficits and their interrelationships (Christensen, 1974). Halstead began his studies by observing the behavior of persons with known brain lesions. He recorded their behavior in many different types of everyday situations and then attempted to translate his observations of deficits into testing procedures that could be administered in a standardized manner.

In terms of formal testing procedures, both investigators used well specified tasks, but Luria strongly objected to any attempts to translate performances into quantitative scores (A.R. Luria, personal communication, 1966). Halstead, on the other hand, made a special effort to develop procedures that would yield quantitative scores either in terms of measured performances or number of errors. In both cases, however, a procedure of examination was established which would provide data about the abilities and deficits of individual subjects.

Luria (1970) proceeded with a subjective type of analysis of the performances of patients with brain lesions, performing what he called a factor analysis. In his analysis he determined the nature of the subject's problems, the constellation of overall difficulties, and determined the underlying "factor" that was responsible for the problems shown by the subject and the particular area of the cerebral cortex that reflected the underlying "factor."

Curiously, Halstead also used factor analysis as the major tool for developing an operational definition of his theory. However, the types of factor analysis employed by these two investigators were totally different. Luria used a subjective and permissive procedure for concluding on the basis of his clinical observations that a particular factor was impaired. Halstead used the statistical procedure referred to as factor analysis in which intercorrelations were obtained between all pairs of variables; the analysis represented extraction of variance in a manner that permitted clustering of variables that presumably had common elements.

In terms of procedure, both investigators depended upon responses of individual subjects with cerebral damage as a basis for generating the data on which their theories were based. Luria believed in examining the patients according to the difficulties that were reported or demonstrated before the examination and that increasingly became apparent as the examination progressed. Halstead believed in administering a standard set of psychological measures which he felt were adequate to reflect the full array of neuropsychological functions, and to administer the same battery to assess brain-behavior relationships of every subject.

Luria believed in a clinical approach, in which his observations of deficits and their interrelationships, together with analysis of the fundamental areas of impairment, were the important data. Halstead believed in a standardized administration of the testing procedure which generated a quantitative score, and the scores for the various tests were then subject to analysis and interpretation.

In brief, the procedure for collection of data was strictly standardized and presumably replicable in Halstead's approach whereas the examination and conclusions for Luria were dependent upon his observations of the subject's deficits.

Although there were differences in the procedures for reaching conclusions about individual subjects, the theories of Luria and Halstead had a number of features in common. It is interesting to note that although both theories identified an energy source for the higher-level aspects of cerebral functioning, these energy sources were remarkably different in terms of their conceptualization. Luria appealed to the ascending reticular activating system and its role in regulating and determining registration of incoming stimulus material at the level of the cerebral cortex, noting that impairment in this energy source would have special significance in reducing the attention, alertness, and character of the material registered in the brain. While evidence has accrued to indicate that the reticular activating system also has modulating influences on response output, Luria emphasized the receptive component.

The reticular activating system had not been described at the time that Halstead was doing his investigations and was therefore not available for incorporation into his theory. Nevertheless, he felt very strongly that the system of brain functions which produced behavior must have some type of energy source. He appealed to the metabolic functions of the brain as this energy source, which he called the *Power Factor,* and related this aspect of brain function particularly to the endocrinological functions of the body. While Luria felt that the ascending reticular activating system regulated the energy level and tone of the cerebral cortex, Halstead tended to relate the Power Factor more strongly to response elements of the system.

Both theories emphasized a sequential series of operations by the brain in subserving neuropsychological functions and a flow through the brain tissue, represented by neuronal interconnections, that was responsible for the behavioral cycle. In this sense, each theory made a functional statement of how the brain works with relation to behavior. Essentially, the theories were similar in terms of a requirement for registration of input through the sensory avenues, complex central processing of this input, and selection and regulation of an appropriate response by the brain. However, these theories differ in the emphasis they place upon sensory input and its analysis and upon the integrative and executive role of the brain in organizing complex responses.

Although hypothetical in nature, Luria's theory is much more detailed in each of these respects. For example, he identified sensory input at the primary receptive areas and postulated that additional analysis and integration of sensory input occurs at secondary and tertiary areas of the cortex. In fact, he postulated that lesions in these various areas result in a different kind and interrelationship of deficit, which can be analyzed in the individual case.

Concerning motor functions, Luria emphasized the importance of the anterior frontal lobes in "executive" functions, believing that this area of the brain is involved in every complex behavioral process. Halstead, on the other hand, tended to separate the factors of biological intelligence, relating the Directional Factor (which was involved in sensory reception as well as motor output) to the other factors of biological intelligence (but in a less specific manner).

Halstead's theory of biological intelligence did not relate specifically to individual areas of higher level functions of the brain and did not explicitly lateralize cerebral functioning to differential abilities. In fact, he considered his theory to be localized in the anterior frontal areas, even though he realized that language functions involved the left cerebral hemisphere to a major extent in areas caudal to the anterior frontal cortex. Halstead's theory did not take into account all of the various types of neuropsychological deficits that are related to the presence of lesions behind the anterior frontal area.

Luria (1970, 1973), on the other hand, paid special attention to integration of language and related verbal symbolic functions into his theory even though, as we have noted above, aspects of this information did not correspond entirely with available facts. Although it has been reported that Luria had begun to consider integration of specialized functions of the right cerebral hemisphere within his theory (Goldberg & Costa, 1981), it must be recognized that for Luria specific higher-level abilities related principally to language and verbal skills.

The central feature of Luria's theory of the way in which the brain was involved in higher level processing related particularly to (1) registration of incoming information through sensory avenues in the primary sensory areas, (2) diffusion and processing of this information through secondary and tertiary areas of the cerebral cortex, and (3) involvement of the anterior frontal areas in selection, organization, and execution of every complex behavioral response.

The central feature of Halstead's theory related particularly to the operation of the Abstraction Factor, which he viewed as the basic element of intelligence. The Abstraction Factor analyzed incoming information and was fundamentally responsible for reality-testing.

Reality-testing, in turn, was related to a feature of Halstead's theory that was unique in the two theories. Halstead postulated the existence of the Central Integrated Field Factor (C Factor), which represented the background, stored information, and essentially the total body of uniqueness of the individual as determined by his interactions with the environment in the past. Halstead felt that the C Factor was dynamic within the individual, and was subject to change through learning and limitation through adverse or pathological involvement of the brain.

The central feature of Halstead's theory was that incoming information was analyzed and rated according to the individual's C Factor, providing a basis for determination of new and old information, common and uncommon information, and the known with respect to the unknown. The interaction of the A Factor and the C Factor provided for the basic intellectual functioning of the individual. These Factors, in turn, were regulated in their efficiency of operation by the degree of energy provided by the Power Factor.

Considering the biological areas of involvement, both Luria and Halstead emphasized the anterior frontal tissue. However, as noted above, Luria developed his theory to relate to primary receptor areas through association tissues with the anterior frontal tissue regulating and mediating responses through the motor system. Halstead felt that his theory of biological intelligence, in terms of its essential features concerning the A and P Factors, were subserved by the anterior frontal areas bilaterally.

Although each theory has its unique elements and includes postulates that have not been documented, they have a number of features in common (as well as certain differences) which stem partly from the initial approach of observing and studying persons with brain lesions and partly from prior knowledge within the area of neurology and neurophysiology, and partly from the methods used to generate the information on which the theories were based.

With respect to this latter point, Halstead used standardized testing procedures that yielded quantitative scores and based his theory on statistical

analyses of the data. Luria eschewed quantitation of defective behaviors resulting from brain damage and used a flexible examining technique that was initiated in the individual case by the patient's own report of his self-observed deficits. Luria adapted his examination according to the responses of the subject as the examination progressed, and both clinical conclusions and theoretical positions were developed on the basis of Luria's insights.

Reitan (1975) has described Luria's methods and procedures as the ultimate disregard for the scientific requirement of cross-validation. In discussing the use of quantitative versus impressionistic methods in developing theories of brain-behavior relationships, Halstead (1947a) noted that "impressionistic methods of observing behavior were the basis of extended controversies."

Luria's theory continues to be discussed and debated whereas, as noted by G. Goldstein (1986), "The concept of biologic intelligence is not widely accepted today . . ." Halstead's use of standardized procedures, rigorously defined methodology, and quantitative analysis — as contrasted with impressionistic observations — may in fact have spared us a generation or more of debate and controversy.

The Reitan-Wolfson Theory of Brain-Behavior Relationships

Reitan and Wolfson (1985a, 1985b, 1986b) have proposed a theory of brain-behavior relationships that grew from detailed evaluation of neuropsychological functions in thousands of persons with various types of brain disease or damage as compared with results obtained on normal control subjects.

Obviously, there is nothing new about basing a theory on such observations. Although Halstead defined his theory through factor analysis, the tests he used as a basis for the factorial solution were primarily developed from his observations of brain-damaged patients as they dealt with problems in everyday living. Luria's theory had a neuropsychological component but was principally based upon his clinical study of many individual patients with brain lesions.

The unique aspect of the approach followed by Reitan and Wolfson was to test the adequacy of the data on which the theory was based through prediction, in the individual case, of the biological status of the brain as discerned through detailed clinical study (including autopsy in many cases) by neurologists, neurosurgeons, and neuropathologists. As we have noted elsewhere, in the early stages of these investigations it was not uncommon for the neuropsychological test results, in individual cases, to inadequately reflect a lesion that was clinically documented. Some patients, for example, with clean surgical excisions of cerebral tissue in certain areas were mistaken for control subjects! Beginning with a presumption that all areas of the cerebral cortex were actually involved in neuropsychological function, it was possible to develop and expand the neuropsychological test battery to the point that the relevant functions were measured. This approach recognized that brain-behavior relationships are extremely complex and that pathological involvement of the brain covers a multitude of dimensions and can be expressed in many different ways.

If the basic approach is to infer normality from measured abnormality through correlation of neuropsychological measurements with definitely known pathological conditions involving the brain, it is imperative that the full range of pathological conditions be considered. In addition, recognizing the problem of individual differences, even given a certain pathological condition, it is necessary to review case after case in order to identify the necessary and critically significant conditions (as contrasted with associated conditions) that characterize the behavioral deviations.

Statistical approaches, based upon interdependent variables, do not differentiate between behavioral manifestations which tend only to be *associated* with the condition and behavioral circumstances that are invariably *caused* by the condition. The only way to learn which variables are basically and fundamentally related to a pathological condition of the brain is to determine which variables permit prediction of the pathological condition in question. This approach may sound familiar to the reader. We were using this approach to determine the ways in which various behavioral measurements were related to the brain, but essentially the same approach, when validly established, constitutes clinical diagnosis.

It is clear that valid clinical diagnosis represented the fundamental criterion in developing our theory, even though the developmental aspects of the studies involved were oriented toward understanding brain-behavior relationships. Halstead recognized the importance of this approach and strongly advised that it be followed when determining which aspects of neuropsychological measurement were of critical (as compared with associated) significance for brain functions. Halstead himself made some effort to follow this procedure, but the range, number, and organization of measurements that he used in his earlier work was insufficient to permit success on a regular basis.

As noted earlier, the great emphasis on the specialized functions of the two cerebral hemispheres has led overwhelmingly to postulation of two-factor theories of cerebral functioning. Halstead (1947a), in his theory of biological intelligence, required four factors (or five factors if the Directional Factor is divided into receptive and expressive units). Luria proposed the existence of three fundamental blocks. Block 1 was particularly concerned with delivery of information to the brain, Block 2 with dispersion and processing of this information in the cerebral cortex, and Block 3 with integrative and executive functions leading toward the individual's response.

Both of these theories considered the processes of information reaching the brain, responses being imposed on the environment, and complex central processing intervening. Luria emphasized the integrative features, occurring particularly within Blocks 2 and 3; Halstead more explicitly recognized the range of experiences representing the uniqueness of the individual, the underlying metabolic functions which provided energy to the system, the basic intellectual function of abstraction and reasoning, and the integration of these factors.

We believe that any theory of brain-behavior relationships must necessarily recognize receptive and expressive aspects of brain functions in terms of the adequacy and efficiency with which the brain receives information and engages in responses. Luria proposed that the ascending reticular activating system represented the electrophysiological basis for the readiness of the brain to register incoming information, but we prefer to avoid postulating any such specific mechanism.

Earlier work on the ascending reticular activating system as an arousal and alerting mechanism for the cerebral cortex, which appeared initially to hold such exciting promise, has not had the clinical impact that was anticipated. Halstead's theory, which predated knowledge of the ascending reticular activating system (Moruzzi and Magoun, 1949), did not relate the energy source to registration of incoming material; instead, Halstead postulated a power source for intellectual functions directly.

We feel that integration of receptive and expressive functions with central processing is important and must be considered within the total context of brain-behavior relationships, but development of detailed knowledge about these functions is probably best left to specialists in sensory and muscle physiology. However, implementation of a neuropsychological theory definitely requires that the functional adequacy of the primary receptive areas of the cerebral cortex be assessed, and to do this assessment a number of tests of simple tactile, auditory, and visual functions are included in the Halstead-Reitan Battery.

Motor functions warrant similar attention, and the Halstead-Reitan Battery includes measures of primary aspects of motor function (Finger Oscillation and Grip Strength) as well as tests of complex integration of motor functions with sensory input and significant problem-solving requirements (Tactual Performance Test). Important as motor and sensory functions may be, the major challenge for a neuropsychological theory of brain-behavior relationships concerns central processing.

The Reitan-Wolfson model of brain-behavior relationships requires initially that information arrive at the cerebral cortex via the various sensory avenues. Primary sensory areas are located in each cerebral hemisphere, indicating that this initial level of central processing is generally represented in the cerebral cortex, but involves the temporal, parietal, and occipital areas particularly.

Neuropsychologically, the first level of central processing involves alertness, attention, registration of incoming information, continued concentration, and screening of incoming information in relation to prior experiences (immediate, intermediate, and remote memory). It is apparent that the adequacy with which incoming information is registered in the brain determines the usefulness of the information and what the brain can do with it. Persons with cerebral damage vary greatly in this respect. Severe and extensive cerebral lesions often cause such generalized impairment of alertness, attention, and concentration that the subject has no prospect of being able to function adequately. Generalized cerebral impairment of this type is frequently identified clinically as a memory loss.

When registration of incoming information is so deficient that the individual is not able to relate it to past experiences, it may appear that memory is the basic deficit. It must be recognized that registration plays a major role in the initial aspects of memory function and memory, in turn, is represented in neuropsychological functioning by reference to the content of the task at hand. For this reason we have chosen to respect "memory" as being represented throughout a broad range of neuropsychological measurements. Memory is depicted as a generalized cerebral function rather than a separate type of function susceptible to measurement by "memory" tests (the approach of experimental psychology).

Persons with severe and striking impairment at this first level of central processing tend to do very poorly on almost any task presented to them. Such subjects fail to show striking patterns and relationships among higher-level test findings (such as differences between Verbal and Performance intelligence), even when a lateralized lesion may be present in addition to diffuse involvement. However, it may be possible to identify *specific* deficits in these patients, which in turn may permit inferences regarding lateralization of focal cerebral damage, but this approach requires methodological implementation through use of specific tests (as compared with general measures) (Reitan, 1986).

The first level of central processing, represented by alertness, attention, concentration, and memory, interacts with the differential functions of the two cerebral hemispheres. For example, persons with generalized involvement as well as severe destructive lesions of the left cerebral hemisphere may be considerably less alert in dealing with verbal and language information than in dealing with visual-spatial problems.

We propose various levels of central processing in our theory of brain-behavior relationships, but it is also important to recognize that an interaction occurs among various levels throughout the model. The first level of central processing is rather generally represented in the cerebral cortex and other functions are more explicitly lateralized or localized, and an interaction occurs between selective deficits (often associated with strictly focal lesions) and generalized impairment (often associated with diffuse damage).

After an initial registration of incoming material the brain proceeds to process verbal information in the left cerebral hemisphere and

visual-spatial information in the right cerebral hemisphere. At this point the specialized functions of the two cerebral hemispheres become operational. Although anatomical pathways representing vision, audition, and tactile perception appear generally to be equivalently represented on the two sides of the brain, verbal information — especially through vision and audition — reaches the left cerebral hemisphere and visual-spatial (and probably temporal-sequential) information is processed by the right cerebral hemisphere.

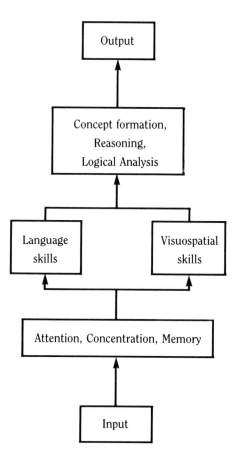

Figure 4-1. A conceptual model of the Reitan-Wolfson Theory of Brain-Behavior Relationships.

Many studies in the literature (as noted elsewhere in this chapter) support the differential dependence of verbal and visual-spatial information on the two cerebral hemispheres, but the exact process by which incoming information is routed to one hemisphere or the other is poorly understood. A considerable amount of evidence suggests that differential routing is less firmly established early in life than when the individual is older, and is apparently dependent upon a maturational development of brain-behavior relationships. There is, however, evidence which suggests that such a predisposition may exist even in infancy (Molfese, 1977).

With normal development of brain-behavior relationships the differential functions of the two cerebral hemispheres are quite distinctly established, as shown by the nearly perfect specialization of verbal functions in the left cerebral hemisphere and the preponderant tendency toward localization of spatial abilities in the right cerebral hemisphere, especially in right-handed persons who have had the advantage of normal development of brain-behavior relationships (Wheeler & Reitan, 1962).

At this point we should note again that clinical observation indiates that higher-level verbal and visual-spatial functions may not show any decided lateralization effect, even in instances of lateralized cerebral lesions, among persons who are grossly impaired at the first level of central processing. These persons have such limited registration of incoming material that the higher-level processing functions, concerned with differential verbal and visual-spatial content, have limited opportunity to function.

In our theory the highest level of central processing is represented by abstraction, reasoning, concept formation, and logical analysis. Research evidence (Doehring & Reitan, 1962) indicates that these functions are also generally represented throughout the cerebral cortex, although particular tasks (depending upon their verbal or visual-spatial content), may establish a lateralizing effect. The best measure of this function in the Halstead-Reitan Battery, the Category Test, does not show any lateralizing effect, even though the content of the test is entirely non-verbal. In addition, the Category Test is *not* exclusively sensitive to anterior frontal lesions as presumed by some investigators. Persons with non-frontal as well as frontal lesions demonstrate definite impairment on this measure.

The sensitivity of the Category Test to cerebral cortical damage, regardless of localization, probably is the reason for the remarkable ability of this test to reflect cerebral damage. The Category Test is definitely a general test of the adequacy of cerebral cortical functioning and any person with such diffuse (generalized) involvement is likely to demonstrate impairment when compared with the performance of control subjects.

Impairment at the highest level of central processing has profound implications concerning the adequacy of neuropsychological functioning. Persons with such impairments have lost a great deal of capability to profit from experiences in a meaningful, logical, and organized manner. In casual contact such persons may appear to be relatively intact. However, because of the close relationship between organized behavior and memory, they often complain of memory deficits and are grossly inefficient in practical, everyday tasks. They are not able to organize their activities properly and frequently direct their energy to elements of the situation that are not appropriate to the nature of the problem.

This non-appropriate activity, together with an eventual withdrawal from attempting to deal with problem situations, constitutes a major component of what is frequently and imprecisely referred to as "personality" change. Upon inquiry such changes are often found to consist of erratic and ill-considered behavior, deterioration of personal hygiene, a lack of concern and understanding for others, etc. When examined neuropsychologically, it is usually found that these behaviors are largely represented by cognitive changes at the highest level of central processing rather than emotional deterioration.

Clinical evaluation of the individual subject with relation to this neuropsychological model requires an understanding of the integrative aspects of central processing at the various levels. The emphasis on the specialized functions of the two cerebral hemispheres has tended to detract from the other levels of central processing which are more generally distributed throughout the cerebral cortex.

For example, a person may have a focal lesion of the left cerebral hemisphere that has resulted in pronounced dysphasic manifestations. If this subject is evaluated only for dysphasia, the generalized aspects of neuropsychological dysfunction may be neglected, regardless of how completely the dysphasic difficulties are assessed and described.

A therapeutic approach that centers only on the specific deficits, neglecting the more general characteristics of impairment, is likely to be grossly inadequate. Speech therapy may improve some aspects of the dysphasic manifestations, but the patient may be so significantly impaired in abstraction, reasoning, and concept formation abilities that it is impossible to reach normal functional levels.

Patients with the entire range of neuropsychological deficits, both with respect to type and severity, as well as corresponding brain lesions, were considered in the development of the Halstead-Reitan Battery, and this process led to an integration of the various aspects of central processing in clinical evaluation. The importance of evaluation and its relationship to all of the elements of neuropsychological functioning cannot be overemphasized when attempting to gain a full understanding of brain-behavior relationships for the individual subject.

The operational definition of this neuropsychological model of brain-behavior relationships is based upon the individual tests in the Halstead-Reitan Battery and clinical implementation depends upon administration and interpretation of the test results. The extremely close relationship between the Halstead-Reitan Battery and the neuropsychological model stems from the fact that the tests were developed in order to reflect the full range of brain functions and their interrelationships and this, in turn, led to description of the model.

Remediation approaches (as represented by REHABIT) also relate explicitly to the theoretical model, its clinical exposition in the individual case with the test results of the Halstead-Reitan Battery, the interdependent interpretation of specific and general deficits, and the organization of training materials as required by the particular deficits of the individual subject within the general framework of brain-behavior relationships.

Similarities and differences between the theories of Luria and Halstead were described earlier. At this point we will pay brief attention to the similarities and differences of the theory proposed by Reitan and Wolfson with relation to those of Luria and Halstead.

As related to central processing, the input and output aspects of the Reitan and Wolfson theory are no more intimately tied to brain functions than the Halstead theory, and not as closely tied in, as was done on a hypothetical basis, by Luria. The basic content areas of the Reitan-Wolfson theory constituted an essential aspect of the model of neuropsychological functioning and placed more emphasis on lateralization of function than either the Halstead theory or Luria theory.

Reitan and Wolfson did not postulate a specific energy source of intellectual functions as Halstead did with his Power Factor and Luria did in relating the ascending reticular activating system to higher-level aspects of brain functions. However, the Reitan and Wolfson theory emphasizes the importance of registration of incoming material, particularly at the first level of central processing, and the process of scanning this material and relating it to prior experiences. This aspect of the Reitan-Wolfson theory relates to the registration in the sensory areas emphasized by Luria and the importance of relating incoming information to past experiences as noted by Halstead (in his proposed interaction between the Abstraction and Central Integrative Field Factors).

As noted above, Halstead's was the only theory among these three to specifically identify an element representing the background of the individual within which immediate intellectual processes of the brain operate. He did this in postulating the Central Integrative Field Factor, which essentially represented the uniqueness of the individual with respect to his range of past experiences.

There can be little doubt that each individual has unique past experiences and that the environment has a very significant influence on determining brain-behavior relationships. It is not likely that Luria would have denied this possibility, and Reitan and Wolfson certainly recognize it. However, in this respect the theories of Luria and Reitan and Wolfson focus more specifically on the immediate operational features and functional aspects of brain-behavior relationships, implicitly recognizing that these operations occur within unique individuals.

The central features of the Reitan-Wolfson theory emphasize (1) registration of incoming material and integration of this material with the individual's past experiences, (2) a second level of processing depending largely upon content of incoming material and organized according to the lateralized functions of the cerebral hemispheres, and (3) a third stage of central processing, especially directed to more complex and difficult tasks and thereby representing perhaps the highest features of human brain functioning, consisting of concept formation, reasoning, and logical analysis.

Although these stages of central processing have a directional organization, we also postulate that a breakdown in neuropsychological functioning may occur at any level, and that interactions between the levels of central processing may occur in either direction, gradually leading to a more competent solution and response. However, some tasks, by their very nature, require careful and detailed registration; other problems will be processed principally by one cerebral hemisphere; and other tasks, depending upon their degree of complexity, will require sorting according to their elements into conceptual categories and careful logical analysis.

The Reitan-Wolfson theory, in terms of its anatomical representation, includes a combination of notions relating to equipotentiality of cerebral cortical tissue and of regional-localization. The first and third stages of central processing relate to the principle of equipotentiality; the middle stages, depending upon lateralization of functions and specialization of abilities, falls within the pervue of a regional-localization hypothesis.

V

CURRENT APPROACHES TO REHABILITATION OF HIGHER-LEVEL BRAIN FUNCTIONS

The Conventional Approach in Rehabilitation Medicine

Recently a chapter by Sell and Rusk entitled "Rehabilitation Following Central Nervous System Lesions" was included in Youmans' six volume treatise, *Neurological Surgery* (1982). Before his death, Dr. Sell was the Acting Clinical Director of the Institute of Rehabilitation Medicine of New York University Medical Center. Dr. Rusk, who is perhaps the best-known medical specialist in rehabilitation, is founder of the Institute of Rehabilitation Medicine.

Neuropsychological rehabilitation of cognitive deficits usually falls administratively within the activities of rehabilitation centers or departments of physical medicine and rehabilitation. It is important that the reader have an opportunity to relate the functions of neuropsychologists who work in the rehabilitation setting to the overall setting in which this work takes place. Obviously, there is some variability between institutions, but the Institute of Rehabilitation of the New York University Medical Center is one of the most well-known facilities and has an outstanding reputation.

Sell and Rusk (1982) begin their review of the comprehensive rehabilitation program by indicating that a highly co-ordinated team approach is required. Secondly, they state that the treatment should be provided in a comprehensive rehabilitation center even though there are many departments in general hospitals that can provide outstanding rehabilitation services. In their review of the functions of the rehabilitation team, these authors (as will be apparent to the reader) concentrate on many very practical activities that are part of the overall rehabilitation program.

Sell and Rusk begin by describing briefly the activities of the *rehabilitation nurse*, noting that he/she has more contact with the patients than anyone else. The nurse must be very familiar with techniques for positioning and turning severely disabled patients and must be able to help the patient understand and adjust to his/her disability as well as cope with problems of incontinence. The rehabilitation nurse must also maintain close contact with the physical and occupational therapists in order "to assure that ability to perform tasks learned in the therapy areas will be carried over."

The *physical therapist* is responsible for maintaining range of motion of all of the patient's joints, thereby preventing contractures. He/she also regularly measures the patient's muscle strength. In addition, the physical therapist must administer exercises for muscle strengthening and use various mechanical devices or techniques which are available for this purpose. The physical therapist also supervises the patient's performance of certain activities of daily living and, in the later stages of rehabilitation, is responsible for providing the patient with training for travel and ambulation in the community.

The *occupational therapist* provides exercises similar to those given by the physical therapist, but the exercises are directed primarily toward developing dexterity and functional capabilities. Sell and Rusk note that the occupational therapist has a primary responsibility for training patients to use their upper extremities and for assisting the patient who has perceptual problems. Training in feeding, grooming, and self-care is initiated as soon as feasible. When appropriate, instruction and supervision in prevocational training is also given.

Sell and Rusk summarize by indicating that the rehabilitation nurse, the physical therapist, and the occupational therapist must combine and co-ordinate their efforts in order to teach the patient techniques such as self-transfer, proper positioning and turning in bed, dressing, safe use of the bathroom, and other necessary tasks.

The fundamental abilities and skills described above represent basic aspects of rehabilitation. The next areas described by Sell and Rusk involve somewhat higher levels of training and fall within the domains of speech therapy and psychology.

The *speech pathologist* assesses speech deficits among patients with aphasia, dysarthria, and other speech disorders; offers speech therapy, either individually or in groups; and monitors the patient's progress. Sell and Rusk emphasize the importance of evaluating speech disorders and providing speech therapy. They recognize the general differentiation between non-fluent (receptive) and fluent (expressive) aphasic disorders, but note that

most of their patients have such severe limitations in all modes of communication that the deficit must be referred to as *global aphasia.* (It is apparent that the patients referred for rehabilitation are frequently among the most severely impaired.)

In addition to a detailed evaluation and classification of the aphasia, the speech therapist also provides therapy either individually or in group sessions. Sell and Rusk point out that the "value of formal speech therapy in global aphasia is still being debated," but that speech therapy nevertheless offers "important psychological support for the patient with a severe communicative disorder." The speech pathologist also informs other members of the rehabilitation team about the patient's deficits in communication and counsels members of the family.

These authors note that every patient who requires intensive rehabilitation as a result of a severe paralysis should also be evaluated in depth by a *psychologist.* The psychologist communicates his/her findings to the rest of the rehabilitation team in order to facilitate proper psychological approaches to the patient in the overall training program. Psychological testing should provide an understanding of perceptual and cognitive problems and permit the psychologist to co-operate with the occupational therapist in tailoring individual programs to meet specific needs. The psychologist is also responsible for providing supportive psychotherapy, especially for persons with reactive depression following impairment of brain functions.

The *social worker* is involved in consultation with the patient and his/her family, in making discharge plans, and in establishing liaisons with appropriate community services. The social worker also assists in such practical matters as securing financial sponsorship for continuing treatment.

The *vocational counselor* uses the information provided in the overall evaluation of the patient to make plans for continuing education or vocational placement. This area is of major importance in attempting to integrate the patient into the community within the framework of constructive and satisfying activities.

As noted by Sell and Rusk, driver training is an important consideration in rehabilitation. Independent mobility is highly valued in our society, and many rehabilitation centers have their own driver's training programs. Most patients are able to learn to drive an automobile even if they have severe physical disabilities, and Sell and Rusk feel that such training should be provided before discharge from the rehabilitation program.

A *home planning consultant* is also valuable in assisting a physically handicapped person to adapt to the requirements of daily living. The home planning consultant visits the patient's home, recommends modifications (or possibly a complete change in living quarters), and instructs the patient in dealing with barriers that may exist within the home.

Finally, Sell and Rusk note that all of the activities and personnel described above must be closely supervised by an experienced *physician* who is a specialist in the field of rehabilitation medicine. In addition to maintaining close contact with the rehabilitation team, this physician will often consult with physicians in other medical specialties. The authors note that these specialties frequently include urology, neurological surgery, neurology, orthopedic surgery, internal medicine, psychiatry, and ophthalmology. In addition, the physiatrist has the final responsibility of informing the patient and the family members about the progress of the rehabilitation process and any problems that may still need to be resolved.

Sell and Rusk turn next to the problem of rehabilitation of patients with intracranial lesions, concentrating particularly on hemiplegia, but also mentioning the rehabilitation requirements of patients with ataxia, extrapyramidal symptoms, and brainstem dysfunction. Many tactical points of information are significant in terms of immediate rehabilitation measures for the hemiplegic patient, including proper positioning in bed, frequency of turning, positioning, etc. These procedures are important in the early care of patients in order to prevent pressure sores, contractures, and deep vein thromboses. Footboards, handboards, and orthotic devices are used according to the particular needs of the patient.

A host of activities may be initiated to facilitate improvement and recovery of function as the patient's neurological function begins to return. Various implements are available to assist patients redevelop co-ordinated use of their upper extremities. Depending upon the deficits of the individual patient, training activities must be designed to develop reciprocal movements of both lower extremities in preambulatory training; attention must be given to strengthening particular muscle groups as needed in order to accomplish functional movements; and the proper orthosis must be selected in accordance with the patient's needs.

It is clear that a major emphasis in rehabilitation is concerned with redevelopment of muscular functions and regaining functional movements. These efforts basically are oriented toward helping the patient to regain the abilities to perform the activities of daily living.

Sell and Rusk address the area of neuropsychology under the heading of "Perceptual Retraining." They note that patients with cerebral lesions have many deficits over and beyond loss of language and related abilities, including disturbances in visual spatial tasks, apathy, impulsivity, hostility, and an unwillingness to acknowledge the nature and severity of their problems. These conditions lead to the need for "perceptual retraining."

First, an initial orientation training is required in which the patient becomes aware of his problems; second, the cognitive deficits must be identified; and third, a highly individualized training program must be devised and implemented, either by a specially trained psychologist or occupational therapist.

Next, Sell and Rusk discuss the significance of an uninhibited neurogenic bowel and/or bladder and the disturbing effect this can have on the patient as well as the interfering effect it may have on the rehabilitation program. The authors note that many techniques have been developed to assist with this problem.

Finally, consideration is given to the equipment that might be needed by an ambulatory hemiplegic patient following discharge from the hospital. A number of devices and pieces of equipment have been developed which can be of special advantage to persons with impaired muscle function.

As noted above, these authors also give brief attention to rehabilitation efforts for patients with ataxia, extrapyramidal symptoms, and brainstem dysfunction, noting the types of training and exercises that are required, procedures that should be taken to ensure the safety of the patient when performing various types of activities, and instances in which electronic devices for basic communication may be advantageous. Most of the remainder of the chapter is concerned with rehabilitation of the patient with spinal cord dysfunction, although brief final considerations are given to the areas of vocational rehabilitation, recreational activities, and patient and family counseling.

It is apparent that rehabilitation centers must be concerned with a broad range of problems that characterize persons with brain lesions. These problems extend from prevention of decubiti to vocational placement. The role of the neuropsychologist is to evaluate the patient's intellectual and cognitive impairment resulting from cerebral damage, determine the patient's emotional status, and attempt to retrain the basic aspects of neuropsychological functions. These assessments and therapy may represent critically important areas, but obviously are rather restricted concerns within the total rehabilitational process.

It should be recognized, however, that the work of Diller and Ben-Yishay, from the same Institute as Sell and Rusk, has been highly significant in the development of this area. Yet, Sell and Rusk devote more space in their review of the rehabilitation process to problems with bladder and bowel control than to restoration of higher-level aspects of brain functioning.

It probably is necessary for us as neuropsychologists to recognize that physiatrists, who generally are in charge of rehabilitation centers, are not overly impressed with our recent efforts in the area of brain retraining, regardless of how exciting it may seem to us. In fact, it appears that an urgent problem faced by neuropsychologists involves recognition by others of the significance of the contribution they can make in the rehabilitation system.

In a recent review of clinical neuropsychology in rehabilitation, Alfano and Finlayson (1987) cite Ben-Yishay (1981), Diller and Gordon (1981), Gianutsos (1980), Goldstein and Ruthven (1983), Prigatano (1986), and Trexler (1982) as sources for their statement that ". . . the field of neuropsychology has undergone considerable change, and there is a growing literature that reflects the attention currently being paid to developing active therapeutic strategies for the remediation of cognitive deficits in brain-injured humans."

These authors go on to say that, "There are those who contend that a major aspect of neuropsychology's future development as a clinical discipline will rest on its capacity to: (1) delineate cognitive strengths and weaknesses as a result of brain injury, (2) predict the extent to which cognition will influence the potential for recovery and improvement, (3) determine the management implications of an individual's cognitive profile and (4) provide treatment directed specifically toward improving areas of neuropsychological deficit," citing McSweeney, Grant, Heaton, Prigatano, and Adams (1985), Miller (1984), and Newcombe (1985). One can only conclude that retraining of cognitive and neuropsychological functions following brain injury is viewed as an area of great significance within the field of clinical neuropsychology, but that the area of rehabilitation medicine has at best only partially concurred with our self-evaluation.

Rehabilitation and Brain Retraining in Neuropsychology

The current interest in rehabilitation of persons with traumatic brain injury is reflected by the numerous volumes and review articles that recently have been published on this subject. Some publications have been devoted to infants, children, and adolescents (James, Anas, & Perkin, 1985; Ylvisaker, 1985) whereas a larger number of publications have focused on adults (Adamovich, Henderson, & Auerbach, 1985; Bach- y-Rita, 1980; Caplan, 1987; Edelstein & Couture, 1984; Goldstein & Ruthven, 1983; Grimm & Bleiberg, 1986; Miller, 1984; Miner & Wagner, 1986; Prigatano & others, 1986; Rosen & Gerring, 1986; Rosenthal, Griffith, Bond, & Miller, 1983; Trexler, 1982.)

These recent publications identify the diversity of problems caused by a head injury and the many difficult factors involved in helping head-injured persons return to a normal, productive life. We will not attempt a complete review of these many publications, but it should be noted that they range from careful and detailed consideration of the theoretical bases of recovery (Bach-y-Rita, 1980) to specific instructions for performing rehabilitation exercises and procedures (Adamovich, Henderson, & Auerbach, 1985). Interestingly, there is even a book of rehabilitation exercises intended specifically to upgrade the functions of the right cerebral hemisphere (Burns, Halper, & Mogil, 1985).

These various publications range in content areas from immediate diagnostic and life-saving surgical care to long-term problems confronting vocational readjustments and the many problems that intervene. The conventional approaches in rehabilitation medicine are frequently covered, but the newly emerging area of retraining the cognitive functions of the brain is also emphasized. A brief review of the topics considered in this literature indicates that the pathophysiology of head injuries as well as immediate treatment procedures are frequently included. Some of the books even include a brief review of neuroanatomy.

Other topics covered in recent publications include the demographic characteristics of the head-injured patient; evaluation using standard and specialized neurological techniques, including evoked responses as well as neuropsychological methods of assessment; procedures and criteria for evaluating the severity of injury; factors involved in the prognosis and assessment of outcome; and review of the many types of disability and deficit associated with head injuries, ranging through deficits of sensory and motor functions, impairment in language and communicational skills, studies of post-traumatic epilepsy, problems of social adjustment, limitations with respect to educational progress, vocational difficulties, associated injuries and medical complications, limitations of both basic and advanced activities of daily living, and effects on the family.

These are important issues that must be considered within the range of problems and factors concerned with rehabilitation of the individual head-injured subject. Because the entire scope of rehabilitation is beyond the framework of the present volume, we will concentrate on a review of (1) psychological disabilities (particularly relating to intellectual and cognitive impairment), (2) various treatment approaches that have been proposed for improving these types of deficits, and (3) selected individual programs that have been described in the literature.

In addition, we will present a detailed description of our own program for retraining the intellectual and cognitive aspects of brain functions which is known as REHABIT (Reitan Evaluation of Hemispheric Abilities and Brain Improvement Training).

Overviews of Neuropsychological Rehabilitation

Goldstein (1984) and Grimm and Bleiberg (1986) have recently published overviews of the area of psychological rehabilitation in which they consider theoretical, methodological, and practical issues. Goldstein emphasized the differences between neuropsychology and other areas of psychology in terms of its development and uniqueness of approach and contribution.

Neuropsychology has consistently made use of cognitive, perceptual, and motor tests for evaluating abilities dependent upon brain functions. The tendency to use tests to obtain data regarding individual subjects has been more predominant in neuropsychology than in clinical psychology. In addition, of course, the particular nature of tests used in neuropsychology has centered on those that most consistently reveal deficits in persons with brain disease or damage.

As many authors who have reviewed the recent history of clinical neuropsychology have done, Goldstein also notes the earlier emphasis on diagnosis of brain damage as the essential mission. He states, "Neuropsychologists are often called on to assist in localization of brain lesions or to offer a general opinion concerning the condition of the patient's brain." He notes that neuropsychologists frequently work with other neurological scientists and indicates that ". . .it would appear that psychometric-laboratory methodologies are currently the best approaches available for diagnosis of brain damage using behavioral methods."

In their review of the development of clinical neuropsychology, Reitan and Wolfson (1985b) perceived a much broader scope of significant contributions. Although there has always been an interest in individual evaluation and diagnosis (not only of brain damage but also of the behavioral consequences of brain damage), the area of clinical neuropsychology emerged as a scientific discipline principally through the efforts of physiological psychologists on the one hand and clinical psychologists on the other. (This statement, as noted in more extensive reviews [such as those by Reitan and Wolfson, 1985b and Rourke and Brown, 1986], differentiates between the areas of clinical neuropsychology and behavioral neurology. Behavioral neurology has developed principally through the efforts of physicians such as Geschwind, Benson, Hécaen, Heilman and Luria.)

The original interest in clinical neuropsychology on the part of clinical psychologists — most of whom functioned in a psychiatric setting — was to effect a differentiation between persons with and without cerebral damage (Reitan, 1966b). Physiological psychologists, however, studied brain-behavior relationships principally in animals and generally had little if any interest in clinical problems. Certain physiological psychologists, such as Ward Halstead, found that they were in fact much more interested in human than animal brain-behavior relationships and focused their research efforts in the human area. These efforts were oriented principally toward discerning scientific information that related the brain to behavior (although practical, clinical use of the information was certainly valued).

At the same time, clinical psychologists tended principally to focus their research efforts on identification of a single test that would differentiate between persons with and without brain damage. They hoped to discover a specific procedure or test that would differentiate between patients with psychiatric problems and neurological difficulties and patients with only psychiatric problems.

Halstead realized immediately that the behavioral manifestations of brain disorders were complex and extensive and that a number of tests would be required to do proper justice to this range of behavioral complexity. In fact, he was trying to lay the groundwork for a fuller understanding of the effects of cerebral damage. Such information would be useful in clinical diagnosis, but also would be valuable in many other aspects of understanding of brain-behavior relationships, including approaches to remediation and brain retraining.

In the early phases of clinical neuropsychology Reitan concentrated his efforts on developing a comprehensive understanding of the way in which results on a battery of neuropsychological tests related specifically to a variety of lesions, and this focus tended to emphasize development of knowledge that would permit neurological diagnoses on the basis of neuropsychological measures.

Current reviewers of these developments often fail to understand that in the initial phases it was necessary to validate psychological tests as *neuropsychological* tests by demonstrating their valid relationship to the biological (pathological) condition of the brain as well as their validity in relating to independent neurological diagnoses. Initially there was a real necessity for establishing the basis of clinical neuropsychology through differentiating between those psychological tests or procedures that actually had a close relationship to the biological condition of the brain and the many aspects of psychology that were much more closely related to environmental determinants of behavior.

Responsiveness to this need, however, scarcely serves as a basis to conclude that a diagnosis *per se* was the only interest of these investigators. In fact, in Reitan's laboratory an effort was made from the very beginning (dating back more than 30 years) to engage in specific brain retraining exercises with individual patients who had relatively chronic and static lesions. Obviously, a desire to gain more information about brain-behavior relationships (even though it was used to assist in specific neurological diagnosis as well as in gaining a full understanding of the consequences of cerebral disease or damage in the individual patient), did not preclude the early interests of many investigators in neuropsychological rehabilitation.

Goldstein (1984) expresses a principal interest in coalescing the methods of neuropsychological assessment with the principles and practices of behavior modification. He discusses at some length the schism that he feels tends to develop between psychologists with a neurological orientation and those who develop a behaviorist theory based on observable stimulus-response relationships, noting particularly that Skinner (1950) did not feel that it was necessary to describe behavior in physiological terms.

Again, we can only comment that in spite of differences in interest and approach by various psychologists, a coalition of methodology and aims is not precluded. It should be entirely possible for a person with an interest in the biological bases of behavior to have an equivalent interest in the redevelopment and application of an approach that emphasizes stimulus-response contingencies. In fact, application of principles of behavior modification have demonstrated a remarkable degree of effectiveness in influencing and changing behavior patterns even of persons with significant mental retardation, which almost certainly represented a significant biological limitation (Spradlin, 1963).

Goldstein expresses a concern about whether behavior modification techniques can possibly have an influence on persons with cerebral damage. Concerns along similar lines have been raised many times regarding persons with cerebral damage, but we must emphasize again that the existence of brain disease or damage in no way rules an individual out of the human race or, as contended by Kurt Goldstein (1939), changes psychological functions fundamentally in kind as compared with degree.

Nevertheless, Gerald Goldstein (1984) states, "The question of whether or not the behavior modification techniques that have been so effective in psychiatric and educational applications will work with brain-damaged patients remains basically unanswered. This question is a major theoretical one for neuropsychology, because if behavior therapy does in fact work it will become necessary to rethink some of our basic assumptions involving brain-behavior relationships." Since this question was, in fact, answered in principal and in practice more than 25 years ago by demonstrating successful behavior modification in brain-damaged mentally retarded subjects (Spradlin, 1963), it is apparent that approaches organized around stimulus-response contingencies can modify behavior even of the lowest organisms, not to mention brain-damaged, psychiatrically disturbed, and normal human beings.

It does not seem to be a question of whether behavior modification approaches can be effective among brain-damaged persons, but rather whether the specificity of stimulus-response contingencies will do more than modify specific behaviors. In some situations, individual behavioral performances are often so highly specific that it is difficult to presume any generalization of the training effect as the environmental circumstances change. Goldstein (1984) considers this problem and notes that, "The role of neuropsychological assessment in the rehabilitation process is that of specifying the behaviors that may serve as appropriate targets for treatment." The basic bridge between clinical neuropsychology and behavior modification requires specification of the deficits that need to be remediated through neuropsychological assessment.

Goldstein states that in terms of rehabilitation planning a test must be quite specific in its identification of any particular deficit in order to be helpful in formulating an appropriate program. As an illustration he notes that a person may perform poorly in copying the designs of the Bender-Gestalt test, but this does not identify whether the basic problem was incorrect perception of the figures, impairment of motor ability needed to perform the drawings, or a defect in the ability to coordinate visual input (observation of the figures) with the movements necessary for drawing. The defective performance, as an end result, is often not sufficient to identify the basic disorder in need of rehabilitation.

Although there is some validity to this point, one must also remember that human behavior always requires input of information to the brain, processing by the brain, and output regulated by the brain in terms of a response. Neuropsychological remediation is dependent upon sensory input and motor output, but in content does not overlap greatly with the areas of sensory physiology (or other approaches in remediation of input deficits, such as the area of physiological optics) or with areas related specifically to motor output (such as physical therapy). Neuropsychological assessment must consider whether information gets to the brain and whether the brain has motor mechanisms available to permit an appropriate response.

Neuropsychological brain retraining, however, must focus on the higher-level aspects of central processing. There is no doubt that a careful evaluation of the higher-level behavioral aspects of brain functions is imperative in designing a program of rehabilitation, and that such a comprehensive evaluation cannot be accomplished through use of a single test (such as the Bender-Gestalt). An appropriately designed battery of tests provides a great deal of information about deficiencies in central processing as compared with limitations of input and output. It would appear that Goldstein's concern in this regard may be answered most adequately by emphasizing the importance of careful and detailed evaluation of both the strengths and weaknesses of an individual's neuropsychological functions.

A question also must be asked about whether the deficits are specific or general in nature. If the deficits are not highly specific and distinct in nature, it may well be a mistake to focus a rehabilitation program on artificial constructs. In many cases retraining of neuropsychological deficits perhaps may be best accomplished by using a relatively broad approach in which major areas of brain-related behavioral deficits are identified rather than using an approach which targets highly specific behaviors.

Identification of specific behavioral targets is required when using behavior modification techniques and is also emphasized in rehabilitation medicine more generally (e.g., activities of daily living). This type of approach, however, may represent one of the limitations of this area for the general upgrading of brain functions in various areas of performance that seem to be needed by most persons with cerebral damage. It is well recognized that neuropsychological deficits cover a range from specific to general (Goodglass & Kaplan, 1979; Reitan & Wolfson, 1985a), and it is probably a mistake to develop rehabilitational programs in neuropsychology on the presumption that the behavioral aspects of brain functions are made up of a host of specific and separate abilities.

Grimm and Bleiberg's Conceptualization of Rehabilitation

Grimm and Bleiberg (1986) have reviewed the area of psychological rehabilitation with special reference to traumatic brain injury and have offered a conceptual framework which falls essentially within the traditional characterization of rehabilitation efforts.

First, these authors emphasize the multiple and diversified disorders frequently experienced by persons with head injury and the necessity for involving persons from many disciplines, including physical therapy, occupational therapy, psychology, medicine, nursing, vocational counseling, biomedical engineering, social work, and recreation therapy. There is no doubt that specialists from these various disciplines can make a significant contribution to the overall aspects of rehabilitation following head injury, but it is equally clear that such a conceptualization reflects an overall approach rather than one describing cognitive remediation or rehabilitation.

Secondly, Grimm and Bleiberg note that the definition of rehabilitation in their view is nebulous, gives rise to varied expectations, and that the results achieved are often disappointing. While the

goal of rehabilitation may be to restore the individual to a "maximal level of functioning," they caution that even when this goal is achieved it may be quite different for different patients, depending upon the severity of the initial deficits and what is realistically possible in terms of rehabilitation.

We must caution, however, that "maximal level of functioning," in terms of what is achieved in the individual case, presumes that rehabilitation efforts routinely are maximally effective. If only relatively modest improvement is achieved in one case and is viewed as reaching the "maximal level of functioning," the end result itself may be the limiting factor for progress.

Nevertheless, Grimm and Bleiberg emphasize that goals must be "adjusted over time in concert with the progress or regress of the individual's functional status," suggesting that failures to achieve initial goals in the rehabilitation process essentially serves as the criterion by which "maximal level of functioning" is defined. Although this definition may be comforting to the rehabilitation specialists (in the sense that achievement of limited progress is all that could have been expected), it may not be equally as comforting for the patient to be told that his "maximal level of functioning" corresponds, by definition, with the outcome (however limited) of the rehabilitation program.

Grimm and Bleiberg (1986) proposed a conceptual framework that is intended to link the various activities that are included in comprehensive rehabilitation. This framework consists of a three-dimensional configuration organized according to levels or types of intervention, intervention objectives, and the stage of treatment ranging from acute to chronic.

Five levels of intervention are identified: (1) *Biological intervention,* consisting of immediate and long-term medical and related procedures, including surgery, infection control, motion exercises, contracture prevention, etc. (2) *Individual intervention* that includes environmental modifications, behavior modification, cognitive retraining, psychotherapy, depression management, crises intervention, possible restructuring of the environment, and education for teaching patients how to minimize their risk of sustaining a future head injury, (3) *Team intervention,* including adaptation of the patient to institutional policies and procedures, stress management training, and specialized training and education to lay the groundwork for eventual employment, (4) *Family intervention,* which includes family therapy, counseling for grief or role redefinement, preparation for role changes within the family, legal and/or homemaking assistance, and home safety modifications, and (5) *Societal intervention,* which may include experiencing sheltered workshop settings, the use of transitional living facilities or arrangement of permanent group or individual living situations, job-coaching assistance, re-entry into the work force, and enactments of legislation regarding safety standards and improved safety in individual behavior.

From this extensive range of levels of intervention and the examples of activities given above, it is apparent that Grimm and Bleiberg have proposed a conceptual framework that goes far beyond the types of activities involved in retraining of cognitive functions dependent upon the biological condition of the brain. Nevertheless, these authors devote a considerable portion of their review to the area of cognitive rehabilitation, noting that many procedures have been suggested and that a standard set of therapeutic activities is generally not employed. Their discussion emphasizes the importance of identifying and describing specific deficits which must be analyzed in terms of their stimulus characteristics and response demands in order to develop training procedures that are specifically pertinent.

Grimm and Bleiberg review various reports of retraining efforts in the areas of visual-perceptual functions and memory, but note that multi-faceted programs may be necessary for persons with traumatic brain injuries because of the complex cognitive, behavioral, and emotional problems that

such patients often display. They note that neuropsychological deficits frequently include "orientation and arousal (attention, concentration, and vigilance), psychomotor skills (eye-hand coordination and dexterity), cognitive perceptual integration (constructional skills), visual information processing skills, verbal ideational skills, memory functions, and general interpersonal and communication skills." They feel that a hierarchy of specific tasks is necessary for training in each of these areas, but conclude that an answer to the question of whether cognitive retraining programs have practical value requires further study and that cognitive retraining, as a therapeutic modality, has "yet to come of age."

Gudeman and Craine's Principles of Cognitive Rehabilitation

The cognitive retraining program established at the Neuropsychology Laboratory of the Hawaii State Hospital was one of the first programs to develop an organized set of training activities applied to the individual subject. The staff at this institution viewed their efforts as a systematic application of psychological and neurological principles to assist individuals in overcoming or adapting to deficits that resulted from brain damage.

This program has been described in a workbook that provides examples of a large number of specific training techniques (Craine & Gudeman, 1981). In turn, a series of principles underlying brain retraining evolved (Craine, 1982).

Craine states the first principle as follows: "The plasticity of function within the central nervous system provides the basis for restructuring neuro training activities to promote and enhance recovery from brain damage." This principle merely states that improvement following brain damage is possible.

Finlayson, Alfano, and Sullivan (1987) state this principle in somewhat different terms, noting that, "There has long existed a myth that damage to the adult brain is irreversible." Obviously, however, the initial principle probably must state that positive effects, of one kind or another, can result from cognitive brain retraining or there would be little point in undertaking the effort. In addition, however, as Finlayson, Alfano, and Sullivan indicate, the previously existing tendency to presume that no improvement following brain damage could occur, in accordance with failure of functional regeneration of neuronal connections within the central nervous system, did in fact lead to rehabilitation philosophies oriented toward "adjustment to loss" strategies rather than toward active remediation.

A more important consideration, over and beyond the fact that improvement occurs in adult subjects following brain damage, concerns the short-term and long-term biological responses to damage that underlie this process. Some of these possible mechanisms have been reviewed in this volume in Chapter I.

Principle two postulates that facilitated recovery (as contrasted with spontaneous recovery) is advantageous. The principle is stated as follows: "The cerebral cortex is a dynamic process of neurological organization that can be completely halted or slowed by injury or by environmental deprivation or it can be greatly increased or heightened by carefully planned environmental stimulation."

There is, of course, abundant evidence to indicate that the human organism is influenced by stimulus-response contingencies emanating from circumstances in the external environment. This process has long been known as *learning*. Obviously impairment may result from injury or environmental deprivation (Riesen & Aarons, 1959; Riesen, 1961), and even special postnatal care and attention, such as stroking, may lead to physical improvement.

The prospect for learning among brain-damaged subjects has already been well established, and Reitan (1959a, 1959b) has shown that the potential for improvement (as contrasted with initial level of performance) is essentially similar among brain-damaged and control subjects. It seems, then, that this principle, which states that impairment may occur and improvement may be facilitated by special training procedures and exercises, is hardly surprising.

The third principle proposed by Gudeman and Craine is scarcely more than a restatement of the second principle. They state principle three as follows: "The organization of learning within the cerebral cortex results from repeated activity on the part of the individual and becomes organized into functional systems of behavior."

In effect, this principle does little more than state that the individual develops behavioral capabilities that were not present before the training was instituted. The presumption that this learning becomes organized "within the cerebral cortex" and "results from repeated activity" does nothing more than presume that the cerebral cortex underlies behavior and that a series of trials is necessary for learning to occur.

Craine goes on to state that, "It is essential to commence the training for any particular task at exactly the right level of difficulty." This statement obviously is presumptive, because criteria do not exist to determine "exactly the right level of difficulty" for the individual subject. Much research data does exist, however, to indicate that it is advantageous to begin training at a level that produces positive rather than negative reinforcement (i.e., a level at which success occurs). Secondly, if the task is obviously too difficult for the individual, little comprehension of the stimulus-response relationships will occur. Although Craine suggests establishing base rates for each of the exercises to be used for the patient, it is more economical to begin training at a level at which success obviously can be achieved and quickly progress to more difficult material.

Craine also feels that this principle involves "the necessity of putting some numbers to all of the training activities." It may be desirable to quantify training activities of the individual subject, but there is no intrinsic necessity to do so.

As far as the subject is concerned, the same effect will be produced regardless of whether the therapist has developed a training procedure that can be reduced to a quantitative number.

Craine points out that it is advantageous to be able to show the subject a graph based upon quantitative aspects of procedure to indicate progress that has been made over time. Depending upon the degree of progress anticipated by the subject, this procedure may have either positive or negative effects.

As we have previously noted in this volume, principles of brain-behavior relationships have a hierarchical (or sequential) organization in terms of nervous system function. Craine invokes a hierarchical organization of behavior, presumably in conjunction with underlying nervous system functions, as the basis for the fourth principle. This principle states: "The activities of training must recapitulate the developmental stages involved in the individual's original acquisition of the learning or skill that is being trained."

Prior investigators (Doman, Spitz, Zucman, et al., 1960) have placed great emphasis on such a principle for rehabilitating brain-damaged children. They insist, for example, that movements of the upper and lower extremities must be practiced at great length before beginning with higher-level activities (such as academic work).

There is no evidence available to support a hypothesis that developing co-ordinated movements *per se* subserve the ability to develop reading and other academic skills. In fact, any statement of a sequential order or hierarchial organization of abilities (extending, for example, from simple to more complex) can be made only approximately and must recognize the existence of many individual exceptions. There are many persons with excellent academic capabilities who early in life suffered from strabismus or "squint." There are others who early in life suffered serious motor disabilities (e.g., poliomyelitis) who never were able to develop coordinated movements of the four extremities but nevertheless manifested excellent higher-level brain functions.

In addition, the exact sequence of ability development, even in terms of fairly specific tasks, has never been rigidly described. It is essentially presumptive to state (Craine, 1982) that, "The idea is simply that the completion of the development of one stage is essential and is a prerequisite to the development of the next stage."

This notion has never been adequately tested in terms of relationships between nervous system development and behavior, primarily because the stages of behavior have never been clearly established in a neuropsychological sense. We do not make these statements to deny that certain stages may be identified. Piaget (1971) felt that there were distinct stages in development of cognitive abilities, even though further investigation appears to indicate that these stages are not at all as clear as Piaget originally postulated. It is important, however, that the individual be carefully assessed for neuropsychological deficits, both generally and in specific areas, and that the training activities begin at an appropriate level and proceed in a sequence of training tasks that gradually increase in level of difficulty.

Principle five presumes that integration of sensory input is a necessary and important aspect of neuropsychological rehabilitation. The principle states: "Complex higher cortical functions represent an integration of multiple sensory modalities which supplement each other in the acquisition of learning."

This principle is reminiscent of the early theories of brain-behavior relationships (described previously in this volume) that were proposed by Munk (1890) and von Monakow (1905). These theories were designated by Halstead (1947a) as *aggregation theories,* in which localized sensory areas within the cerebral cortex are joined functionally by a large number of intracortical connections, the aggregate effect being one of integrating comprehension of sensory stimuli from the external environment and resulting in intelligent behavior. Of course, this principle also relates closely to Luria's theory in which primary, secondary, and tertiary sensory areas represent comprehension of the external environment.

It must be noted that the integration of multiple sensory modalities is a conceptualization which has not been well documented or established through formal research investigations. It is entirely possible that integration of sensory activities at the level of the cerebral cortex is important to develop a full understanding and appreciation of situations and circumstances that surround the individual. However, to view this appreciation only as an integration of sensory input seems somewhat limited. This type of appreciation obviously requires abstraction, reasoning, logical analysis, and concept formation skills.

Rather than emphasize the lowest common denominator (sensory input), it might be better (in terms of higher-level cognitive rehabilitation) to recognize directly that concept formation, abstraction, and reasoning abilities — which are generally represented in the cerebral cortex (Doehring & Reitan, 1962) — are the significant targets for rehabilitation. In fact, Craine describes a procedure in which retraining of impaired tactile finger recognition can be facilitated by pairing a *tactile* stimulus to a particular finger with a *visual* stimulus. In this case the remaining ability to identify the visual stimulus and pair it with the tactile stimulus is presumed to provide a basis for improving tactile finger recognition.

This example, in its own right, illustrates the limited objectives that emanate from an orientation directed toward the lowest common denominator (in this case, primary sensory input). Although there may be some advantage in training the individual in tactile finger recognition, this skill is so specific in nature that it has been used principally as a diagnostic test in neuropsychology rather than a target for training. Brain retraining procedures should be oriented toward achieving

effects of a much broader nature than those represented by the specific (as contrasted with the general) neuropsychological tests that are required for diagnostic evaluation of the biological condition of the brain.

The basic procedure in neuropsychological rehabilitation obviously requires identification of the most significant aspects of neuropsychological deficit for the individual subject and development of a training program that is pertinent in retraining areas of function that are fundamental to adaptation to problems in living. One could seriously question whether training in tactile finger localization would have any generalization effect in terms of meeting the complex problems that are involved in meaningful aspects of daily living.

The sixth principle is oriented toward a more general type of brain retraining and is concerned with developing capabilities of a general nature in meeting everyday problems. This principle is stated as follows: "The primary objective of neuro training is to promote and develop the processes underlying learning and is concerned with the dynamics of learning rather than the specific content of any area."

We would strongly agree that such general training is necessary; however, it is important to specify the types of training activities and the target abilities that are involved in this type of training. Many college professors state that the principal objective of their courses is to teach the student to "think." However, when one investigates the content of the courses and the pedagogical procedures, one finds that the purpose was to teach the student to "memorize" specific points of information. Obviously, the procedures implied by this principle would scarcely include training the subject to identify fingers through touch, but it would be necessary to identify procedures that would be effective in developing "the processes underlying learning."

The seventh principle is highly pertinent in retraining of neuropsychological functions dependent upon the brains of human beings. This principle emphasizes that training should be given in accordance with the needs of the subject. The alternative to this principle states that training should be given in areas of strength rather than weakness so that the individual can in some manner develop compensatory mechanisms which employ the remaining strengths (rather than being limited by areas of weakness) in practical aspects of living.

Rourke, Bakker, Fisk, and Strang (1983) have critically evaluated rehabilitation approaches oriented toward areas of deficit rather than areas of strength. Our own research has strongly indicated that spontaneous recovery occurs in the areas of initial deficit. If one wishes to utilize spontaneous recovery following brain injury as part of the brain retraining program, one presumably would emphasize the areas of initial deficit. Over and beyond this consideration, however, it seems perfectly reasonable to provide help where help is needed rather than to use an "adjustment to loss" strategy in which remaining abilities presumably can serve as some type of prosthetic device in overcoming the areas of deficit. Gudeman and Craine state this principle as follows: "The effectiveness of neuro training activities is dependent upon and relative to the degree to which the deficits can be specified for an individual patient." This principle makes it quite clear that a careful and adequate assessment of the individual subject is necessary in order to prescribe an appropriate training program.

Finally, principle eight in Gudeman and Craine's framework emphasizes the importance of providing the subject with information regarding any progress that is made. They state this principle as follows: "Consistent and direct feedback to the patients about their performance is a crucial aspect of neuro training."

In our experience the training procedures themselves make it quite clear to the individual whether progress is being accomplished. The greatest positive reinforcement is provided intrinsically when the subject realizes that he/she has learned to do something that he/she previously was not able to do. We feel that feedback (or positive reinforcement) should be intrinsic in the training procedures; it is not sufficient for the rehabilitation therapist only to say kind and encouraging words. It is imperative that the subject make some actual progress in use of the training procedures. This does require that the training activities be separate and discrete, and composed of individual units so that the subject will be able to comprehend the fact that he/she has mastered a particular problem.

Alfano, Finlayson, and Sullivan's Overview of Neuropsychological Rehabilitation

Alfano and Finlayson (1987) note that "Rehabilitation programs continue to concentrate heavily, if not exclusively, on 'improving physical disability.'" These authors have recently presented a review of the role of clinical neuropsychology in rehabilitation. Earlier approaches had focused primarily on counseling or psychotherapeutic intervention with the principal aim being one of assisting the brain-damaged and neuropsychologically impaired person to adjust to his/her deficits.

The current and future role of clinical neuropsychology in rehabilitation of brain-damaged persons, as conceptualized by these investigators, can be summarized in four points: (1) Delineation of cognitive strengths and weaknesses that result from brain injury, (2) Development of further knowledge of cognitive ability structure which will permit prediction of the potential for recovery and improvement of the individual brain-damaged subject, (3) Determination, on the basis of the individual's cognitive profile, of the management implications of neuropsychological deficit, and (4) Development and use of procedures that are specifically oriented toward providing treatment and rehabilitation in areas of neuropsychological deficit.

These authors provide a brief description of theories, processes, and mechanisms that may subserve spontaneous recovery in patients who have relatively static and chronic conditions of brain damage. They also note, however, that biological aspects of brain functions may be influenced by environmental factors. They cite the evidence that an enriched environment may contribute significantly to various aspects of behavioral development and performance (Davenport & Greenough, 1976; Petit & Alfano, 1979; Rosenzweig, 1984). Although spontaneous recovery often occurs, facilitated recovery, through the use of cognitive remediation procedures, may result in even further improvement which in turn may also be represented by biological changes in brain function.

Alfano and Finlayson cite evidence that cognitive impairment itself is a significant variable in determining the outcome following rehabilitative treatment. It might well be expected that impairment of perceptual and motor abilities would be a significant factor in determining the eventual adequacy of the individual in self-care skills. However, Finlayson, Gowland and Basmajian (1986) have also reported that abstraction and reasoning abilities, as measured by the Category Test, were significantly related to the degree of improvement of upper limb functions in stroke patients. These results strongly suggest that cognitive impairment, at least in certain areas of function, may be a significant factor in determining the potential of the brain for redeveloping adaptive abilities, even in terms of primary aspects of movement.

Alfano and Finlayson review various approaches to cognitive remediation that have been proposed in the literature and note that these approaches generally are oriented toward a conceptualization of brain-behavior relationships that is rather oversimplified in nature. The history of neuropsychological assessment progressed from single-factor to multi-factor explanations of the behavioral correlates of brain functions. The original simplified notions of the essential nature of neuropsychological impairment following brain damage

gradually evolved into a much more complex characterization of brain functions related to behavior. It appears that a similar pattern is developing for the neuropsychological models of cognitive retraining.

Up to this point the methods of brain retraining have focused primarily on a delimited and rather restricted set of abilities, apparently based on the presumption that the neuropsychological effects of brain damage are relatively specific and homogeneous in nature. The treatment procedures have been directed toward rather specific types of problems. Alfano and Finlayson emphasize that it is important to recognize not only the specific deficits that result from brain damage but the general deficits as well. This point was clearly stated by Goodglass and Kaplan (1979) in their discussion of the need for both general and specific neuropsychological tests in the assessment procedure.

Alfano and Finlayson review the neuropsychological model of brain-behavior relationships proposed by Reitan and Wolfson (1985a, 1986b, and this volume) and its relationship to development of a treatment plan using REHABIT (see the case report in this volume that exemplifies this approach using REHABIT). They stress the importance of neuropsychological evaluation as the first step to rehabilitation because of the importance of characterizing the brain-related strengths and weaknesses of the individual subject as a basis for designing a program of cognitive retraining. This comprehensive evaluation serves to identify areas of strengths and weakness across the entire range of neuropsychological functioning and permits the development of understanding of the particular needs of the individual subject. This is in contrast to using existing procedures that engage in a "routine implementation of a standard set of techniques designed to address an array of cognitive deficits presumed to be characteristic of, or present in, all cases of brain damage."

In this paper Alfano and Finlayson review and evaluate many basic considerations in cognitive retraining. They identify what they consider to be the basic aims and requirements of neuropsychological rehabilitation; discuss theories, processes, and mechanisms that may underlie spontaneous recovery; review evidence which suggests that neuropsychological impairment may be an integral factor in the potential of the individual for recovery even of physical deficits; review evidence which indicates that environmental influences may bring about biological changes in brain structure and function which in turn subserve eventual neuropsychological recovery; and discuss current models of neuropsychological deficits and the importance of a complete assessment of strengths and weaknesses of the individual subject (in contrast to a presumption of homogeneous impairment in all cases of brain damage) as a basis for devising and implementing neuropsychological treatment procedures that fit the needs of individual subjects. Finally, a recent publication by Finlayson, Alfano, and Sullivan (1987) described a case report in which their particular neuropsychological approach to the principles and practice of cognitive remediation are illustrated.

Practical Problems and Considerations
Regarding Neuropsychological Rehabilitation

The approach to retraining neuropsychological functions in the brain-damaged individual is determined not only by general conceptualizations but also by highly practical questions concerning the procedure to be followed. The authors who write on this topic regularly stress the importance of doing an evaluation to learn about areas of strength and areas of deficit as a basis for devising (prescribing) a training program that is suitable for the individual subject.

In the past there was a strong tendency to emphasize only the training materials rather than an interaction of training materials *and* the individual subject, presuming that these materials would be advantageous and effective for every brain-damaged person. This orientation stemmed from a presumption that brain damage had relatively constant and invariable effects on higher level functions from one person to another. Research over the last 40 years has clearly dispelled this notion and has led to at least a partial recognition of the complexity of brain-behavior relationships and the fact that brain damage results in highly varied combinations of deficits for the individual. Next, it is clear that a unique brain retraining program, at least in terms of emphasis and application of various training activities, is needed for each person.

When a complete neuropsychological evaluation has been performed and the strengths and weaknesses of the individual subject identified, a procedural question arises concerning the ways in which the training should proceed. Should the remaining strengths be utilized, either as a vehicle for approaching the training of the areas of deficit or as a basis for compensating for impaired function? Or should the areas of impairment be addressed directly and specifically, based upon the presumption that these are the areas that need retraining (as contrasted with the abilities that were not initially impaired)? Would a combination of these two practical approaches be effective? Rourke, Bakker, Fisk, and Strang (1983) have given careful consideration to the arguments for and against each of these approaches. Even though their interests focused on the area of child neuropsychology, the basic considerations concerning this question are essentially similar for children and adults.

Arguments for Brain Retraining
Using Unimpaired Functions

Several arguments have been advanced in support of a brain retraining approach that is oriented toward areas of competence (unimpaired abilities). Some writers seem to feel that impairment due to brain damage is essentially permanent (or at least not susceptible to significant improvement) and, as a result, they feel that there is little use in expending efforts to attempt to achieve recovery of these impaired functions.

This conclusion is seriously misguided and incorrect. In this volume we have given many examples of spontaneous recovery and discussed the biological bases of the recovery process; the basic theme of this volume is facilitated recovery through brain retraining. We have emphasized and illustrated repeatedly in evaluation of individual cases that the process of spontaneous recovery following brain injury is characterized neuropsychologically by improvement in the areas of deficit.

Nevertheless, some authors recommend that the brain-damaged subject be trained deliberately to use his areas of competence in attempting to deal with practical problems in everyday living in order to avoid failures that would occur if the areas of deficit were used. Many examples of this kind of approach can be cited. For example, if a person has sustained significant damage of the speech and language area of the left cerebral hemisphere and is dysphasic, the recommendation would be that in meeting problems in living the subject orient his lifestyle in such a manner that verbal communication and use of language functions would be minimized and that the activities of the individual would be oriented toward non-verbal activities. In a vocational application, such a person would be directed toward manual types of tasks that required psychomotor and manipulatory abilities rather than verbal or communicative skills.

This type of approach obviously limits the potential of the individual for using the full range of human capabilities in developing a lifestyle or pattern of behavior and would tend to reduce the quality of the individual's life as a result of neglecting the fundamental (though impaired) aspects of higher brain functions. Certainly an approach to neuropsychological rehabilitation that neglects or disregards certain abilities that are subserved by normal brain functions can hardly be considered adequate. Instead, it is imperative that

an attempt be made to restore impaired brain functions, regardless of any effort that is made to use retained functions as a compensatory mechanism.

Sometimes a recommendation is made to use remaining abilities as vehicles to train areas of deficit. For example, if a brain injury has resulted in severe dyslexia, even to the point that the individual demonstrates visual letter and number dysgnosia, it may be difficult to teach the subject to recognize, differentiate, and understand the symbolic significance of individual letters and numbers through the visual avenue. However, it is obvious that reading involves rapid and accurate processing of individual letters. Without such ability, the individual would be significantly and seriously impaired in regaining reading skills.

Tactile form recognition might be relatively intact in such a person even though visual recognition of numbers and letters was seriously impaired. In practice, however, it is likely that a complete neuropsychological examination would show that tactile form recognition with the right hand was more significantly impaired than with the left hand because the damage responsible for visual letter dysgnosia and dyslexia very likely would be in the left cerebral hemisphere and also cause right-sided impairment in simple tactile cognitive tasks.

In such a case recommendations have been made that the subject be trained through touch to recognize and differentiate individual block letters that are placed in the left hand. The rationale behind this recommendation is that tactile form recognition of the left hand, being relatively intact, can be utilized as an avenue to permit input to the brain of the relevant stimulus material needed to redevelop an appreciation and understanding of individual letters.

It is important, however, to consider such a recommendation and practice in conjunction with knowledge of how the brain is organized. As noted above, if the patient had a significant left cerebral lesion that impaired visual letter recognition and reading ability, it is likely that tactile form recognition with the right hand would also be significantly impaired (Hom & Reitan, 1982). This was the rationale for using the unimpaired left hand for learning to appreciate the spatial configurations represented by the stimulus material. However, tactile information coming to the brain through the left hand would arrive in the right parietal area. The right parietal area emphasizes appreciation of visual-spatial configurations rather than the symbolic meaning of verbal material. In effect, the training task would be one of trying to teach the right cerebral hemisphere to understand the symbolic meaning of letters and to develop basic reading skills. Since the right cerebral hemisphere in adults is minimally involved in such activities even under normal conditions, it would be questionable whether this hemisphere would be able to acquire such abilities in the brain retraining process.

As noted in an earlier section of this volume, it seems likely that in adults there is relatively little sharing of function of the two cerebral hemispheres (even though this process does appear to be operational for children during the early developmental years). If the aim were to train the subject to appreciate language symbols, it would hardly seem appropriate to direct the training to the right cerebral hemisphere. It is likely that the damaged left cerebral hemisphere is still the appropriate training target and that restoration of abilities in dealing with language symbols, to the extent that it will occur, will be a result of a return of function in the left cerebral hemisphere.

In practice, it is often difficult to devise a brain retraining program that permits use of unimpaired abilities to compensate for impaired abilities, even in the training process, because of the dependence of various abilities on determined areas of the cerebral cortex as well as the complexity of deficits resulting from cerebral damage.

Obviously, the aim of using one sensory input avenue to facilitate the functional capability of another input avenue is not addressed by this particular argument. It may be quite useful to teach the individual to recognize block letters using his right hand, even though tactile form recognition is impaired, in conjunction with attempting to teach the subject to recognize letters through the visual avenue. Intersensory integration in training procedures has been recommended, and its value is definitely implied by certain research findings (Birch & Lefford, 1964). However, an approach of this type must recognize the anatomical and neuropsychological organization of brain-related abilities rather than to fractionate this information. In other words, it is not sufficient to identify a particular intact function and to presume that that function then can be used for any type of training, regardless of the areas of deficit shown by the individual subject and the relationship of the training efforts to the way in which the brain is organized with relation to behavior.

An essentially similar problem is encountered in the case of children. Sometimes a child has specific difficulty in learning to recognize individual letters through vision and a recommendation is made to teach the child to recognize letters through tactile recognition. In many such cases the brain lesion is not specifically lateralized or restricted to a particular area and tactile form recognition is not significantly more impaired on one side than on the other.

The problems cited above would apparently be circumvented because the child could receive incoming tactile information from both sides, even though information from the left hand might be interpreted by the brain principally with respect to visual-form characteristics of the stimulus material and incoming tactile information from the right hand might be more closely related to the verbal and symbolic aspects of the material. Presumably, however, both the verbal-symbolic and the visual-form aspects of the stimulus material would complement each other in effecting a complete understanding and comprehension by the brain.

The problem in this case, though, often is that in children with conditions of brain dysfunctions that cause this type of problem, detailed neuropsychological assessment reveals that the deficit is not exclusively in the areas of visual recognition and appreciation of the symbolic aspects of the stimulus material; instead it is also frequently represented by a deficit in appreciation and understanding of spatial configurations and relationships. In fact, in many children the underlying deficit is complex and diversified, involving numerous interrelated neuropsychological aspects of brain functions. Problems and deficits of this nature, however, can be discerned by careful and complete neuropsychological examination using a standard battery that evaluates both strengths and weaknesses and permits an organized understanding of the ability structure of the individual subject.

Many writers in this area refer to areas of competence that may be used to facilitate training of impaired areas or to compensate for the tactical deficiencies in behavior that would relate to the impaired areas. Rather than emphasizing specific abilities or mechanisms, the consideration relates to a complex of abilities subsumed under a general designation. The most prominent example of this approach is represented by references to memory impairment. There is general agreement that memory is not a specific or unitary type of function, but instead is a complex and diversified ability in terms of its neuropsychological conceptualization as well as its relation to the biological status of various areas of the cerebral cortex.

It can be seen, then, that to identify a subject as having a "memory" disorder provides information of limited usefulness for brain retraining. In such persons it is not uncommon to find both strengths and weaknesses in memory tasks, depending upon the particular content of the memory problem. Persons with left cerebral lesions

have notoriously poor memory for verbal and related symbolic material; persons with right cerebral lesions have defective memory for visual-spatial and temporally oriented material; and persons with generalized impairment of brain functions frequently complain of severe memory problems when their difficulty is one of organization, abstraction, and recognition of the pertinence of material to be remembered with relation to the overall situation.

Researchers who recommend that "areas of competence" be identified so that they can be used for compensatory functions or so that they can be related to specific activities in everyday living often fail to recognize the complexity of underlying neuropsychological abilities which in total represent the "area of competence." It is important to remember that brain-behavior relationships are extremely complex and have tremendous variability among individuals. Even with verbal functions, for example, the traditional differentiation between fluent and non-fluent aphasia characterizes the selective nature of aphasic losses, even though most individuals with aphasia show evidence of both types.

Considerations of this type again emphasize the importance of careful and complete neuropsychological evaluation for each individual subject so that any selective impairment can be identified and deficits in general aspects of neuropsychological functioning can be documented. In fact, in developing the Halstead-Reitan Battery it was necessary to experiment with a considerable number of measures, even including ones which appeared in many instances to produce redundant information. For example, finger tapping speed and grip strength are both measures of primary motor functions. In many cases these measures agree in the way they demonstrate a deficit, but in some instances they do not agree and thereby provide evidence of more selective losses.

In examining for tactile-perceptual skills, we found it necessary to retain in the Battery tests of tactile form recognition, tactile finger localization, and finger-tip number writing perception, even though in many cases they produce similar and confirming results. In some cases, however, a person may show little deficit in finger-tip number writing recognition but significant (and even lateralized) losses in tactile finger recognition. Our clinical experience has indicated that in this particular configuration, losses in finger recognition assume added reliability for their neurological implications.

It is apparent that a neuropsychological test battery by itself is not enough to provide an adequate understanding of brain-behavior relationships for the individual subject; equal or greater significance must be attached to the neuropsychological competence and knowledge of the neuropsychologist who analyzes and interprets the results. A survey of brain-behavior relationships may be provided by the test results, but the adequacy of the brain retraining program that is prescribed for the individual subject, even when organized training material is available (such as REHABIT), depends upon the understanding of the neuropsychologist who interprets the data.

Another reason for emphasizing areas of neuropsychological competence in the brain retraining program relates not to a positive advantage, but instead to a negative effect resulting from the alternative procedure in which areas of deficit are confronted directly. Anyone who has attempted to retrain the brain of a significantly impaired subject has observed the stress and frustration that is felt by the subject when he/she is required to continually work with tasks that are in his/her weakest ability area. It is much more pleasant to select tasks that the individual can perform satisfactorily, will be enjoyable to perform and provide a feeling of personal satisfaction and accomplishment. Most therapists prefer to have the brain-damaged subject perform in his areas of strength than in his areas of weakness. In fact, the frustration that arises from finding even an essentially simple task

to be impossible to perform is sufficient in many cases to cause the subject to break down in tears. Neuropsychological rehabilitation therapists frequently wonder why it is necessary to inflict such emotional trauma on the brain-damaged person as often becomes apparent and is manifested when using training materials that were deliberately selected to provide practice in the subject's areas of greatest weakness.

Nearly everyone is familiar with the dislike, negative reactions, and even fear that many children develop for academic activities and the classroom situation generally because of the negative experiences (even approaching punishment) that they suffer. In the interests of human civility and kindness (not to mention respect for the psychological dictum of positive reinforcement), an argument is offered that the brain-damaged person should not be forced to work on tasks that depend upon abilities in which the subject is obviously deficient.

There is no easy answer to this problem unless a decision is made to train the areas of strength and neglect the areas of weakness. If the areas of strength are trained, one is in effect ignoring the consequences of brain damage and, if anything, only creating further disparity between impaired and intact abilities. When attempting to train areas of weakness, a great deal depends upon the neuropsychological rehabilitation therapist or neuropsychologist who works with the impaired individual. Liberal encouragement and understanding must be given to the person who is struggling with retraining tasks in his/her areas of greatest deficiency, and there is no doubt that a great deal of emotional support is required. However, even a little progress is often recognized and warmly welcomed by the brain-damaged person and serves as strong encouragement for continuing with the task.

The frustration and discouragement experienced by many subjects as a result of training in areas of deficiency provides the strongest argument for a one-to-one relationship in the training program. The child in the classroom who is embarrassed by failure rarely receives the kind of individual attention that would dissipate the adverse emotional reaction. In brain retraining, however, a very close interaction and bond develops between the therapist and the patient. Frustration and disappointment can be dissipated to an extent through this interaction, and many subjects manage to continue their retraining program over extended periods with intact motivation and interest.

Rourke, Bakker, Fisk, and Strang (1983) note that an approach emphasizing areas of strength as opposed to weakness may be appropriate and helpful when the subject exhibits dense deficits which are extremely resistive to training. Dysphasia, represented by severe, extensive, and even global language loss, is often cited as such a condition. However, it is clear that other areas of function, such as the ability to deal with visual-spatial relationships or ability in the area of abstraction, reasoning, and logical analysis, may also be very strikingly impaired in individual cases.

Research results (Dikmen, Reitan, & Temkin, 1983) have shown clearly that more severe neuropsychological deficits do not recover spontaneously to the level shown by less severe deficits, but the absolute degree of spontaneous recovery is actually greater when the initial deficit is more severe. Research findings do not suggest that deficits, because of their severity, are necessarily resistive to either spontaneous or facilitated recovery. The degree of recovery may be much more closely related to the biological condition of the rest of the cerebral hemispheres, excluding the area of principal damage. If the brain in general is in good biological condition, even very severe deficits resulting from a focal lesion and being fairly specific in nature may show remarkable recovery.

A case in point is a 35-year-old man, a high school graduate, who suffered a discrete vascular lesion in the posterior part of the language area of the left cerebral hemisphere (case C.H. described in Reitan & Wolfson, 1985a). It was discovered that C.H. had a defective kidney which had caused extreme elevation of his blood pressure and this in turn had resulted in bleeding of a cerebral vessel.

This man had a profound aphasic deficit, principally characterized by auditory language receptive deficits (auditory verbal dysgnosia). The lesion appeared to have very discrete effects, since C.H.'s finger tapping speed with his left hand was in the normal relationship to the speed achieved with the right (preferred) hand and his performances on the Tactual Performance Test were not seriously impaired and in the expected relationship. The most striking finding in this case was that C.H. had a Category Test score of only 8 errors. These results, in the presence of severe dysphasia, obviously are highly unusual. However, they stem from a highly discrete lesion and are entirely consistent with the neurological conclusion of the location of the lesion (posterior temporal-parietal area).

The neuropsychological test results suggested that C.H.'s brain was generally in excellent biological condition, with the aphasic manifestations relating to the specific area of damage rather than the extent of involvement. It would seem that C.H. had an excellent brain with which to recover from his neuropsychological deficits, even though the deficits themselves were quite severe. In fact, C.H. showed an absolutely remarkable recovery which progressed rapidly and consistently following removal of his damaged kidney and reduction of blood pressure. Two weeks after the operation he had no signs of residual dysphasia.

Results in this instance, supplemented by clinical observations as correlated with neuropsychological findings in many other cases, suggest that recovery potential is not only related to the specific area of damage and the severity of neuropsychological deficit, but also to the biological condition of the rest of the brain. When cerebral cortical damage results in severe neuropsychological deficits and the brain is generally compromised in its biological status, the prospect of recovery is considerably limited. However, it is not sufficient to conceptualize this problem only in terms of deficits that are "resistive to training." The reasons why the deficits are resistive in this respect must be considered, and the overall condition of the brain, in conjunction with specific or focal involvement, appears to be highly significant.

Rourke, Bakker, Fisk, and Strang (1983) also suggest that it may be important to provide training in areas of strengths "simply to enhance his/her already relatively well-developed behavioral capabilities." The reasoning behind this recommendation is that neuropsychological deficiencies, especially for children, may be "constantly challenged" in the classroom situation whereas other abilities, even though relatively unimpaired or well-developed, may go essentially without challenge. Among traumatically brain-injured persons it is likely that the areas of principal deficit are subjected to more critical challenges by the requirements of the general environment than unimpaired abilities, but it would hardly seem reasonable to deliberately train unimpaired abilities just because the environment did not stress or tax these abilities as much as those in the area of impairment.

Judging from the comments of Rourke et al., it would appear that these authors also feel that directing training efforts to the unimpaired or well-developed neuropsychological abilities of the subject serves a useful purpose in improving morale, motivation, and self image. This may be a valid and useful postulate. In fact, as noted earlier, it is sometimes discouraging, disheartening, and depressing for the head-injured individual constantly to face tasks in his/her principal areas of neuropsychological deficit. In our rehabilitation program we have successfully used training material in the area of an individual's strengths, not for purposes of upgrading unimpaired abilities, but instead explicitly for improving morale and self-image.

Still another reason cited by Rourke et al. for offering training in the the area of neuropsychological strengths is that further development of these areas may lead to additional abilities through opening avenues for general cognitive development. In other words, developing one ability may lay the groundwork for developing other abilities and the overall process leads to a generalized improvement of ability structure.

It is, of course, likely that there is a sequential process in development of ability structure, but the neuropsychological status of the individual subject must be considered carefully in such a situation. One of the debilitating effects of brain damage is that the ability structure is characterized by much more variability than among normal persons. In other words, some abilities remain at the pre-injury level and others sustain significant impairment. This leads to a situation in which there are "peaks" and "valleys." Since most manifestations of practical intelligence in everyday situations involve a variety of abilities, the retained (unimpaired) skills frequently are of limited value in constructive accomplishment or reaction to problem situations and the impaired abilities play a major role in limiting the overall response effectiveness.

In one sense, the competence of the individual tends to be determined by the least common denominator. Therefore, it may be disadvantageous to offer training that augments the range of abilities (i.e., makes the "peaks" even higher with relation to the "valleys"). Rather than attempt to augment neuropsychological strengths to prepare for future development of ability structure, it would appear to be more advantageous to orient training efforts toward eliminating the areas of weakness and thereby achieve a better integrated and less variable ability structure.

Finally, Rourke et al. indicate that there may be instances in which a subject should be encouraged to utilize strong areas of neuropsychological performance in order to facilitate planning, organization, and strategies for performing more effectively in areas of deficit. As a specific example, when language abilities are essentially unimpaired but there are deficits in the ability to deal with spatial and temporal-sequential problems and problems in utilizing abstraction, planning, and logical analysis skills, it may be possible to use verbal strategies to facilitate improved performances in the areas of deficit. In other words, techniques of verbal mediation could, in such an instance, be of advantage. This procedure, however, focuses primarily on remediation of the area of weakness, with the area of strength being involved essentially only as a means for effecting such training.

Arguments for Brain Retraining Directed Toward Neuropsychological Deficits

Insofar as brain retraining is necessary at all, it would seem obvious that the need is determined by areas of weakness or deficit. On this basis, the brain retraining program would be directed toward the areas of need. The training program actually becomes necessary because there are brain-related deficits, not because there are brain-related strengths. (It is likely that there are variable degrees of adequacy of brain-related abilities even among persons who have not sustained any damage to the brain and that training weaker areas [or areas of comparative deficit] in such persons would also be advantageous.)

In our judgment, emulation of the natural response to the effects of brain injury (or spontaneous improvement) constitutes the best argument for directing training to the areas of weakness. Longitudinal studies of persons who have sustained neuropsychological impairment due to brain injury demonstrate unequivocally that the areas of impairment are the areas that show recovery on retesting. It seems eminently reasonable, in terms of general biological considerations, that healing occurs in the area of the wound rather than in an area that was not injured or impaired.

In terms of the treatment procedure, it is obvious that one would attempt to be pertinent to the area of need. One would scarcely treat an unimpaired part of the body when the injury was elsewhere, and it would seem reasonable to direct cognitive rehabilitation treatment to the impaired aspect of ability structure rather than to the unimpaired abilities.

In addition to formal research results (Dikmen & Reitan, 1976; Dikmen, Reitan, & Temkin, 1983) which on retesting show recovery of impaired functions and relatively little change of unimpaired functions, this volume contains many clinical examples which demonstrate this phenomenon. Perhaps it is not surprising that nature remediates the area of deficit, considering the fact that the deficits due to brain trauma represent the only functions one could possibly expect to improve following brain trauma. In other words, there is nothing about brain trauma that serves to facilitate or improve the abilities that were spared by the brain injury.

There are definite problems implicit in undertaking a retraining program for a person who has suffered neuropsychological impairment and many of these difficulties have been outlined above. It seems eminently reasonable, however, to attempt directly to retrain the area of impairment, and thereby restore ability structure to its premorbid status, than to direct training attention to the unimpaired areas, and thus create even greater variability and disparity in ability structure.

In individual cases of discrete and selective neuropsychological deficits a question of approach scarcely arises. We have seen instances in which visual form discrimination was significantly impaired but other aspects of neuropsychological functioning were good to excellent. In such a case one obviously would not feel the need to retrain the excellent areas of abilities but would attempt to deal with the specific problem of visual form discrimination.

In other instances we have seen examples of retention of prior high Verbal and Performance IQ values, excellent verbal communicational skills, high levels of competence in specific tasks that involved visual-spatial and manipulatory functions, but striking deficits in the area of abstraction, reasoning, and logical analysis. Although this pattern of results frequently elicits a knee-jerk conclusion of "frontal lobe damage," we must comment that this response is usually expressed by those psychologists who have had limited opportunity for comprehensive neuropsychological evaluation of persons with focal lesions in both non-frontal and frontal locations.

In fact, this particular pattern is not at all uncommon among persons suffering from the effects of closed head injuries. Selective deficits, particularly in the area of abstraction and reasoning, may occur in persons with either generalized or focal damage, although when damage is focal more specific neuropsychological deficits are also present in many cases. In such cases the apparent significance of the deficit for practical performances (particularly in vocational and professional settings) may be strikingly apparent. This occurs particularly because of the area of distinct weakness with relation to the general retention of neuropsychological strengths. A direct approach toward remediation of the area of deficit may have dramatic effects even in the short term training situation. In cases with severe, generalized, neuropsychological impairment (when the entire ability structure must be elevated), the retraining task is much more difficult.

When Should Brain Retraining Begin?

In practical terms, a question frequently arises about when neuropsychological brain retraining should begin. Our experience suggests that it is advantageous to begin the training program as soon as possible. Obviously, as we have emphasized repeatedly, neuropsychological evaluation is necessary in order to identify the ability structure of the individual and to draw inferences concerning brain-behavior relationships. However, the main reason to prescribe a training program and to begin training as soon as possible (which necessarily must follow neuropsychological assessment) is to integrate the training exercises with spontaneous recovery of neuropsychological functions.

Research studies have suggested that the major degree of spontaneous recovery occurs in the early months following the head injury. In fact, Jennett and Teasdale (1981) postulate that essentially all spontaneous recovery occurs within the first six months following injury. Our data (this volume) indicates that a substantial degree of recovery occurs during the first 12 months following injury and that, on the average, relatively little further recovery occurs beyond that point. (We should note, however, that in individual instances we have seen improvement continue for considerably longer periods of time.)

It is a tremendous advantage, in terms of motivation, interest, and morale of the patient to observe his/her improvement. This improvement may very probably be due both to brain retraining exercises (facilitated recovery) and spontaneous recovery, but the improvement itself is very gratifying to the patient, family members and others closely involved, as well as to the neuropsychological rehabilitation therapist. On later evaluations it may be impossible to dissociate the effects of spontaneous recovery and facilitated recovery, but this is a relatively unimportant problem compared to achieving the best possible clinical outcome. (If one wishes to differentiate spontaneous from facilitated recovery, the effort must be made by comparing one group with another in an appropriate research design.)

The head-injured individual's deficits are most pronounced shortly after the injury, before any significant spontaneous recovery has taken place, and the subject may be quite shocked to experience the cognitive impairment to the degree that it exists. Nevertheless, it is important to begin the training program as soon as the subject has recovered sufficiently to be given a full neuropsychological examination.

There are other advantages to beginning training as soon as possible. Some persons with significant impairment in particular areas following brain injury may develop patterns of behavior or behavioral styles that tend to neglect the area of deficit. It is likely that the environment of the subject will set the requirements in terms of necessary behavioral responses, but in some instances, particularly with specific deficits, the subject may attempt to circumvent his/her deficits by avoiding situations that are likely to expose his/her limitations. It would be advantageous to remediate these areas of deficit in the initial phases rather than to permit them to alter the behavioral patterns of the subject and possibly introduce maladaptive behavior.

A principal reason to begin brain retraining as soon as possible relates to the hierarchical organization of the neuropsychological ability structure. In describing our model of neuropsychological functioning, we have emphasized that appreciation of input material through attention, concentration, and memory is fundamental to higher-level intellectual functions.

Among those subjects who have sustained serious impairment in attention and concentration, it would be necessary to address training activities to redevelopment of these areas in order to begin to deal effectively with more complex intellectual tasks. Although there is an interaction between all levels of central processing, it is necessary initially to register material satisfactorily in the brain if the higher-level capabilities of the brain are to deal effectively with the material in producing an integrated response cycle.

In addition, understanding the relationship between an individual's brain-related deficiencies and strengths is imperative in order to design a training program that is specific for the needs of the individual subject. Therefore, the prescription for brain retraining should be developed soon after neuropsychological testing is completed and implemented promptly.

The Nature of Neuropsychological Deficits Resulting from Brain Trauma

Recent publications have reviewed studies of neuropsychological deficit resulting from brain trauma. Levin, Benton, and Grossman (1982) have thoroughly reviewed the literature on closed head injuries and research investigations dealing with open and penetrating head injuries. In addition, Groher (1983) has reviewed communication deficits, Ben-Yishay and Diller (1983) have reported on cognitive deficits, Brooks (1983) has reviewed memory losses, and Rosenthal (1983) has reported on studies of behavioral sequelae in traumatic brain injury.

In the first volume of *Traumatic Brain Injury* Reitan and Wolfson devoted a chapter to the review of neuropsychological studies of the effects of brain trauma, organizing the chapter essentially with respect to the Reitan-Wolfson neuropsychological model of brain-behavior relationships. Following this guide, studies were reviewed under categories of alertness, vigilance, and rate of information processing; visual-perceptual skills and manipulatory abilities; verbal and language function; memory disorders; impairment of abstraction, reasoning, logical analysis, planning, and executive abilities; selected specific aspects of behavioral dysfunction; and emotional and personality deviations following head injury. Citation of these relatively recent reviews may be important in identifying content areas representing deficits needing rehabilitation or retraining in cases of brain trauma.

Neuropsychological investigations of the consequences of craniocerebral trauma indicate clearly that any or all of the intellectual, cognitive, and personality characteristics of brain function may be impaired with brain injury. This is particularly true when considering the widespread damage that the brain may sustain, including both primary and secondary effects as well as focal and diffuse involvement. Therefore, the reader should be aware that there is nothing unique about the particular characteristics of neuropsychological deficit following brain injury.

Comparative studies of traumatic brain injury and other conditions (such as neoplastic involvement and stroke) certainly suggest that in cases of intrinsic neoplasms and strokes the deficits are generally somewhat more profound and severe, but the general nature of psychological impairment is not fundamentally different (see the Neuropsychological Deficit Scale comparisons reported in Chapter III and Hom & Reitan, 1982). Therefore, in cases of head injury a program oriented toward rehabilitation or brain retraining must be adequately extensive to cover the entire range of neuropsychological deficits. It is equally obvious that some head injuries cause severe deficits and other injuries result in much milder impairment, and a training program must also be designed to be appropriate in retraining across the entire severity range.

Since most persons who are referred for neuropsychological rehabilitation have very significant, serious, and widespread neuropsychological impairment, most training programs are designed to remediate relatively profound deficits. Recent attention, however, has been directed to the adverse consequences of relatively mild head injuries, and there is a growing recognition that even mild brain trauma may result in impairment that seriously disrupts the ability to resume vocational responsibilities as well as the head-injured individual's general quality of life.

In fact, as we have previously noted, many persons who show significant neuropsychological impairment on the Halstead-Reitan Battery (especially in the area of abstraction, reasoning, judgment, and planning abilities) are not even recognized in many rehabilitation centers as having any problems. As a result, there is no planning for neuropsychological rehabilitation of these persons

and no training programs available. However, this situation is gradually changing as programs such as REHABIT are introduced. In cases of this kind it is not sufficient to depend only upon the complaints of the head-injured subject as a basis for identifying the areas of deficit or for developing a brain retraining program. It is imperative that neuropsychological testing methods be used to determine the nature of the deficit and establish a basis for prescribing a program of brain rehabilitation.

In many rehabilitation centers there is a growing realization that a head-injured person may have significant cognitive impairment even when he/she appears to be relatively normal on casual observation. In these cases brain retraining is particularly important because critically needed training may be given that can make the difference between serious vocational failure and psychiatric problems and the ability to return to a relatively normal life.

It is especially important that intellectual and cognitive deficits be assessed with relation to what are termed "behavioral sequelae." Rosenthal (1983) characterizes the behavioral manifestations of head injury as perhaps the most difficult to understand, measure, predict, and treat. He feels that rehabilitation staff members as well as the relatives of head-injured patients consider these types of problems to be the greatest obstacle to successful rehabilitation and resumption of a productive status within the family and community.

Rosenthal defines these problems as "those overt actions that result in socially maladapted interactions between the patient and the environment," consisting essentially of "emotional or personality changes that result from head injury." He differentiates changes of this kind from cognitive and intellectual deficits that would include impairment in thinking, information processing, learning ability, memory, visual perception, etc. Although he recognizes that cognitive deficits may contribute to socially maladaptive behaviors, the cognitive and emotional disorders resulting from head injury are considered to be basically separate.

The problem with the orientation proposed by Rosenthal is that many of the higher-level neuropsychological deficits, particularly in the area of abstraction, reasoning, and logical analysis, often are unrecognized as cognitive deficits and are treated as emotional sequelae of head trauma. Over the years we have examined many persons who have been referred for psychiatric evaluation and treatment following a head injury and who, upon testing with the Halstead-Reitan Battery, were shown to have neuropsychological deficits that were of obvious significance even though not subject to identification through casual observation.

An example of such a case was a young man with a Master's degree in Business Administration who was viewed as one of the promising young executives of his firm. His position in the firm required him to collect and organize all relevant information concerning identified problems of an operational nature, present an analysis of these problems together with recommendations for improvements and corrections to a committee made up of officers of the firm, and to communicate the conclusions of this committee to appropriate department heads for action. Prior to sustaining a severe closed head injury he had been quite successful in performing this job.

Following his discharge from the hospital he resumed his vocational responsibilities but performed much more poorly. Often he neglected to include relevant aspects of the total situation which were obvious to the members of the committee to which he reported. They began to reach a conclusion that this employee was either grossly careless or had lost interest in performing well, with a private opinion being expressed that he was "using his head injury as an excuse for neglecting his duties." The head-injured subject, of course, was aware of the difficulties that he was encountering but could not understand why he was performing so poorly. In many instances he himself would recognize that he had neglected essential features of the problem that he was supposed to analyze, could not understand why he was not organizing his work better, and felt a great deal of anxiety and depression. Finally, he was referred for evaluation to a psychiatrist who was thoroughly familiar with the types of deficits often revealed by the Halstead-Reitan Battery and after a single interview recommended neuropsychological testing.

The results of the Halstead-Reitan Battery indicated that the subject had IQ values that fell in the superior range; however, he was grossly defective in performing the Category Test. It was apparent that he was significantly impaired in his ability to observe recurring similarities and dissimilarities in stimulus material, select the relevant and critical aspects of the situation that needed attention, and implement responses that would be appropriate in solving the problem.

In this man's case subtle and unrecognized neuropsychological deficits were impairing his ability to perform successfully and led directly to what Rosenthal would classify as "behavioral sequelae." Although many experts in the area of head injury recognize that neuropsychological deficits can give rise to emotional problems of adjustment, there remains a need to effect a closer integration between these areas.

A Selective Review
of Neuropsychological Rehabilitation Programs

The great interest among neuropsychologists in retraining brain functions, particularly among persons with traumatic brain injury, has led to the development of cognitive rehabilitation programs in many rehabilitation centers and brain injury units. Probably the program that has been established for the longest period of time is at the Institute of Rehabilitation Medicine, New York University Medical Center. Other well-known centers for neuropsychological rehabilitation include the Brain Injury Rehabilitation Unit of the Veteran's Administration Medical Center in Palo Alto, California; the Community Hospital in Indianapolis,

Indiana; the Braintree Hospital in Braintree, Massachusetts; the Medical College of Virginia in Richmond, Virginia; and Rancho Los Amigos in Downey, California.

A number of other centers have been established and the organizational and procedural aspects of these centers show a considerable degree of variability. In each case, however, the focus is on preparing the brain-injured person to return to the most normally functioning existence possible for him/her.

It is important to recognize that interest in retraining brain functions is not new, even though there has been a great proliferation of interest and activity in the last ten to fifteen years. During World War II army hospitals established head-injury centers specifically for the purpose of neurological, psychological and vocational evaluation and rehabilitation. Although the efforts were somewhat unsophisticated in the field of psychology and retraining efforts were limited essentially to the area of occupational therapy, the basic purpose and intent was much the same as it is today.

Patients were admitted to these centers when there was evidence of a significant head injury. A medical and neurological evaluation was performed, psychological testing was done using instruments such as the Wechsler Scale, the Shipley-Hartford Retreat Conceptual Quotient, the Hunt-Minnesota Test for Organic Brain Damage, the Trail Making Test, and Rorschach's Test (Aita, Reitan & Ruth, 1947; Aita, Armitage, Reitan, & Rabinovitz, 1947; Aita & Reitan, 1948).

The personal involvement of one of us (RMR) in these efforts indicated quite clearly that a substantial degree of improvement occurred in individual cases, even though little was known of the mechanisms of repair of tissue or recovery. Nevertheless, it was fascinating to observe essentially spontaneous recovery of language functions as well as other problem-solving capabilities and manifestations of general efficiency in meeting practical problems. Neurological findings, the results of psychological testing, and evaluations by vocational counselors were integrated in an attempt to provide guidance to individual brain-damaged soldiers and to assist them in achieving as adequate a post-injury adjustment as possible in civilian life.

These early observations of recovery from cerebral damage led to a continuing interest for one of us (RMR) to attempt to facilitate the spontaneous recovery process. Efforts were undertaken with individual patients to provide brain retraining as early as the 1950's, working not only with persons who had sustained a traumatic brain injury but also with persons who had vascular lesions and viral infections of the brain. Some of these experiences with individual subjects and a description of the approaches taken toward brain retraining have previously been recounted (Reitan, 1979).

It became quite clear that when the general neuropsychological aspects of brain functioning were relatively intact, even though a focal lesion and relatively specific deficits might be present, there was a good potential for spontaneous improvement. Stroke patients did not seem to show the same degree of general improvement that was customarily observed in patients with traumatic brain injury, possibly because the stroke patients had more serious general involvement of the brain resulting from cerebral vascular disease (over and beyond the specific focal lesion) and aging effects.

Even in the individual case of traumatic injury, however, the potential for full recovery seemed to be limited by the severity of the general deficits as well as the specific neuropsychological impairment. Although in many cases we were able to make excellent progress in brain retraining, we observed that emotional stress arising from circumstances not directly associated with the brain damage or the effects of systemic illness caused a regression of abilities in areas in which a degree of recovery had previously occurred. Nevertheless, the results were encouraging, even in cases of severe neuropsychological deficit.

The importance of detailed and complete neuropsychological evaluation was clearly demonstrated when developing a program of brain retraining that was specific and appropriate for the individual subject. I (RMR) shared with many of these brain-injured patients the discouragement, frustration, and even exasperation that resulted from their neuropsychological impairment.

For example, a man with a serious right cerebral lesion, a patient we had previously examined, came to me one day almost in tears, telling me about the difficulty he had experienced trying to change the tire of his son's bicycle. His verbal intelligence was still in the superior range, but he was not able to perform simple tasks that involved manipulatory skills and spatial relationships. He felt even more frustrated in his inability to perform the manipulations of catheterization procedures required in his work as a cardiologist.

Together we tried to remediate his deficits, working initially with very simple kinds of toys that were designed for children in kindergarten and progressing to more difficult types of manipulatory tasks. Fortunately, in this case the neuropsychological deficits were rather specific in nature. The physician retained excellent abilities in abstraction, reasoning, and logical analysis in spite of the fact that sparing of these functions rarely occurs. He was able to understand his problem in a rather broad context and to realize the importance of continued efforts toward redeveloping his skills. He was able to continue with his faculty appointment in a medical school, even though it was necessary for him to restrict many of his functions initially and he needed help in many respects.

Eventually this man redeveloped his skills and finally reached the point where he could function efficiently and without restrictions in all of the activities in his professional work. Although we can identify individual cases dating back many years in which it was possible to achieve successful

outcomes, the existence of formal programs especially developed to facilitate recovery of neuropsychological functions in persons with cerebral damage constitutes significant progress.

Organization and Operational Procedures of a Neuropsychological Rehabilitation Program

Although cognitive retraining programs have a considerable degree of variability, we felt that it might be helpful to the reader if we included a description of an actual program.

Dr. William Lynch has spent a number of years developing the Brain Injury Rehabilitation Unit (BIRU) of the Palo Alto Veteran's Administration Medical Center (Lynch, 1987).

The Unit serves outpatients, most of whom have sustained head injuries. After admitting a patient to the Unit a detailed review of records is made and supplemented by further evaluation as necessary. Although the rehabilitation efforts of the Unit center around neuropsychological retraining, the evaluation is oriented toward a multidisciplinary approach, including neurology, psychiatry, speech/language and audiology, occupational therapy, physical therapy, neuroradiology, and psychosocial evaluation.

In addition to using the techniques available in these areas, which provide a relatively complete description of the individual, a detailed neuropsychological evaluation is also performed using a variety of tests, including the Wechsler Adult Intelligence Scale-Revised, the Wechsler Memory Scale, measures of academic achievement, the Minnesota Multiphasic Personality Inventory, and parts of the Halstead-Reitan Neuropsychological Test Battery. Additional tests are also used depending upon the particular problems of each patient or the results generated by the standard examination.

In addition to evaluation of the patient, specialists from the various disciplines mentioned above may be working concurrently with the individual patient. Integration of the activities and progress made in neuropsychological brain retraining with therapeutic efforts from other areas is emphasized.

A special effort is made to obtain information regarding the extent to which the patient is impaired in independent activities of living. The Brain Injury Rehabilitation Unit (BIRU) uses the Rating of Patient's Independence (Porch & Collins, 1974) which provides evaluation in areas of self-care, socialization, and communication. Self-care ratings relate to dressing, grooming, toilet activities, ambulation, and eating. The socialization ratings include assessment of health awareness, memory, scheduling, interpersonal activities, transportation, occupation or avocation, personal business, and housing. The communication section is concerned with rating of speech, understanding, reading, writing, and gestural communication. This rating form is completed two times, first upon admission and again at discharge from the Unit. The results of this rating scale assist in structuring the treatment plan, focusing treatment activities, and evaluating outcome.

In addition, the BIRU has developed a Problem List that is completed for the individual subject, based upon all of the sources of prior information and evaluational procedures, in order to provide a systematic review of any difficulties that may be present. Ratings are generally made at intake, one month, three months, in preparation for discharge, and at the time of discharge.

The Problem List includes nine areas: (1) memory difficulty, (2) impaired language processing, (3) difficulty with mathematical computations, (4) impaired sensory functions, (5) impaired motor functions, (6) pertinent medical conditions or illnesses, (7) emotional problems, (8) social problems, and (9) cognitive deficits.

Finally, treatment objectives are organized in a structured manner using the Goal Attainment Follow Up Guide (Kiresuk & Sherman, 1968). For each problem area shown by the patient, possible

outcomes are specified and ranges of behavior that would represent outcomes that were less favorable or more favorable than expected.

The first stage of the treatment process is viewed as a period of orientation and lasts about four weeks. During this time additional evaluations are performed and the patient is exposed at least briefly to a number of treatment procedures. During this orientation period a check list is used for further evaluation and is directed toward rather specific aspects of (1) *Self care* (Is the subject continent? Able to feed himself? Able to groom himself? Able to maintain adequate personal hygiene? Able to dress himself? Able to make coffee? Able to get his own lunch? etc.); (2) *Ambulation* (Needs a wheelchair? Can he/she manage the wheelchair properly? Walk safely? Can he/she manage stairways? etc.); and (3) *Orientation to the hospital community* (Can he/she find his way to the Unit? to the dining room? to the canteen? Can he/she use the shuttle bus?).

It is apparent that these aspects of the program follow the traditional procedure in most rehabilitation centers of identifying rather highly specific behaviors as a basis for devising a treatment program and assessing outcome.

The major aspect of the neuropsychological rehabilitation program is divided into a basic phase, an advanced phase, and a transitional phase. The basic phase emphasizes individual treatment sessions (with group therapy being used sparingly) and a general discussion group, composed of up to twelve patients, that meets twice weekly. The individual treatment sessions are designed to emphasize various areas, including individual relaxation, assertiveness, social skills, language, memory, and computer-assisted cognitive retraining.

Relaxation training is conducted by a licensed vocational nurse, provided during weekly one-hour sessions, and focuses particularly on the use of relaxation tapes and the patient's progress during the previous week. Copies of the relaxation tapes are eventually supplied to the patient for home use. Evaluation of the effectiveness is based upon the patient's own report as well as measures of pulse rate and blood pressure.

Training in assertiveness and communicational skills is also offered individually or in small group sessions for one-hour periods each week. The licensed vocational nurse who leads the group discusses the role of assertiveness in everyday living, describes situations that call for assertive responses, and requests solutions from the patients.

Social skills are taught in one-hour weekly sessions and deal with appropriate appearance, dress, conversation, and responses to others. These discussions are supplemented by monthly field trips either to locations within the hospital or other nearby locations.

Language training is provided in group sessions for patients who demonstrate evidence of dysphasia or dysarthria and is intended to supplement individual speech/language therapy offered by the speech pathologist. Emphasis is placed upon group exercises which deal with effective listening, writing, spelling, and speaking.

A specific effort is made to provide memory training either in a basic group (which involves discussions and demonstrations, such as verbal rehearsal, use of mnemonic devices, or note taking) or an advanced group (which uses complex visualization techniques, mnemonic lists, and discussions intended to test and improve reading comprehension). Common aids to memory, particularly involving strategies of associations, are also used and practiced.

Computer-assisted cognitive retraining is customarily provided only for one to two hours per week for each patient because of limitations in staff and equipment. The procedure involves use of a microcomputer or video game system to improve alertness, attention, concentration, motor responsiveness, memory, academic abilities (such as spelling and reading), and word finding. Results of each session are recorded and converted to graphic form in order to demonstrate the progress that is made.

The training offered at the basic level emphasizes close supervision and is intended for patients who have limited independence and lack the capability to interact in group treatment sessions. Patients may therefore remain in the basic phase for several months or, when they do not show much improvement, may not progress to the advanced phase.

In the advanced phase there is greater emphasis upon group treatments, with specific sessions oriented toward general discussion, social skills, assertiveness, relaxation, current events, memory, and language. In addition, patients are given direction in independent study in preparation for eventual vocational or educational activities. Those patients who show evidence of gross confusion, aggressive outbursts, irrelevant verbalizations, or other behaviors that are disruptive in group settings are not included in the advanced phase.

At this point we can comment that the BIRU apparently serves patients who at least initially are much more impaired than persons who can profit from REHABIT. Of course, it is relatively traditional for rehabilitation centers to include only patients with quite serious and even profound neuropsychological deficit rather than individuals who have very subtle types of deficits (which often are not discernible even on casual observation).

The final phase of the BIRU treatment program, called the transitional phase, coincides with the period during which discharge planning is underway. The patient enters this phase when a judgement is made that maximum benefits have been achieved from the basic and advanced phases of treatment. The formal program of the Unit is strikingly reduced and these subjects attend only a session called "transition group" which meets biweekly. During this period the patient may work part-time in a competitive or sheltered workshop environment or resume educational activities (at least on a limited basis). The emphasis in the transitional phase is to effect a transfer from the hospital environment and the treatment program to real-life activities.

After discharge from the transitional phase an attempt is made to follow the patient for at least one year, either by clinic or home visits, telephone contact, or correspondence. A family support group meets twice a month and patients and family members typically discuss issues such as finances, emotional problems, difficulties in dealing with the patient, etc.

Lynch concludes the description of the BIRU program by discussing the advantages of microcomputers in rehabilitation. He notes that computers can present information rapidly, reliably, and repetitively, with speed and precision in stimulus presentation. There are a large number of computer programs that either have an educational theme or have been written especially for rehabilitation use. Lynch emphasizes the variety of ways in which the patient may interact with the computer and this is sometimes an advantage to

a person with significant motor deficits. These interactional devices include customized paddle controllers, joysticks, or keyboards. The patient may also use a light pen or, in newer systems, merely touch the screen with his fingertip.

(We have tended to view the limitation of motor responsiveness, with relation to solution of the problems, as a disadvantage in use of computer training. It seems much more effective for the subject to be required to deal with the actual stimulus material in three-dimensional space and to engage in the manipulations required for solving the problem.)

Lynch also notes advantages which include the storage and retrieval of data which can be gathered routinely and with minimal effort, the relatively low cost of complete computer systems at the current time, and the interest and enjoyment of the activity shown by many patients. He concludes by stating that he believes that use of microcomputers has potential as an adjunct to traditional modes of treatment but that at present they should not be thought of as replacements for standard treatment procedures.

VI

REHABIT: A STRUCTURED PROGRAM FOR RETRAINING NEUROPSYCHOLOGICAL ABILITIES

REHABIT
Reitan Evaluation of Hemispheric Abilities and Brain Improvement Training

Many specific procedures for training children as well as adults have been developed over the years, but these training programs have not been organized around a meaningful conceptualization of human brain-behavior relationships. The Halstead-Reitan Neuropsychological Test Batteries provide a solution to this problem by identifying an individual's impaired or deficient neuropsychological functions in the framework of a model of brain-behavior relationships. In other words, the Halstead-Reitan Battery provides a diagnosis on which to prescribe a remediation program. This procedure makes it possible to offer the specific types of training needed by the individual person..

Training of both children and adults is viewed within this same framework. Differences in neuropsychological evaluation of children and adults must be recognized, largely due to the fact that children are in a developmental phase of achieving brain-related abilities. However, if they suffer impairment in a particular area, the basic area tends to be the same as the area in which an adult may have deficiencies. The training program materials for children and adults are essentially similar, except that in many instances the training begins at a more simple level for the child.

Verbal and language functions are customarily related to the integrity of the left cerebral hemisphere; visual-spatial and manipulatory skills are dependent on the status of the right cerebral hemisphere. Recent investigations, in fact, have emphasized the specialization of brain functions in association with the cerebral hemisphere involved. However, the non-specialized types of abilities, which are dependent upon the brain *generally,* have been relatively neglected. Because they involve all cerebral tissue rather than representing specialized capabilities, it might be reasonable to postulate that the abilities that characterize brain functions generally might be more important than the abilities that are represented by only one-half or even a lesser proportion of the brain.

The area noted above, which covers the broad range of abstraction abilities, represents cerebral cortical functioning generally and, in terms of its representation in the brain, it can be postulated that abstraction, reasoning, and logical analysis abilities may be more fundamental than the specialized skills. This is an interesting point to consider in evaluating the criteria that contribute to our customary educational values which emphasize, to such a great degree, the functions of the left cerebral hemisphere. The REHABIT training program does not use a "shotgun" approach to brain retraining; instead, it has specifically been organized to remediate the individual's neuropsychological deficits, as determined by an evaluation with the Halstead-Reitan Battery.

Considering the importance of abstraction abilities and their central role in brain training, five tracks of training materials have been established in REHABIT:

1. *Track A* contains equipment and procedures that are specifically designed for developing expressive and receptive language and verbal skills and related academic abilities.

2. *Track B* also specializes in language and verbal materials, but deliberately includes an element of abstraction, reasoning, logical analysis, and organization.

3. *Track C* includes various tasks that do not depend upon particular content as much as reasoning, organization, planning, and abstraction skills.

4. *Track D* also emphasizes abstraction but its content focuses on material that requires the subject to use visual-spatial, sequential, and manipulatory skills.

5. *Track E* specializes in tasks and materials that require the subject to exercise fundamental aspects of visual-spatial and manipulatory abilities.

Regardless of the content of the training materials being used for the individual subject, every effort is made to emphasize the basic neuropsychological functions of attention, concentration and memory.

With many children and adults it is necessary to give training in each of these five tracks. In some instances, one area should be emphasized much more than the other areas. The decision for prescribing training should be based upon the results of testing with the Halstead-Reitan Battery.

The REHABIT program has recently been revised and expanded and now includes over 250 training items.

TRACK A

Track A of REHABIT consists of training materials that are intended to develop cognitive abilities in the area of verbal, language and academic competence. A considerable amount of emphasis is placed upon developing familiarity with basic aspects of academic performance, especially in reading, writing, and arithmetic. We have not emphasized rote training in spelling, but many aspects of Track A provide the opportunity for spelling exercises and, if the subject has particular problems in spelling, the rehabilitation therapist should use the material to engage in such exercises and training.

The basic segments of Track A include (1) the development of preliminary reading skills (learning the alphabet; developing familiarity with consonant and vowel sounds; phonetics; vocabulary building; practice with word beginnings, word endings, and the use of contractions; compound words; synonyms, antonyms, and homonyms; practice in the use of words in sentences; and an introduction to simple reading), (2) extensive materials for developing reading skills, (3) training in both printing and cursive writing, (4) more advanced training in word-building exercises, and (5) an introduction to familiarity with numbers, number concepts, counting, addition, subtraction, and other basic arithmetical exercises up to the sixth grade level.

Finally, Track A includes material specifically developed for retraining aphasic subjects, concentrating on the areas of word-finding, reading, writing, arithmetic, and verbal comprehension and memory.

Prior to using any of these training exercises, we strongly recommend that careful consideration be given to offering detailed instruction in the area of auditory verbal comprehension. Many children (and some adults), especially those with subtle dysfunction of the left cerebral hemisphere, have great difficulty in auditory verbal comprehension. As noted, this type of deficit is common among aphasic adults.

Obviously, if the subject fails to understand the verbal information coming into the brain, it becomes very difficult to respond appropriately. Initial training in perception and understanding of auditory verbal communications is a prerequisite for additional training in this area. Of course, appreciation of visual input material is equally important, but this is emphasized in the materials oriented toward reading-readiness training as well as training in reading and arithmetical procedures.

Materials for Developing Auditory Verbal Comprehension and Integration with Appropriate and Responsive Performances

Impairment in the area of auditory verbal comprehension is prominently documented among aphasic patients. In fact, one of the major categories of aphasia includes fluent aphasic deficits that are closely related to specific impairment in the ability to understand spoken language. Curiously, however, in programs of remediation and rehabilitation the expressive components of language functions seem to be principally emphasized. For example, among school children with learning deficiencies, it is not uncommon to refer to difficulties in spelling, writing, and reading as if the deficits were entirely related to failures in expression.

In our conceptualization of the neuropsychological behavioral model we have emphasized that input, central processing, and output are necessary to describe the neuropsychological behavioral cycle. Nevertheless, the subject with a reading deficiency is often described as if reading output is his/her only limitation, when input mechanisms through the visual avenue and central processing deficits may in fact represent the major limitation. It must be recognized, therefore, that impaired appreciation of input or receptive material, coming to the brain, can have a very limiting effect upon the adequacy of responses in any behavioral situation.

This input deficit frequently occurs in the auditory avenue as well as in the visual modality, and it is not at all uncommon to encounter complaints from parents that "Johnny just won't listen." In a great number of instances in which complaints of this nature are prominent we have found on neuropsychological examination that the child shows substantial (though perhaps subtle) indications of left cerebral dysfunction. Although the deficits are not sufficiently pronounced to be identified as "fluent aphasia," they are still quite clearly brain-related and represent a significant receptive problem.

In many such instances the child is blamed for having a poor attitude, not being properly motivated, being uncooperative, and perhaps even having personality problems. In instances of this kind we often have found that the child has never received even routine training in listening skills and the unrecognized impairment of left cerebral receptive functions has created a special problem, even though the child may be of average intelligence or above.

As we have remarked previously, the neuropsychological behavioral cycle begins with input of material to the brain as the first step. Following this it is necessary for the brain to comprehend the input material before an appropriate response is possible. Because of this sequential relationship we elected to begin REHABIT with specific training in the area of auditory verbal comprehension. It is only reasonable to teach the subject to understand incoming material fully and adequately before asking for comprehension of the material and/or an appropriate response. Impairment of input (receptive) skills often goes unrecognized in the classroom situation or in the home and, as mentioned above, creates problems that frequently are interpreted as lack of co-operation on the part of the child, impaired motivation, or personality problems.

It is important initially to perform a complete neuropsychological evaluation of brain-behavior relationships because many children will show evidence of mild left cerebral dysfunction. These children frequently have auditory verbal comprehension problems and difficulties in making satisfactory academic progress. Even when there have not been specific complaints regarding auditory verbal comprehension or academic progress, we find that children with mild left cerebral dysfunction frequently show difficulties of this nature upon investigation, which turn out to be significant regarding the overall clinical problem.

We recommend that every child who has difficulties with academic subject matter (or who demonstrates evidence of learning disabilities that appear on neuropsychological examination to be brain-related) receive specific training with the initial materials in Track A in order to increase the child's capability to appreciate the symbolic significance of auditory verbal communications.

Track A begins with three tape cassettes which tell simple stories that include a number of details. The subject is asked to listen to the story and explicit instructions are given for responses which are to be entered on an answer sheet.

In the first story, for example, a child goes to the grocery store with her mother and they buy four items. The sequence in which these items are purchased must be recorded by the child by drawing crayon lines around various pictures. Next, the subject is instructed to cut out these pictures and to paste them on another page in the answer form, putting each item in the proper position. Finally, the subject is shown a picture of a toy store and a picture of a food store. Twelve objects are also shown and the subject is instructed to identify the objects that can be purchased at the food store and the items that can be purchased at the toy store.

A similar format is used with the two additional tape cassettes. It is often necessary to use these cassettes a number of times before the subject develops a full understanding and recollection of the stimulus material, and the tapes should be interspersed with other training materials that are included in Track A.

The second set of items in Track A consists of six books in which the subject is given instructions and asked to carry them out. The books range from ones that contain relatively simple sets of instructions to ones that are more complex. Many of the responses require dealing with visual-spatial relationships and the subject responds through performing an activity rather than responding verbally. The tasks therefore provide an opportunity for integrating right hemisphere functions with left hemisphere instructions. The responses require tracing and coloring of figures, free-hand drawing, drawing of figures according to printed instructions, and cutting out figures.

Adults and older children who already have the ability to read may use these books independently; younger children may need to have the rehabilitation therapist read the instructions to them.

The third set of training materials in Track A consists of numerous tape cassettes that are designed to give the subject experience in responding to an extensive range of verbal communications perceived through hearing. The principal requirement is for the subject to listen carefully and follow the instructions.

The first set of 18 cassettes provides verbal instructions concerning motor activities. The second set of 15 cassettes is concerned particularly with memory and auditory verbal perception.

The material is organized according to difficulty level for the auditory instructions that are communicated. The most simple level in the Auditory Memory series begins by presenting a pair of pictures and the subject is instructed to draw a line of a particular color through the picture identified either first or last. The task progresses in complexity to include three pictures and the response requires drawing a line above the picture identified first, second, or third, etc. The subject must not only comprehend the instructions given but must remember the instructions with relation to the specific aspects of the required response.

The third set of training materials included in this sequence requires the subject to deal with figure-ground relationships among auditory stimuli. In other words, background noises are present that interfere with perception of the stimulus material, mask the stimulus sound, and distract the subject. This set of training tapes consists of 22 cassettes. Extensive experience is available for the subject to focus his auditory attention on the stimulus even though the background provides distraction. Again, relatively simple responses are required which establish that the subject has understood the verbal communication. The principal requirement, however, concentrates on auditory verbal perception.

The next set of 17 cassettes begins with a procedure that requires the subject to identify pictures (using various methods of response) with the sound delivered on the tape. As a simple example, if the tape presents the sound of ringing bells, the subject is required to identify a picture of the bell. These procedures gradually become more difficult and complicated as the task proceeds.

A second phase of the stimulus material is concerned with identification and differential selection of initial and final consonants. Training and recognition of consonants is particularly important in speech-sound perception because the consonants (as contrasted with vowels) carry the major communicational information.

The next set of materials in this set requires the subject to identify consonant sounds and blends and indicate whether they occur at the beginning, middle, or end of each given word. At this point, the training material has progressed from more general verbal communication to perception of details of individual words.

The final set of nine cassettes presents a verbal description of an object and the subject is required to listen carefully and select the target object from various alternatives that are presented. The training material continues with this type of problem through three levels of difficulty and requires auditory comprehension of the verbal material communicated, visual scanning of the stimulus material, recognition and differentiation of visual-spatial configurations, and correlation of the verbal description with the visual-spatial material. The input requirements relate to auditory verbal comprehension functions of the left cerebral hemisphere whereas the output (or response) requirements are designed to depend principally on right cerebral functions.

The overall training activities obviously effect an integration of right and left cerebral functions, giving the subject not only training and experience in integration of brain functions generally but an opportunity to demonstrate through performance his/her understanding of the verbal communications.

The amount of material provided under this general heading of *Auditory Verbal Comprehension* is quite extensive and ranges from very simple procedures to tasks that are relatively complex. In addition, the material is sufficiently extensive to provide an opportunity for varied presentation. Although it is desirable to repeat exercises that the subject has not performed adequately, it is not necessary to repeat them so frequently that positive practice-effect becomes a significant factor. Nevertheless, it is advisable for the rehabilitation therapist to keep a record of the adequacy of the subject's responses so that the types of activities that are particularly difficult for an individual subject may be repeated until a satisfactory level of skill is achieved.

Academic Readiness Training

The second set of materials in Track A is concerned with a large number of procedures and exercises that are aimed toward establishing the foundation for developing skills in reading, spelling, and writing. Despite its routine nature, it is necessary initially in every area of endeavor to begin by communicating rotely some basic information. In other words, if a subject is going to learn to recognize the symbolic significance of letters of the alphabet, it is necessary that he/she gain familiarity with the differential spatial configurations represented by the various letters.

As the subject begins to develop competence in identifying individual letters, it is important that the "sound" of the letter be communicated. Therefore, the first item in this section uses alphabet flash cards that depict upper and lower case letters of the alphabet together with a picture of an object that begins with the letter shown. The opposite side of the card includes several words that begin with the target letter and one word that begins with a different letter. This material may be used when the subject has developed some skill in reading words. Some of the flash cards include upper case letters on one side and lower case letters on the other side. Cards that present the entire alphabetical series are also included.

Since a subject is able to identify pictures by name earlier than being able to recognize letters of the alphabet or be aware of their sounds, it is important to begin with verbal identification of the picture. At this point the rehabilitation therapist should communicate to the subject the name of the letter and associate the sound of the letter with the picture. This material can thereby serve as an introduction to phonics.

After the subject has learned to identify the letter and the letter-sound in association with the picture of an object, the rehabilitation therapist should use flash cards that contain only the target letters and no pictures. For subjects who have developed preliminary reading skills, the reverse side of the cards can also be used to identify the words and to select the word that begins with a different letter.

There is a considerable degree of variability among subjects concerning the amount of training needed to learn consistently to identify letters of the alphabet correctly. The rehabilitation therapist should remember that the letters of the alphabet represent an extensive series of spatial configurations, and for the beginner in this task (or the severely brain-damaged subject) the problem is not only one of learning the symbolic association but also of learning to differentiate various spatial representations.

It is not uncommon for some persons with excellent verbal capabilities to have difficulty with this task because of the visual form perception requirements. Instances have been observed of extreme disparities between abilities in the individual child with, for example, a high verbal IQ who fails to learn to read because of difficulty in visual processing of spatial configurations represented by letters of the alphabet. The initial phase of reading requires the subject to learn to recognize individual letters and a considerable degree of overtraining is necessary.

The next set of materials consists of six cassettes with a total of 34 lessons that are each approximately five minutes in length. These cassettes provide instructions to the subject (intended to improve auditory verbal comprehension) and a response sheet. The first 20 lessons are devoted to developing an appreciation and understanding of consonant sounds. Four additional cassettes deal with digraph sounds, and the final 10 lessons are intended to develop an appreciation and understanding of long and short vowel sounds. This material serves basically as an introduction to phonics. In our training procedures we emphasize the importance of a serial progression from initial to more advanced skills in developing reading ability.

We included a considerable diversity of material to be used in helping the subject develop familiarity with letters of the alphabet and their sounds. In this way it is possible to move from one item to another in order to give the subject the experience of dealing with different material, even though the basic intent is the same.

One of the items, for example, consists of a box that contains 50 levers, each of which may be depressed individually. Depression of the lever marked "A," for example, causes a display in which the letter "A," the word APPLE, and a picture of an apple appear. In addition to the 26 letters of the alphabet, certain digraphs are also presented in the same manner and colors as well as numbers are included.

The material is presented in an interesting format and provides the subject with an opportunity to develop familiarity with both upper and lower case presentations of letters of the alphabet, selected digraphs, colors, and words.

An even simpler procedure uses a rubber inlay puzzle for both upper and lower case letters. The subject's task is to fit the letters into their proper spaces. Vowels are presented in one color and consonants in a different color. This material helps the subject to become familiar with the shape of letters of the alphabet, to differentiate vowels from consonants, and to learn the sounds associated with each letter. In addition, the tactile element of the task assists the subject in gaining appreciation of the difference between letters in terms of touch as well as vision.

Finally, fitting the objects into their appropriate spaces provides additional practice and experience in tasks that require a degree of motor co-ordination. In fact, in order to reinforce the tactile experience of the spatial configuration represented by the letters, it is a worthwhile exercise to have the subject place the letters in their proper positions without the use of vision (either with the eyes closed or while wearing a blindfold).

As we have noted previously, the stimulus material has been selected to represent an integration of the specific content of each item with brain functions more generally, and in the training process we encourage the rehabilitation therapist to relate the specific content to various sensory avenues and also to engage manipulatory skills and performance activities (right cerebral hemisphere) and abstraction and reasoning activities (general aspects of cerebral cortical functions) in exercises using the particular stimulus material (in this case letters of the alphabet).

The remaining training material selected for laying the groundwork for development of academic skills consists of various phonetic exercises to give the subject a further introduction to vowel and consonant sounds, short words and somewhat more difficult words that use only a single vowel but with varying consonant combinations, familiarity with words that use blends, consonant digraphs, and finally, simple reading.

Additional material provides training in use of contractions, compound words, synonyms, antonyms, and homonyms. Emphasis has also been given to vocabulary building, based upon selection of words from lists of the most commonly used words. These words are also presented individually, so the subject can select words needed to express a thought and thereby learn to build sentences.

This same material can be used with persons who have already developed preliminary academic skills by selecting words that represent certain parts of speech or words that must be used in conjunction with the punctuation included.

High-use words are also presented, together with pictures, to teach the dual meanings of common homonyms. Additional stimulus material is oriented toward developing an appreciation of synonyms, using the same appropriate picture to establish pairs of words that have essentially the same meaning.

Within each set of exercise materials, the content extends from simple to more complex with the material ranging from preschool activities to higher levels. It is the responsibility of the rehabilitation therapist to select appropriate material.

For example, an older child or adult might have developed basic skills in academic subject matter but still have a personal deficiency in vocabulary. Much of this teaching material can be used at the higher levels for such subjects.

Many adults with cerebral damage resulting in impairment of basic language and verbal skills will review these simple materials quite quickly. However, such subjects often have specific lacunae in their language structure and sometimes encounter unexpected difficulties with apparently simple items.

Finally, the material in this section includes books (as contrasted with the audio-cassettes described earlier) to assist in developing auditory discrimination, reception, association, and memory. These materials provide exercises in the area of verbal reasoning using comprehension types of questions, inferences regarding what must necessarily have occurred between the beginning and end-point based on information provided, answering who, when, where, what, and why questions, and other exercises to help the subject to not only comprehend verbal material but to use verbalizations in giving meaningful explanations. All of these exercises lead up to the point where the subject will be able to begin using simple Dolch-type books to read stories for individual entertainment.

Material for Developing Reading Skills

The items in this section of Track A were selected specifically to develop reading skills. Some of the material overlaps with items in the preceding section, but is at a somewhat more advanced level.

The material begins with a series of eight books designed to facilitate reading comprehension, beginning at the first grade level and extending through the fourth grade. Two books for study are provided at each grade level so that rather extensive material is available. In addition, a teacher's guide is provided for the books at each grade level and placement tests are also given to evaluate the subject's progress.

The workbooks are organized in a very similar manner. Within each book the difficulty level gradually increases through a series of 42 lessons. The material is organized to facilitate reading comprehension through a systematic approach that consists of finding the main ideas, understanding details, understanding where, understanding when, understanding why, understanding how things are alike or different, reading between the lines, reading many kinds of writing, reading new words, and finally reading for purposes of studying.

This section also includes another book that presents more advanced material concerned with vocabulary development. This book is divided into 42 lessons, each of which concentrates on the definition of 12 essential words. In succeeding lessons the words previously studied are repeated in order to consolidate the subject's understanding of them. In total, 504 words are high-lighted in order to be sure that the student has a basic vocabulary. However, these words are relatively advanced and are appropriate for training at the high school level.

As additional basic training in reading we have included within REHABIT the seven areas of instruction that compose the Wordshop Reading Cassette Program. Each section is accompanied by a workbook which contains worksheets for use by the subject.

The training material begins with reading readiness exercises and continues to develop familiarity with consonants, vowels, initial blends, initial digraphs, and final digraphs; fundamental aspects of word building, familiarity with the role of vowels and silent consonants in words, together with other rules; development of spelling skills; and recognition of sentences and the use of punctuation.

This material is quite extensive and provides a great deal of basic training. The Reading Readiness section consists of six cassette tapes, each about 12 minutes in length, answer sheets, a pencil, and colored crayons. The material is organized in such a way that the subject is required to make frequent responses using the answer sheets. For example, the first cassette, which is concerned with developing familiarity of rhyming words, begins by instructing the subject to draw a green crayon line from a picture of a fish to a picture of a dish, from a goat to a boat, and so on. The recorded material thereby gives the subject additional experience in auditory verbal comprehension. These activities all focus on developing familiarity with verbal content necessary for establishing reading skills.

The remaining cassettes continue with a great deal of additional material oriented toward developing further familiarity with words as a preparation for learning reading skills.

Practice in word-building is important as a basis for developing an understanding of both simple and complex verbal communication. Some of the word-building material included in REHABIT consists merely of individual letters from which the subject can make selections to form particular words. Other word-building materials are designed to develop familiarity with beginning and ending consonant blends.

Such material can be presented in relatively simple form. For example, one of the items included in this section consists of 24 pictures. Twelve of the pictures have the first two letters of the object pictured (e.g., a picture of a duck with the letters "du" printed below). For this particular picture the subject must search through additional materials on which letters are printed, find the item that has the letters "ck," and add these to the picture to complete the word. Other pictures do not include either the beginning or ending consonant blends and the subject must find the blends (either beginning or ending consonant blends) to go with the picture.

Finally, one of the sections of the Wordshop materials is devoted to word building. The material consists of nine cassette tapes, each tape having two lessons. The subject uses an answer form to complete each lesson.

This material begins with a definition of root words and illustrates how prefixes and suffixes can be added. The second lesson provides practice in learning to add "s," "ed," and "ing" to make new words. Additional lessons demonstrate how the sounds of "-ed" at the end of words may differ, how dropping of a final "e" from the root word and adding a suffix that begins with a vowel is performed (e.g., "place" and "placing"), adding suffixes to make new words (e.g., "sun" and "sunny"), and practice in forming plurals, using prefixes, identifying and writing compound words, contractions, and singular and plural nouns that show possession, etc.

It can be seen that the word-building exercises included in REHABIT extend from such simple procedures as combining two letters to form a word to understanding of relatively complex word forms. This very extensive material provides the subject not only with the basic knowledge necessary to develop skill in reading but also in verbal expression much more generally.

As an example of the extensive content, the final set of materials, which consists of six 12-minute cassette tapes, is concerned with rules of punctuation. The material included in only this single area covers recognizing sentences; working with subjects and predicates in sentences; using pauses to show meaning; using pitch to show meaning; understanding end punctuation marks; writing conversation; using commas as clues to meaning; conventions of punctuation in use of the comma; punctuation involving the period, question mark, exclamation point, and quotation mark; further conventions of punctuation using the apostrophe, punctuating friendly letters, and punctuating business letters.

It is obvious that this material extends beyond the preliminary grades and in fact is intended to go up to the 6th grade. However, the material as a whole provides a systematic and organized method to communicate a great deal of information and training to subjects who need increased familiarity with various aspects of verbal communication.

Although the Wordshop Reading Cassette Program includes nine cassette tapes that are concerned with spelling generalizations, the instructional material is more heavily oriented toward study of word structure, phonetic elements, and the use of syllables than with rote training in spelling. The Wordshop cassettes were structured with the idea that basic familiarity with generalizations that relate to spelling would contribute to spelling ability. However, rote practice in spelling is also necessary. Therefore, we have included a number of workbooks, extending from the 3rd through the 8th grade level, that concentrate specifically on spelling of individual words.

The material in this section is quite extensive. It includes three books, each covering two grade levels. Each book consists of 30 lessons together with review lessons. Within each book the words proceed from simple to more complex. Each of the 30 lessons in each book is presented in a standard manner.

Initially, the rehabilitation therapist reads the spelling words for the lesson and the subject writes them as well as he/she is able. Words that are misspelled are identified and must be written correctly. The next step is for the subject to use the spelling words for the lesson in an appropriate manner in sentences that are given. Next, the subject repeats the words from dictation and writes them. Then, the subject alphabetizes the spelling words for each lesson and writes them down correctly. Finally, the spelling words for the particular lesson are again read to the subject and written. These procedures provide a considerable amount of practice and rehearsal with individual selected words that increase in complexity.

Development of Skills
in Printing and Cursive Writing

Track A also includes several training materials to facilitate development of printing and writing skills. The initial set of items includes laminated plastic cards that can be written on with a crayon and wiped clean. Each card contains a capital letter of the alphabet. The initial procedure is to have the subject trace over the letter to give practice in learning to make the letter. In addition, each card includes an indented representation of the letter so the subject can use his/her finger to draw the shape of the letter, following the indentations as a guide. Finally, space is provided on the card for the subject to write the letter independently, attempting to copy the letter as shown.

The second set of materials includes identical material except that the letters of the alphabet are written in cursive script. Similar materials are present for numbers ranging from 0–9. Other training material presents the stimulus items in the form of manuscript capital letters and manuscript lower case letters. This material serves as an excellent introduction to developing initial skill in writing and printing letters of the alphabet. In addition, the rehabilitation therapist can encourage the subject to learn the names of the letters as well as the sounds represented by the various letters. Practice of this kind is very useful as an introduction to independent writing of letters and, eventually, words.

Training in Number Concepts
and Arithmetical Skills

This section of Track A includes an extensive set of materials for training in arithmetic-readiness activities and provides specific training in addition, subtraction, multiplication, and division. The training in arithmetic-readiness uses a number of procedures for communicating the symbolic significance of numbers and for developing an understanding of number concepts and relationships.

Additional training material concentrates on combinations of stimulus configurations in order to provide training in counting and to develop basic concepts of addition. A number of procedures are included to teach the concept of fractions. Training material includes various geometric figures (such as squares and circles), subdivided into component parts, in order to establish a basic understanding of the concepts involved in the arithmetical operations of addition, subtraction, multiplication, and division.

Following this basic training in readiness for arithmetical procedures, the material provides specific exercises in arithmetical operations extending from the first through the sixth grade. Flash cards that cover the basics in addition, subtraction, multiplication, and division are included to consolidate the subject's understanding of arithmetical procedures and to develop memory functions to the point that the basic functions become automatic and ingrained.

The arithmetic-readiness procedures begin with a set of posters that identify numbers from one to ten and associate the numbers with an appropriate number of pictorial objects as well as the written number. This material is useful in establishing the notion of quantity with the symbolic representation of the number.

The training material includes additional items that provide opportunities for counting. The items provided for practice in using the sequence of numbers, such as counting pennies and the addition of pennies to identify nickels. The procedures continue with games that are based upon numbers, quantities, and sums.

In this section we have also included the Hainstock Blocks, which permit association of numerical figures with the number of plastic balls in each cell. The subject can shake the board, dividing the number of plastic balls into two segments for each number. For example, in one instance there may be six balls in one section and one ball in the other section that correspond with the number "7." When the board is shaken a second time, there may be four balls in one section and three in the other. The subject is thereby able to discern that the number "7" corresponds with seven balls, regardless of their particular division. The training material goes on with specific tasks involved in addition, initially using sums only through 10.

The arithmetic-readiness material also includes a number of items that encourage the subject to develop an appreciation of fractions, extending from whole figures up to fractions of one-sixth. Manipulation of this material, together with use of counting skills, demonstrates that the whole figure may consist of one or more parts, depending upon how the figure is subdivided. Exercises with this set of stimulus figures lays the groundwork, using pictorial representations, for learning to "take away" or subtract.

Following this arithmetic-readiness material, the training materials in this section of Track A continue with specific training in arithmetical procedures. These are subdivided according to grade level and extend from grade one through grade six.

Four books are available for grades one and two and these are devoted basically to exercises consolidating counting activities and rehearsing the groundwork for addition and subtraction. Remaining manuals in this section of REHABIT extend through the full range of problems involved in basic arithmetic, including adding, subtracting, multiplying, and dividing fractional and mixed numbers, applying these arithmetical procedures with decimals, and finding percentages and dealing with problems which involve percentages. The material gradually extends from simple to more complex arithmetical procedures, divided into half-grade levels.

As noted above, sets of flash cards are also used to consolidate basic skills in addition, subtraction, multiplication, and division by establishing rote memorization of the basic and fundamental facts. The subject's response to flash cards can often be used as a diagnostic procedure in order to identify areas of arithmetical function that require additional training and rehearsal. In addition, brief presentation of stimulus material may in some instances identify those persons who have difficulty with visual form discrimination. It is, of course, obviously important that the subject be able to recognize each number immediately and without difficulty in order to perform arithmetical operations.

These types of problems often require training with materials included in Tracks D and E in order to establish basic abilities in differentiating spatial configurations as a prelude to developing arithmetical skills.

The final material included in Track A was intended for persons who had developed language and numerical skills but who, as a result of cerebral damage, had lost these abilities and become aphasic. The material is organized in much the same way as the training material used for teaching young children.

The training material in Track A (previously described) can be used for aphasic adults in a manner similar to the way that it is used for initial training of children. However, a careful evaluation and analysis of the aphasic subject's deficits is necessary in order to identify the particular training materials that will be necessary.

A basic difference between children and adults concerns deficiencies of initial acquisition (among children) and a loss of previously acquired abilities (among adults). This difference requires determination of comparative deficits, or neuropsychological needs, of impaired vs. unimpaired abilities among adults. Thus, a complete neuropsychological evaluation is imperative for both children and adults, but the specific content of training material is often identical.

The training material in this final section, even though devised for adult aphasia rehabilitation, may be useful for both children and adults as review material and for consolidation of basic abilities that were previously developed.

TRACK B

Items included in Track B were carefully selected to emphasize tasks with verbal and language content. It includes material which ranges from very simple to complex tasks. The items are related to the material in Track A, but require a certain degree of more general problem-solving, abstraction, reasoning, and memory skills.

Track B begins with a very simple procedure in which numbers are associated with pictures which vary with respect to the number of objects depicted. The numbers themselves are locked into sequence by being pieces of a jigsaw puzzle. As the subject solves the jigsaw puzzle he/she can be instructed about the word that identifies each number (what the number is called) and the sequence of numbers from 1 to 10 according to the way in which they fit into the puzzle.

The next step is to dissemble the jigsaw puzzle made up of numbers, placing each number on the appropriate picture according to the number of objects shown. For example, the number "1" would be placed on the picture of a pail, the number "2" is placed on the picture of two teddy bears, the number "3" on the picture of three balloons, and so on. This exercise helps the subject to associate the symbolic representation of numbers with the number of objects depicted, contributing to an appreciation of the quantitative significance of the numerical symbols.

The second item in Track B is also oriented toward developing an association between printed numbers and the number of objects depicted. However, a somewhat different approach is used. The subject is provided with the individual pieces of a jigsaw puzzle. The clues for solving the puzzle are represented not only by the pictorial material but also by the sequence of numbers from 1 to 10. When the puzzle is solved, the subject can be instructed to observe that the number "1" is beside a single scarecrow, the number "2" is beside two sunflowers, the number "5" is beside five rabbits, etc.

In addition to providing information about the sequence of numbers from one to ten and their quantitative representation, this task exercises brain functions more generally through the use of the jigsaw puzzle. In order to solve the puzzle the subject must learn to observe pictorial elements in detail and relate them in a meaningful way through use of spatial configurations. Besides numerical content the task involves recognition of non-numerical objects and integration between visual-spatial representations and the symbolic meaning of numerals.

The second part of this particular item in Track B involves the same type of task with letters of the alphabet as the significant content. It consists of a jigsaw puzzle in which the solution is dependent upon clues received from non-verbal pictorial representations and letters of the alphabet. When the puzzle is solved the subject will discover that the letter "A" is next to a picture of ants, the letter "B" is next to a bear, the letter "L" is next to a lion, and so on. This task is designed to develop familiarity with individual letters of the alphabet and their sequence and to serve as an introduction to phonics through association with pictures.

The training material in this section gradually increases in complexity. For example, the third item in Track B provides training in recognition and identification of various geometric configurations after a delay interval that may vary in length. On one side of the booklet a circle and a plus sign may serve as the stimulus figure. After the subject has had an opportunity to view this particular spatial configuration, the stimulus configuration is covered and, after an interval, the subject is asked to identify the particular configuration from a set of four configurations shown on another page.

The tasks increase in difficulty to the point that a series of five geometric shapes must be registered initially and identified not only according to the five different shapes involved but also ascending to the sequence in which they appeared.

Although it may seem that training in the ability to identify sequences of geometric shapes is principally a right hemisphere activity, it is important to recognize that verbal and numerical symbols also are represented by various types of spatial configurations. This task, therefore, proceeds to use letters of the alphabet in the same role that geometric shapes had previously been used. The subject is required to look at a configuration of letters and, after an elected interval, to identify the letters that have been observed on a page that includes a number of alternative configurations. The training material then moves on to using words as the stimulus configuration.

Obviously, if the subject has developed simple reading ability and can conceptualize the set of letters as a word, identification of the corresponding word becomes much easier. In fact, the rehabilitation therapist can use this type of material to provide an introduction to initial phases of reading. The stimulus configuration "trace," for example, must be identified after initially seeing the word among four alternatives consisting of "crate," "trace," "react," and "cater."

The material can be made more difficult by increasing the interval between exposure of the stimulus configuration and exposure of the alternative items from which selection is to be made. The stimulus material itself continues with various combinations of letters of the alphabet and words in cursive writing. The entire process in this item permits an extension from initial registration and recognition of sequence of non-verbal geometric configurations to printed letters of the alphabet, printed words, cursive letters of the alphabet, and cursive words.

The material in Track B contains progressively more difficult verbal material, with the tasks selected according to a theme that requires more complex abstraction and reasoning abilities. For example, one of the items is made up of a series of sentences with a key word omitted. Four alternatives are given for each of the missing words. Sometimes more than one word is missing in a sentence and the subject must read the sentence and select the appropriate word among the four alternatives for completion of the sentence.

As an illustration, one sentence consists of "The chair was (MADE CUT PAINTED LIFTED) green." The correct response would be to underline PAINTED. This task requires the subject to identify the appropriate word in the context of the sentence, a simplified version of the task-requirements of the Word Finding Test (Reitan, Hom, & Wolfson, in press) which has been found to be very sensitive to brain damage, especially of the left cerebral hemisphere.

An important and practical aspect of having developed familiarity with the symbolic significance of numbers relates to telling time; therefore, two of the items included in Track B are specifically concerned with learning to tell time. One of these items consists of an extensive group of cards on which clock faces are depicted. The face of the clock is identical in each picture but on each card the background appearance of the clock surrounding the face is different. The subject must learn to tell the time shown on the face of the clock regardless of the variability of the rest of the configuration. The material is organized so that the subject is able to write his/her answer below each clock-face and, upon completing the task, to turn the card over and check whether his/her answer corresponds with the printed answer.

The second item concerned with telling time consists of a clock-face with a red hour hand and a black minute hand that are movable and can be manipulated by either the subject or the rehabilitation therapist. The full combination of twelve hours and sixty minutes can be utilized. In using this procedure we recommend that the subject be taught not only how to tell time from a clock-face but that activities which normally occur at various times of the day be associated with the particular times depicted.

The material included in Track B was selected to require a degree of reasoning and logical analysis in association with verbal and pictorial material. As an additional example of this procedure, one of the items includes 30 pictures in 15 pairs representing cause-and-effect relationships.

For example, one picture may show a man diving into a body of water with his clothes on,

and the printed question on the back of the card asks, "Why is the man diving into the water with his clothes on?" The subject's task is to sort through additional cards until he finds a picture that appears to provide an appropriate answer. The correct picture is of the man swimming to rescue another person. On the back of the second card is the statement, "The man is diving into the water because he wants to help the person who's drowning."

This set of materials can be used initially either through use of the pictures alone, the printed sentences alone, or finally, through an integration of the pictures and the printed sentences. Although the material is intended to help develop language skills and vocabulary, the approach is through establishing cause-and-effect relationships as well as a description of sequential aspects of behavior. The desired outcome is not only to assist in developing verbal abilities, but to integrate verbal abilities with pictorial representations in a manner designed to promote skills in logical thinking.

The material included in Track B also was selected to train the subject in quantitative relationships as a basis for developing a more sophisticated understanding of the meaning of numbers and fractions. One of the items intended for this purpose uses cuisenaire rods. The material consists of a large number of plastic figures. The smallest are cubes, the next figures are doubled in length, and progress to figures that are ten times as long as the cubes. The rods also vary in color. This material allows for a great number of activities, all directed toward developing concepts of size and quantitative relationships.

As a simple procedure, the rods can be organized in length from the shortest to the tallest. The subject can then determine how many shorter rods are required to match the length of a longer rod, and the concept of fractions can be introduced. Combinations of rods can be assembled to demonstrate that two-fourths are equal to one-half, for example, and that three-fourths plus one-fourth equals the full extent of a given figure.

The material can be used at a very simple level, in terms of matching, and can teach the basic concepts of addition, multiplication, division, and fractions.

In accordance with our desire to increase motivation by including games or game-like activities in REHABIT, one of the items in Track B is a game called Tri-Ominos. This is essentially a game of dominos, in which the figures are represented by triangles and must be matched in accordance with the two numbers along each side.

For example, if a "4" and a "1" were printed along one side of the triangular figure, it would be necessary to match with a figure that has the same number. The game requires the subject to observe the available stimulus material, organize it as needed for selection, and relate the stimulus material to the configuration that is being formed in the process of the game.

It is obvious that many of the tasks in Track B do not relate exclusively to left cerebral functions. This type of item selection was done quite deliberately because the materials included in this Track were intended to extend in two directions, relating on the one hand to materials in Track A and on the other to materials in Tracks C, D, and E. Besides including elements of numerical or verbal symbols, the material frequently requires a degree of logical analysis and reasoning as well as solution of problems involving spatial and sequential elements.

In Track B we have emphasized especially the association of pictorial (non-verbal) material with numerical and verbal symbols in order to achieve a degree of integration between these various tracks. In accordance with our aim of promoting an integration of neuropsychological functions, many of the individual items include requirements of a perceptual or performance nature that extend across the entire range of the neuropsychological behavioral model described above.

TRACK C
Sorting, Classification, Reasoning, Logical Analysis, Planning and Abstraction

Many investigators of intelligence, including some who related intellectual impairment to cerebral damage, have concluded after years of study that abstraction and reasoning abilities represent the fundamental nature of intelligence. Although one might question how thoroughly such abilities are represented by the Stanford-Binet Intelligence Scale, Terman assigned abstraction, reasoning, and concept formation a central role in his definition of intelligence. Gelb, Goldstein and others, in the clinical tradition of evaluation of brain-behavior relationships, reached the conclusion that abstract (as contrasted with concrete) thinking was the essential characteristic of normal brain functions.

In fact, Goldstein carried this distinction to the point that he was far less interested in whether a task could be completed successfully than in the manner in which the task was done. Even if the task was successfully completed through use of concrete thinking approaches, he characterized the performance as defective. He felt that (1) there was no overlap between the abstract and the concrete approach, (2) they were essentially different processes, and (3) one represented normal and the other represented impaired brain functioning.

Halstead, in his theory of biological intelligence, assigned abstraction the principal role in central processing by the brain. His theory consisted essentially of input from the environment, output to the environment after brain processing had been completed, and abstraction, reasoning, and logical analysis as the essential features of central processing. He included an additional factor in his theory of biological intelligence, but this represented the Power Factor or the energy available for brain functioning. In his four-factor theory of neuropsychological functioning, abstraction, reasoning, and logical analysis was integrated with input and output to constitute intellectual functioning.

Through years of research and clinical evaluation of individual subjects with and without cerebral damage, our experiences have led to a similar conclusion. In the Reitan-Wolfson neuropsychological model of brain functions we have assigned abstraction and reasoning the highest level of cognitive functioning, but it is important to recognize that these abilities are integrally associated with the specialized functions of the two cerebral hemispheres.

In other words, the specialized functions relate principally to content of the material being processed (verbal and language functions versus manipulatory skills and spatial relationships) which in turn must be analyzed, organized, and understood through abstraction processes. This conceptualization is further supported by evidence of the differential specialized functions of the two cerebral hemispheres (Sperry, 1974; Wheeler & Reitan, 1962) as contrasted with the experimental finding that abstraction abilities are represented in all parts of the cerebral cortex, including the parts in each hemisphere that are principally involved in the specialized functions (Doehring & Reitan, 1962).

As we have noted previously, REHABIT as a brain retraining program must deal with the specialized neuropsychological abilities of the brain but in addition must effect an integration of these specialized abilities with the general functions of abstraction, reasoning, and logical analysis. Therefore, Track C represents a central feature of REHABIT, concentrating on basic abilities in abstraction and reasoning but attempting to establish linkage with verbal and language skills for the left cerebral hemisphere and spatial and manipulatory abilities with the right cerebral hemisphere. The training materials included in Track C were selected to emphasize abstraction and reasoning abilities with lesser emphasis being placed upon the content of the task.

Because impairment of abstraction, reasoning, concept formation, and analytical abilities is such a common feature among persons with impaired brain functions, it is often necessary to begin brain training using the materials found in Track C. Our experience indicates that training of the general aspects of brain functions is a prerequisite to training in the specifics.

Many children with learning disabilities demonstrate generalized impairment of brain functions even though the child's limitations appear to fall in the area of academic proficiency and progress. However, it is important to recognize that in many instances the area of academic competence is the only area that is tested. The child performs poorly in the classroom, but when his brain functions are assessed more generally through neuropsychological testing, he also shows many brain-related deficiencies.

In the individual case any aspect of impaired brain functions may be significant to cause limited academic ability, but failure in the area of abstraction and reasoning is often of major importance. The child needs the ability to understand the general context in which he is trying to master specific skills in order for the specific training to have meaning.

It is often stated that individual children have *specific* learning disabilities but, on examination with the Halstead-Reitan Battery, by far the majority of children have *general* as well as specific deficits. Until the child develops sufficient ability in the area of abstraction and reasoning and has a general ability to understand complex situations, it frequently is of limited value to attempt to accomplish training in the basics of academic skills.

One can teach the child rote behavior related to language and numerical symbols, but the potential for development, growth, and generalization of these experiences may be limited. We have found that initial training with Track C is frequently required, with an approach to the more specific skills represented in Tracks A and E coming about only through an integrative approach using Tracks B and D.

Content of Track C

As in the other Tracks, the items in Track C extend from very simple materials to tasks that are relatively complex. However, especially in Track C, it is important to recognize that even very simple material can be used for training of relatively complex skills in abstraction and reasoning.

The initial step required to develop abilities in this area depends upon careful and accurate observation of recurring similarities and differences in stimulus material. The basic processes of sorting and classifying depend upon such observations. However, even using only a few physical stimulus dimensions, it is possible to develop relatively complicated problems. Even the very simple items at the beginning of Track C can be used for rather high-level training.

We will try to indicate some of the ways in which this can be accomplished, but we would also appeal to the ingenuity of the rehabilitation therapist in developing varied uses for each item. The therapist should keep in mind that a particular item may be used at a very simple level of training in one point in the training process and that the same item may be used at a later point in a much more complicated format.

Track C begins with bead stringing activities and the material consists of 15 beads and two stringers. There are five different shapes of beads in five different colors. This material is described as being appropriate for children age 2 through 5 years and was intended by the manufacturers as a preschool activity. The item certainly can be used in this manner, essentially to develop motor and manipulatory skills, but it can also be used in a much more complex way.

The first step in using this item should be to instruct the subject to string the beads through the stringer in order to develop initial familiarity with the material. Since the beads come in five shapes and five colors, a number of additional activities are possible. The next step would be for the rehabilitation therapist to string a set of beads, using one of the stringers, and to have the subject emulate this procedure using another stringer. Gradually, as the subject develops confidence and familiarity, principles of organization can be introduced.

One procedure might be to sort the beads by color and string all beads of a certain color before another color is added. Another procedure might be to sort the beads by shape, and string all beads of one shape before another shape is started. Another principle might be to string the beads in a sequence so that no two beads of the same color are adjacent to each other. This notion can be further complicated by stringing the beads in a specific color sequence so that yellow, red, green, orange, and blue are repeated in consecutive series.

From these few illustrations it is apparent that a considerable range of sorting and organizing activities is possible. Although the rehabilitation therapist should provide examples for the child (or severely impaired adult) initially and guide the subject in using different principles for sorting and stringing the beads, it is desirable to encourage the subject to initiate and develop principles of sorting and to carry out these principles independently whenever possible.

A final activity using this item should lead to comprehension of a principle and recapitulation of a performance in accordance with the principle rather than having to depend upon specific memories. For example, the rehabilitation therapist can string beads according to a principle communicated to the subject as the beads are being strung. Then, after having completed the activity, the therapist removes the stimulus material. At this point the subject should be given an opportunity to repeat the performance of the examiner. Help should be given as necessary to relate the principle involved to the actual activities in order to guide the subject's performance.

The initial phases of this kind of training should be quite simple in nature and adapted to the abilities of the subject. For example, the stringing process might call for the use of two beads of the same color, followed by two other beads of a different color, and so on. The rehabilitation therapist should discuss the principle with the subject when the beads are being sorted into their proper groups as well as during the stringing activity. Finally, after the subject has completed the task, the string of beads completed initially by the examiner should be brought out for careful comparison with the string completed by the subject.

It is apparent that even such a simple procedure as stringing beads, intended for preschool children, can be used quite effectively with older children and even with adults by increasing the organizational complexity of the task. The rehabilitation therapist may wish to use beads and stringers at a very simple level in one instance but return to the task at a more complex level when the subject has progressed to a higher ability level. Much of the material in Track C is of such a nature that the ingenuity of the rehabilitation therapist can be exercised in this manner.

Another item in Track C uses various booklets to provide exercise in visual perceptual discrimination and categorization of objects. One booklet provides line-drawings with several of the objects in a row being identical except for one of the objects being turned in the wrong position. The subject must identify the identical figures as well as the one that is different from the others. Using this material, he/she is given an opportunity to observe the significance of minor differences in similar spatial configurations and develops an appreciation of the directionality of the figures depicted. In addition, the material provides preliminary training in grouping and classification through questioning the subject about the ways

in which the pictures are different and the ways in which they are alike.

Another simple training exercise consists of 30 cards, depicting 15 pairs of things that go together (such as a hammer and nail, a bat and ball, and a lock and key). When these cards are spread out before the subject, they provide an opportunity for careful inspection and review of the details of the picture, followed by selection of pictures that go together. In this exercise the subject should be questioned about the rationale for associating the two objects, regardless of whether the answer is correct or incorrect.

In addition, this material can also be used to facilitate the development of vocabulary and verbal communicational skills. For example, when the subject selects the two pictures that depict a hammer and nails, he/she should be asked questions such as, "What is a hammer used for?" As the child or dysphasic adult develops familiarity with the stimulus material, a memory aspect of the task may be introduced. The subject can be presented, for example, with a picture of a bat and asked to recall by name the object with which the bat is associated and then proceed to find the correct picture.

A somewhat more complicated task involves discerning the missing object in a given picture. One task, for example, consists of eight stimulus cards with three types of objects depicted in each of the four quadrants on each card. However, each quadrant is missing one object because a total of four objects is used. In one quadrant a picture may be shown of a lemon, an apple, and a nut. However, the four objects used in total also include berries. In this particular quadrant the berries are missing. To solve the problem the subject must inspect each of the quadrants, determine the missing item from observation of the content in other quadrants, and select from a series of cards the missing item.

On other cards four items are included in each quadrant but one of the items clearly does not belong with the others. It often is easier for a young child, or a person with impaired abstraction and grouping abilities, to respond to an inappropriate item than it is to respond to a missing item. However, this material provides excellent practice in exercises of this type, going from quite simple to somewhat more complex problems.

Using this same item, a memory component may be introduced, using the white circles that are included with the material. One of the circles can be used to conceal or block out individual items in the pictures. When a particular object, such as an apple or a lemon, is covered, the subject can be asked to discern from the content of other pictures on the same card which object is missing. These exercises encourage close observation of visual material, identification of the pictures with respect to meaning, and logical reasoning, based upon observation of additional pictures, to effect grouping of objects into meaningful categories.

Another type of organizing procedure that we have found helpful requires the subject to use cues to place objects appropriately in a printed grid. One item, for example, consists of a board with 16 squares with a margin around the entire grid. Additional stimulus material consists of hundreds of cards that vary in color and content. Some of these cards are marked with an outside black border and these cards are used as the "cue" cards to be placed in the margin around the grid.

Such a card containing a blue spot might occupy a certain position and all of the figures that were included in the corresponding row of squares would have to contain the color blue. The additional details relating to a particular square on the grid would require consideration of the co-ordinates involved. If a cue card in a particular row was identified by the number "3" and a corresponding cue card above a particular column was represented by a flower, the subject would have to find a card that contained three flowers to place in the intersecting square.

In this task the variability of the "cue" cards is quite extensive, permitting a great number of organizing possibilities. The material extends from quite simple to relatively complex tasks and is useful in training preschool children with normal brain functions, as well as older children and adults who have impaired abstraction and reasoning abilities.

Track C also contains a considerable amount of material that requires the subject to establish associations between pictures according to their content. Simple sorting activities require the subject to group pictures into various categories on the basis of their content. Other procedures require the subject to identify pictures that do not belong with others considering the category represented by the group.

Still other pictures depict activities, divided into two phases. For example, the first card may show a picture of a particular type of activity and a second card must be selected to complete the activity. Selection of pairs of pictures, in accordance with the activity involved, assists the subject to develop a logical association between the pictures in terms of content and action.

Other material in Track C consists of rubber inlay formboards. These formboards use identical shapes but are graduated in size in one instance and according to geometric shapes in another instance. Young children may use this material for developing the concept of size. For older or more advanced children, we recommend that the subject learn to place the objects in the correct place either with the eyes closed or blindfolded.

With many children it is necessary to let them practice on material of this kind with their eyes open initially in order to learn to appreciate the general configuration of the material and the formboard. However, comprehension through tactile perception of the orderly representation of figures from smallest to largest, represents an excellent training activity in integration of the aims of Track C with right hemisphere functions.

Some of the training materials in Track C are composed principally of a large number of stimulus materials that can be sorted, classified, and grouped in various ways. One item, for example, consists of 15 cartons of hundreds of stimulus figures and three sorting trays. The figures vary in color (red, green, blue, yellow, and purple) and shape (beads, discs, and animal figures). It is possible to sort the figures according to any number of principles, based upon single characteristics or combinations of characteristics. In addition, these objects can be used to integrate the purposes of Track C with those of Track A for purposes of counting and learning basic addition and subtraction principles.

A number of the items in Track C use pegs and pegboards. Because the pegs vary in shape, color, and size, it is possible to arrange the pegs on the board in various configurations. As an example, the subject could place pegs of the same color in each row, pegs of the same color according to graduated height in each row, alternation of graduated height of pegs in adjacent rows, alternation of pegs so that a progression of colors was represented, etc.

In addition to organizational activities of this kind that are permitted by these sets of pegs and boards, it is possible to organize an arrangement of pegs according to pre-determined principles and have the subject reproduce the design, not by remembering where each individual peg went, but instead by following the principles involved. Obviously, this kind of activity can extend from very simple to quite complex tasks. It is necessary for the rehabilitation therapist to work closely with the subject in developing an understanding of the principles involved in each instance.

This material is intended basically to develop conceptual skills and the ability to organize stimulus material in accordance with a known principle, but it obviously includes practice in motor and manipulatory skills as well as in dealing with spatial relationships. This aspect of Track C is therefore oriented toward integrating abstraction and reasoning skills with the right-hemisphere activities emphasized in Tracks D and E.

One of the items in Track C is organized specifically to facilitate memory. However, the material can be used to develop memory in conjunction with underlying principles of organization. The material itself consists of 70 small objects of various colors and shapes. A memory tray is included that has four different compartments, each of which may be covered by a lid. This material permits the subject to engage in numerous exercises, such as (1) selection of objects through memory of a specific object, and (2) selection of objects to complement completion of groups included in the memory box according to principles (e.g., the objects must all differ from each other in one respect or another, etc.).

These exercises can range from very simple memory procedures to tasks that are relatively complex. The basic purpose of the material, however, is to permit development of problem-situations for the subject to solve according to an organizing principle. This material is intended to provide training in memory tasks that are integrated with organizing principles in order to permit deduction to facilitate the memory process.

Finally, a considerable number of tasks are included in Track C to use with persons who are impaired in maintaining alertness and attention. The basic mechanism in central processing is oriented toward registration of incoming material and relating the incoming material to prior experience and skill (as well as memory of previous experiences).

The first exercise of this type is to underline the number "4" whenever it appears on a page of numbers. It is necessary for the subject to proceed in an orderly fashion, and be alert continuously to identify the number "4." The exercise can also be performed using different numbers (or combinations of numbers) which are selected for the individual exercise. The subject should repeat this task many times in total, with practice being distributed over various training sessions. Gradually, even the brain-impaired subject who initially has great difficulty paying attention to specific stimulus material will begin to develop improved skills (unless, perhaps, there is an underlying disease process that causes progressive pathological deterioration of the brain).

Additional training material is provided for the same type of task using geometric figures, nonsense designs, complex designs, letters of the alphabet, combinations of letters in meaningless configurations, and combinations of letters to form simple words. Obviously, the material extends from simple to complex content requirements, but is consistently organized in a manner that requires alertness, close attention, and continuous concentration. These abilities are fundamental to eventually be able to successfully use the higher skills in central processing, but are often impaired in persons with compromised brain functions. The rehabilitation therapist may time each performance in order to gain a quantitative record of improved efficiency as practice progresses.

It may be necessary to use these focused activities for improvement of alertness and concentration as initial or early training exercises for some persons. This determination can usually be made by considering the results of the Speech-sounds Perception Test and the Seashore Rhythm Test in the context of other results of the Halstead-Reitan Battery.

In applying REHABIT it is important to keep in mind the sequential nature of central processing activities of the brain as represented in our neuropsychological behavioral model. Incoming material requires attention and concentration for initial registration before the specialized or higher aspects of brain function can effectively be used.

TRACK D

Track D emphasizes the importance of right hemisphere functions in development of abilities that we believe are important in the practical aspects of everyday living. These functions center particularly around visual-spatial, tactile-spatial, and sequential tasks. While the specialized functions of the left cerebral hemisphere facilitate and abet communicational skills, the functions of the right cerebral hemisphere permit the individual to function efficiently in space and time.

Although the academic orientation of our society places great value on verbal, language, and communicational skills, individual efficiency of performance, in a practical sense, is heavily dependent upon right cerebral functioning. Nevertheless, the role of the right cerebral hemisphere in behavior seems to be relatively neglected (and probably undervalued) in our society, apparently because of the strong emphasis on proficiencies related to academic training and language. (Obviously, many of the types of training available in an academic setting relate to right hemisphere activities as well, but priority appears to have been given to left hemisphere skills.)

A question has sometimes been raised about whether left or right cerebral lesions are more disabling in human beings. As with many either-or questions, the answer may be relatively meaningless because of the different functions subserved by each cerebral hemisphere. In other words, the answer may well be "both." A question of this type probably cannot be answered unless a procedure was available for assigning equal weight and relevance to the functions subserved by each cerebral hemisphere. The Halstead-Reitan Neuropsychological Test Battery was devised according to procedures which might achieve this end, and in the individual case the lateralized Neuropsychological Deficit Scales provide a practical answer.

The Battery was developed through examination of thousands of patients with brain lesions that varied in their location, severity, type, and status. The criterion was that the results of the Battery be adequate to identify brain dysfunction regardless of lateralization, location, or other dimensions.

The General Neuropsychological Deficit Scale (described in Chapter III) appears to be the best single index of severity of overall neuropsychological impairment following brain damage. It is interesting to note that lateralized lesions, involving either the left or right cerebral hemisphere, appear to have closely comparable General Neuropsychological Deficit Scale scores, both falling well within the range characteristic of brain damage. These results suggest that the two cerebral hemispheres are of equivalent overall significance with respect to intellectual, cognitive, and adaptive functions. In turn, the results emphasize the significance of right as well as left cerebral functions and underline the importance of considering and including impairment of specialized abilities due to right cerebral damage in brain retraining programs.

For reasons that recognize the importance of the right cerebral hemisphere, we have taken great care to develop Track D in considerable detail. The ordinary academic setting appears to do little to develop abstraction and reasoning abilities in the context of visual-spatial tasks, tasks that involve sequential elements, and performance types of problem-solving activities.

The types of training activities included in Track D are relatively familiar to most professionals, either through their use in various psychological tests of a performance nature or in training and rehabilitation activities. In fact, some of the types of items included in Track D are similar or even identical to certain items previously described, although they are used in a different manner.

The emphasis in Track D is on the visual-spatial requirements of these tasks in a context of abstraction, reasoning, and logical analysis, rather than on development of, for example, numerical concepts. Because of the general familiarity with many of the tasks included, a detailed description of each item is not necessary. However, the reader should note that nearly every item permits development of skills in naming of shapes and colors, counting, sorting and grouping, and reproduction,

after an interval, to stress the integration of memory and principles of visual-spatial organization.

Despite the selective nature of the material in Track D, we again emphasize the importance of using the material in as broad a manner as possible, depending upon the apparent needs of the individual subject. In other words, if the subject has difficulties in counting or naming, the stimulus material should be used to assist in developing these abilities. In addition, the difficulty level of the task can often be sharply increased by requiring the subject to duplicate various items from memory.

If the item had been constructed initially according to well-defined principles, the use of these principles to facilitate the reproduction provides exercise in a very fundamental and practical aspect of memory. Memory that is facilitated by principles of organization for the activities involved often serves as a fundamental basis for achieving efficiency of performance. Therefore, throughout the material in Track D the training technician should be aware of the opportunities for naming, counting, sorting, and grouping, as well as reproduction according to established principles, rehearsal of those principles, and facilitation of delayed reproduction through use of organizing principles as well as strict memory processes.

Track D is intended to accomplish a close integration between the content of the visual-spatial training material and the use of abstraction, reasoning, logical analysis, and principles of organization.

A large part of the content of Track D makes use of block-design types of tasks. In these tasks the subject is provided with blocks that have different colors or designs on each side and is instructed to reproduce a pictured design or pattern using the blocks. Standard block-design tasks are represented, and the training material goes on to include not only two but three-dimensional block design tasks as well. Some of the material extends to picture designs in which various surfaces of the block contain parts of a picture which must be assembled in order to reproduce the whole picture.

Other block-design tasks use blocks in the shape of various geometric forms rather than cubes, and these must be combined to reproduce the entire configuration. Items of this type include the familiar parquetry figures and designs that have frequently been used in rehabilitation and brain retraining programs, thereby extending the content and configurations into many kinds of constructional tasks that go well beyond designs formed with standard cubes.

Track D also makes extensive use of formboard puzzles of various types. For more impaired or younger subjects we recommend that these form-boards be performed with the use of vision. How-ever, as with the Tactual Performance Test in the Halstead-Reitan Battery, it is very instructive for many subjects to solve the formboard, placing the appropriate pieces in their proper spaces, with eyes closed or while wearing a blindfold. This latter procedure also emphasizes the integration of tac-tile perception and problem-solving of a spatial nature.

As with the other tracks, the training material is generally organized from simple to more com-plex tasks. However, in Track D we have included a number of training tasks in which a single type of training material progresses from quite simple to more complex tasks.

Sequential picture cards, for example, are used quite extensively in Track D. These tasks involve sets of pictures that must be organized in sequence in order to depict an unfolding activity or succes-sive aspects of a story. They are basically similar to the Picture Arrangement subtest of the Wechs-ler Scales.

In order to maintain organization of the ma-terial, a single item in Track D includes several sets of such pictures, extending from very simple problems to ones that are considerably more com-plex. The training technician should recognize that the very simple materials should be used with sig-nificantly or seriously impaired persons and that

the more difficult materials in the same item might well be reserved for use at a later stage in the training program.

Arrangement of pictures in sequence accord-ing to a logical principal or analysis of the stimulus material is a very important training activity be-cause of the extent to which it requires detailed analysis of visual-spatial information and logical thinking.

A number of items in Track D make use of beads and laces because, as noted in description of materials included in Track B, a great range and variety of organization of stimulus material can be accomplished with these simple materials. The most important use of this material in Track D relates to organizing the beads in a sequence that accords with a given principle and, after a delay, exercising the understanding of the principle as a mnemonic device for reproduction of the initial effort.

The same type of activities can be performed using a stand with several poles and rings or beads that fit over the poles. Several items include this type of material and, again, we recommend that the rings or beads be placed over the poles in a sequence that represents a principle such as grad-uated size, alternating colors, or more complex sequences as might be needed for the individual subject.

Track D also includes jigsaw puzzles as a train-ing aid in the use of cues involving various types of spatial relationships to facilitate right hemi-sphere abilities. One of these jigsaw puzzles, which is relatively simple in nature, must be fitted to-gether in a sequence of pieces that tell a story, integrating an understanding of spatial relation-ships and sequential organization.

Mazes are also included to provide still another type of training activity in dealing with spatial re-lationships. Some items include "attribute" blocks that vary in color, shape, size, and thickness. While most of the stimulus materials vary in color, shape, and size, thickness adds a less usual variable that can be quite helpful in providing an additional physical dimension of the stimulus material for sorting and grouping purposes.

Several items were included for specific interest or for areas of training that do not require extensive repetition. One of these, for example, provides training in understanding positions of objects in space (up-down, over-under, behind-in front of, on-off, in-out, open-closed, left-right, and between two other objects). Young children or severely impaired persons sometimes require training in such basic relationships, but an extensive set of materials, represented in multiple training items, is not needed.

Another set of stimulus materials essentially consists of a building set. Various plastic pieces can be fit together to form configurations, designs, and representations or actual objects. This material can be used quite extensively and repeatedly because of its flexibility.

We also included a game which emphasizes memory for designs. This is a "lotto" type of game in which the subject is permitted to turn up two cards at a time and observe the designs on each card. The aim of the game is to be able to turn up two cards that have identical designs. In order to accomplish this aim it is necessary for the subject to remember designs that he has seen before and their location. This game requires that the subject pay close attention to the individual designs in terms of their similarities and differences, as well as remembering their location in the spatial distribution of the cards. This task is especially useful for persons who have receptive deficits in the visual-spatial area, a type of impairment that often accompanies lesions in the posterior part of the right cerebral hemisphere.

Track D also includes several workbooks that provide a wide range of exercises in dealing with spatial relationships. We feel strongly that actual manipulation of objects is important in brain training and that workbooks alone do not provide the range of flexibility that is required. However, workbooks do have the advantage of providing an extensive range of exercises and are particularly useful in providing material for visual form perception.

A final aspect of Track D emphasizes visual-spatial input (or receptive functions) in specific detail. Every item in Track D requires perception of the stimulus material, a degree of central processing, and expression of a response. However, since so many training items emphasize the response aspect (in terms of drawing, manipulating objects, forming and completing designs with objects, etc.), we deliberately included several tasks that depend mainly upon visual form perception. This type of training is particularly important for some children in development of basic skills necessary for the visual form discrimination requirements in reading.

One of these tasks requires the subject to sort objects in accordance with a guide that is provided. The subject must examine each object carefully, determine whether it is the same or different as compared with a number of objects used as guides, and accomplish the sorting on this basis.

Another procedure requires the subject to view complex designs and select from alternatives the design that matches the target figure.

Finally, a particular procedure requires the subject to view similar pictures, searching for differences in pairs of pictures, and identifying the differences. This task requires attention to specific details of the overall visual-spatial configuration represented by the picture.

As noted above, some of the items in Track D that have a similar content are included in the same section of the training materials, and even though they progress from rather simple to much more complex tasks, they provide for variability in training activities. It is the responsibility of the rehabilitation therapist to become familiar with the material and to use it in a flexible manner that fits the ability level of the subject.

In this respect it is important to keep in mind the basic operating principle that it is far better to have the subject work on something that is easy for him than to work on something that is too hard. The corollary of this principle is that the subject should be given the opportunity to derive a feeling of satisfaction induced by successful performance rather than a feeling of unhappiness produced by failure.

TRACK E

Track E contains training materials that were selected to provide basic experience in the fundamentals of spatial relationships. Problem-solving activities in the context of spatial relationships is not emphasized (the problem-solving element was extensively represented in Track D). Much of the material in Track E is relatively simple in nature, although some of the items explore relatively complex aspects of spatial configurations.

Track E includes a variety of materials for training purposes. An item for persons who have extremely limited ability in dealing with spatial relationships consists of a hardwood box that has various shapes cut out of the cover and 10 hardwood forms that fit through these various shapes. The shapes are a circle, square, triangle, and two rectangles of different sizes.

The task merely is to place the blocks through their proper shapes on the cover of the box. The task provides basic and preliminary experience in appreciation of shapes through both the visual and tactile avenues as well as experience in simple manipulation of objects.

This task is very simple in nature, but it can be complicated in various ways by organizing the sequence in which objects are placed within the box. Integration with Tracks A and B can also be achieved through naming of the figures.

Additional items provide the opportunity for learning to draw various shapes. For this purpose plastic wipe-off cards and plastic crayon markers are used. For persons with very limited drawing abilities, the wipe-off cards reproduce a target figure using broken lines, and the subject merely has to draw over these lines. In other instances the subject has to independently reproduce the figure as exactly as possible. The training material can also be used for drawing figures and designs for which a target figure (sample) has not been provided.

The receptive aspects of visual-spatial relationships are also emphasized in Track E. One of the items includes a fairly extensive set of materials for sorting stimulus cards into appropriate slots in a box depending upon cues given for the appropriate placement of each card. This activity requires close observation of the stimulus material on each card and an opportunity is available to check the accuracy of responses by opening the box and checking to see if only the appropriate cards are included.

This exercise was devised to develop an appreciation of shape, color, quantity and numbers, directionality, depicted emotional responses (laughing versus crying), ordering, and matching according to given codes of varying complexity. Although the procedures are not difficult, many subjects with impaired right cerebral functioning need specific training in these basic aspects of visual form perception.

Another item uses a set of 30 cards to illustrate 10 spatial relationships of a relatively simple nature, including over and under (or above and below), on and off, next to or beside, in front of, in back of or behind, between objects, through objects, and within objects. Adults usually have no difficulty with simple relationships of this kind unless there is severe damage of the right cerebral hemisphere. In young children, however, rehearsal of these relationships is sometimes highly desirable.

Additional items include bead-stringing activities to match the patterns shown on individual cards. While such material can be used in a much more complex manner, as described in Tracks C and D, it is valuable within Track E to emphasize the spatial characteristics of the stimulus material as well as the sequential organization of the patterns.

Track E also includes a considerable amount of material for basic practice in block-design activities and in solution of simple jigsaw puzzles. As we have noted previously, the puzzles can be solved through use of vision among persons who are quite limited in their ability to deal with spatial relationships, but solving the puzzles with the eyes closed or blindfolded has special advantages for the more advanced subject or as the subject progresses in development of skills through training.

Pegboard activities are also provided, using pegboards with a large number of holes and variously colored pegs. Pattern cards are provided for purposes of duplication of the configuration, although the training technician may find it valuable in many cases to devise patterns on the pegboard, have the subject observe and review the pattern carefully in order to discern underlying principles, and reproduce the pattern after a delay.

Some of the material was selected to provide training in visual perception of details. In one item nine laminated cards are presented, each depicting a scene that includes a great number of details. Target details are identified for the subject and he/she must search each card in order to find them. This activity is intended to develop ability in visual form perception and attention to individual details in the context of distracting figures.

Many years ago Strauss and Werner (1941) emphasized the importance of impairment in appreciation of figure-ground relationships among brain-damaged children. Although this is only one of the many ways in which impaired brain functions may be manifested behaviorally, it does represent an important area of visual perception.

Finally, simple material is included in the form of geometric figures from which larger geometric figures can be formed. This material ranges from simple to fairly complex problems. However, the material can be used in quite an extensive manner. For example, two triangles can be used to form a larger triangle, or the same two triangles can be used to form a rectangle. In another instance, for example, two triangles can be used to form a right-angle triangle that represents half of a square, and smaller triangles, a square, and a parallelogram can be combined to form the other half of the square. Developing competence in manipulation of these geometric figures can be very helpful to persons with posterior right cerebral lesions in regaining a basic understanding of spatial relationships.

As noted above, the materials in Track E can be used for sorting, grouping, organizing according to principles, and memory exercises. The intent in selecting materials for Track E was to provide basic instruction in the area of spatial relationships, but the rehabilitation therapist should not hesitate to use the material creatively in order to increase complexity as well as to relate the tasks to problems in abstraction, reasoning, and problem-solving generally.

Illustrative Case

Volume I of *Traumatic Brain Injury* (Reitan & Wolfson, 1986b) was concerned with communicating an understanding of the pathophysiological and neuropsychological consequences of traumatic brain injury. Volume II has focused on the after-effects of brain injury, concentrating on biological processes of repair of damaged tissue, prognosis, outcome, spontaneous recovery, and brain retraining. Although it was necessary to effect a subdivision of content matter in the two Volumes, it is important to recognize that all of these areas are relevant as far as the individual patient is concerned. We demonstrated the process of neuropsychological evaluation using the Halstead-Reitan Battery in an extensive and varied series of cases in Volume I, but commented only briefly on the approach that would be used in retraining higher-level brain functions.

The detailed description of REHABIT on the preceding pages permits us to be much more detailed with regard to the specific aspects of brain retraining that would be followed. In order to emphasize the relevance of the entire range of information as applied to the individual patient (pathophysiology, neuropsychological evaluation, spontaneous recovery, and facilitated recovery or brain retraining), we will select a patient used in Volume I for these detailed considerations regarding retraining of higher-level brain functions. We will not repeat the entire description of the neuropathology nor the neuropsychological evaluation. Instead, we will again present the results of the Halstead-Reitan Battery, summarize the major aspects of neuropsychological ability structure (including the nature and areas of deficits as well as strengths), determine the needs of the subject, and proceed with a description of the training exercises that should be used.

ILLUSTRATIVE CASE

Name:	W.C.	Sex:	Male
Age:	30	Handedness:	Right
Education:	12	Occupation:	Mechanic & Restaurant owner

A detailed presentation of the head injury sustained by this man, the neurological findings, and the neuropsychological evaluation and diagnosis was presented in *Traumatic Brain Injury Volume I.* In brief, W.C. was in a moving vehicle accident two and one-half months before the neuropsychological examination. He sustained a head injury and was unconscious for about three hours and confused for several additional hours before he began to recognize others, communicate verbally, and understand his situation. He was discharged after four days of hospitalization but was somewhat impaired and confused; he returned to the hospital and remained there for another 18 days.

Neurological examination was done immediately preceding the neuropsychological testing and the findings (including EEG) were essentially within normal limits. However, the neurologist felt that the patient showed evidence of impaired alertness and some degree of confusion. The neuropsychological test results for W.C. are presented so that the interested reader may refer to them directly.

The detailed interpretation of these results was presented in Volume I. However, before prescribing a retraining program using REHABIT it is important to review and summarize the test results in order to understand precisely the nature of the problem and the neuropsychological deficits that are in need of remediation.

W.C. earned a General Neuropsychological Deficit Scale (G-NDS) score of 55, a value that falls in the range of moderate impairment (Chapter III). Comparison of the contributions of the four sections of the G-NDs (level of performance, specific deficits, patterns and relationships, and right-left comparisons) indicates that W.C. accumulated more points in the section concerned with level of performance and somewhat fewer points in the section concerned with specific deficits than for the overall brain-damaged group.

THE HALSTEAD-REITAN
NEUROPSYCHOLOGICAL TEST BATTERY

Patient **W.C.** Age **30** Sex **M** Education **12** Handedness **R**

WECHSLER-BELLEVUE SCALE

VIQ	101
PIQ	89
FS IQ	95

Information	8
Comprehension	9
Digit Span	11
Arithmetic	10
Similarities	9
Vocabulary	7

Picture Arrangement	3
Picture Completion	8
Block Design	8
Object Assembly	11
Digit Symbol	7

TRAIL MAKING TEST

Part A: **35** seconds
Part B: **312** seconds

REITAN-KLØVE TACTILE FORM RECOGNITION TEST

Dominant hand: **9** seconds; **0** errors
Non-dominant hand: **10** seconds; **0** errors

REITAN-KLØVE SENSORY-PERCEPTUAL EXAM

				Error Totals	
RH ___ LH ___	Both H:	RH **1** LH ___		RH **1** LH ___	
RH ___ LF ___	Both H/F:	RH **4** LF ___		RH **4** LF ___	
LH ___ RF ___	Both H/F:	LH ___ RF ___		RF ___ LH ___	
RE ___ LE ___	Both E:	RE ___ LE **2**		RE ___ LE **2**	
RV ___ LV ___	Both:	RV ___ LV ___		RV ___ LV ___	

TACTILE FINGER RECOGNITION

R 1 ___ 2 ___ 3 ___ 4 **1** 5 **1**   R **2** / **20**
L 1 ___ 2 ___ 3 **1** 4 ___ 5 ___   L **1** / **20**

FINGER-TIP NUMBER WRITING

R 1 **1** 2 **1** 3 **3** 4 **3** 5 **4**   R **12** / **20**
L 1 **3** 2 **3** 3 **1** 4 **1** 5 **1**   L **9** / **20**

HALSTEAD'S NEUROPSYCHOLOGICAL TEST BATTERY

Category Test	86

Tactual Performance Test

Dominant hand:	6.4		
Non-dominant hand:	5.8		
Both hands:	3.1		
		Total Time	15.3
		Memory	5
		Localization	3

Seashore Rhythm Test

Number Correct	14	10

Speech-sounds Perception Test

Number of Errors		14

Finger Oscillation Test

Dominant hand:	45	45
Non-dominant hand:	43	

Impairment Index **0.9**

MINNESOTA MULTIPHASIC PERSONALITY INVENTORY

		Hs	77
		D	53
?	50	Hy	64
L	46	Pd	46
F	60	Mf	59
K	48	Pa	50
		Pt	52
		Sc	73
		Ma	55

REITAN-KLØVE LATERAL-DOMINANCE EXAM

Show me how you:
throw a ball	R
hammer a nail	R
cut with a knife	R
turn a door knob	R
use scissors	R
use an eraser	R
write your name	R

Record time used for spontaneous name-writing:
Preferred hand	**12** seconds
Non-preferred hand	**29** seconds

Show me how you:
kick a football	R
step on a bug	R

REITAN-INDIANA APHASIA SCREENING TEST

Form for Adults and Older Children

Name: _____W. C._____ Age: __30___

Copy SQUARE	Repeat TRIANGLE
Name SQUARE	Repeat MASSACHUSETTS "Massachusses"
Spell SQUARE	Repeat METHODIST EPISCOPAL "Method Epicopol"
Copy CROSS	Write SQUARE
Name CROSS	Read SEVEN
Spell CROSS	Repeat SEVEN
Copy TRIANGLE	Repeat/Explain HE SHOUTED THE WARNING.
Name TRIANGLE	Write HE SHOUTED THE WARNING.
Spell TRIANGLE	Compute 85 – 27 =
Name BABY	Compute 17 X 3 =
Write CLOCK	Name KEY
Name FORK	Demonstrate use of KEY
Read 7 SIX 2	Draw KEY
Read MGW	Read PLACE LEFT HAND TO RIGHT EAR.
Reading I	Place LEFT HAND TO RIGHT EAR
Reading II	Place LEFT HAND TO LEFT ELBOW

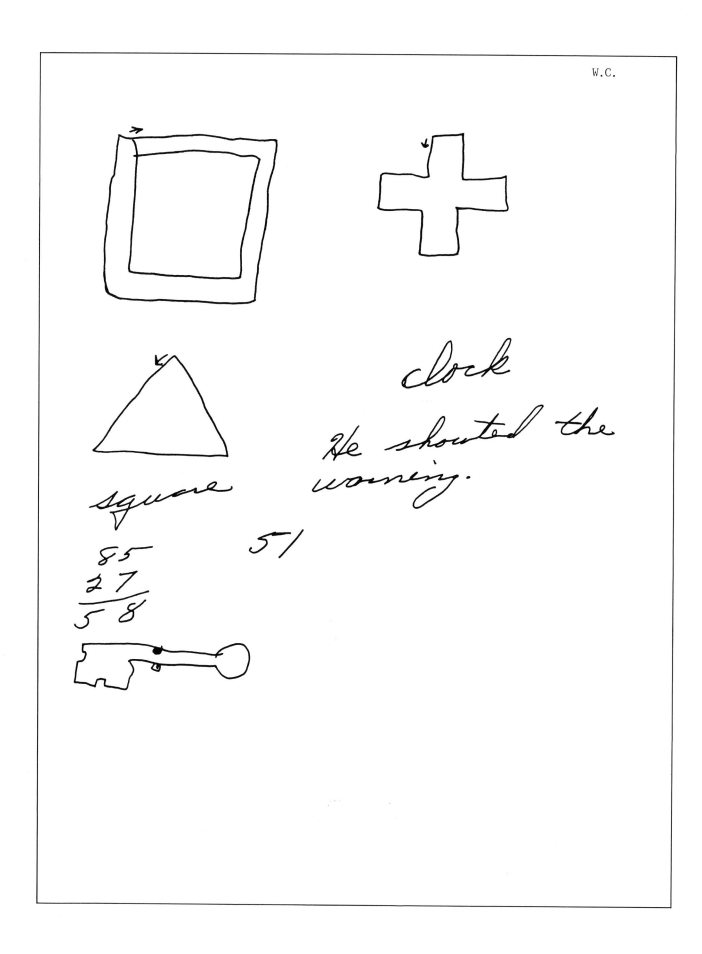

clock

He shouted the warning.

square

$$\begin{array}{r} 85 \\ 27 \\ \hline 5\ 8 \end{array}$$

51

W.C.'s Left-Neuropsychological Deficit Score (L-NDS) score was 8 and his Right-Neuropsychological Deficit Score (R-NDS) was 9. Each of these values was sufficiently high to suggest the presence of involvement of the left and right cerebral hemispheres, but the fact that the two values were nearly equal argued against a conclusion that the cerebral damage was lateralized.

Evaluation of the test results made it quite clear that the most pronounced evidence of impairment was derived from general rather than specific indicators, although indications of impairment were present in both areas. W.C. earned an Impairment Index of 0.9 (indicating that about 90% of the tests included in this Index had scores in the brain-damaged range). He performed particularly poorly in the area of abstraction, reasoning, and flexibility and alertness in his thought processes. This significant impairment was demonstrated by his performances on Part B of the Trail Making Test and on the Category Test.

In addition, several scores suggested that W.C.'s alertness and ability to concentrate, in a general sense, were defective. He performed poorly on the Seashore Rhythm Test (a score of 14 correct) and made 14 errors on the Speech-sounds Perception Test. It is also probable that the extremely poor performances on both hands in finger-tip number writing perception (especially as contrasted with his considerably better scores in tactile finger recognition) reflected some impairment in the ability to focus his attention and concentration to the specific task at hand.

Specific indicators reflected evidence of damage to both cerebral hemispheres. The patient had difficulty enunciating METHODIST EPISCOPAL, demonstrating mild central dysarthria. His relatively poor score on the Speech-sounds Perception Test, particularly when considered with relation to his average Verbal IQ, suggests that he may have some difficulty in receptive aspects of auditory verbal comprehension.

Right hemisphere deficits were indicated by the very low score on the Picture Arrangement subtest and relatively low score on the Block Design subtest of the Wechsler Scale as well as by deficits in the ability to copy simple spatial configurations (especially the key).

These results indicate that the principal deficits are general rather than specific and that an approach must be taken to upgrade overall alertness together with his ability in abstraction, reasoning, and flexibility of thought processes. Although use of Tracks A and E might be useful in the long-term brain retraining process, it is clear that initial emphasis should be placed on training with Tracks C, D, and B.

In the process of retraining W.C.'s brain functions it will be necessary for the rehabilitation therapist to engage in communication with him. It would be important to keep in mind that this man may have possible problems in both expressive and receptive aspects of language functions and he should be encouraged to state any confusion he might have in this regard.

In addition, it would be important to ask W.C. regularly to express, in his own words, what he is attempting to do and what the nature of the problem is. In this process it would be important to have the patient practice enunciation by repeating after the examiner any words that were not correctly pronounced and, in addition, to emphasize auditory verbal comprehension. Observation of deficits in these areas might, in fact, provide a basis for deciding to use the rather extensive materials in Track A for retraining in the area of auditory verbal comprehension.

The rehabilitation therapist should use a general approach that emphasizes the importance of attention and concentration over time. Many of the training exercises can be used in a manner that emphasizes registration of initial observations, not only on a rote basis but also in terms of how the various materials are arranged and organized. Every opportunity should be taken to encourage W.C. to observe the systematic and orderly organization and arrangement of stimulus materials, to comment on these and describe the principles involved, and to use these principles as a basis for replicating the material at a later point in time.

We would recommend that items from Track C be used initially for specific training purposes. Item C-1 (Big Wood Beads) could be used very effectively. This material consists of 15 wood beads representing five shapes and five colors as well as two stringers. This man has sufficient motor skills to be able to string the beads on the stringer without difficulty. However, his poor scores on the Category Test and Part B of the Trail Making Test suggest that he has serious deficiencies in understanding even simple organizational principles.

The therapist could suggest to W.C. that he follow a sequence relating to color (such as yellow, red, green, and blue beads) and repeat these in a successive series. He could be encouraged to state the principle that he was following verbally and to demonstrate the principle through his actions.

A second principle might be to string the beads according to a color principle that required that two beads of the same color never be placed next to each other. The same principles could be applied with respect to the shape of the beads involved, with variations extending from requiring a different shape with each successive bead to principles that required a replication of the same shape (even though not the same color) before another shape could be strung.

In following these activities using stimulus material as simple as wooden beads, it would be important to exercise memory with respect to the performance. For example, the therapist could string the beads according to a preselected principle, perhaps using a principle that was familiar to the subject through his prior activities. W.C. should be encouraged to observe the stimulus material and discern the principle prior to removing the beads. He should then be encouraged to repeat the stringing, even of an extensive number of beads, not through rote memory but instead by use of the principle itself.

It is important to recognize that stimulus material does not necessarily have to be very complex in nature in order to engage the subject in relatively complex abstraction, reasoning, and logical analysis tasks. This point is made abundantly clear by considering the content of the Category Test. The stimulus material is quite simple in nature, but the principles underlying the organization of the material may be relatively complex.

Item C-3 could also be used effectively with W.C. This material consists of eight stimulus cards, each of which contains pictures of four objects with only three objects represented in each quarter of the card. The subject's task is to find the missing item among the three identified objects in each quarter of the card, select that item from the available picture cards, and place it with its appropriate group.

This task requires not only grouping in accordance with items that fall in the same category, but careful observation of what is present and what is missing. It is more difficult for a person with impaired abstraction abilities to identify a missing item than it is to identify a given item that does not belong with others in its category.

Item C-3 can be used in this latter manner also. For example, the subject is given a picture that includes several items, one of which does not go with the others. The subject's task is to identify this item and to block it out by covering it with a white circle.

Item C-3 can also be used in terms of training observations, observing and stating organizational principles, and using immediate memory facilitated by not only direct observation but by the underlying principle.

Item C-15 (Cylinder Peg-Board) could also be used very effectively in giving W.C. the kind of training required in terms of his neuropsychological deficits. This item consists of a peg-board and 55 pegs, all of the same size but represented by 10 different colors. Among the 55 pegs, 10 pegs have one color, 9 pegs another color, 8 pegs still another color, and so on down to only 1 peg of the final color. The peg-board consists of rows of spaces that extend from 10 to 1.

W.C. should be asked first to organize the pegs with relation to the holes, trying to sort them in some way that effects a meaningful organization. As the subject works with this task he will gradually discover that he can place 10 pegs of the same color in the row of 10 holes, 9 of the same color in the row with 9 holes, and so on completing the board.

Various other designs can be worked out in terms of distribution of colored pegs in the various holes. In fact, the rehabilitation therapist should make up various designs, show the organization of the material to W.C., discuss the nature of the design and any organizing principles that relate to it, and finally remove the pegs and have W.C. reproduce the design.

This kind of activity not only provides training in observation and application of rules of organization of stimulus material, but it is also important in developing a basic understanding and appreciation of spatial relationships. W.C. demonstrated some degree of impairment in tasks of this kind (Block Design and his difficulty in copying simple spatial configurations).

Item C-16 (Shape Peg-Board) provides additional materials that can be used in much the same way as item C-15. The Shape Peg Board consists of 54 figures of six different colors and nine different shapes. A board is also included on which there are nine spindles approximately 2½ inches high. Seven figures will fit on each spindle.

This stimulus material permits organization of the 54 figures in a variety of ways according to color and shape. Figures of the same shape could be placed over a single peg in a sequential order of color, with the sequence being reproduced for each different figure.

Following completion of this task, the figures could be removed in a standard sequence that would effect a new organization in sets of nine

figures (because there are nine spindles on the board). W.C. should then be questioned to express verbally the relationship between the original organization of the figures and the resulting organization that occurred as a result of removal of the figures in the pre-determined sequence. This task provides another example of the way in which relatively simple stimulus material can be used in quite a complex manner with respect to training abstraction and reasoning abilities. Track C consists of many additional items that can be used in much the same manner as those previously illustrated.

W.C.'s neuropsychological test results make it quite clear that he needs training in Tracks D and B as well as C. His basic deficits were in the area of general (as opposed to specific) indicators, and his major problems related to impairment of alertness, concentration, abstraction, reasoning, and flexibility in thinking. However, in his particular case, it would be important to extend the basic training in abstraction and reasoning abilities to the content areas represented by functions of both the right and left cerebral hemispheres. In other words, W.C. needs to extend his abstraction and reasoning to visual- spatial and sequential content material (Track D) as well as to verbal problem-solving procedures (Track B).

W.C. demonstrated a striking deficit on the Picture Arrangement subtest of the Wechsler Scale (a score of 3). We have emphasized repeatedly in this Volume that the course of spontaneous recovery is characterized by improvement in the areas of initial deficit. This finding has been shown in longitudinal studies (Dikmen & Reitan, 1976) as well as in clinical evaluation of individual cases (Reitan & Wolfson, 1986b). Of course, it is obvious that the areas of deficit are the areas that need rehabilitation. In attempting to remediate the impairment caused by head injury, obviously there is little point in directing retraining efforts to abilities that were not impaired.

In considering practical application of this set of circumstances, it seems entirely reasonable to use training procedures that are essentially similar to the tasks that originally identified the deficits. A great deal of research and clinical effort has been invested over the years to develop standardized neuropsychological tests that reflect the full range of impairment experienced following brain injury. These very tests probably most clearly and precisely identify the kind of impairment sustained and the kind of retraining that is required.

Nevertheless, Barth and Boll (1981) identify a problem that emanates from this procedure, noting that outcome measures of cognitive retraining often closely resemble the training tasks themselves. If one were to use a standard neuropsychological test battery for initial diagnosis of deficits, model the training program in accordance with the deficits measured, and then use the same test battery for assessment of outcome, a problem of circularity in procedure could be present. A question would exist about the generalized ability of the training. As noted by Grimm and Bleiberg (1986), such a procedure is "simply not sufficient, and further research is needed to determine if one is actually restoring "cognition" or merely training a specific behavioral facsimile."

These considerations must be evaluated with relation to the purpose of brain retraining. If the purpose is to improve the neuropsychological deficits of the impaired subject, it seems perfectly appropriate to use training tasks that are relevant to the type of impairment sustained. If, on the other hand, the purpose is to demonstrate "improvement" on specific neuropsychological tests, training the person to perform the specific tests may well demonstrate "improvement" in the score but nevertheless leave unanswered the question of generalized ability of the training.

To some extent a conflict inescapably exists in the attempt to achieve these two purposes, but the principle value obviously centers on the value of the procedures to the patient. Since the neuropsychological tests have been developed to reflect the basic and fundamental deficits associated with

brain damage, they presumably represent ability measures that would have a degree of general significance for other classes of behavior.

Next, in practical terms we recommend that the training program attempt to emulate the effects achieved, in part, by spontaneous recovery (or the natural recovery process) and that the training activities be deliberately selected for their appropriateness to the deficits manifested by the subject. Noting that W.C. did very poorly on Picture Arrangement, we would elect to use training tasks designed to bring about improvement in this fundamental ability.

Track D of REHABIT includes a number of procedures that require the subject to place picture cards in a proper sequence in order to tell a story. Item D-33 (Sequence Picture Cards) is organized to present tasks of this kind at different levels of difficulty.

The simplest task begins with only two cards and the subject must decide on the basis of his inspection and comprehension of the pictorial material which card comes first. Instead of merely asking the subject to arrange the cards in sequence (as done in formal psychological testing), the training procedure should require the subject to explain his observations of each picture and to relate these explanations to each other with regard to the sequential organization.

Items in D-33 progress to three and four cards per problem up to as many as ten cards in a sequence. As the subject begins to develop skill in this task, we have found it advantageous to complicate the problem by including irrelevant pictures.

Another variation is to include two or more sets of pictures. The subject is then required to sort the pictures in accordance with similarity of subject matter before arranging the pictures in proper sequence.

While this type of training may be viewed by many as doing nothing more than teaching the subject to do the Picture Arrangement subtest of the Wechsler Scale, it is important to keep in mind that this particular test has distinct relevance to the functional adequacy of an identified part of the cerebral cortex (right anterior temporal area) and if this area is damaged the resulting fundamental deficits must be addressed.

Although scores on Picture Arrangement and Block Design show a tendency to dissociate depending upon whether the lesion involves the right anterior temporal lobe or more posterior parts of the right cerebral hemisphere, the differentiation probably relates to sequential organization of visual-spatial (pictorial) material as contrasted with spatial organization alone. These types of tasks may be brought closer together in terms of their requirements by using training materials that require a sequential procedure in terms of completing a complex spatial organization.

In the case of W.C. we would also recommend the use of D-28 (Pyramid Puzzles). This item consists of nine plastic laminated pattern cards on which are printed strip-patterns utilizing various colors. The subject is required to reproduce the pattern card using a set of 18 strips of rubber-like material which are 1 inch wide and vary in length from 1 inch to 12 inches.

For subjects with severe impairment, it is possible to construct the pattern by actually placing the strips according to color and size in their appropriate places on the pattern card.

As with most simple materials, it is possible to complicate the task and make it considerably more difficult. For example, in the training procedure W.C. should be shown a pattern card and have time to inspect it very carefully. Then the rehabilitation therapist should remove the pattern card before W.C. proceeds to reproduce it with the colored strips. Intermediary steps can be taken in which the subject is permitted to organize the stimulus material while observing the pattern card, selecting and placing the pieces in order in terms of how he plans to use them, and then reconstructing the design after the pattern card has been removed.

W.C. showed evidence of right hemisphere difficulties not only in terms of the poor Picture Arrangement score but also with respect to mild difficulties in copying simple spatial configurations. The type of training offered by the prior item would be of value in its own right in the attempt to improve ability to deal with spatial relationships over and beyond training in sequential procedures.

We would also recommend item D-22 (Large Parquetry and Patterns) for additional training in learning to deal with spatial configurations. This item consists of 16 plastic laminated design cards and 156 parquetry pieces that come in eight colors. The design cards range from fairly easy configurations to ones that are rather complex and difficult.

This material can be used to train ability in dealing with visual-spatial tasks at a moderately difficult level. In addition, of course, the materials can be used in a "memory" mode, in which the subject is shown a design and asked to reproduce it. The task can be made much more difficult by requiring the subject to select the parquetry pieces needed to reproduce the design from a larger number of pieces than are actually needed.

A final procedure that can be used, depending upon the rapport with the patient and the patient's frustration tolerance level, is to present an impossible task. Some subjects, who have excellent abilities in dealing with spatial problems of this type quickly recognize that an essential piece is missing and that the problem cannot be solved with the pieces provided.

However, persons with significant residual impairment have great difficulty with such tasks. W.C. would not be a good candidate for this latter procedure (at least in the early stages of training) because of the very significant impairment he showed on measures such as the Category Test and Part B of the Trail Making Test. His fundamental ability in structuring problems and defining their nature would preclude his recognition of the fact that the problem was insoluble, and probably only lead to a significant degree of frustration and discouragement.

Item D-30 (Pattern Blocks and Pattern Blocks Task Cards) is another item that would be helpful in retraining W.C. This material consists of 250 plastic blocks that represent six shapes and six colors. Twenty-two laminated pattern cards are included that extend from rather simple to relatively complex problems.

The subject's task is to select the blocks necessary to complete various designs shown on the pattern cards. Many of the pattern cards include printed instructions, so it is possible for the subject to proceed independently. In many instances it is necessary to locate missing blocks and to effect a continuation of the pattern that has already been started.

In addition to training in dealing with spatial relationships, this material can be used by the rehabilitation therapist to develop skills in dealing with fractions, measurement of area and the perimeter of configurations, and even to establish basic principles in geometry.

W.C. also showed certain findings that indicate that his left cerebral hemisphere was involved. His finger tapping speed was a little slow with his right hand as compared with his left hand, he had definite difficulties perceiving a tactile stimulus to the right side when it was given in competition with a stimulus to the left side, he had somewhat more difficulty in finger-tip number writing perception on his right hand than his left hand, and he showed evidence of central dysarthria.

Although he did not demonstrate specific deficits that would lead to a conclusion that he was aphasic, it is very probable that these indications of left cerebral damage have some significance for a degree of impairment in dealing with language symbols for communicational purposes. These indications of left cerebral damage must be considered in conjunction with the findings of serious general deficits as manifested by the four most sensitive indicators in the Battery (Impairment Index, Category Test, Part B of the Trail Making Test,

and the Localization component of the Tactual Performance Test).

As we noted earlier, W.C. has his major difficulties in tasks that require general and integrative neuropsychological functions rather than in the area of specific deficits. Therefore, when training is offered in tasks that involve verbal and language skills, it must always be kept in mind that the patient must at the same time receive training in the areas of abstraction, reasoning, organization of stimulus material, and integration of the elements of the problem. In fact, Track B was developed for just this purpose, since so many persons with cerebral damage show evidence of significant impairment in abstraction, reasoning, and integrative functions.

We would recommend that item B-12 (Why? Because!) be used in the training program together with many other items from Track B. Item B-12 consists of 16 pairs of pictures. Each pair of pictures can be associated in terms of meaningful relationships.

For example, one picture shows a girl dropping a plate and another shows a broken plate. The first step in using this item is to have W.C. sort the pictures in accordance with similarity of content. The next step is to organize the principles with respect to sequence involved. Finally, W.C. should be questioned about the relationship between the pictures.

On the back of the first picture in each pair is a written question and on the back of the second picture is the answer establishing the cause-and-effect relationship. For example, the question in one instance might be "Why is the policeman stopping the motorcyclists?" and on the back of the companion picture, as is shown in the picture itself, is the statement, "Because one of them is not wearing a helmet." This may appear to be rather simple material, but for a person (like W.C.) who demonstrates such significant impairment in the area of understanding organizational stimulus material and cause-and-effect relationships, it is probable that he would have some difficulty and would profit from the training.

Item B-16 (Triominos) would also be of value to W.C. This item consists of a game of dominos in which the figures are represented by triangles and must be matched in accordance with the total of two numbers on each side of the triangle. The arithmetical requirements are relatively simple, but it is necessary for the subject to observe the available stimulus material and organize it for selection as needed. In addition, the task promotes development of basic abilities in spatial relationships through having to deal with the triangular configuration. The principle purpose for using this item with W.C. would be to encourage him to view the available stimulus material, organize it, and select it as needed in solution of the problem.

Finally, most people with left cerebral involvement have difficulty with receptive aspects of verbal communication (auditory verbal comprehension) as well as with expressive verbal abilities. Probably more recognition and emphasis is placed upon expressive functions than receptive functions, but it must be remembered that difficulty in comprehending verbal communications through the auditory avenue can constitute a very significant deficit in practical aspects of living.

In working with W.C. in his overall brain retraining, we would strongly recommend that some time be taken to be sure that he has reasonably adequate abilities in understanding verbal communications. Track A devotes a considerable amount of material to the area of auditory verbal comprehension.

For example, Item A-1 consists of three tape cassettes which tell simple stories that are fairly detailed. The subject is asked to listen to the story and to provide answers to various questions concerning it. Item A-2 consists of a set of six books in which the subject is given increasingly complicated instructions and asked to carry them out.

Further training of this type is given by item A-3 which includes additional tape cassettes that give explicit instructions for carrying out certain tasks. The communications are presented at three levels of difficulty, through an extensive series of lessons at each level, and in increasing degrees of difficulty.

Additional tape cassettes are presented in items A-4 through A-7 which emphasize different aspects of auditory comprehension. One set of tapes emphasizes memory functions. Another set uses background noises that serve to mask a stimulus sound, interfere with comprehension, and distract the subject from the auditory verbal communication. Training with these tapes is particularly helpful to the brain-damaged subject because of difficulties that are often present in differentiating the verbal communications from background distractions.

Other tapes concentrate on auditory discrimination, particularly concentrating on identification and selection of consonant sounds and blends which occur at the beginning, middle, or at the end of given words.

In nearly every subject with left cerebral damage, even though definite dysphasia may not be present, it is advisable to provide brief training in the area of auditory verbal comprehension if for no other reason than to determine whether or not the subject has particular difficulties of this type. Auditory receptive problems are particularly common in children with left hemisphere deficits and often go unrecognized.

Preliminary Research on the Effectiveness of REHABIT

As is true in many areas of psychology that have practical significance, formal research studies using proper controls have been slow to appear in validating the usefulness of REHABIT as a brain retraining procedure. Of course, many encouraging and even exciting reports of clinical improvements in individual cases have been made both among children and adults. Observations of this kind may be convincing to those who have actually seen the changes in individual brain-injured subjects, but they do not constitute adequate scientific evidence.

Dr. David Sena collected neuropsychological test results before and after use of REHABIT for brain retraining of individual subjects. He showed results on the subjects to one of us (RMR), wondering whether the apparent improvement in neuropsychological functioning might have any particular meaning. It was apparent that many of the changes went well beyond expectation either as a result of spontaneous improvement following brain injury or as a result of positive practice-effects. In some of the cases, however, individual patients had shown no improvement whatsoever.

It was apparent that some brain-injured subjects were gaining a remarkable recovery of neuropsychological functions, even though this was not happening in every case. The results were impressive in individual cases, but it was apparent that a considerable amount of investigation would be necessary in order to establish the validity of the findings.

Sena had tested his subjects initially, gave them 12 months of training with REHABIT, and then tested them again. Even though improvement had frequently occurred in the test scores, it would be necessary first to establish that this improvement extended beyond expected practice-effects and, secondly, that the improvement was greater than that expected as a result of spontaneous recovery.

In order to study these questions it would be necessary to compose two control groups: (a) normal subjects that had been tested initially and tested again 12 months later — to study positive practice-effects resulting from taking the same tests a second time, and (2) a group of brain-injured subjects who had been tested initially and had been tested 12 months later but who had not received any exposure to REHABIT or any other cognitive retraining program — to study spontaneous recovery of neuropsychological functions.

Fortunately, I (RMR) did have such groups in my files and Sena and I were able to devise a preliminary study (Reitan & Sena, 1983).

The results indicated that substantial improvement had occurred for the subjects who had been trained with REHABIT in comparison with the other two groups. The results reached levels of statistical significance on a number of variables (even considering the small number of subjects). The original investigation suggested that cognitive brain retraining using REHABIT was a definite advantage in terms of facilitating the recovery process.

Sena and his associates have continued investigation of the use of REHABIT, coupled with retraining procedures that have included ATARI games and specialized computer software. The initial study conducted by Sena (1985) evaluated a group of only 12 subjects who had sustained brain injury an average of 18.4 months before the initial evaluation. Spontaneous recovery would have been largely completed before the subjects were enrolled in the study. In addition, retesting 12 months after the initial examination may well have represented a long enough interval to minimize positive practice-effects.

The retest results indicated that these subjects showed statistically significant improvement on 31 of 39 measures, covering a broad range of neuropsychological functions. However, additional evaluation was necessary to make direct comparisons of persons who had undergone treatment with REHABIT as compared with those who had not received such treatment.

Sena and Sena (1986b) reported results in which 13 subjects had been trained with two to three sessions of REHABIT per week for one year or more and compared initial and retest results with a group of 8 subjects who had similar brain injuries but had received no cognitive retraining. Initial testing indicated that neuropsychological functions of the two groups were essentially similar before training with REHABIT was begun.

They were also similar with respect to age, education, and gender distribution. Therefore, the only known difference between the groups related to cognitive training given two to three times a week for one of the groups.

Neuropsychological re-evaluation was done for both groups 12 months after the initial examination. The group that had received no treatment showed little change in test results on retesting, earning scores essentially similar to those that were obtained initially. However, the group that had been subject to brain retraining showed significant improvement on 18 of 30 measures.

These studies also included 6 subjects who had continued cognitive brain retraining over a second year. Improvement in neuropsychological test scores from year one to year two continued on 42% of the measures, yielding evidence of statistically significant improvement on 90% of the tests in the Battery used for assessment over the two-year period. Sena and Sena (1986c) drew some inferences regarding areas of improvement during the first as compared with the second year of training, but conclusions of this nature may be premature, considering the small number of subjects involved. It does appear clear, however, that subjects with a brain injury may be retrained in basic neuropsychological functions and that the effectiveness of retraining is definite when compared with brain-injured control subjects who do not have the benefit of retraining with REHABIT.

Sena and Sena (1986a, 1986b, 1986c) have done fairly detailed studies of their groups who received and did not receive training with RE-HABIT and found essentially that there were no differences in age, gender, education, ethnic background, distribution of preferred vs. non-preferred hands, type of injury, and post-injury interval before training was begun.

Sena, Sena, and Sunde (1986a) administered an extensive range of neuropsychological tests to family members of the brain-injured sample in order to assess changes at a 12-month interval. They found that the family members who had not sustained brain damage or disease showed minimal changes in the initial test results and those obtained 12 months later.

A second study (Sena, Sena, & Sunde, 1986b) compared the changes shown by the brain-injured subjects and those of the family members, and found that the brain-injured subjects who had received cognitive retraining showed substantially more improvement than their family members.

Sena, Rakoff-Sunde, Sena and Bracken (1987) administered the Neurobehavioral Rating Scale that was developed by Levin, Overall, Goethe, High, and Sisson (unpublished manuscript, 1985) to 18 brain-damaged subjects who had received at least a year of cognitive retraining and to non-brain-injured family members. The brain-injured subjects rated only themselves in the initial phases of treatment and again after six months to one year of treatment; the family members performed self-ratings as well as ratings of the brain-injured subjects.

The initial ratings indicated that family members perceived some evidence of behavioral difficulties in the brain-injured subject but little in themselves, and the self-ratings of the brain-injured subjects were essentially similar to the ratings given to them by their family members. Self-ratings of the brain-injured subjects, made after brain-retraining had been given, showed little evidence of change. However, family members perceived more improvement in the behavior of the patients than the patients saw in themselves.

When doing self-ratings on the second evaluation, the patient's family members rated themselves as being essentially similar to the results of the first rating, although there was a trend toward a decline in the adequacy of their adjustments. These results, although based on small numbers of subjects, suggest that brain-injured individuals actually improve in their behavioral adjustments, as indicated by ratings of their family-members, but that they have little insight or understanding of this improvement (as indicated by minimal changes in their own self-ratings).

In summary, this series of studies supports a conclusion that cognitive retraining is of value in facilitating the recovery process in persons with brain injury. Of course, results presented earlier in this volume indicate clearly that spontaneous recovery following brain trauma definitely occurs during the first 12 months following the insult and is more pronounced, in terms of absolute degree of improvement, among persons who were initially more seriously impaired.

Alfano and Meyerink (1986) and Meyerink, Pendleton, Hughes and Thompson (1985) have also reported a greater degree of improvement of neuropsychological functions in brain-injured persons (N = 9) who received training oriented toward remediation of measured deficits as compared with a matched control group, most of whom had received only traditional rehabilitation therapies such as speech therapy, occupational therapy, and/ or physical therapy.

VII

THE USE OF COMPUTERS IN CLINICAL NEUROPSYCHOLOGY

A question is often raised about using computers for administration, scoring, and interpretation of the Halstead-Reitan Neuropsychological Test Battery. Two factors recommend computer-assisted interpretation: (1) the growing availability and flexibility of computers, and (2) the straightforward, original, and logical approach used in the interpretation of the test results. Except for scoring and computational procedures, we wish to caution the reader about a number of problems that exist in this area. It appears that scoring the tests and computing variables such as the Neuropsychological Deficit Scale score represent procedures for which computer application is eminently reasonable.

Two functions are currently beyond computer ability: (1) the necessary interaction between the subject and examiner in administration of the Halstead-Reitan Battery, and (2) the interpretation of the complexities and subtleties of the data for individual subjects. For this reason we have provided detailed instructions for administration of the tests (Reitan & Wolfson, 1985a) and in Volumes I and II of *Traumatic Brain Injury* we have given an extensive set of examples of clinical interpretation.

We recognize that there is great variability among neuropsychologists in their experience and competence in clinical interpretation of the data and that computers can produce general guidelines; however, computer programs which generate reports and evaluations cannot be used satisfactorily at the present time, especially considering the importance and ramifications of conclusions regarding brain-behavior relationships for the individual subject.

Mainly through the influences of Meehl (1954), a general impression has developed that statistical prediction is superior to clinical interpretation in many situations and instances. However, in clinical neuropsychological evaluation of the Halstead-Reitan Battery, clinical interpretation has regularly proved superior to statistical prediction using multivariate statistical methods (Reitan, 1964). Even a consideration of the clinical interpretations offered in Volumes I and II of *Traumatic Brain Injury* should convince the reader that much more detailed inferences can be reached by using competent clinical interpretation rather than statistical methods of classification and prediction. In clinical neuropsychology evaluation and conclusions for the individual subject appear to contradict the trends that statistical prediction is superior to clinical prediction.

The reason for this probably relates to the use of tests as a *battery* rather than as individual predictors. As we have observed repeatedly (Reitan, 1966b), a particular relationship between scores might initially suggest a lesion of one cerebral hemisphere, but at a later point in the interpretation this relationship might be too weak to support such a conclusion in the context of the other test scores. Therefore, a deficit in a particular direction might be used quite validly for an initial hypothesis, but because of its lack of power have equal validity for a later differential prediction.

In any case, it is apparent that a considerable degree of sophistication can be developed in clinical interpretation of the Halstead-Reitan Battery and it would appear that the responsible aim should be toward encouraging the widespread development of such skills among clinicians who use the Battery, rather than to run the risk of settling for a computer program which at this point in time almost certainly represents an inadequate degree of clinical expertise.

In this regard we should also note that clinical responsibility and ethics require that the psychologist who is responsible for communicating computer-generated conclusions must necessarily be in a position to evaluate the validity of these conclusions and to support them in clinical practice.

Even though there are many questions about the use of computer technology in psychological assessment, there can be no question that computers have both a present and a future in this area. A special series of articles on computerized psychological assessment was included in a 1985 issue of the *Journal of Consulting and Clinical Psychology,* and several of these articles will be referred to below. Adams and Heaton (1985) have included an article in this series that is concerned particularly with neuropsychological test data and Adams and Brown (1986) have evaluated the role of the computer in neuropsychological assessment. Interest in this area obviously is strong

among clinicians, probably stemming from the limited time they have available for administration, scoring, and interpretation of psychological test data.

Erdman, Klein, and Greist (1985) have reviewed the use of the computer in interviewing, behavioral assessment, psychiatric diagnosis, and psychotherapy. There are definite potential advantages for computers in activities that are routine and repetitive, require rapid computation, and are readily subject to simple quantification. Although a considerable amount of the patient's time may be required to answer computer-presented questions about history information, a great deal of material can be examined in this manner and easily assembled for review.

Erdman, Klein, and Greist (1985) point out that Angle, Ellinwood, and Carroll (1978) and Angle, Ellinwood, Hay, Johnsen, and Hay (1977) developed a computer system that used 3,450 questions in 29 problem areas to cover behavioral assessment in considerable detail. It required about four to eight hours for the patient to complete this interview. Although some patients may prefer to interact with a person rather than a computer, studies have suggested that patients either had no preference or actually preferred the impersonal aspect of a computer interview.

Mathematical and logical models for computer decision-making for psychiatric diagnosis also have been studied (Fleiss, Spitzer, Cohen, & Endicott, 1972) and substituting a computer for a person in psychotherapy has been explored by a number of investigators (Marks, 1978; Selmi, Klein, Greist, Johnson, & Harris, 1982; Slack & Slack, 1977; Wagman, 1980; Wagman & Kerber, 1980). These procedures have used computer programs developed for rather delimited areas of content, such as treatment of specific phobias, dilemma counseling, and treatment of depression.

A problem in this area concerns the limited capability of computers to use natural language systems and ask open-ended questions. However, it is possible to program the computer to ask a series of standard questions about psychological difficulties in selected areas and to encourage the subject to talk about specific problems after they have been identified. There is a technique to detect whether the patient is speaking and, during pauses by the patient, the computer can be programmed to make comments along the lines of encouragement and the need for additional explanation. In fact, investigations have indicated that many subjects accept this interaction with a computer and are quite willing to divulge their emotional problems and difficulties when answering computer-generated questions. Erdman, Klein, & Greist (1985), while noting the potential usefulness of such programs, also comment that it would seem possible that ethical and effective use of such programs will require the patient to have initial as well as ongoing interaction with a therapist.

Educational programs can also be presented by a computer. One study, for example, has shown that in collecting urine specimens fewer contaminating bacteria were present in the urine samples of subjects who received computer instructions than in the specimens of subjects who received either written or verbal instructions from a medical student (Fisher, Johnson, Porter, Bleich, & Slack, 1977).

Computer scoring and clinical evaluation have been used extensively in investigating personality and emotional problems of adjustment. Hofer and Green (1985) indicate that the most commonly computerized test of this kind is the Minnesota Multiphasic Personality Inventory (MMPI). Programs have been developed for interpreting many other tests in this area, including the 16 Personality Factor Questionnaire (Karson & O'Dell, 1975), the Rorschach Test (Exner, 1974; Piotrowski, 1980), the Personality Inventory for Children (Lachar, 1982; Wirt, Lachar, Klinedinst, & Seat, 1984), and the Millon Clinical Multiaxial Inventory (National Computer Systems, 1984).

Erdman, Klein, and Greist (1985) and Butcher, Keller, and Bacon (1985) review the relatively long

history of computer use in personality assessment, the frequent use of computers for clerical tasks (such as scoring and test administration), and computer-generated interpretations of the data produced by individual subjects. The clinical use of interpretations for individual patients has attracted a considerable degree of concern. In fact, Matarazzo (1983), noting the marginal involvement that is necessary for the clinician in these situations, expressed concern about the degree of responsibility that would routinely be assumed by the clinician and the problems that might accompany the clinical use of computer-generated reports by persons unqualified to use the tests properly.

Hofer and Green (1985) have reviewed many issues concerned with competent practice in the use of computerized test administration and interpretation. They note that the mode of presentation of many tests changes when they are transferred from the form in which they have been validated to computer presentation, and that very little attention has been paid to the possible effects of such changes. Frequently no studies are done to determine the equivalence of the computer-presented and the clinically-presented forms of the tests, even though it is quite likely that such differences will occur and require computation of new norms and cutting scores. At this point it should be noted that the problems cited by Hofer and Green apply not only to transformation of tests from clinical to computer presentation, but also to development of alternate forms of neuropsychological tests (such as the Category Test and the Tactual Performance Test).

Hofer and Green (1985) note that factors required in computerized administration may possibly affect test performances sufficiently that "people would not receive the same score when tested by computer than they would have received if they had been tested conventionally." They note that differences in results may occur when the subject faces a computer instead of a person in test administration, and that these differences might be related to ethnicity, gender, age, and socioeconomic status. Preliminary studies have indicated that Blacks did relatively better on a computerized version of an intelligence test although the scores for Caucasians were unchanged.

These authors conclude that careful attention must be paid to the equipment, procedures, and conditions of testing to be certain that computerized and clinical presentation of the tests yield equivalent results. The alternative would be to develop new norms and bases for interpretation of the computerized version of the test. Such steps are rarely taken, and Hofer and Green point out that the inferences made from test scores based on conventional versions of the tests are uncritically transferred to the results generated by computer administration. They note that if plausible reasons exist to doubt the equivalence of conventional and computer administered forms of a test that it will be necessary to develop new validation, normative, and cutting score data from the computerized version in order to use the test properly and ethically.

In neuropsychological testing these problems become more pronounced than when using the type of paper-and-pencil tests discussed by Hofer and Green. The examiner plays an integral role in generation of data when administering the Halstead-Reitan Battery, because the aim consistently is to elicit the best performance of which the subject's brain is capable.

Many years ago we experimented with the Category Test and automatically produced the bell (for correct responses) or the buzzer (for incorrect responses). In other words, it was not necessary for the examiner to set the controls regulating the bell or buzzer for each response. Observation of testing under these circumstances indicated that in time the examiner became less involved in the testing procedure, did not pay close attention on an item-by-item basis to the performances of the subject, and subjects appeared to develop an approach to

the test items that represented decreased concern. We did not design and carry out a study to compare results obtained with the two procedures, but our observations were sufficient to suggest strongly that we should maintain the standard procedure and have the examiner involved, item-by-item, in controlling not only the presentation of items but the bell or buzzer elicited by the patient's response.

There appears to have been a tendency in administering of psychometric instruments to permit the subject complete leeway in the degree of effort he/she invests in the test. As an extreme example of this situation, one of us (RMR) once observed a person trained in physiological and comparative psychology administer a paper-and-pencil test to a subject. The examiner observed protocol very strictly in a number of respects (wearing a white lab coat and reading the instructions from a card because "the test had always been administered in this manner"), but left the subject alone to work on the test for the allotted time. When asked what would happen if the subject sat and looked out of the window instead of working on the test, the bemused psychologist smiled and said, "She would get a low score."

In neuropsychological testing, using the Halstead-Reitan Battery, we have not been willing to presume (especially among brain-damaged patients) that an adequate degree of effort will be invested volitionally in the task at hand. It is the examiner's responsibility to make certain that the subject pays close attention to the stimulus material and makes a continuing effort to perform as well as possible.

Even those psychologists who have the most limited experience with brain-damaged subjects (or with normal subjects, for that matter) realize that a tremendous degree of variability exists among subjects in terms of their intrinsic interest, application of effort, and desire to do well. Variability in test scores will inevitably be due to such motivational factors (at least in part), but when using the Halstead-Reitan Battery it is the responsibility of the examiner to minimize such influences. It is likely that the computer will simulate the role of the comparative and physiological psychologist mentioned above to a greater extent than it will simulate a properly trained examiner.

Even without considering differences of this kind between computers and human beings in psychological test administration, Hofer and Green state (p. 836) that, "There is no substitute for the development of specific techniques of validation and evaluation appropriate to the new tests" and they correctly admonish the psychologist not to "apply a new test to real-life decisions without some kind of justifiable validity evidence. Even if the old models of validation do not apply in a straightforward way, the general idea behind construct validation, an analysis of the content of test questions, and the relation of individual differences, however represented, to criteria will provide some basis for gathering evidence showing that performance on the test is valid for making an interpretation."

Computer-Assisted Neuropsychological Evaluation

Adams and Heaton (1985) and Adams and Brown (1986) have given special attention to computer-assisted procedures in neuropsychological testing and interpretation. In addition to administrative uses, Adams and Brown point out that the computer is very useful for calculation of various parameters of the patient's performance and can readily be programmed to compute values such as IQ's and other variables. They indicate that this is the area for computer use that has the greatest promise, but at the same time appears to be the least well developed in application.

Despite the developments of computer capabilities for test administration, these authors feel that administering tests by computer changes the nature of the tests, influences the patient's perception of the procedure, and therefore changes

the testing situation. These are the types of circumstances that Hofer and Green (1985) warned about, indicating that new normative data, validational studies, and cut-off points may be required. Adams and Brown conclude (p. 89) that, "currently available programs sold along with proprietary computers for test administration are uniformly less effective or useful than their promoters suggest."

Adams and Brown indicate that there are three major approaches to computer classification or diagnosis in neuropsychology. The *taxonomic approach* identifies characteristics of the performances of the subject and uses these findings to classify the individual subject within a framework that already has been constructed. For example, if a number of syndromes or categories had been identified within the field of neuropsychology, the particular characteristics of individual neuropsychological protocols that qualify the results of an individual for these categories could be identified. If the purpose were to classify the individual according to other categories (e.g., medical or neurological diagnosis), the neuropsychological characteristics that represent the diagnostic categories could be used as a basis for classifying the individual subject.

Adams and Brown identify the neuropsychological "key" approach developed by Russell, Neuringer, and Goldstein (1970) as an example of this category. Two problems that create difficulties with the key approach concern (1) the lack of clarity in the criteria of the key, and (2) failure, in the individual instance, for the data to fit perfectly into a particular category.

A second approach identified by Adams and Brown is the *geometric/geographic procedure*. In this approach an attempt is made to develop mathematical or graphic criteria for particular classifications and to determine how well the neuropsychological findings for an individual subject fit these criteria. The procedure requires identification of characteristic cases of patients who fall in a particular category and determination of whether the results on any particular subject more closely correlate with one category or another. The geometric/geographic approach basically concerns determination of the "goodness of fit" of the individual neuropsychological protocol and classical cases which represent categories of interest. These authors identify the neuropsychological program developed by Swiercinsky (1978) as an example of this approach.

The third approach is represented by attempts to *simulate the cognitive activity of the clinician* in the analysis of neuropsychological data. Adams and Brown classify Adams' Revised Program and Brain I, the program developed by Finkelstein (1977), as examples in this category. One could question the "pureness" of these various computerized approaches for their differentiated categorization, considering the degree of overlap that actually exists among them.

Adams and Heaton identify four obstacles to automated test interpretation of neuropsychological data. First, they note that clinical neuropsychology has not yet developed to the point that there is general agreement regarding the diagnostic decisions that should be made, and that these decisions vary considerably from one patient to another.

Second, the knowledge concerning brain-behavior relationships and the application of research findings to clinical decision-making is incomplete. It is clear that in many instances research results can serve as general guides, but competence in clinical interpretation necessarily depends upon a great deal of experience with individual patients. The problem here is not concerned with possible invalidity either of research findings or of clinical interpretation; it is concerned with the uniqueness of the individual subject and limitations inherent in the generalizations that result from use of formal research methods.

Adams and Heaton identify a third obstacle which stems from the influence of demographic and other variables that influence test performances but are not related to known aspects of cerebral function or dysfunction. Such variables have been identified as age, education, and, in terms of primary motor functions, gender. Other variables that may complicate interpretation are "low innate intelligence and specific learning disabilities." Although such factors may be "obstacles" in interpretation to some persons, for neuropsychologists who are familiar with the influence of these variables on tests in the entire Battery, such factors represent an opportunity for a more detailed explanation of brain-behavior relationships.

Adams and Heaton point out that Matthews (1974) has shown that persons with low IQ's (below 80) are likely to score poorly on neuropsychological tests even though they do not have acquired cerebral disorders. There is no doubt that this is true. However, it should first be noted that there is no magic cutting point (such as an IQ of 80). Second, an orientation of this type seems limited to the aim of identifying "acquired cerebral disorders" through neuropsychological testing. IQ values can be influenced by environmental factors as well as biological factors, but it is quite possible to identify such differential influences and thereby learn more (rather than less) about the subject's ability structure.

We should also note that neuropsychological tests are essentially similar to general intelligence tests in their reflection of limited capabilities. On neuropsychological tests many people of limited ability are able to do relatively less well than persons of higher abilities; exactly this same fact applies to measures of general intelligence. Because very limited performances translate into low IQ scores in the instance of intelligence measures does not change the fact that a limited sampling of behavior was obtained.

The final point made by Adams and Heaton about the limitations of automated test interpretation is a corollary of our incomplete knowledge of the determinants of neuropsychological test performances. They caution that our limited knowledge predisposes the clinical deployment of computer programs to be premature and potentially unethical at the present time. They feel that any use of such programs must be closely supervised by a competent neuropsychologist and should be identified as *experimental.*

The existing programs, mentioned above under the three categories representing the approaches used, in fact are not able to provide any type of detailed neuropsychological interpretation. They tend to classify patients only as brain-damaged or non-brain-damaged, state which hemisphere is involved, give an opinion about whether the lesion is static or progressive, and postulate an etiology.

Answers to these questions have often been determined by a physician using neurological procedures (e.g., CT scan) before the patient is even referred to the neuropsychologist. Obviously, there is much more to neuropsychological evaluation than categorizing patients into these neurological types of categories. The basic aim in neuropsychological evaluation is to identify and assess the significance of deviations in ability structure that have consequences for adaptation to problems in living, and relate these particular deviations to biological determinants.

In their evaluation of automated interpretation of neuropsychological data Adams and Brown conclude that the three computer programs mentioned above are "inadequate as comprehensive neuropsychological experts." They view the clinical value of any of these programs as limited, and the subtleties or individual differences in lesion location, type, and severity compromise the clinical validity of the programs.

Adams and Heaton conclude that the "output of computerized interpretation programs should contain a clear disclaimer that they are *experimental* research documents and should not be considered as a substitute for a clinical report from a qualified neuropsychologist" (emphasis added). They also say that, "No responsible neuropsychologist would use any of the currently available programs for the Halstead-Reitan or LNNB as the sole basis to produce interpretations and/or reports." In fact, noting the potential for misuse of "canned neuropsychological report programs by unqualified nonpsychologists," Adams and Heaton suggest that "exclusive reliance on automated reports may never be desirable."

Although additional study certainly may lead to further refinements in their demonstrated validity, it is apparent that at this time computer-assisted procedures in neuropsychology are far from ready for ethical clinical application. In Volumes I and II of this book we have presented a number of individual case protocols and interpretations of the test results because it is imperative for neuropsychologists to develop clinical competence. In order to do this, one must study numerous cases in sufficient detail so that the interrelationships of test results and their meaning become clear.

While the cases in these two volumes involve instances of traumatic brain injury and their neuropsychological consequences, we must also remind the reader that no one can achieve expertise in clinical interpretation of the Halstead-Reitan Battery unless the consequences of other types of brain involvement (including neuropsychological deficit with unknown cause) are understood equally as well. An appreciation of the neuropsychological deficits that are characteristic of traumatic brain injury obviously requires an understanding of the deficits that characterize other conditions of brain damage as well as the neuropsychological deficits that are common to brain damage regardless of etiology.

VIII

INTERPRETATION OF INDIVIDUAL CASES

A great deal of variability in type, location, and extent of cerebral damage occurs among head-injured persons and there is corresponding variability in the resulting neuropsychological deficits. There is no way to summarize or communicate this interindividual variability except by providing extensive illustration with individual cases. Statistical constants which summarize results on groups of individuals obviously are inadequate. Presentation of a series of individual cases is the only approach that can communicate at least some of the degree of this variability that exists. Clinical skills in neuropsychological interpretation presumes an understanding of the differences as well as the similarities among persons who have sustained a traumatic brain injury, and a careful study of neuropsychological findings can serve effectively to establish the groundwork for gaining such skill.

In *Traumatic Brain Injury Volume II* we have deliberately attempted to complement the cases presented in Volume I. In addition, we have also tried to review (at least briefly) the full range of pathophysiology represented in brain injury. The cases we have presented represent mild and severe head injuries, concussion and documented tissue damage (penetrating brain injuries and contusions), men and women, and older and younger adults. The subjects also represent a range of education and occupations.

Although some of the cases included in Volume I presented results of serial examinations, all of the subjects included in Volume II were given serial examinations on a predetermined time schedule. Each subject was (1) initially examined following the brain injury, (2) re-examined 12 months after the initial examination, and (3) examined with the entire Battery a third time 18 months after the initial examination. In addition, physical neurological examinations and electroencephalograms were also done on a predetermined schedule.

Except as indicated in the case reports, none of the patients was enrolled in a formal rehabilitation program. Comparisons of the three neuropsychological examinations for each subject therefore permit an opportunity to assess and evaluate *spontaneous* neuropsychological recovery following brain injury. Serial neurological or neuropsychological evaluations in the ordinary clinical setting are often performed on subjects who have special problems and continue to be under medical care because of these problems (rather than on those individuals who recover well and do not require clinical follow-up). In this instance, however, each subject was enrolled in a formal research study and was followed regardless of his/her clinical course. The findings on these particular subjects are therefore unbiased.

We would call the reader's attention to the fact that nearly every subject shows substantial and significant improvement during the interval between the initial examination and the 12-month examination, with the individual interpretations demonstrating the clinical assessment that corresponds with group-data presented in Chapter III. The reader will also note the clinical evidence of deterioration of previously recovered abilities that occurs in many patients between the 12th and 18th month following head injury. It is important to realize the significance of the neuropsychological data obtained at later examinations for assessing impairment that was not clearly documented at the time of the initial examination. In many instances the substantial recovery shown at a later examination provides the strongest evidence to document the impairment that was present initially.

The standard sequence of serial examinations used for each of the case examples presented in this Volume provides an opportunity for the reader to identify areas of neuropsychological deficit and to assess any spontaneous improvement (or deterioration) that is demonstrated on successive examinations. As noted, these subjects were not involved in any formal program of cognitive retraining and any improvement is essentially a matter of spontaneous recovery. More specifically, the improvement may be viewed as a reflection of the natural course of recovery following head injury.

We call the reader's attention to the observation that the area of initial deficit is generally the area that shows recovery. Thus, nature's plan appears to be one of healing the wound. Although there have been many discussions of focusing rehabilitation programs on the areas of strengths (rather than the areas of deficit), it probably is important to observe that the natural course of recovery focuses on improving the areas of deficit.

Whether it is possible to improve on nature may be debated, but our recommendation is that the natural course of recovery be facilitated with cognitive retraining programs. On the face of it there seems to be little point in concentrating on areas of function that were not impaired initially (and are therefore, presumably, in no particular need of retraining), or in trying to use these areas of function to overcome, in one way or another, the area of deficit. Our experience has been that the abilities subserved by the adult brain, or its fundamental neuropsychological functions, do not have a degree of flexibility that permits substitution of one ability for another in terms of practical effectiveness of meeting problems of everyday living.

The reader will note that spontaneous recovery (nature's plan) is far from perfect in the sense that the recovery process is not absolutely continuous. In fact, the recovery process appears to be biphasic. While recovery almost invariably occurs in the area of initial deficit, the systematically organized data presented in this Volume (Chapter III) demonstrates for the first time that in the long-term process there appears to be a significant degree of deterioration of previously recovered neuropsychological functions. More specifically, some patients show deterioration of previously recovered abilities during the 12th-month to 18th-month interval following the initial examination. This finding is particularly pertinent to the programs of cognitive retraining for the individual subject. Anticipation of deterioration following initial recovery as part of the natural process emphasizes the importance of attempting to preclude this deterioration through long-term cognitive retraining efforts.

Although we have tried to be comprehensive in our interpretation of results for individual subjects, we have presumed that the reader will have at least an introductory level of clinical competence in interpretation of the Halstead-Reitan Battery. Some of the finer points of interpretation of the neuropsychological data will be unclear or perhaps entirely missed by the reader who has not had some prior experience. Obviously, the reader must be thoroughly familiar with the tests, their score ranges, and the expected inter-relationships among the variables, but explicit experience in interpretation is also recommended.

For the reader who has not had such an introduction, we strongly recommend *The Halstead-Reitan Neuropsychological Test Battery: Theory and Clinical Interpretation* (Reitan & Wolfson, 1985a), with special reference to the chapters on Guidelines to Interpretation of the Halstead-Reitan Test Battery and Normative Data as well as the clinical interpretations of individual cases. In presenting case interpretations in this Volume we have been somewhat repetitious in order to deal with each case as a complete unit. Repetition of certain points in interpretation, however, may also be advantageous inasmuch as the entire configuration of test results is different for every case.

As we have noted above, the only way to communicate the full range of information as it applies to the individual subject and assist the reader in developing skill in clinical interpretation is to provide case illustrations. In our teaching we have learned that a student's learning in this area is greatly facilitated by following a fixed procedure.

As the first step in each case evaluation we recommend that the reader review, analyze, and organize the test results. Then, before reading the history information, the neurological findings, or the interpretation of the neuropsychological data that is given in the text, we recommend that the reader study the neuropsychological test results in careful detail and attempt to determine (1) whether the individual has normal brain functions, (2) the type of neuropsychological deficits that are present and their implications concerning areas of damage in the cerebral hemispheres, and (3) whether the lesion occurred recently or enough time has elapsed for the brain to reach a degree of stable organization.

We realize that the fourteen cases presented in this Volume cannot provide comprehensive instruction in all of the neuropsychological effects of traumatic brain injury. We suggest that the reader study these cases carefully in conjunction with those presented in Volume I (Reitan & Wolfson, 1986b). An even more systematic approach to clinical interpretation would be to first study the neuropsychological results on a range of patients with various types of lesions, since different types of involvement of the brain yield at least somewhat different neuropsychological findings. The reader will become aware of the subtleties of interpretation for a particular disease entity as he/she progresses through the case illustrations.

Case #1

Name:　　C.D.

Age:　　26

Education:　10

Sex:　　　Male

Handedness:　Right

Occupation:　Truck driver

Background Information

C.D. was a 26-year-old man who was involved in a domestic fight and received gunshot wounds to the head and neck with a .22 caliber rifle. The neck wounds were not severe, but one of the bullets entered the left side of the head about 1 inch anterior to the left external ear canal. X-rays demonstrated a bullet tract extending from the left anterior temporal area to the left occipital region with two larger terminal bullet fragments lodged in the left occipital lobe.

Neurological Examination

C.D. received emergency treatment at a local hospital and within two hours of the injury was transferred to a major medical center. At that time he was in a light coma and showed evidence of disconjugate gaze. His deep tendon reflexes were symmetrical and within normal limits. He was able to move all of his extremities but had impaired motion in his right hand and arm. He did not respond to verbal commands but did respond appropriately to painful stimulation.

C.D. was taken to surgery shortly after being admitted to the medical center hospital. In addition to repair of the various neck wounds, a left subtemporal decompression and a partial anterior temporal lobectomy were performed. The patient was comatose and totally non-communicative for the next five days. On the sixth post-operative day he showed some improvement and his physician felt that he was able to understand verbal communication to some extent and possibly even perceive objects visually.

On the seventh post-operative day C.D. was restless and did not seem to be aware of his environment. However, he gradually began to improve and ten days after the injury he was able to be up in a chair. He was beginning to eat, but still did not communicate verbally in any respect. Twenty-one days after the injury he was more alert and active, but it was apparent that he was severely aphasic. He was discharged twenty-five days after the injury. At that time he was alert and seemed oriented, but he was able to speak only a few phrases.

The neurological examination done at the time of discharge demonstrated a right homonymous visual field defect with no evidence of nystagmus. The extraocular movements were intact, his muscle strength and tone were normal and equal bilaterally, and his coordination was good. However, C.D. had a pronounced expressive aphasia and it was difficult to judge his overall intellectual competence. An electroencephalogram done at this time showed evidence of severe disturbances of brain function, centering in the left anterior and mid-temporal area with variable spread to the adjacent parietal and posterior temporal areas.

Neuropsychological Examination

The initial neuropsychological examination was done seven and one-half weeks after the injury. It was not possible to obtain any information from

THE HALSTEAD-REITAN
NEUROPSYCHOLOGICAL TEST BATTERY

Patient **C.D. (I)**　Age **26**　Sex **M**　Education **10**　Handedness **R**

WECHSLER-BELLEVUE SCALE

VIQ	<50
PIQ	84
FS IQ	62
Information	1
Comprehension	0
Digit Span	0
Arithmetic	0
Similarities	2
Vocabulary	1
Picture Arrangement	10
Picture Completion	8
Block Design	8
Object Assembly	5
Digit Symbol	5

NEUROPSYCHOLOGICAL DEFICIT SCALE

Level of Performance	46
Pathognomonic Signs	26
Patterns	3
Right-Left Differences	7
Total NDS Score	82

HALSTEAD'S NEUROPSYCHOLOGICAL TEST BATTERY

Category Test	102

Tactual Performance Test

Dominant hand:	8.7
Non-dominant hand:	6.0
Both hands:	2.9

Total Time	17.6
Memory	6
Localization	3

Seashore Rhythm Test

Number Correct	16	10

Speech-sounds Perception Test

Number of Errors	(Could not do)

Finger Oscillation Test

Dominant hand:	38	38
Non-dominant hand:	36	

Impairment Index 　 **0.9**

TRAIL MAKING TEST

Part A: **70** seconds
Part B: **247** seconds
Discontinued at 6 (Circled #11)

STRENGTH OF GRIP

Dominant hand: **54.0** kilograms
Non-dominant hand: **47.5** kilograms

REITAN-KLØVE TACTILE FORM RECOGNITION TEST

Dominant hand: **18** seconds; **0** errors
Non-dominant hand: **18** seconds; **0** errors

REITAN-KLØVE SENSORY-PERCEPTUAL EXAM

			Error Totals	
RH___ LH___	Both H:	RH___ LH___	RH___ LH___	
RH___ LF___	Both H/F:	RH___ LF___	RH___ LF___	
LH___ RF___	Both H/F:	LH **1** RF **1**	RF **1** LH **1**	
RE___ LE___	Both E:	RE___ LE___	RE___ LE___	
RV **4** LV **0**	Both:	RV **4** LV___	RV **9** LV___	
4　　**0**		**4**		
0　　**0**		**1**		

TACTILE FINGER RECOGNITION

R 1___ 2___ 3 **1** 4 **2** 5___　R **3** / 20
L 1___ 2 **1** 3___ 4___ 5___　L **1** / 20

FINGER-TIP NUMBER WRITING

R 1 **1** 2 **1** 3 **1** 4 **4** 5 **2**　R **9** / 20
L 1 **1** 2 **1** 3 **2** 4 **2** 5 **1**　L **7** / 20

MINNESOTA MULTIPHASIC PERSONALITY INVENTORY } NOT GIVEN. PATIE~~NT~~ COULD NOT READ

		Hs	___
		D	___
?	___	Hy	___
L	___	Pd	___
F	___	Mf	___
K	___	Pa	___
		Pt	___
		Sc	___
		Ma	___

REITAN-KLØVE LATERAL-DOMINANCE EXAM

Show me how you:

throw a ball	R
hammer a nail	R
cut with a knife	R
turn a door knob	R
use scissors	R
use an eraser	R
write your name	R

Record time used for spontaneous name-writing:

Preferred hand	22	seconds
Non-preferred hand	40	seconds

Show me how you:

kick a football	R
step on a bug	R

RIGHT HOMONYMOUS VISUAL FIELD LOSS, MAINLY INVOLVING THE UPPER QUADRANTS.

REITAN-INDIANA APHASIA SCREENING TEST

Form for Adults and Older Children

Name: _____C. D. (I)_____ Age: __26__

Copy SQUARE Patient had great difficulty understanding instructions.	Repeat TRIANGLE "Tri-egg-sus"
Name SQUARE "Like a house you mean? Well it's black and it's white. You could lay it down underneath the water."	Repeat MASSACHUSETTS "Doggaggis"
Spell SQUARE Patient kept on saying, "Strayed" after being told the name. "T," wrote an A in the air, "R-W."	Repeat METHODIST EPISCOPAL "Mek-ed, it is."
Copy CROSS	Write SQUARE
Name CROSS "I just can't think --. It's people that live there -- the other people help people go up. If someone gets hurt, they fix you up."	Read SEVEN "C - S --"
Spell CROSS "T-R-Y---E-D"	Repeat SEVEN
Copy TRIANGLE	Repeat/Explain HE SHOUTED THE WARNING Repeat-"He shouted de ducket." Explain-"I can't think about that."
Name TRIANGLE "Guys used to be dead inside that, but I can't tell you right now."	Write HE SHOUTED THE WARNING.
Spell TRIANGLE "T-R-Y---E-D-, T-R-Y-E-D."	Compute 85 – 27 = "92." Examiner gave 56-32 and patient solved correctly.
Name BABY "Me, but small. She's waving at the left one." Examiner questioned. "Oh, a duffer?"	Compute 17 X 3 = Couldn't understand instructions. Finally said, "Oh I couldn't do that one." Examiner gave 13x3("16"); (see below)*
Write CLOCK Talked about drawing a picture of the clock, but wrote "11:00."	Name KEY "A house - put it in to turn so you're opening it."
Name FORK "That is eating, I can't say it right now."	Demonstrate use of KEY
Read 7 SIX 2 "H, six, oh, I didn't see that one, two."	Draw KEY
Read MGW "H-C-W"	Read PLACE LEFT HAND TO RIGHT EAR. "Bulk lees are his ed. No! Hayd he li-ed lees dot."
Reading I "See the because boy -- It walks around."	Place LEFT HAND TO RIGHT EAR Held up left hand - did not know where to place it.
Reading II "The-- he is a four is be. The is he a his --- that's all I can say."	Place LEFT HAND TO LEFT ELBOW Placed left hand to left ear; then, left hand to right ear.

* 4x6("101") and 2x3("12").

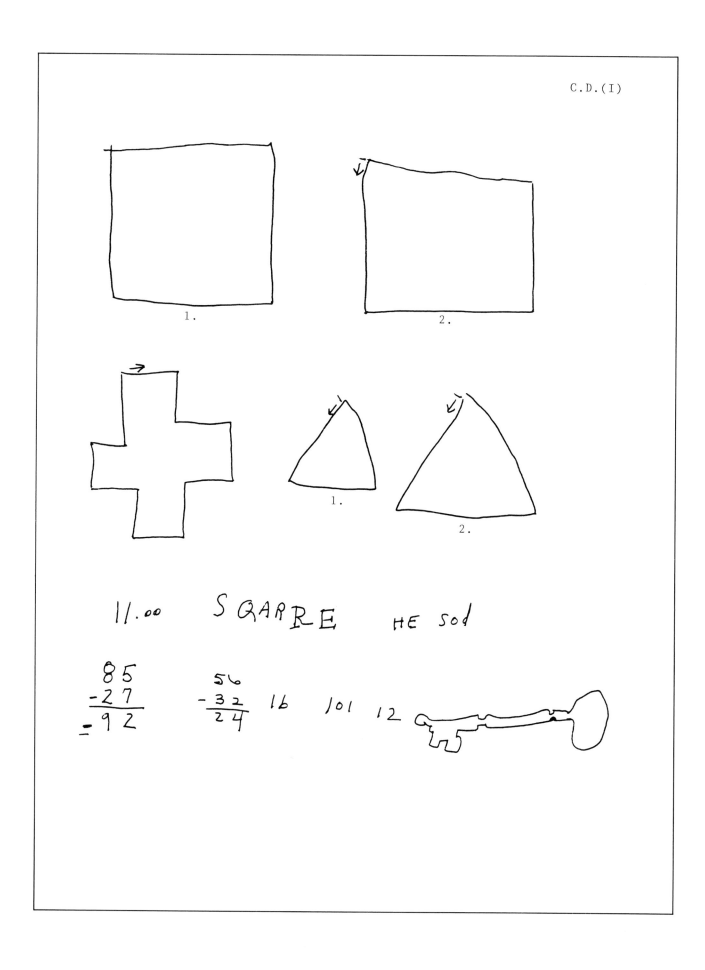

1.

2.

1.

2.

11.00   SQARRE   HE SOd

85
-27
= 92

56
-32
24   16   101   12

C.D. concerning his own assessment of his problems because of his difficulties in verbal communication. An attempt was made to obtain answers to the items on the Cornell Medical Index Health Questionnaire, but C.D. could not read the items and was not able to understand the statements when they were read to him.

In reviewing the test results for this man it may be instructive to keep in mind the nature and location of the brain lesion. The bullet was from a small calibre weapon, and information derived from x-rays as well as surgery indicated that the damage principally involved the left temporal lobe and extended to the left occipital area. Only the EEG — which showed the most prominent disturbances in the anterior and mid-temporal areas with a spread to adjacent tissue in the parietal area as well as the posterior temporal area — suggested that the lesion had more extensive biological significance. Although clearly destructive, the wound was relatively well-defined and caused by a rather discreetly penetrating missile (bullet). One might presume, then, that this lesion was better contained than a lesion caused by penetration of a larger and more generally destructive missile.

With an injury of the type that C.D. sustained, one might expect (1) profound impairment in the use of language symbols for communicational purposes, (2) distinct deficits on tasks that are sensitive to damage in any part of the cerebral cortex, (3) relative sparing of motor functions on the right side of the body, (4) comparable sparing of tactile-perceptual functions on the left side of the body (although there might be more deficits involving tactile-perceptual abilities than motor skills, considering the evidence of some possible impairment of the lower part of the parietal area), and (5) homonymous visual field losses (since the left occipital lobe was definitely damaged and bullet fragments still remained in that area).

The Wechsler Scale results indicated that C.D. showed very definite evidence of impairment, especially involving verbal intelligence. He was

aphasic, had great difficulty with expressive verbal communication, and could hardly be expected to perform normally on tests of verbal intelligence. Nevertheless, in clinical examination of the individual subject it is important to actually administer the tests, because some patients with aphasia perform much better than others and it is necessary to assess the degree of deficit for each patient. In other words, the practice sometimes adopted by certain neuropsychologists and speech pathologists of failing to measure verbal intelligence because verbal deficits are clinically obvious is not supported by findings of variability in results on individual patients.

Although C.D. earned a Performance IQ that fell in the Low Average range (84) and exceeded only about 14% of his age peers, it would be difficult to discern confidently that any impairment was present. However, the low score (5) on Digit Symbol may represent cognitive deficit, since this test is generally sensitive to cerebral damage regardless of lateralization or location. The patient had an equivalent score (5) on Object Assembly, but results on this subtest are often quite variable (probably due to the few number of items included in the subtest and the element of "luck" that differs from one person to another). Therefore, it is difficult to be certain that the low score on this measure is due specifically to cerebral damage.

Results obtained on the G-NDS (82) fell in the range of Severe Impairment and the four most sensitive indicators in the Halstead-Reitan Battery (Impairment Index, Category Test, Trails B, and Localization of the TPT) also make it quite clear that C.D. had significant impairment of generalized neuropsychological abilities. He earned an Impairment Index of 0.9 (about 90% of Halstead's tests had scores in the brain-damaged range). The only score that did not contribute to the Impairment Index was the Memory score (6) of the Tactual Performance Test. C.D. performed extremely poorly on the Category Test (102 errors) and this result cannot be attributed to the presence of aphasia. Reitan (1960) compared patients with distinct and severe aphasia with patients who had comparable brain lesions but no evidence of aphasia and found that their mean scores on the Category Test were nearly identical. Thus, the significant impairment in ability to formulate possibilities, develop hypotheses on the basis of observations, and draw meaningful conclusions (the processes involved in logical analysis) constituted a separate and very significant deficit.

C.D. demonstrated this same kind of confusion and difficulty on Part B of the Trail Making Test (247 sec), but in this instance the symbolic content of the stimulus material (numbers and letters of the alphabet) may have imposed on the area of function represented by aphasic deficits (Reitan, 1960). C.D.'s best performance on the four most sensitive general indicators was on the Localization component of the Tactual Performance Test, but even this score (3) was definitely in the range characteristic of persons with cerebral damage.

Although we can never be absolutely positive of the precise localization of cerebral damage in any case, it would appear that C.D. had sustained discrete damage principally in the left temporal area, a condition which would be expected to produce impairment on the general indicators in addition to any specific deficits.

C.D. showed serious impairment even on simple tasks that required abilities at the basic level of central processing (the ability to pay attention to specific stimulus material and maintain concentrated attention over time). One such task, the Speech-sounds Perception Test, was undoubtedly limited by C.D.'s specific manifestations of aphasia. However, he performed scarcely better than chance on the Seashore Rhythm Test (16 correct), indicating the presence of significant impairment in the test's basic requirement of paying attention over time. This indication, however, was attenuated (at least in part) by results on the Tactual Performance Test. In fact, C.D. performed quite well on the third trial of the TPT (when using both hands) and was able to remember fairly well the different shapes that were used in the test.

Except for the evidence of a right homonymous visual field loss that mainly involved the upper quadrants (corresponding with temporal lobe damage to a greater extent than parietal lobe damage), motor and sensory-perceptual skills (output and input functions) showed relatively mild impairment. Grip strength was adequate on both sides and approximately in the expected relationship (although C.D. may have been just a little weaker with his left hand than would normally have been expected). Conversely, his finger tapping speed was somewhat slow on both sides and just a little slow with the right hand (38) as compared with the left hand (36). On the Tactual Performance Test relationships between performances with the dominant hand (first trial, 8.7 min) and non-dominant hand (second trial, 6.0 min) did not deviate greatly from normal expectancy. Thus, the test results relating to motor functions confirmed the information derived from the medical evaluation and neurological surgery which suggested that the motor strip of the frontal lobe was not significantly damaged.

C.D. was somewhat slow on certain tactile-perceptual tests. On the Tactile Form Recognition Test he required a considerable amount of time to identify the figures with each hand but this may have been due to a deficit in central processing rather than tactile perception. He made two mistakes in tests of bilateral simultaneous tactile stimulation; one occurred on the left side of the body and the other was on the right side.

One might well have expected evidence of difficulty in perception of bilateral simultaneous auditory stimuli, but the patient had no difficulty with this test. This finding emphasizes one of the basic rules in neuropsychological interpretation of specific deficits: When such deficits do occur they can be depended upon to represent underlying cerebral damage; when they do not occur one is left essentially with little or no information. One cannot draw positive conclusions on the basis of negative evidence when using the "sign" approach. Therefore, the fact that this man had no difficulty perceiving bilateral auditory stimuli in no way rules out the significance of the other findings that definitely implicate the left temporal area.

Loss of visual perception, particularly in the middle and upper part of the right visual field for both eyes, precluded the ability to obtain normal results with tests for bilateral simultaneous visual stimulation. The findings, of course, were highly significant for implicating the geniculostriate pathway in the left cerebral hemisphere. As noted above, the fact that the primary visual restriction was more prominent in the upper quadrant than lower quadrant also provides positive evidence of more serious damage in the left temporal area than the left parietal area.

Finally, results of the Reitan-Kløve Sensory-perceptual Examination indicate that C.D. had mild difficulty in tactile finger localization that was more definite on the right hand (3 errors) than on the left hand (1 error). The patient also made more mistakes in finger-tip number writing perception on the right hand (9 errors) than on the left hand (7 errors), but the greater number of total errors diminished the significance of the proportional difference between the two hands (the greater number of errors may well have related to the requirement for closer attention in finger-tip number writing than in tactile finger recognition). Thus, C.D. had relatively mild impairment of motor and tactile-perceptual functions on the right side of the body as compared with the left side, essentially the results one would expect from the medical and pathological description of the lesion. Except for evidence of the right homonymous visual field loss, one might actually have had difficulty using this data to draw a definite conclusion regarding left cerebral damage.

Results of the Aphasia Screening Test yielded definite and unequivocal evidence of left cerebral damage. Before reviewing the specific findings, it would first be worth noting that C.D. is quite typical of patients with severe aphasic deficits: he showed an admixture of input (receptive) and output (expressive) deficits. In fact, in evaluating his individual responses, it often was difficult to determine the extent to which the impaired performance was due to a recognition of the stimulus material, an expression of what the patient's brain had recognized, or a combination of both.

Second, in evaluating the individual responses, it is clear that C.D. did not show discrete, separate, and specific deficits; rather, he had a general problem in dealing with the symbolic aspects of language and verbal material for communicational purposes. Despite the fact that most treatises on aphasia identify specific and discrete types of difficulties among aphasic patients, the findings noted above and characterized by this rather typical aphasic patient indicate the difficulties encountered in assigning aphasic symptoms of a specific nature to the individual subject on the basis of defective performances.

Nevertheless, theories of aphasia emphasize a great number of specific types of aphasic deficits as well as types of aphasia. The theoretical and anatomical significance of specific deficits, and even the significance of the presence of one specific deficit without another (dissociation syndrome), have been marshalled as fundamental aspects of aphasiology, despite the fact that it is hardly ever possible to effect such discrete discriminations in the individual case. Although there are unusual and quite rare cases that show highly specific losses, any tendency to base the theory and content of a discipline on unusual and rare cases (as contrasted with more typical findings) can scarcely improve the relevance of the discipline to clinically meaningful applications. For a more detailed evaluation of the theory and content of aphasiology the reader is referred to Reitan (1984).

The contention and aim underlying the evaluation of aphasia, as included in the Halstead-Reitan Battery, is to obtain meaningful information for the individual person which, in turn, is subject to integration with other data in developing an understanding of the individual's brain-behavior relationships. In this context one must also consider the particular examination for aphasia that one uses and its purpose and construction. Many of the comprehensive assessment procedures currently in use are essentially tests of verbal intelligence rather than evaluations of the subject's ability to use verbal material for communicational purposes. Admittedly, there is often a degree of overlap in these areas. In general, however, there are two approaches to the evaluation of aphasia. The first approach is concerned with an expression of level of performance on the verbal tasks, rated along the normal probability distribution in terms of adequacy of performance. The second approach is oriented toward the identification of particular deficits on simple verbal tasks (the types of errors that should not be made by a person with a normal brain). In terms of practical evaluation there is a tremendous difference in these approaches.

The Halstead-Reitan Battery utilizes both of these approaches. In this case, for example, C.D. demonstrated extremely limited verbal intelligence as measured under the formal procedures of the Wechsler Scale and, at the same time, showed a wide range of deficits on the Aphasia Screening Test. In many cases, however, the separate natures of verbal intelligence and aphasic deficits are quite clear and both areas should be evaluated in assessing the individual patient. These various issues have been discussed elsewhere in the context of a more extensive evaluation of theories of aphasia and methods for evaluating aphasia (Reitan, 1984).

A review of C.D.'s responses on the Aphasia Screening Test will substantiate the above comments. First, it is important to use the test instructions themselves, as given by the examiner, as a basis for evaluating the auditory receptive capabilities of the patient. When C.D. was asked to copy the square he had great difficulty understanding what he was being asked to do. The examiner's notation of these problems was important in identifying the presence of impaired auditory verbal comprehension (Wernicke's aphasia and also an essential feature of "fluent" aphasia).

However, C.D.'s expressive (non-fluent) aphasia became apparent when he was asked to name the SQUARE. His response ("Like a house you mean? Well it's black and it's white. You could lay it down underneath the water") is difficult to comprehend. One could not conclude from C.D.'s verbalization that he had any idea of the name of the figure. It was necessary to tell him the name of the square in order to ask him to spell the name. He was not able to repeat the word "square," but kept saying the word "strayed." Finally he began using letters but was unable to state them in a sequence that had any relation to the spelling of the word.

C.D.'s naming difficulty (dysnomia) was demonstrated quite clearly when he was asked to give the name of the CROSS. In this case his response suggested that he did understand the symbolic nature of the figure but was not able to give its name. However, he was not able to identify any of the correct letters when attempting to spell CROSS. In fact, it appeared that he was making an effort to spell TRIANGLE, although he had not yet seen this figure. His attempt to name TRIANGLE was not really comprehensible, but it was obvious that he could not give the name. In spelling TRIANGLE he began correctly with the first two letters, but then became entirely confused. His naming deficit was clear when he was asked to give the name of the baby. Possibly the patient also demonstrated some degree of right-left confusion when he said "She's waiving at the left one."

C.D. manifested further difficulty in auditory verbal comprehension when he was asked to look at the picture of the clock and write its name. As is true for many persons having left cerebral lesions and impairment in use of verbal symbols for communicational purposes, C.D. had a tendency to draw a picture of the clock. However, he only talked in very vague terms about drawing the clock and finally wrote, "11:00." It was apparent that he knew what the fork was, but was not able to give the name. He had the same kind of problem when attempting to read 7 SIX 2. Finally, he was not able to identify individual letters of the alphabet correctly. His prior responses suggested that he would have great difficulty reading either SEE THE BLACK DOG or HE IS A FRIENDLY ANIMAL, A FAMOUS WINNER OF DOG SHOWS, and this was confirmed by his attempt.

C.D. was also significantly impaired in his ability to enunciate various words. The criterion for central dysarthria is the addition, omission, or transposition of syllabic sounds in repetition of the given words. C.D. could scarcely reproduce any of the syllabic sounds involved in repeating TRIANGLE, MASSACHUSETTS, and METHODIST EPISCOPAL.

Patients who do not register verbal information well through the auditory avenue are often unable to reproduce such information. Thus, C.D.'s impairment in repeating the sentence HE SHOUTED THE WARNING is probably representative of impaired registration or a deficit in auditory verbal comprehension (auditory verbal dysgnosia). It is difficult to discern whether his inability to explain the sentence reflected the auditory verbal dysgnosia or a problem in verbal expression. All C.D. was able to say was, "I can't think about that." In either case, whether the deficit was receptive or expressive, the results are clearly indicative of impairment in the area of using language symbols for communicational purposes. In fact, C.D.'s difficulty is probably a valid indication of the admixture of input and output deficits that are commonly demonstrated by patients with aphasic losses.

In adult subjects impairment in dealing with simple arithmetical processes and confusion in the symbolic significance of numbers has been found to occur about four times more frequently in persons with left cerebral damage than persons with right cerebral damage (Wheeler & Reitan, 1962). Even though he was correct in one instance, C.D. obviously was confused when trying to perform simple arithmetical problems. These difficulties clearly manifest the presence of dyscalculia.

It was apparent that C.D. knew what a key was, but his response made it equally apparent that he was not able to identify it by name. This is quite typical of patients with a significant naming problem.

C.D. again manifested his difficulty in reading when asked to read PLACE LEFT HAND TO RIGHT EAR. From his response it is difficult to know whether he had any conception of the symbolic significance of the printed material (a significant receptive loss) or whether his problem was in saying the words that demonstrated his understanding (an expressive loss). Because it is necessary for the individual subject to both register the material as well as respond to it, with central processing serving as an intermediary, it is often difficult to determine precisely where the deficit lies for the individual patient. In fact, in many patients with aphasia, it is very likely that both receptive and expressive losses are present simultaneously.

C.D. demonstrated an inability to recognize body parts (body dysgnosia). Again, a problem exists in differentiating between impairment in auditory verbal comprehension (auditory verbal dysgnosia) and confusion regarding body parts (body dysgnosia). On the next item, however, C.D. seemed definitely to confuse body parts as well as right and left sides. As shown by Wheeler and Reitan (1962), right-left confusion and body dysgnosia both relate principally to left cerebral damage.

Finally, C.D.'s difficulty in writing and arithmetic (principally left cerebral dysfunctions) are apparent. He also showed significant impairment in the ability to copy simple spatial configurations, a deficit manifested particularly by the disparity of the extremities in his drawing of the cross and in the confusion with the spatial representation of details of the key.

Difficulties in drawing customarily are related to right cerebral hemisphere dysfunction rather than left cerebral damage; however, Wheeler and Reitan (1962) found that a significant proportion of persons with left cerebral lesions also had problems with drawing simple figures. Further analysis of these cases indicated that when aphasic difficulties were obviously present in conjunction with significant impairment in drawing simple spatial configurations, the lesion was more likely to be in the left cerebral hemisphere than the right. In fact, aphasic patients who demonstrate particular difficulty in drawing simple spatial configurations in addition to their language problems tend to have lesions in the posterior part of the language area. Thus, in this case, we would be inclined to attribute C.D.'s drawing difficulties to involvement of the posterior temporal areas, taking into consideration the very pronounced additional indications of impairment in the use of language symbols for communicational purposes. In other words, in this particular instance, the difficulties with reproducing simple figures, considered in conjunction with the aphasic manifestations, do not require postulation of a specific lesion in the posterior part of the right cerebral hemisphere.

Considering the deficits shown by C.D. and the neurological (as well as behavioral) evidence that the frontal lobe was probably minimally involved and the parietal area was relatively spared, it is of interest to review C.D.'s deficits. He had very pronounced losses of both a receptive and expressive nature in terms of language communicational skills. The deficits relating to auditory verbal comprehension, well recognized in the literature, probably relate to damage in the posterior language area of the left cerebral hemisphere. Expressive verbal deficits (such as dysnomia) have often been attributed to involvement in the posterior-inferior part of the left frontal lobe (Broca's area). There

has been a remarkable persistence among aphasiologists in attribution of expressive aphasic deficits to Broca's area, even though Broca's own patients had lesions that were considerably more extensive, and in fact involved the temporal lobe. While Broca's area is of definite significance with respect to expressive language disorders, it is important to recognize that this area does not necessarily need to be involved and that similar kinds of expressive aphasic manifestations may occur even among patients with anterior left temporal lobe damage (Reitan, 1984).

To summarize C.D.'s performances on the Aphasia Screening Test, we would note that C.D. had demonstrated (1) a failure to be able to understand verbal communications through the auditory avenue — a sign of damage in the posterior part of the language area *(auditory verbal dysgnosia)*, (2) obvious difficulty in giving the names of common objects *(dysnomia)*, (3) confusion about using letters in their proper sequence to represent the spelling of words *(spelling dyspraxia)*, (4) confusion in identification of individual letters of the alphabet *(visual letter dysgnosia)*, (5) inability to read simple material *(dyslexia)*, (6) inability to repeat various words and enunciate certain sounds *(central dysarthria)*, (7) inability to perform arithmetical operations and recognize the symbolic significance of numbers *(dyscalculia)*, (8) inability to recognize parts of the body *(body dysgnosia)*, (9) *right/left confusion*, and (10) inability to copy simple shapes *(constructional dyspraxia)*.

Three months after the initial neuropsychological testing C.D. was again given a physical neurological examination and an electroencephalogram was done. He continued to demonstrate severe aphasia, with more expressive than receptive difficulty. Confrontational testing of the visual fields still showed a right homonymous hemianopia. It was not possible to elicit definite evidence of motor dysfunction, but the deep tendon reflexes were greater in the right upper extremity than the left, and when walking the patient showed evidence of a greater spontaneous swinging of the left arm than the right arm and the right fingers were held in a more flexed position. The examiner also noted that C.D. seemed to be rather anxious, laughed often, and in fact appeared "silly" in his general responsiveness.

At this time the electroencephalogram was very similar to the tracings obtained at the time of the first neuropsychological examination. C.D. continued to show very severe disturbance of brain function, principally involving the anterior and middle areas of the left temporal lobe, with lesser abnormalities extending through the temporal lobe to the posterior parts of the left cerebral hemisphere. When compared with the tracings obtained earlier, this EEG showed slight improvement.

By the time of the 12-month examination, C.D. had developed epilepsy and had experienced five major motor seizures. He reported that he experienced a "loud noise in his head" before these seizures began. He had had this same kind of "loud noise" on several other occasions, but the aura was not always followed by convulsive activity.

The neurological examination showed evidence of a very mild hyperreflexia on the right side, pronounced expressive aphasia, mild receptive aphasia, and a right homonymous hemianopia. Although the neurologist felt that this right homonymous visual field defect was present, confrontational mapping of the visual fields during the neuropsychological examination was judged to be unreliable. In addition, the patient manifested no difficulty in tests of bilateral simultaneous visual stimulation, correctly responding above eye level, at eye level, and below eye level with both unilateral stimulation and bilateral simultaneous stimulation. Thus, C.D.'s ability to respond correctly to stimuli in the complete visual fields would suggest that the prior evidence of right homonymous hemianopia had shown significant evidence of improvement.

EEG tracings at the time of the 12-month examination showed definite improvement even though there was still a very severe widespread disturbance of brain function, principally involving the left anterior and middle temporal areas. When questioned, C.D. indicated that there were no major or significant changes in his life during the past year. He had been unable to return to any type of regular work and said that he spent his time around the house and yard doing minor jobs and working on his car.

A review of the test findings for the second neuropsychological examination indicates that C.D. had (1) a much lower Verbal IQ (50) than Performance IQ (90), (2) pronounced aphasic deficits of both a receptive and expressive nature, (3) serious impairment of higher-level aspects of brain functions, and (4) relatively minimal involvement of motor and sensory-perceptual skills. Even though definite evidence of brain damage was still present, the G-NDS score had decreased from 82 (severe impairment) to 60 (moderate impairment).

It was clear to the neuropsychological examiner that C.D. had significant difficulties understanding the test instructions and it was frequently necessary for the examiner to repeat the instructions. C.D. understood that he should interrupt the examiner and insist on receiving further information if anything was unclear to him. However, we followed strict adherence to Wechsler's procedure in administration of the Wechsler-Bellevue Scale and under these circumstances the patient was able to make very little progress on the Verbal subtests. This was partly due to his impaired ability to comprehend the verbal communications from the examiner during the formal test, partly due to his own difficulty in responding verbally, and partly due to the actual impairment in the area of central processing of verbal symbols. C.D.'s Performance IQ (90) probably also reflected a degree of impairment resulting from cerebral damage, but it would be difficult to draw this conclusion confidently from the distribution of Performance subtest scores alone.

THE HALSTEAD-REITAN
NEUROPSYCHOLOGICAL TEST BATTERY

Patient ___C.D. (II)___ Age __27__ Sex __M__ Education __10__ Handedness __R__

WECHSLER-BELLEVUE SCALE

VIQ	50
PIQ	90
FS IQ	67

Information	2
Comprehension	1
Digit Span	0
Arithmetic	1
Similarities	1
Vocabulary	0

Picture Arrangement	8
Picture Completion	7
Block Design	9
Object Assembly	10
Digit Symbol	7

NEUROPSYCHOLOGICAL DEFICIT SCALE

Level of Performance	34
Pathognomonic Signs	18
Patterns	3
Right-Left Differences	5
Total NDS Score	60

TRAIL MAKING TEST

Part A: __75__ seconds
Part B: __252__ seconds

STRENGTH OF GRIP

Dominant hand: __68.5__ kilograms
Non-dominant hand: __64.0__ kilograms

REITAN-KLØVE TACTILE FORM RECOGNITION TEST

Dominant hand: __14__ seconds; __0__ errors
Non-dominant hand: __11__ seconds; __0__ errors

REITAN-KLØVE SENSORY-PERCEPTUAL EXAM — No errors

Error Totals

RH ___ LH ___	Both H: RH ___ LH ___	RH ___ LH ___
RH ___ LF ___	Both H/F: RH ___ LF ___	RH ___ LF ___
LH ___ RF ___	Both H/F: LH ___ RF ___	RF ___ LH ___
RE ___ LE ___	Both E: RE ___ LE ___	RE ___ LE ___
RV ___ LV ___	Both: RV ___ LV ___	RV ___ LV ___

TACTILE FINGER RECOGNITION

R 1___ 2___ 3___ 4___ 5___ R __0__ / __20__
L 1___ 2___ 3___ 4___ 5___ L __0__ / __20__

FINGER-TIP NUMBER WRITING

R 1___ 2___ 3___ 4___ 5___ R __0__ / __20__
L 1___ 2___ 3___ 4 _2_ 5___ L __2__ / __20__

(PATIENT USED A MULTIPLE-CHOICE METHOD TO
POINT TO THE NUMBER REPRESENTING HIS ANSWER)

VISUAL FIELD MAPPING WAS UNRELIABLE.

HALSTEAD'S NEUROPSYCHOLOGICAL TEST BATTERY

Category Test		94

Tactual Performance Test

Dominant hand:	11.6	
Non-dominant hand:	7.0	
Both hands:	5.2	
	Total Time	23.8
	Memory	6
	Localization	0

Seashore Rhythm Test

Number Correct	12	10

Speech-sounds Perception Test

Number of Errors	34

Finger Oscillation Test

Dominant hand:	43	43
Non-dominant hand:	38	

Impairment Index	0.9

MINNESOTA MULTIPHASIC PERSONALITY INVENTORY

NOT GIVEN. P
COULD NOT R

		Hs	___
		D	___
?	___	Hy	___
L	___	Pd	___
F	___	Mf	___
K	___	Pa	___
		Pt	___
		Sc	___
		Ma	___

REITAN-KLØVE LATERAL-DOMINANCE EXAM

Show me how you:
throw a ball	R
hammer a nail	R
cut with a knife	R
turn a door knob	R
use scissors	R
use an eraser	R
write your name	R

Record time used for spontaneous name-writing:
Preferred hand	13 seconds
Non-preferred hand	31 seconds

Show me how you:
kick a football	R
step on a bug	R

REITAN-INDIANA APHASIA SCREENING TEST

Form for Adults and Older Children

Name: _____ C. D. (II) _____ Age: __27__

Copy SQUARE	Repeat TRIANGLE
Name SQUARE	Repeat MASSACHUSETTS "Monkachess"
Spell SQUARE "Four different sides." Had difficulty understanding instructions. Then "Q-A-R." Finally, "E."	Repeat METHODIST EPISCOPAL "Mensacussis"
Copy CROSS	Write SQUARE
Name CROSS "Is it a Q? I know what it used to be."	Read SEVEN
Spell CROSS "C----- or G,P." Clearly confused. Then, C-R-O-S-E."	Repeat SEVEN
Copy TRIANGLE	Repeat/Explain HE SHOUTED THE WARNING. Repeat: "He shouted at -- sun." Could not explain.
Name TRIANGLE "Is it a V? They had three of them."	Write HE SHOUTED THE WARNING. Could not write. Examiner had to repeat each word individually.
Spell TRIANGLE "T-R-" could not go on and wanted to write. See attempt.	Compute 85 – 27 = Didn't know the meaning of minus or equal sign. Asked, "Take away?"
Name BABY "A young one -- a he and she."	Compute 17 X 3 = Responded verbally, "21." Attempted computation and wrote incorrectly. Given 10 x 2 and done correctly.
Write CLOCK Could not think of how to write. Said, "Quack -- Quack" -- then "clock."	Name KEY "Lock or open?" Couldn"t name.
Name FORK " Eat with it."	Demonstrate use of KEY
Read 7 SIX 2 " 7-6. Oh, excuse me -- 7-6-2."	Draw KEY
Read MGW	Read PLACE LEFT HAND TO RIGHT EAR. "Place let hand to right ear."
Reading I	Place LEFT HAND TO RIGHT EAR Raised left hand Didn't know what else to do. Finally put left hand on right palm.
Reading II "He is a furno anno, a fãmõs winner of dog. " Patient didn't see SHOWS. Examiner pointed out and patient said "show."	Place LEFT HAND TO LEFT ELBOW Placed left hand on right thigh.

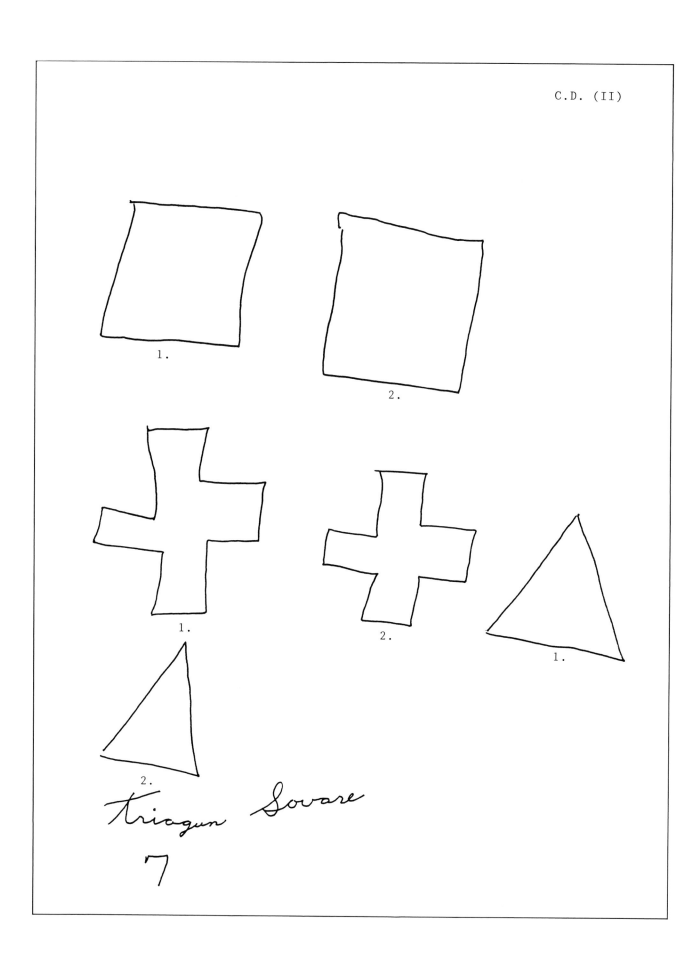

Ite shoting the worning.

$$\begin{array}{r} 85 \\ -27 \\ \hline 58 \end{array} \quad = \quad \frac{\times 7}{\times 5}$$

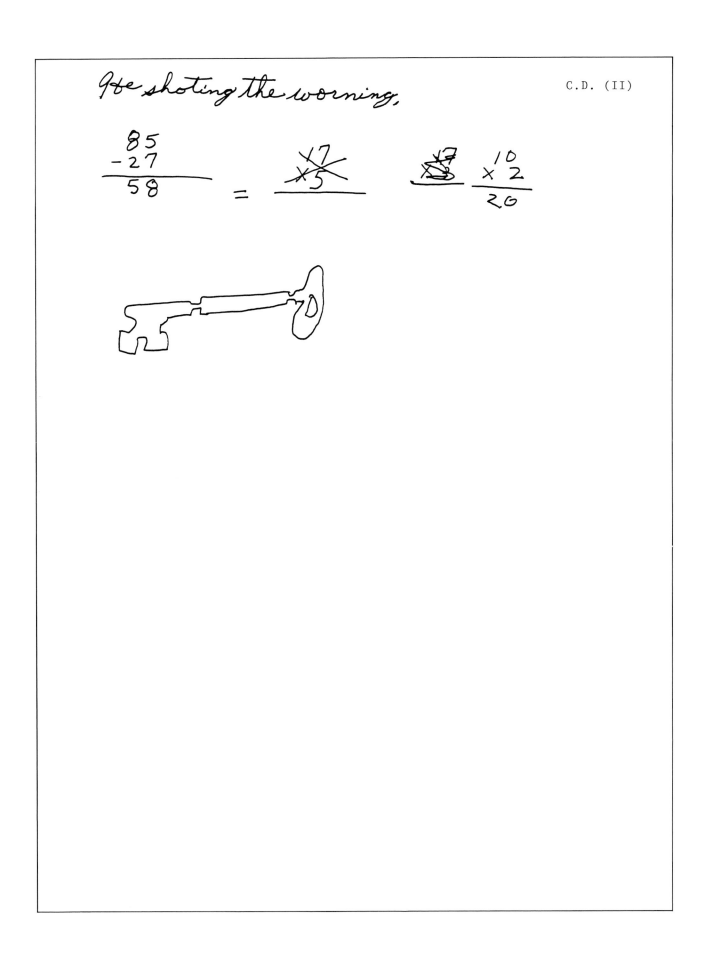

C.D.'s generalized deficits were pronounced, as indicated by the G-NDS score of 60, an Impairment Index of 0.9, 94 errors on the Category Test, a score of 252 seconds on Part B of the Trail Making Test, and an inability to localize any of the figures used in the Tactual Performance Test. In fact, we would judge that the patient was significantly impaired even in the fundamental requirement of central processing that relates to ability to focus attention to specific stimulus material and maintain concentration over time.

C.D.'s aphasic manifestations were also pronounced. A review of his attempts to name common objects indicated that he had a severe dysnomia. Auditory verbal dysgnosia was apparent to the examiner when she attempted to give instructions for the various procedures and C.D. also revealed his difficulty in registering simple verbal material in various ways throughout the test. C.D. demonstrated an inability to produce appropriate letters for spelling words (spelling dyspraxia), and even though he was able to do very simple reading, he easily became confused and demonstrated dyslexia.

Certain responses suggest that C.D. had a tendency to fail to perceive the right side of stimulus configurations. When he was asked to read "7 SIX 2" he responded initially only to "7" and "SIX" before recognizing that the complete response included the "2." On the second reading item he obviously was confused (probably both on a receptive and expressive basis), but he did not respond to the last word in the sequence. It appeared to the examiner that he did not notice the word "SHOWS," which falls to the far right of the bottom line. When the examiner pointed out this word the patient appeared to be somewhat surprised and said "show." It is not at all uncommon for patients with right cerebral lesions to have difficulties perceiving the left side of stimulus configurations, but this type of difficulty, relating to perception of the right side of space in patients with left cerebral lesions, is seen much less frequently. The fact that such difficulties can in fact happen on the right side of spatial configurations in persons with left cerebral lesions is documented by the results shown by this man.

C.D. showed definite evidence of central dysarthria in his attempts to repeat MASSACHU-SETTS and METHODIST EPISCOPAL. His difficulty in registering verbal material through the auditory avenue (auditory verbal dysgnosia) was apparent when he tried to repeat and explain HE SHOUTED THE WARNING. Because C.D.'s writing ability was limited by poor spelling it is somewhat difficult to judge whether he manifested evidence of dysgraphia. A judgment of this kind is not of specific significance concerning diagnostic conclusions because both spelling dyspraxia and dysgraphia have similar implications for left cerebral damage.

Note that C.D. also demonstrated obvious dyscalculia, body dysgnosia (confusing his elbow and his thigh), and right/left confusion. Each of these deficits also has significance for left cerebral damage rather than right cerebral damage. Right-left confusion is often present in patients with relatively mild left cerebral deficits but body dysgnosia usually implies the presence of a wider range of deficits of greater severity.

Finally, C.D. showed evidence of mild constructional dyspraxia, but, as mentioned earlier, his difficulties in this respect may well have been due to involvement of the posterior part of the language area. His level of ability to copy simple spatial configurations was roughly equivalent to that demonstrated at the initial examination.

A direct comparison of the initial examination and 12-month testing indicated that C.D. showed improvement in a number of respects, as manifested by the change in the G-NDS from 82 to 60, but he continued to perform at the same level in other areas and was somewhat worse on some measures. General indicators showing improvement included Part B of the Trail Making Test and possibly the Category Test (although this measure may have benefitted only from positive practice-effect). Motor and sensory-perceptual functions were improved bilaterally (especially with the right hand). The improvement in grip strength probably was due to a general increase in activity level.

C.D. was somewhat quicker in tactile form recognition (especially with the left hand) and showed very significant improvement (particularly with the right hand) in tactile finger localization and finger-tip number writing perception. As mentioned above, conflicting evidence was present for the right homonymous hemianopia, but it is likely that the patient's visual fields had improved significantly. He also performed somewhat better on the Speech-sounds Perception Test, improving from complete inability to perform the task to earning a score of 34 (which still represents significant impairment). In addition, C.D. may have shown marginal improvement, over and beyond positive practice-effect, on the IQ measures.

Despite evidence of a degree of improvement, some of the tests reflected changes that go beyond chance variation and indicate deterioration. These findings were most apparent on various aspects of the Tactual Performance Test. C.D. required significantly more time on the first trial (right hand) and the third trial (both hands), and these changes were reflected in an increased Total Time score. In addition, while he had been able to localize three of the figures correctly in his first drawing, he was not able to localize any at all on the second examination. Finally, although he had achieved essentially only a chance performance on the Seashore Rhythm Test on the first examination, his present score (12 correct) was somewhat worse than would be expected even on a chance basis.

In summary, the overall results for this man, who had significant and serious damage of left cerebral cortical tissue, showed improvements in certain respects and some evidence of deterioration. Twelve months after the initial neuropsychological examination C.D. demonstrated continued serious neuropsychological deficits.

Between the 12-month and the 18-month examinations C.D. had two additional major motor seizures. He continued to identify a strange sensation in his head which preceded these seizures, but also said that he had this sensation on other occasions. The neurologist was impressed with C.D.'s improved affective state, feeling that C.D. was behaving in a much more appropriate (i.e., less silly) manner.

C.D. continued to demonstrate expressive aphasia (which the neurologist judged to be considerably improved) and receptive aphasia (which was considered to be at about the same relatively mild level). The neuropsychological examiner found evidence of right homonymous hemianopia. An electroencephalogram done at this time continued to show wide-spread abnormalities which were most prominent in the middle and posterior areas of the left cerebral hemisphere. A comparison with the previous tracings indicated definite improvement.

Upon questioning, C.D. said that over the past six months there had been no particular changes in his living pattern and that things were about the same. Although it was still necessary to communicate with him very carefully when giving the instructions for the various neuropsychological tests, it seemed possible to perform the examinations validly.

The general configuration of the test results on the 18-month examination was essentially similar to the findings obtained earlier. C.D. had a limited Verbal IQ (55) as compared with his Performance IQ (89), showed significant impairment on indicators of the general adequacy of cerebral functioning, had pronounced aphasic deficits, and demonstrated some signs of impairment on the right side of the body when compared with the left side of the body. Thus, the findings continued to be indicative of much more severe impairment of the left cerebral hemisphere than the right cerebral hemisphere.

THE HALSTEAD-REITAN
NEUROPSYCHOLOGICAL TEST BATTERY

Patient __C.D. (III)__ Age __28__ Sex __M__ Education __10__ Handedness __R__

WECHSLER-BELLEVUE SCALE

VIQ	55
PIQ	89
FS IQ	69
Information	3
Comprehension	1
Digit Span	3
Arithmetic	0
Similarities	2
Vocabulary	5
Picture Arrangement	11
Picture Completion	7
Block Design	8
Object Assembly	9
Digit Symbol	5

NEUROPSYCHOLOGICAL DEFICIT SCALE

Level of Performance	40
Pathognomonic Signs	26
Patterns	3
Right-Left Differences	13
Total NDS Score	82

HALSTEAD'S NEUROPSYCHOLOGICAL TEST BATTERY

Category Test	85

Tactual Performance Test

Dominant hand:	17.5
Non-dominant hand:	9.7
Both hands:	11.9
Total Time	39.1
Memory	9
Localization	4

Seashore Rhythm Test

Number Correct	20	10

Speech-sounds Perception Test

Number of Errors	42

Finger Oscillation Test

Dominant hand:	44	44
Non-dominant hand:	37	

Impairment Index __0.9__

TRAIL MAKING TEST

Part A: __56__ seconds
Part B: __207__ seconds

STRENGTH OF GRIP

Dominant hand: __51.0__ kilograms
Non-dominant hand: __58.0__ kilograms

REITAN-KLØVE TACTILE FORM RECOGNITION TEST

Dominant hand: __15__ seconds; __0__ errors
Non-dominant hand: __13__ seconds; __0__ errors

REITAN-KLØVE SENSORY-PERCEPTUAL EXAM

		Error Totals
RH ___ LH ___	Both H: RH ___ LH ___	RH ___ LH ___
RH ___ LF ___	Both H/F: RH _2_ LF ___	RH _2_ LF ___
LH ___ RF ___	Both H/F: LH ___ RF ___	RF ___ LH ___
RE ___ LE ___	Both E: RE ___ LE ___	RE ___ LE ___
RV _4_ LV _0_	Both: RV _4_ LV ___	RV _4_ LV ___
0 0		
0 0		

TACTILE FINGER RECOGNITION

R 1___ 2 _1_ 3___ 4___ 5___   R _1_ / 20
L 1___ 2___ 3___ 4 _2_ 5___   L _2_ / 20

FINGER-TIP NUMBER WRITING

R 1 _1_ 2 _2_ 3 _1_ 4 _1_ 5 _1_   R _6_ / 20
L 1 _2_ 2___ 3 _1_ 4___ 5 _2_   L _5_ / 20

MINNESOTA MULTIPHASIC PERSONALITY INVENTORY
NOT GIVEN. PA[T] COULD NOT RE[AD]

?	___	Hs	___
L	___	D	___
F	___	Hy	___
K	___	Pd	___
		Mf	___
		Pa	___
		Pt	___
		Sc	___
		Ma	___

REITAN-KLØVE LATERAL-DOMINANCE EXAM

Show me how you:
throw a ball	R
hammer a nail	R
cut with a knife	R
turn a door knob	R
use scissors	R
use an eraser	R
write your name	R

Record time used for spontaneous name-writing:
Preferred hand	16 seconds
Non-preferred hand	58 seconds

Show me how you:
kick a football	R
step on a bug	R

A DEFECT WAS APPARENT IN EACH RIGHT
UPPER QUADRANT.

REITAN-INDIANA APHASIA SCREENING TEST

Form for Adults and Older Children

Name: _C. D. (III)_   Age: _28_

Copy SQUARE	Repeat TRIANGLE "Dri-tri-ang."
Name SQUARE	Repeat MASSACHUSETTS "Mit-al-etshetts-mitchaloss"
Spell SQUARE "G-no, S--no wait, I left out some in the middle. (Long pause) "H-E-R."	Repeat METHODIST EPISCOPAL
Copy CROSS	Write SQUARE
Name CROSS "I've driven those. There's one in Bremerton. I know what they are."	Read SEVEN
Spell CROSS "G-R-O-S-S"	Repeat SEVEN
Copy TRIANGLE	Repeat/Explain HE SHOUTED THE WARNING. Asked to have the sentence repeated. Then, OK. Explanation-SEE BELOW *
Name TRIANGLE "X-no --." (Could not think of name and told Triangle.) "That's right!"	Write HE SHOUTED THE WARNING. "Say the last one, warling." Could not write.
Spell TRIANGLE Asked examiner to repeat the same several times. Finally said, "Say it again and I'll write it." See his attempts.	Compute 85 − 27 = "60." See.
Name BABY "That's a young one."	Compute 17 X 3 = "21." See.
Write CLOCK Patient made a few movements over the paper, but was not able to write.	Name KEY "That's open a door - and I can't say the name."
Name FORK "When he was eating." Then drew the table setting.	Demonstrate use of KEY
Read 7 SIX 2 "Seven, sink, no-psych, no-psych-two."	Draw KEY
Read MGW "W-G-W." Corrected quickly and said, "I said that dumb - stupid - different."	Read PLACE LEFT HAND TO RIGHT EAR. "Placet let hand do rigth - right, rig - the last one - ear."
Reading I	Place LEFT HAND TO RIGHT EAR "I know what ear is." Pulled right ear and then left ear, both with right hand. Then put right index finger in right ear.
Reading II "He is a fidelly-fiddel amil-and after that its wax, waxer, wixer-none of those are right-of dog show-shove,shoves."	Place LEFT HAND TO LEFT ELBOW SEE BELOW **

* "In other words it could be real loud like 1,2,3,4,5,6 or working out in the house tree(then put his hand to his mouth as if he were shouting).

* Asked examiner to repeat instructions several times. Couldn't comprehend what was wanted.

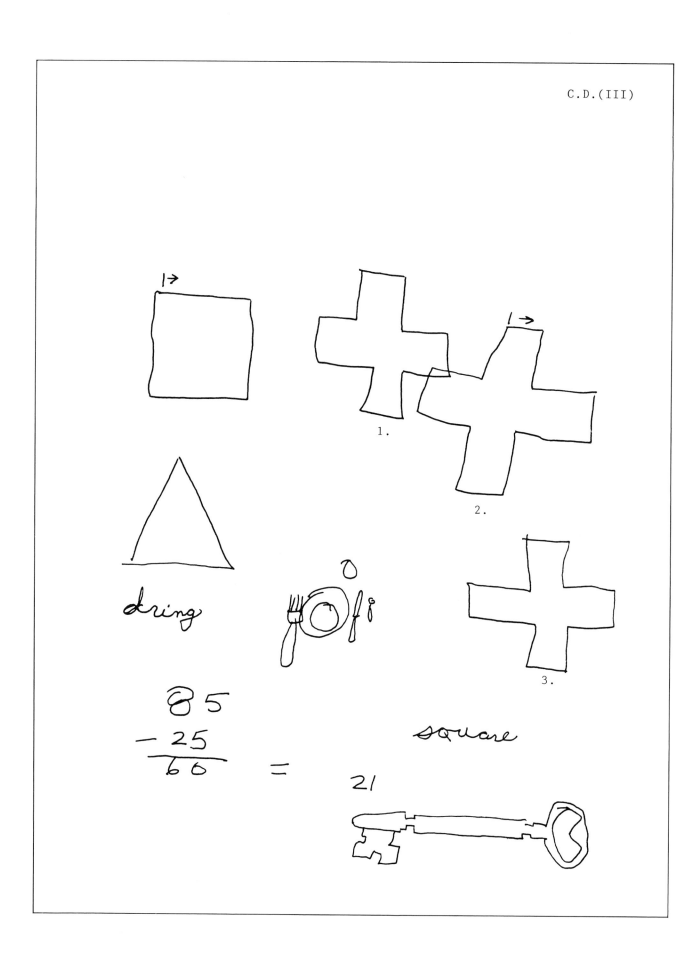

1.

2.

3.

dring

square

85
− 25
───
66   =

21

The four most sensitive general indicators and the G-NDS all had scores within the range of brain-damaged performances. C.D. earned a G-NDS score of 82 and an Impairment Index of 0.9, with only the Memory component of the Tactual Performance Test (9) falling in the normal range. The general indicators therefore demonstrate the presence of significant and serious impairment of abilities dependent upon brain functions.

Even though C.D. did not perform particularly well on the Performance subtests, the lateralizing indicators would include the significantly impaired Verbal IQ value. Undoubtedly, the impairment on the Verbal IQ is due, at least in part, to specific deficits (aphasia) in use of language symbols for communicational purposes.

In addition, lateralizing indicators were also present on comparisons of performances on the two sides of the body. On the Tactual Performance Test C.D. performed quite poorly with his right hand (17.5 min) as compared with his left hand (9.7 min). It is also of significance to observe that the third trial, using both hands, was done worse (11.9 min) than the second trial, using only the left hand (9.7 min). It would appear that using the impaired (right) upper extremity in the third trial actually interfered with the efficiency of performance in placing the blocks.

Other lateralizing signs implicating the left cerebral hemisphere included a grip strength that was significantly less with the right side (51 kg) than the left side (58 kg), impairment in perception of a tactile stimulus to the right hand when a stimulus was given simultaneously to the left face, and a loss in the upper part of the right visual field for each eye (right homonymous quadrantanopsia).

No lateralizing signs of any significance were present to implicate the right cerebral hemisphere. C.D. was somewhat slow in finger tapping speed with his left hand (37) as compared with his right hand (44), but this finding considered by itself cannot be used as a basis for postulating significant impairment of the right cerebral hemisphere.

In summary, the general indicators showed quite clearly that C.D. had significant impairment of adaptive abilities dependent upon brain functions. The lateralizing indicators, including the evidence of significant and severe dysphasia, made it quite clear that the left cerebral hemisphere was primarily involved. In fact, on the basis of the present findings, one would principally implicate the left temporal lobe (on the basis of the strong expressive and receptive aphasic deficits), but it is also likely that other areas might be involved: the posterior part of the frontal lobe (reduced grip strength with the right upper extremity), the left parietal area (impaired perception of a tactile stimulus to the right hand when given simultaneously with a stimulus to the left face), and the geniculostriate tract as it courses through the white matter of the left temporal lobe (right homonymous quadrantanopsia). Thus, the neuropsychological test results continued to reflect the initial information concerning the location of cerebral damage resulting from the gunshot wound.

Direct comparison of the 18-month examination results with the findings obtained previously showed improvement on some measures, similar scores on other tests, and definite deterioration on a number of tasks. Overall, the change in G-NDS scores from 60 to 82 indicates a significant degree of deterioration. Even though his Verbal IQ continued to be very low (55), we would estimate that C.D. had shown some improvement on the Verbal subtests of the Wechsler Scale. He also was a little quicker, suggesting more alertness on Part B of the Trail Making Test (from 252 sec to 207 sec). He definitely improved his Memory score (from 6 to 9) and Localization score (from 0 to 4) on the Tactual Performance Test and was considerably better in differentiating between rhythmic pairs of beats on the Seashore Rhythm Test (20 correct). We would estimate that he showed no significant changes on the Performance IQ subtests, that the mildly improved score (from 94 to 85) on the Category Test was probably due only to positive practice-effect, and that finger tapping speeds were essentially similar with both hands.

There were, however, other changes in the test results that led to an overall evaluation of progressive impairment rather than improvement. C.D. required much more time in total on the Tactual Performance Test than he had at the 12-month examination (from 23.8 min to 39.1 min) and he had shown some additional impairment on this measure from the initial examination to the 12-month examination (from 17.6 min to 23.8 min). Thus, C.D. demonstrated a progressive pattern of overall impairment on this task. He performed more poorly on each of the three trials, but manifested striking deficits with his right upper extremity. His right hand was being used in both the first and third trials, and these were the two trials that were particularly poorly done in comparison with results obtained at the 12-month examination.

C.D.'s grip strength also was reduced, especially with the right upper extremity (from 68.5 kg to 51.0 kg). On the second examination he had shown no evidence of impairment in perception of bilateral simultaneous stimuli, but at the 18-month examination he again found it difficult to perceive a tactile stimulus to his right hand when it was given simultaneously with a stimulus to the left face. It should also be noted that the number of errors made on the Speech-sounds Perception Test increased from 34 to 42. All of these findings suggest some degree of deterioration in the functional status of the left cerebral hemisphere, reflected by a change on the Right-Left section of the G-NDS which deteriorated from 5 to 13 points.

It is difficult to judge whether C.D. showed more significant or serious dysphasia on the 18-month examination than on the 12-month examination. An overall evaluation of the results suggests that the third examination may demonstrate more significant dysphasia, but it must be remembered that on successive individual examinations the same aphasic patient still not uncommonly shows some degree of variability in the specific results obtained, even though the overall interpretation would be essentially similar (Head, 1926; Reitan, 1984). There can be no question, however, that the overall results of the third neuropsychological testing indicate progressive deterioration (at least in certain respects) of left cerebral functioning.

It should also be noted that C.D. also did worse on measures of tactile finger localization and finger-tip number writing perception, although the additional impairment on these measures did not have any particular lateralizing significance.

In summary, C.D., who sustained significant structural damage (particularly in the left temporal and occipital areas), showed marked deficits in line with expectations on the initial examination. On the 12-month examination he improved on a number of tests but also showed some evidence of progressive impairment on other measures (with a general finding of more improvement than impairment). On the 18-month examination he reversed this trend, showing improvement on some measures but deterioration on a greater number of measures. The overall set of results on the 18-month examination clearly indicated that the recovery process was not continuous; rather, it suggested further deterioration of the underlying biological stratum of the brain during the interval between the 12-month and 18-month testings. These results are consistent with and exemplary of the deterioration that often occurs during the 12 to 18 month interval following structural damage of brain tissue (as documented statistically in Chapter III).

Case #2

Name: D.D.

Age: 19

Education: 12

Sex: Male

Handedness: Right

Occupation: Tire repairman

Background Information

This 19-year-old man was changing a tire when the rim flew off and struck him in the head. He sustained deep lacerations on his face and hands and was immediately rendered unconscious by the blow. D.D. was taken directly to a hospital where more careful examination of the facial laceration indicated a 1 cm depression above the left supraorbital ridge, exuding cerebrospinal fluid and exposing brain tissue.

D.D. was immediately taken to surgery for repair of his injuries. The surgical report indicated that the frontal compound depressed skull fracture involved the frontal and ethmoidal sinuses and the medial wall of the right orbit and nasal bone. In addition, D.D. had a left frontal lobe laceration and contusion and it was necessary to surgically remove some necrotic cortical tissue from the left frontal pole. The right frontal pole was also exposed but no gross evidence of damage was apparent. The patient was totally unconscious for four days following the injury and did not regain full orientation for about seven days.

Neurological Examination

Neurological examination at the time of discharge from the hospital (two weeks after the injury) revealed that D.D. was fully alert and oriented with no amnesia for events preceding the injury or after regaining orientation. The examination yielded no evidence of aphasia. D.D.'s visual fields were full but he had a continuous diplopia, caused in part by a lateral displacement of the medial wall of the right orbit and a paresis of both right and left medial rectus muscles and the right superior oblique muscle. No other neurological abnormalities were noted.

In summary, this man had a penetrating injury of the brain with contusion of the left frontal pole that required removal of necrotic cortex. The first neuropsychological examination was done the day following full recovery of orientation (one week post-injury).

Neuropsychological Examination

The tests results indicate that D.D. (1) had probably developed intelligence levels within the range of normal variation, (2) may have experienced some impairment on certain subtests of the Wechsler Scale, (3) showed generalized impairment of neuropsychological functions, (4) had findings implicating left cerebral hemisphere dysfunction, and (5) had indications of right cerebral damage.

Considering the fact that the cortex of the left frontal pole had been lacerated and necrotic tissue had been removed, one may have expected more striking evidence of left cerebral damage. On the other hand, it is possible that the damage in the left frontal area was discrete and well-contained and that the major manifestations of neuropsychological deficit would reflect the more general effects of the head trauma.

D.D. earned a Verbal IQ (95) in the lower part of the Average range (exceeding 37% of his age

THE HALSTEAD-REITAN
NEUROPSYCHOLOGICAL TEST BATTERY

Patient **D.D. (I)** Age **19** Sex **M** Education **12** Handedness **R**

WECHSLER-BELLEVUE SCALE

VIQ	95
PIQ	89
FS IQ	92
Information	8
Comprehension	7
Digit Span	4
Arithmetic	13
Similarities	11
Vocabulary	8
Picture Arrangement	8
Picture Completion	10
Block Design	10
Object Assembly	10
Digit Symbol	6

NEUROPSYCHOLOGICAL DEFICIT SCALE

Level of Performance	27
Pathognomonic Signs	4
Patterns	2
Right-Left Differences	13
Total NDS Score	46

HALSTEAD'S NEUROPSYCHOLOGICAL TEST BATTERY

Category Test — 58

Tactual Performance Test

Dominant hand:	16.3
Non-dominant hand:	8.0
Both hands:	4.8

Total Time	29.1
Memory	8
Localization	5

Seashore Rhythm Test

Number Correct **21** — 10

Speech-sounds Perception Test

Number of Errors — 12

Finger Oscillation Test

Dominant hand:	49	49
Non-dominant hand:	42	

Impairment Index 0.7

TRAIL MAKING TEST

Part A: **49** seconds
Part B: **120** seconds

STRENGTH OF GRIP

Dominant hand: **18.5** kilograms
Non-dominant hand: **51.0** kilograms (HAND INJURY)

REITAN-KLØVE TACTILE FORM RECOGNITION TEST

Dominant hand: **16.5** seconds; **1** errors
Non-dominant hand: **10.5** seconds; **0** errors

REITAN-KLØVE SENSORY-PERCEPTUAL EXAM

			Error Totals	
RH___ LH ___	Both H: RH___ LH ___	RH___ LH ___		
RH___ LF ___	Both H/F: RH___ LF ___	RH___ LF ___		
LH___ RF ___	Both H/F: LH___ RF ___	RF___ LH ___		
RE___ LE ___	Both E: RE___ LE ___	RE___ LE ___		
RV___ LV ___	Both: RV___ LV ___	RV___ LV ___	NOT DONE DUE TO DIPLOPIA	

TACTILE FINGER RECOGNITION

R 1___ 2___ 3___ 4___ 5___ R **0 / 20**
L 1___ 2___ 3___ 4___ 5___ L **0 / 20**

FINGER-TIP NUMBER WRITING

R 1 **2** 2 **1** 3 **1** 4 ___ 5 ___ R **4 / 20**
L 1 **3** 2 **2** 3 **3** 4 **1** 5 **1** L **10 / 20**

MINNESOTA MULTIPHASIC PERSONALITY INVENTORY

		Hs	53
		D	63
?	50	Hy	51
L	40	Pd	62
F	62	Mf	55
K	55	Pa	50
		Pt	60
		Sc	80
		Ma	58

REITAN-KLØVE LATERAL-DOMINANCE EXAM

Show me how you:

throw a ball	R
hammer a nail	R
cut with a knife	R
turn a door knob	R
use scissors	R
use an eraser	R
write your name	R

Record time used for spontaneous name-writing:

Preferred hand	**12** seconds
Non-preferred hand	**49** seconds

Show me how you:

kick a football	R
step on a bug	R

REITAN-INDIANA APHASIA SCREENING TEST

Form for Adults and Older Children

ame: _____ D. D. (I) _____ Age: ___19___

Copy SQUARE	Repeat TRIANGLE
Name SQUARE	Repeat MASSACHUSETTS
Spell SQUARE	Repeat METHODIST EPISCOPAL
Copy CROSS	Write SQUARE
Name CROSS	Read SEVEN
Spell CROSS "C-R-O-S-E"	Repeat SEVEN
Copy TRIANGLE	Repeat/Explain HE SHOUTED THE WARNING.
Name TRIANGLE "Pyramid." Examiner questioned. "Square."	Write HE SHOUTED THE WARNING.
Spell TRIANGLE	Compute 85 – 27 =
Name BABY	Compute 17 X 3 =
Write CLOCK	Name KEY
Name FORK	Demonstrate use of KEY
Read 7 SIX 2	Draw KEY
Read MGW	Read PLACE LEFT HAND TO RIGHT EAR.
Reading I	Place LEFT HAND TO RIGHT EAR
Reading II "He is a family animal, a famous winner of dog shows."	Place LEFT HAND TO LEFT ELBOW

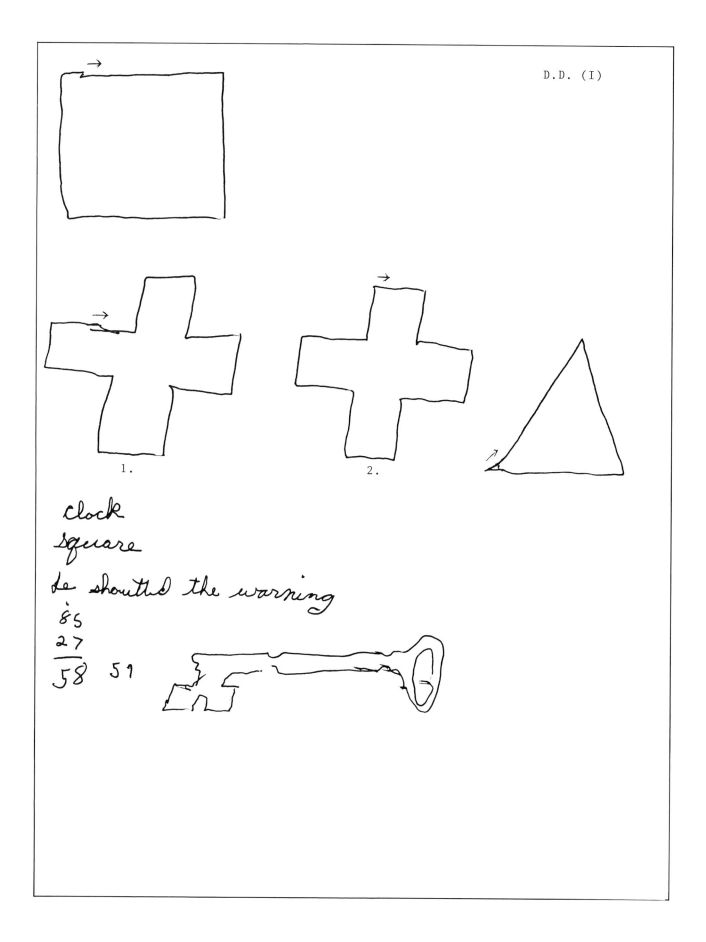

1.

2.

clock

square

he shouted the warning

85
27
----
58   51

peers) and a Performance IQ (89) in the upper part of the Low Average range (exceeding 23%). These values yielded a Full Scale IQ (92) in the lower part of the Average range (exceeding 30%). The subtest scores indicate that D.D. performed somewhat poorly on the Digit Span (4) and Digit Symbol (6) subtests. It is not unusual to find low scores on the Digit Span subtest in hospitalized patients, including persons without cerebral disease or damage. However, for this man, the low Digit Symbol score is probably a valid reflection of brain damage. It is unusual to see such a good Arithmetic score (13) in a person with cerebral damage; however, as we have previously remarked, even though the Arithmetic subtest is probably the most sensitive of the Verbal subtests, it is not a particularly good indicator of cerebral dysfunction. Therefore, the Wechsler Scale does not provide a very comprehensive description of the neuropsychological functions dependent upon the biological condition of the brain and, of course, was never developed with such a specific purpose in mind.

D.D. performed relatively poorly on the four most sensitive indicators in the Halstead-Reitan Battery. He earned an Impairment Index of 0.7 (about 70% of the tests had scores in the brain-damaged range). He also performed almost as poorly as the average brain-damaged subject on the Category Test (58). Although his score on Part B of the Trail Making Test (120 sec) was deficient, his score (5) on the Localization component of the Tactual Performance Test was surprisingly good. However, an inspection of the actual drawing of the TPT board indicates that D.D. was somewhat confused about the spatial configuration represented by the board and blocks and, in fact, drew the board in a horizontal (rather than vertical) position. Usually this kind of confusion contributes to a low Localization score, but in this case the patient had a somewhat fortuitous arrangement of the figures.

D.D.'s degree of general alertness, represented by his scores on the Seashore Rhythm Test (21 correct) and Speech-sounds Perception Test (12 errors), was adequate, even though both scores were in the impaired range and contributed to the Impairment Index.

Lateralizing indicators were present to implicate each cerebral hemisphere. D.D.'s grip strength was quite poor with his right hand (18.5 kg) compared with his left (51.0 kg), but it was apparent that it was painful for him to squeeze the dynamometer because of the laceration on his hand; the examiner noted that the results did not reflect the patient's actual muscular strength. Although D.D. was not noticeably impaired on other tests that required motor functions of the right upper extremity, he performed quite poorly with the right hand (16.3 min) compared with the left (8.0 min) on the Tactual Performance Test. But note also that this lateralized deficit was not limited to motor performances; it was also clearly manifested by impairment of the right hand (16.5 sec) compared with the left (10.5 sec) on the Tactile Form Recognition Test.

The patient demonstrated mild deficits on the Aphasia Screening Test. He was confused in spelling CROSS and writing SHOUTED. When asked to give the name of the TRIANGLE, he first responded by saying "Pyramid." After the examiner asked for another possible name he responded "square." Finally, D.D. manifested a mild confusion in reading HE IS A FRIENDLY ANIMAL, A FAMOUS WINNER OF DOG SHOWS. For some reason, it is not unusual for persons with a left-hemisphere limitation of reading skills to substitute the word FAMILY for FRIENDLY in reading this sentence. Although D.D. showed no gross indications of aphasia (confirming the findings of the neurological examination), he demonstrated some mild difficulties in the ability to deal with language symbols for communicational purposes when his responses were compared to those of thousands of patients with brain lesions as well as control subjects to whom the same standardized procedures had been administered.

Even though the indications of right cerebral dysfunction were relatively mild, they were nevertheless quite definite. Probably the most reliable indicator occurred on the test for finger-tip number writing perception. D.D. had some difficulty on his right hand (4 errors), which may have reflected damage of the left cerebral hemisphere, but he made many more errors (10) on the left hand. The results of this particular test indicated that D.D. had more significant difficulty in the parietal area of the right cerebral hemisphere than in the homologous area on the left cerebral hemisphere. He also was somewhat slow in finger tapping speed with his left hand (42) compared with his right (49) and had difficulty copying simple spatial configurations (even though constructional dyspraxia was not scored on the G-NDS).

We would postulate that D.D. had also sustained damage in the middle part of his right cerebral hemisphere in addition to having dysfunction in the left cerebral hemisphere. Therefore, the overall results are quite characteristic of persons with craniocerebral trauma: reasonably adequate IQ levels, evidence of general impairment, and lateralizing indicators that implicate each cerebral hemisphere.

The G-NDS recapitulated these conclusions with a score of 46 points, which falls in the range of Moderate Impairment. In addition to the 27 points contributed by the Level of Performance indicators (versus 11.95 points for the average control subject), D.D. also accrued 4 points on the Pathognomonic Signs section (even though we conservatively elected not to classify his drawing difficulties as constructional dyspraxia) and 13 points on Right-Left Differences (versus 3.37 points for the average control subject).

On the Cornell Medical Index Health Questionnaire D.D. had relatively few complaints in total. However, he did indicate that he tends to get nervous and shaky when approached by a superior, that strange people and places frighten him, that it bothers him to eat anywhere except in his own home, that he often feels sad, alone, unhappy, and depressed, and often cries, that his feelings are easily hurt, that he is misunderstood by others and upset by criticism, that he must be on guard even with his friends, that people often annoy and irritate him, and that it makes him angry to have anyone tell him what to do. These responses go beyond the complaints of most control subjects but it is difficult to be certain that they have any direct relationship to the effects of the brain injury.

Except for the elevated score (80) on the Schizophrenia scale, the scores on the Minnesota Multiphasic Personality Inventory were essentially within the normal range. From these findings it would seem possible that D.D. has some deviant attitudes about himself and others, that he may be somewhat confused in terms of his immediate perceptions of his environment, and may be mildly depressed.

As is true for most persons with craniocerebral trauma, D.D.'s deficits were fairly widely distributed in terms of their reference to various areas of the brain and neuropsychological functions. In his rehabilitation, D.D. should receive training in (1) using language symbols for communicational purposes, (2) redeveloping his alertness to specific stimulus material and his ability to maintain concentrated attention over time, (3) dealing with tasks that require abstraction, reasoning, logical analysis skills and the ability to keep several elements of a situation in mind at the same time, and (4) dealing with tasks that involve visual-spatial relationships. With neuropsychological deficits involving both cerebral hemispheres, it would appear that the full range of higher-level training activities included in REHABIT should be undertaken. Even though spontaneous recovery almost certainly will take place, it is always advantageous to add specific brain retraining procedures, especially in the areas of the individual's particular needs, in order to facilitate the total recovery process.

The same extensive battery of neuropsychological tests was readministered to this man 12

THE HALSTEAD-REITAN
NEUROPSYCHOLOGICAL TEST BATTERY

Patient __D.D. (II)__ Age __20__ Sex __M__ Education __12__ Handedness __R__

WECHSLER-BELLEVUE SCALE

VIQ	114
PIQ	121
FS IQ	119
Information	11
Comprehension	9
Digit Span	13
Arithmetic	13
Similarities	13
Vocabulary	8
Picture Arrangement	15
Picture Completion	14
Block Design	12
Object Assembly	12
Digit Symbol	13

NEUROPSYCHOLOGICAL DEFICIT SCALE

Level of Performance	7
Pathognomonic Signs	0
Patterns	1
Right-Left Differences	4
Total NDS Score	12

TRAIL MAKING TEST

Part A: __26__ seconds
Part B: __76__ seconds

STRENGTH OF GRIP

Dominant hand: __57.5__ kilograms
Non-dominant hand: __54.5__ kilograms

REITAN-KLØVE TACTILE FORM RECOGNITION TEST

Dominant hand: __7.0__ seconds; __0__ errors
Non-dominant hand: __7.5__ seconds; __0__ errors

REITAN-KLØVE SENSORY-PERCEPTUAL EXAM — No errors

Error Totals

RH___LH___	Both H:	RH___LH___	RH___LH___		
RH___LF___	Both H/F:	RH___LF___	RH___LF___		
LH___RF___	Both H/F:	LH___RF___	RF___LH___		
RE___LE___	Both E:	RE___LE___	RE___LE___		
RV___LV___	Both:	RV___LV___	RV___LV___		

TACTILE FINGER RECOGNITION

R 1___ 2___ 3___ 4___ 5___   R __0__ / 20
L 1___ 2___ 3___ 4 _1_ 5___   L __1__ / 20

FINGER-TIP NUMBER WRITING

R 1___ 2___ 3___ 4 _1_ 5___   R __1__ / 20
L 1___ 2___ 3___ 4___ 5___   L __0__ / 20

HALSTEAD'S NEUROPSYCHOLOGICAL TEST BATTERY

Category Test		25

Tactual Performance Test

Dominant hand:	5.4	
Non-dominant hand:	3.8	
Both hands:	1.6	
	Total Time	10.8
	Memory	7
	Localization	2

Seashore Rhythm Test

Number Correct	25	6

Speech-sounds Perception Test

Number of Errors	4

Finger Oscillation Test

Dominant hand:	58	58
Non-dominant hand:	49	

Impairment Index __0.1__

MINNESOTA MULTIPHASIC PERSONALITY INVENTORY

		Hs	44
		D	64
?	50	Hy	55
L	43	Pd	58
F	46	Mf	47
K	51	Pa	68
		Pt	57
		Sc	53
		Ma	55

REITAN-KLØVE LATERAL-DOMINANCE EXAM

Show me how you:
throw a ball	R
hammer a nail	R
cut with a knife	R
turn a door knob	R
use scissors	R
use an eraser	R
write your name	R

Record time used for spontaneous name-writing:
Preferred hand	10	seconds
Non-preferred hand	41	seconds

Show me how you:
kick a football	R
step on a bug	R

NO APHASIC SYMPTOMS.

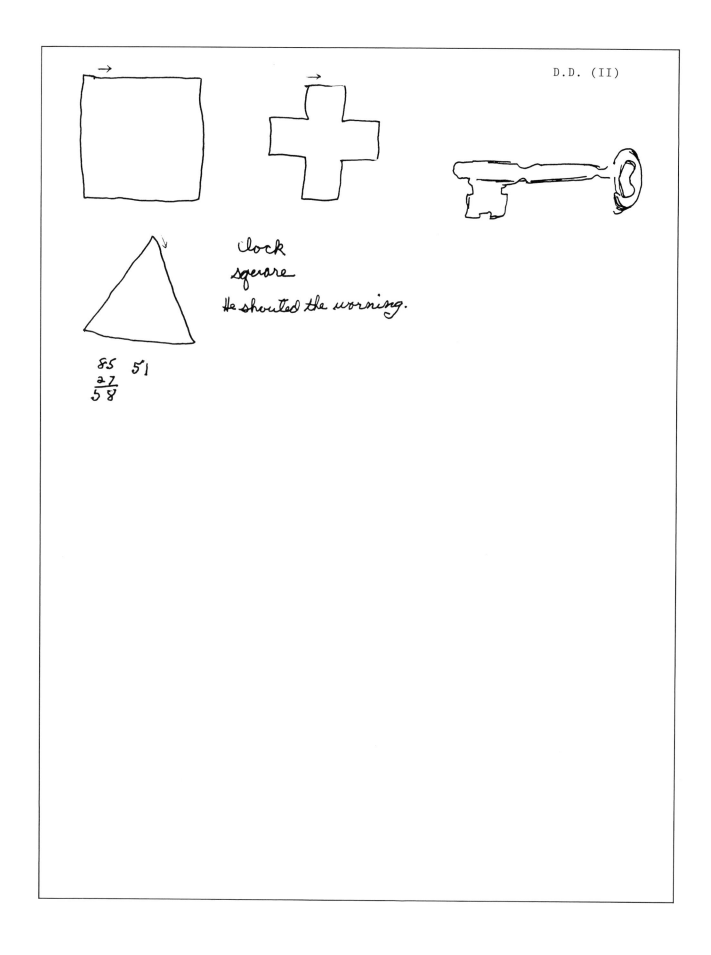

clock

square

He shouted the warning.

85   51
27
58

months after the initial examination. Before directly comparing the results of the two testings we will review the second set of findings, keeping in mind that some degree of positive practice-effect may have occurred.

D.D. earned a Verbal IQ of 114 , which falls in the middle part of the High Average range and a Performance IQ (121) just within the limits of the Superior range. Various studies have indicated that practice-effects cause an increment of about three points on Verbal IQ and five points on Performance IQ when a subject is retested. Therefore, in this case, these IQ values are probably an overestimate of the patient's actual general intelligence levels. Nevertheless, D.D. showed striking improvement in both Verbal and Performance IQ values.

D.D. performed relatively well on the general indicators of cerebral functioning, earning scores within the normal range on the Impairment Index (0.1), the Category Test (25), and Part B of the Trail Making Test (76 sec). On the Tactual Performance Test his Total Time (10.8 min) was well within the normal limits and he performed satisfactorily on the Memory component (7). However, he did not do well on the Localization component (2).

D.D.'s general alertness and his ability to focus his attention was adequate, as indicated by his scores on the Seashore Rhythm Test (25 correct) and the Speech-sounds Perception Test (4 errors). He was also able to pay close attention in tests of tactile finger localization and finger-tip number writing perception and made very few errors. In summary, the general results suggest that D.D. had adequate capabilities on measures of general intelligence as well as on tests of adaptive abilities dependent upon immediate problem-solving capabilities of the brain. This conclusion was convincingly reflected by a change on the Level of Performance indicators of the G-NDS from 27 points on the initial testing to 7 points on the 12-month examination.

Lateralizing deficits on the second examination were not impressive. D.D. demonstrated no aphasia and the only indicator that might possibly implicate the left cerebral hemisphere was a somewhat decreased grip strength with the right hand (57.5 kg) compared with the left (54.5 kg). However, the implications of this finding for cerebral damage are lessened by the fact that the patient was obviously strong on both sides of his body. Except for a somewhat slow finger tapping speed with the left hand (49) compared with the right (58) there were no indications of specific right cerebral dysfunction. The patient's drawings were also within normal limits. He showed no deficits on the Performance intelligence measures, and in the context of the other test results it would be clinically incorrect to judge that the somewhat slow finger tapping speed with the left hand is an indication of right cerebral dysfunction. These results were reflected by normal scores on the additional sections of the G-NDS.

Overall, the test results for this man obtained 12 months after he sustained cerebral damage were essentially within the range of normal variation. It is possible, of course, that some of the scores might still reflect a degree of impairment from pre-morbid levels, but this conclusion cannot be drawn from the current findings.

Looking at the changes that occurred on the results between the first and second neuropsychological testings, we see that D.D. consistently performed better on the second examination. His Verbal IQ increased 19 points, his Performance IQ gained 32 points, and his Impairment Index improved from 0.7 to 0.1. He made only 25 errors on the Category Test (compared with 58), reduced the time required on Trails B from 120 seconds to 76 seconds, and indicated that he was more alert by improving his Seashore Rhythm Test score from 21 correct responses to 25. It is also possible that on the Speech-sounds Perception Test the reduction of errors from 12 to four may have represented some improved left cerebral functioning. The patient's score on the Schizophrenia scale of the MMPI was reduced from 80 to 53.

The only score that showed a worse performance was the Localization score on the Tactual Performance Test. D.D. was able to localize five figures correctly on the first examination and presently could correctly localize only two figures. Despite a lower score on this measure, the patient's drawing actually appeared to be better organized and more realistic on the second examination. The Localization score on the first testing had been viewed as being artificially inflated because of fortuitous relationships among the figures in the drawing. The present result on this test may represent some residual deficit, but in the context of the rest of the test results, certainly does not constitute evidence of significant generalized impairment.

D.D. initially demonstrated positive signs of cerebral damage to each cerebral hemisphere. However, the results on the second Aphasia Screening Test demonstrated no evidence of aphasic disorders. Facility in Tactile Form Recognition had improved with each hand (principally with the right), and grip strength had increased remarkably with the right upper extremity (although the initial deficit was probably due to the injury of the hand rather than left cerebral damage). D.D. had also shown so much improvement in his drawings that they were now within normal limits. The number of errors in finger-tip number writing perception decreased on each hand (especially the right). Finally, although he continued to demonstrate somewhat slow finger tapping speed with the left hand (49) compared with the right (58), D.D. improved his finger tapping speed with each hand.

We had originally concluded that the test results indicated generalized impairment of neuropsychological functions and suggested that D.D. had sustained damage in each cerebral hemisphere. On the second examination D.D. demonstrated improvement quite consistently on

nearly all measures and it would appear that he showed generalized improvement of neuropsychological functions. The scores on the second examination were well beyond improvement expected from positive practice-effect and, since there is no evidence to support a hypothesis that cerebral damage is therapeutic or is likely to produce a sudden improvement in brain-related abilities, it is likely that the patient initially had higher ability levels than he demonstrated on the initial testing and that general recovery of neuropsychological functions had occurred in the interval between examinations.

D.D. was given the same battery of tests 18 months after the original examination. At this time he was thinking about enrolling in college and had no particular complaints.

Although D.D. had shown a striking increase in both Verbal and Performance IQ values between the first two testings, he showed minimal change on these measures on the 18-month (third) examination. He also demonstrated very similar results on the Impairment Index and the Category Test, but showed greater alertness and quickness on Part B of the Trail Making Test and performed significantly better on the Localization component of the Tactual Performance Test. It would appear, then, that the patient either was holding his own or perhaps improving somewhat in terms of general indicators of neuropsychological abilities.

Notice, though, that certain test results raise a question of whether there may have been some mild deterioration of brain functions. Except for a somewhat slow finger tapping speed with the left hand compared with the right, there had been essentially no significant lateralizing indicators in the prior set of test results. However, there were some unusual findings on the third examination that implicate the left cerebral hemisphere. For example, the patient's grip strength with his right upper extremity (55.5 kg) was essentially no better than with his left upper extremity (55.0 kg) and on the Finger-tip Number Writing Perception Test

THE HALSTEAD-REITAN
NEUROPSYCHOLOGICAL TEST BATTERY

Patient __D.D. (III)__ Age __20__ Sex __M__ Education __12__ Handedness __R__

WECHSLER-BELLEVUE SCALE

VIQ	114
PIQ	122
FS IQ	120
Information	11
Comprehension	11
Digit Span	14
Arithmetic	13
Similarities	10
Vocabulary	8
Picture Arrangement	14
Picture Completion	13
Block Design	13
Object Assembly	14
Digit Symbol	13

NEUROPSYCHOLOGICAL DEFICIT SCALE

Level of Performance	3
Pathognomonic Signs	0
Patterns	1
Right-Left Differences	6
Total NDS Score	10

TRAIL MAKING TEST

Part A: __23__ seconds
Part B: __48__ seconds

STRENGTH OF GRIP

Dominant hand: __55.5__ kilograms
Non-dominant hand: __55.0__ kilograms

REITAN-KLØVE TACTILE FORM RECOGNITION TEST

Dominant hand: __12__ seconds; __0__ errors
Non-dominant hand: __11__ seconds; __0__ errors

REITAN-KLØVE SENSORY-PERCEPTUAL EXAM — No errors

Error Totals

RH___ LH___	Both H:	RH___ LH___	RH___ LH___		
RH___ LF___	Both H/F:	RH___ LF___	RH___ LF___		
LH___ RF___	Both H/F:	LH___ RF___	RF___ LH___		
RE___ LE___	Both E:	RE___ LE___	RE___ LE___		
RV___ LV___	Both:	RV___ LV___	RV___ LV___		

TACTILE FINGER RECOGNITION

R 1___ 2___ 3___ 4___ 5___ R __0__ / __20__
L 1___ 2___ 3___ 4___ 5___ L __0__ / __20__

FINGER-TIP NUMBER WRITING

R 1 __2__ 2 __1__ 3___ 4___ 5___ R __3__ / __20__
L 1___ 2___ 3___ 4___ 5___ L __0__ / __20__

HALSTEAD'S NEUROPSYCHOLOGICAL TEST BATTERY

Category Test __23__

Tactual Performance Test

Dominant hand: __5.4__
Non-dominant hand: __4.3__
Both hands: __2.1__

Total Time	11.8
Memory	9
Localization	8

Seashore Rhythm Test

Number Correct __25__ __6__

Speech-sounds Perception Test

Number of Errors __4__

Finger Oscillation Test

Dominant hand: __56__ __56__
Non-dominant hand: __51__

Impairment Index __0.1__

MINNESOTA MULTIPHASIC PERSONALITY INVENTORY

		Hs	39
		D	56
?	50	Hy	40
L	43	Pd	69
F	55	Mf	45
K	49	Pa	65
		Pt	48
		Sc	59
		Ma	43

REITAN-KLØVE LATERAL-DOMINANCE EXAM

Show me how you:

throw a ball	R
hammer a nail	R
cut with a knife	R
turn a door knob	R
use scissors	R
use an eraser	R
write your name	R

Record time used for spontaneous name-writing:

Preferred hand	10 seconds
Non-preferred hand	32 seconds

Show me how you:

kick a football	R
step on a bug	R

REITAN-INDIANA APHASIA SCREENING TEST

Form for Adults and Older Children

Name: D. D. (III)   Age: 20

Copy SQUARE	Repeat TRIANGLE
Name SQUARE	Repeat MASSACHUSETTS
Spell SQUARE	Repeat METHODIST EPISCOPAL
Copy CROSS	Write SQUARE
Name CROSS	Read SEVEN
Spell CROSS	Repeat SEVEN
Copy TRIANGLE	Repeat/Explain HE SHOUTED THE WARNING.
Name TRIANGLE	Write HE SHOUTED THE WARNING.
Spell TRIANGLE	Compute 85 − 27 =
Name BABY	Compute 17 X 3 =
Write CLOCK	Name KEY
Name FORK	Demonstrate use of KEY
Read 7 SIX 2	Draw KEY
Read MGW	Read PLACE LEFT HAND TO RIGHT EAR.
Reading I	Place LEFT HAND TO RIGHT EAR
Reading II "He is a friendly animal, a famous winner of a dog shows."	Place LEFT HAND TO LEFT ELBOW

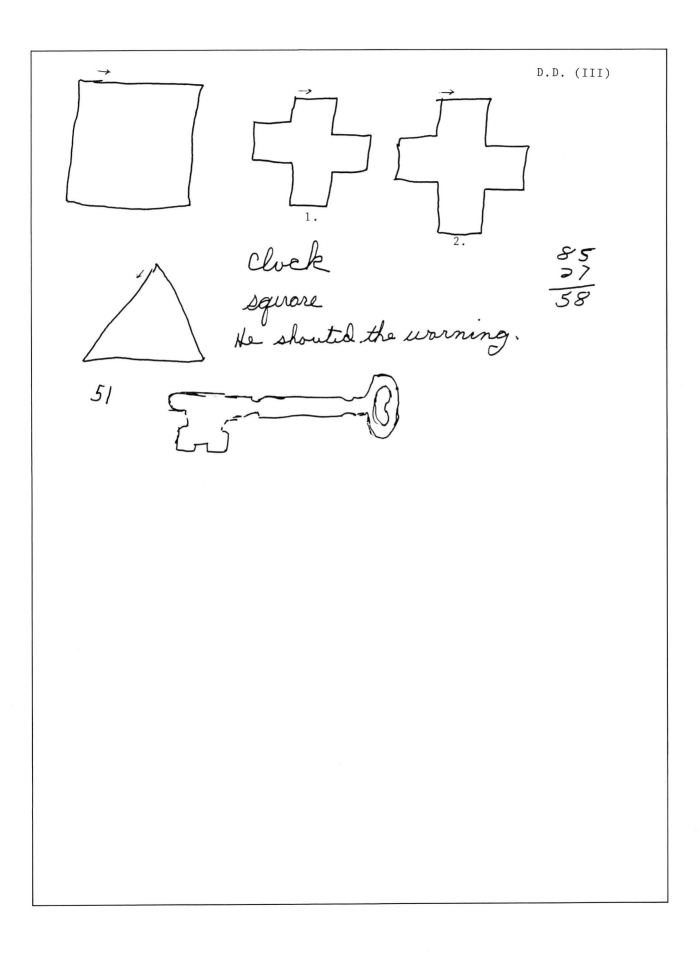

1.

2.

clock

square

He shouted the warning.

51

85
27
‾‾
58

he made three mistakes in twenty trials with his right hand but, as in the second testing, made no mistakes with his left hand.

Finally, D.D. had some difficulty reading HE IS A FRIENDLY ANIMAL, A FAMOUS WINNER OF DOG SHOWS and demonstrated a little confusion with the last phrase. The reader might postulate that these minor errors are due only to chance variation, and this is definitely a possibility. Nevertheless, this particular reading error is fairly typical of persons with left cerebral dysfunction and it is definitely unusual to find both motor and tactile-perceptual deficits on the same side of the body as a result of chance variation. Thus, it would appear that D.D. may have experienced some mild deterioration of certain aspects of left cerebral functioning despite the improvement in general alertness and immediate memory he demonstrated on certain tests. One could also wonder whether his drawings of the cross were as adequate on this examination as on former testings. The first drawing particularly suggests mild right cerebral dysfunction by the disparity in symmetry of the lateral extremities (an error which continues to be demonstrated in the second attempt). Finally, D.D.'s

responses on the Tactile Form Recognition Test were not as quick as they had been previously, but this difficulty was equivalent for the two hands. These changes were too subtle to be reflected on the G-NDS, and indicate the need for careful clinical evaluation of the results over and beyond the use of summary scores.

Although this man had shown striking and consistent improvement between the initial examination and the testing done one year after injury, the results on the 18-month evaluation suggested mild improvement in certain general respects and possible mild deterioration of both left and right cerebral hemisphere functions on other measures. However, the evidence of deterioration was certainly not very pronounced and may have limited significance with respect to adaptations to general problems in everyday living. It should be noted that this patient sustained actual structural tissue damage and in these cases one often sees evidence of more definite deterioration, at least on some measures, during the 12 to 18 month interval following brain injury.

Case #3

Name: P.E.

Age: 42

Education: 12

Sex: Male

Handedness: Right

Occupation: Seaman

Background Information

P.E. was a seaman who was injured when he fell about 40 feet from the mast of a barge. He was immediately rendered unconscious, but by the time he reached the hospital emergency room he seemed to be alert, oriented, and able to respond appropriately in conversation.

Shortly after being admitted to the hospital P.E. relapsed into a coma and responded only to painful stimuli. Seventeen days elapsed before he regained full orientation and was normally responsive and alert. During this interval he had some rational periods but was frequently disoriented, confused, lethargic, and irritable.

Neurological Examination

The neurological examination, performed shortly after P.E. was admitted to the hospital, showed right facial paralysis and hypesthesia. His pupils were constricted and the right pupil was 1 mm larger than the left. Both pupils reacted normally to light and there was no impairment of extraocular movements. A Babinski sign was equivocally present on each side. The remainder of the neurological examination was within normal limits.

In addition to sustaining a head injury, the patient also suffered a dislocation of the right shoulder and fractures of the right scapula, the right femur, and two ribs on the right side.

An EEG done two days after the injury showed marked generalized abnormalities. An EEG done three weeks later demonstrated improvement but bilateral disturbances of the inferior frontal, anterior temporal, and mid-temporal areas were still present and more pronounced on the right. The EEG tracings suggested a cerebral contusion and possible brain stem contusion.

At the time of discharge (three weeks post-injury) the neurological examination revealed only right facial weakness. However, radioisotopic brain scans done immediately after the injury as well as at the time of discharge showed widespread cortical contusions. The second scan showed that some resolution had occurred since the initial scan was taken. The final neurological diagnosis was severe cortical contusions, gradually resolving.

Neuropsychological Examination

The first neuropsychological examination was performed about 11 weeks after the injury. At this time the EEG continued to show marked disturbances of the frontal-temporal areas bilaterally and more pronounced on the right side. On the Cornell Medical Index Health Questionnaire the patient had absolutely no somatic or emotional complaints.

As a general summary statement, we can say that the test results indicate that P.E. (1) had general intelligence levels well above the average, (2) showed evidence of some inflexibility in his thought processes but performed relatively well on most of the neuropsychological tests, and (3) demonstrated certain findings implicating both

THE HALSTEAD-REITAN
NEUROPSYCHOLOGICAL TEST BATTERY

Patient **P.E. (I)** Age **42** Sex **M** Education **12** Handedness **R**

WECHSLER-BELLEVUE SCALE
VIQ	124
PIQ	109
FS IQ	118
Information	15
Comprehension	15
Digit Span	6
Arithmetic	16
Similarities	14
Vocabulary	14
Picture Arrangement	8
Picture Completion	13
Block Design	11
Object Assembly	10
Digit Symbol	5

NEUROPSYCHOLOGICAL DEFICIT SCALE
Level of Performance	20
Pathognomonic Signs	0
Patterns	2
Right-Left Differences	11
Total NDS Score	33

HALSTEAD'S NEUROPSYCHOLOGICAL TEST BATTERY
Category Test   28

Tactual Performance Test
Left hand: 4.7
Left hand: 8.5
Left hand: 4.2

Total Time	17.4
Memory	9
Localization	4

Seashore Rhythm Test
Number Correct   29   1

Speech-sounds Perception Test
Number of Errors   7

Finger Oscillation Test
Dominant hand: 47   47
Non-dominant hand: 41

Impairment Index   0.4

TRAIL MAKING TEST
Part A: **63** seconds
Part B: **147** seconds

STRENGTH OF GRIP
Dominant hand: **38.5** kilograms
Non-dominant hand: **46.0** kilograms

REITAN-KLØVE TACTILE FORM RECOGNITION TEST
Dominant hand: **15** seconds; **0** errors
Non-dominant hand: **15** seconds; **0** errors

REITAN-KLØVE SENSORY-PERCEPTUAL EXAM — No errors
Error Totals

RH___ LH___	Both H:	RH___ LH___	RH___ LH___			
RH___ LF___	Both H/F:	RH___ LF___	RH___ LF___			
LH___ RF___	Both H/F:	LH___ RF___	RF___ LH___			
RE___ LE___	Both E:	RE___ LE___	RE___ LE___			
RV___ LV___	Both:	RV___ LV___	RV___ LV___			

TACTILE FINGER RECOGNITION
R 1___ 2___ 3___ 4___ 5___   R **0** / 20
L 1___ 2___ 3 **1** 4___ 5___   L **1** / 20

FINGER-TIP NUMBER WRITING
R 1 **2** 2 **1** 3___ 4 **1** 5 **1**   R **5** / 20
L 1___ 2___ 3___ 4___ 5___   L **0** / 20

MINNESOTA MULTIPHASIC PERSONALITY INVENTORY
		Hs	57
		D	58
?	50	Hy	60
L	53	Pd	65
F	50	Mf	35
K	68	Pa	45
		Pt	50
		Sc	63
		Ma	60

REITAN-KLØVE LATERAL-DOMINANCE EXAM
Show me how you:
throw a ball	R
hammer a nail	R
cut with a knife	R
turn a door knob	R
use scissors	R
use an eraser	R
write your name	R

Record time used for spontaneous name-writing:
Preferred hand	**12** seconds
Non-preferred hand	**47** seconds

Show me how you:
kick a football	R
step on a bug	R

NO APHASIC SYMPTOMS.

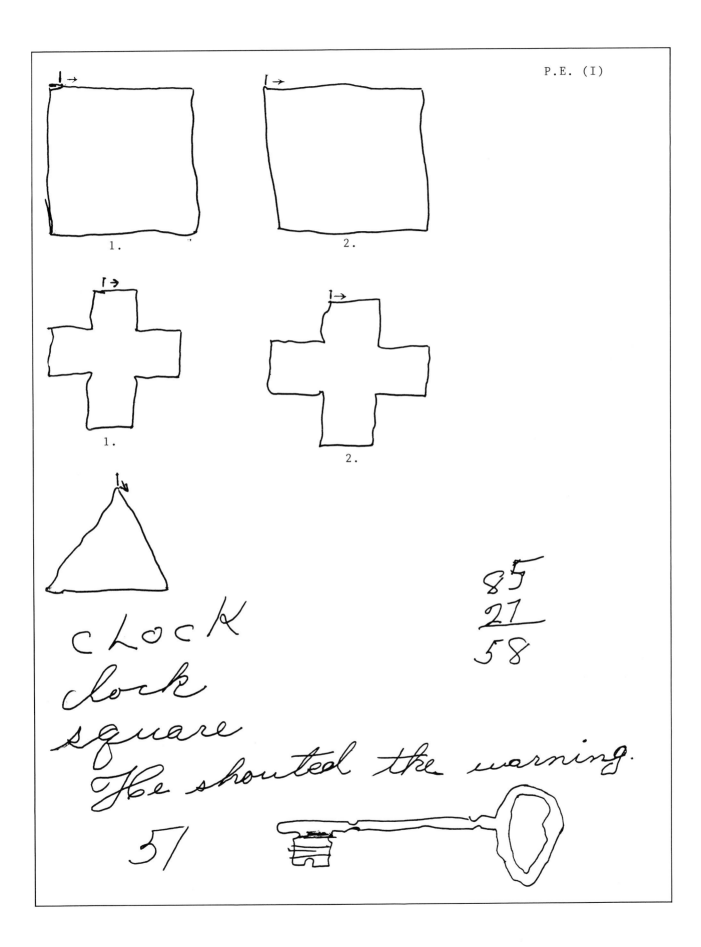

1.

2.

1.

2.

CLOCK

clock

square

He shouted the warning.

51

85
27
58

the left and right cerebral hemispheres. Nevertheless, as we will see, his neuropsychological impairment appeared to be relatively selective in nature.

P.E. earned a Verbal IQ (124) in the Superior range, exceeding about 95% of his age peers. Except for Digit Span (6), he consistently performed well on the Verbal subtests. Many patients facing stressful circumstances (including hospitalization) perform poorly on Digit Span; consequently, a below-average performance on this subtest does not usually have any specific diagnostic significance for impaired brain functions. Considering P.E.'s other scores, though, this low score may have some clinical significance.

P.E. performed considerably worse on the Performance subtests than on the Verbal subtests, earning a Performance IQ (109) 15 points lower than his Verbal IQ and falling in the upper part of the Average range (exceeding about 73% of his age peers). The distribution of scores on the Performance subtests suggests some impairment of cognitive functions. Digit Symbol is generally the most sensitive subtest in the Wechsler Scale and in the context of his other scores, P.E.'s score of 5 on this measure almost certainly indicates some degree of cerebral dysfunction. In addition, we would postulate that the Picture Arrangement score (8) might reflect damage to the right anterior temporal area. Thus, although we cannot use the results of the Wechsler Scale to derive an overall picture of brain-related strengths and weaknesses, we can say that P.E.'s scores suggest that he may have experienced some impairment of brain functions.

In general, P.E. performed relatively well on tests in the Halstead-Reitan Battery, earning an Impairment Index of 0.4 (about 40% of Halstead's tests had scores in the brain-damaged range). The tests contributing to the Impairment Index included (1) the Total Time on the Tactual Performance Test (17.4 min), (2) the Localization component (4) of the Tactual Performance Test, and (3) finger tapping speed of the preferred (right) hand (47).

P.E. scored quite well on the Category Test (28), indicating his good ability in abstraction, reasoning, and logical analysis skills. He was quite slow on both parts of the Trail Making Test, and particularly poor on Part B (147 sec). In fact, this score was definitely the worst of the four indicators most sensitive to the biological condition of the brain. The Impairment Index was a borderline score, the Localization component of the Tactual Performance Test was just within the brain-damaged range, and the Category Test was done well. Part B of the Trail Making Test was performed very poorly; apparently the patient had a great deal of difficulty keeping both the alphabetical and numerical sequences in mind at the same time.

Judging from the scores on the Speech-sounds Perception Test (7 errors) and the Seashore Rhythm Test (29 correct), the basis for P.E.'s deficit was not an inability to attend to specific and well-defined stimulus material. It is safe to conclude that the basic level of central processing — the ability to attend to stimulus material and maintain concentration over time — is relatively intact in this man. Although P.E.'s deficits are relatively selective in nature, they appear to represent higher-level neuropsychological problems.

We should also note that although he made no mistakes, P.E. was somewhat slow in making the decisions required on the Tactile Form Recognition Test. Overall, it appears that he had relatively little difficulty on "power" tests and was able to reach the correct conclusions when given an unlimited amount of time. His worst performances occurred on tests that required efficiency of function and decision-making when time was a limited commodity (e.g. Digit Symbol, Total Time on the Tactual Performance Test, response time on the Tactile Form Recognition Test, judgments regarding the sequence of numbers and letters on the Trail Making Test, and finger tapping speed). Quickness and efficiency in performance are important and significant aspects of normal brain functioning, and P.E.'s performances on these measures represented mild, though significant, impairment of cerebral functions. These deficits were succinctly represented by the Level of Performance section score of 20 on the G-NDS, a value clearly exceeding the mean score of 11.95 for control subjects.

The lateralizing indicators showed deficits involving each cerebral hemisphere. P.E.'s grip strength was definitely reduced with his right upper extremity (38.5 kg) compared with his left (46.0 kg). As mentioned earlier, he dislocated his right shoulder and fractured his right scapula, and it is always necessary to remember that a deficit may be a manifestation of either peripheral damage or cerebral damage. This patient did all three trials of the Tactual Performance Test with his left hand because he had some limitation of shoulder movement on the right side. It is possible that the reduction of grip strength in the right upper extremity may have also been associated with the shoulder injury.

The results obtained on the Finger-tip Number Writing Perception Test help resolve the question of the source of P.E.'s deficits. He made five mistakes in 20 trials on his right hand but made no mistakes on his left hand. Therefore, on the left side, he had both tactile-perceptual difficulties and impaired motor strength. When there are both input *and* output deficits it becomes much more probable that the lesion responsible for the dysfunction is at the cerebral level rather than at the peripheral level. It certainly would not be possible to rule out some concomitant motor limitation of the right upper extremity, but it is likely that the isolated tactile-perceptual deficit is related to impaired brain functions.

Note also that P.E. showed no evidence of aphasia and performed quite satisfactorily on the Speech-sounds Perception Test (7 errors). Considering the overall context of the test results, these relatively good scores indicate that the left cerebral damage is chronic-static in nature rather than progressively destructive.

Indications of right hemisphere damage were not entirely convincing, although certain findings were probably valid indicators of cerebral dysfunction. P.E. was just a little slow in finger tapping speed with his left hand (41) compared with his right (47); however, if this were an isolated finding, it would have minimal lateralizing significance. Remember, though, that P.E. performed quite poorly on the Picture Arrangement subtest of the Wechsler Scale, which might reflect right anterior temporal lobe dysfunction.

The patient's drawing of the key may also be a reflection of cognitive impairment, particularly if we consider the comparative size of the teeth and the handle (however, we conservatively did not give P.E. points for constructional dyspraxia on the G-NDS). The key by itself does not necessarily implicate the right cerebral hemisphere; in terms of clinical judgement, though, this man probably should have been able to do better, considering the overall ability levels that he demonstrated on other tests. In this sense it is even possible that the 15-point difference between the Verbal and Performance IQ values may indicate right cerebral damage.

The G-NDS reflects these deficits, even though clinical interpretation permits greater flexibility and sensitivity in their integrated evaluation. P.E. had a G-NDS score of 33, a value falling in the range of Mild Neuropsychological Impairment with the major contributions coming from the sections on Level of Performance and Right-Left Differences.

We see, then, that the overall test results include some indications of both left and right cerebral hemisphere damage as well as selective deficits in higher-level aspects of central processing. It is somewhat unusual to see such definite left hemisphere indicators in a person who does as well as P.E. on some of the other measures (e.g., the Category Test and Seashore Rhythm Test). Results such as these, however, almost certainly indicate that his deficits were caused by a direct insult to the brain rather than an intrinsic, focal, progressive type of lesion or disease process. In other words, it is likely that this man had a normal brain that sustained an insult and incurred certain deficits as a result. Progressive lesions (such as intrinsic tumors and strokes) customarily have focal neuropsychological concomitants, but also impair brain functions more generally and cause poor scores on the general as well as the specific neuropsychological indicators (Reitan & Wolfson, 1985a).

The results on the Minnesota Multiphasic Personality Inventory reflect the behavioral characteristics, patterns, and inclinations of this man, but they are probably not significant regarding his impaired brain functions.

P.E. was re-examined 12 months after the first neuropsychological examination. He had no particular complaints and believed that he was progressing satisfactorily. An EEG done six weeks after the first neuropsychological examination had again shown bilateral frontal-temporal disturbances which were pronounced on the right side but slightly improved. An EEG done at the time of the second neuropsychological examination showed the same abnormalities with a slight degree of improvement.

First we will evaluate the test results without referring to the previous findings or considering practice-effects. P.E. earned a Verbal IQ (129) in the Superior range (exceeding 97% of his age peers) and a Performance IQ (118) in the upper part of the High Average range (exceeding 89%). These values yielded a Full Scale IQ (126) in the Superior range (exceeding 96%). The distribution of subtest scores suggested that P.E. performed rather poorly on the Digit Span (9), Picture Arrangement (8), and Digit Symbol (9) subtests. Scores on these latter two subtests may reflect some degree of brain impairment.

P.E. performed quite well on tests in the Halstead-Reitan Battery, earning an Impairment Index of 0.3 (about 30% of the tests had scores in the brain-damaged range). The tests contributing to the Impairment Index were the Localization component (3) of the Tactual Performance Test and the Finger Oscillation Test (49). It is apparent that the patient did not demonstrate any striking impairment on these measures; however, he did perform somewhat poorly on Part B of the Trail Making Test (92 sec).

In the context of lateralizing indicators, it appears that P.E. has some residual neuropsychological deficits. His grip strength was no greater with his right hand than with his left (50.5 kg) and he demonstrated some confusion performing the arithmetic problem $85 - 27 =$. Initially he wrote "78" as his answer, then changed it to "58." Although these results certainly do not provide a convincing basis for concluding that left cerebral damage was present (and were not assigned deficit scores on the G-NDS), they do have some supportive value.

More definite evidence was present to implicate the right cerebral hemisphere. P.E.'s finger tapping speed was definitely slow with the left hand (39) compared with the right (49), and he had more difficulty with his left hand (2.4 min) than his right hand (1.7 min) on the Tactual Performance Test. This particular configuration of test results — deficits with the left hand in finger tapping speed and on the Tactual Performance Test in conjunction with apparent difficulties on the Picture Arrangement subtest of the Wechsler Scale — is a fairly definite implication of right anterior temporal lobe damage.

The patient's drawings also raise a question of right cerebral dysfunction. The drawing of the key does not have any specific deficits of significance, but the loss of symmetry in the lateral extremities of the cross probably reflects a mild degree of impairment in dealing with simple spatial configurations. While comparisons of performances on the two sides of the body are represented by a score of 8 on the Right-Left Differences section of the G-NDS (the average score for control subjects is

THE HALSTEAD-REITAN
NEUROPSYCHOLOGICAL TEST BATTERY

Patient __P.E. (II)__ Age __43__ Sex __M__ Education __12__ Handedness __R__

WECHSLER-BELLEVUE SCALE

VIQ	129
PIQ	118
FS IQ	126
Information	15
Comprehension	14
Digit Span	9
Arithmetic	16
Similarities	17
Vocabulary	14
Picture Arrangement	8
Picture Completion	14
Block Design	12
Object Assembly	12
Digit Symbol	9

NEUROPSYCHOLOGICAL DEFICIT SCALE

Level of Performance	15
Pathognomonic Signs	0
Patterns	2
Right-Left Differences	8
Total NDS Score	25

HALSTEAD'S NEUROPSYCHOLOGICAL TEST BATTERY

Category Test	31

Tactual Performance Test

Dominant hand:	1.7
Non-dominant hand:	2.4
Both hands:	1.5
Total Time	5.6
Memory	7
Localization	3

Seashore Rhythm Test

Number Correct	26	5

Speech-sounds Perception Test

Number of Errors	4

Finger Oscillation Test

Dominant hand:	49	49
Non-dominant hand:	39	

Impairment Index __0.3__

TRAIL MAKING TEST

Part A: __57__ seconds
Part B: __92__ seconds

STRENGTH OF GRIP

Dominant hand: __50.5__ kilograms
Non-dominant hand: __50.5__ kilograms

REITAN-KLØVE TACTILE FORM RECOGNITION TEST

Dominant hand: __8__ seconds; __0__ errors
Non-dominant hand: __7__ seconds; __0__ errors

REITAN-KLØVE SENSORY-PERCEPTUAL EXAM — No errors

		Error Totals	
RH___ LH___	Both H: RH___ LH___	RH___ LH___
RH___ LF___	Both H/F: RH___ LF___	RH___ LF___
LH___ RF___	Both H/F: LH___ RF___	RF___ LH___
RE___ LE___	Both E: RE___ LE___	RE___ LE___
RV___ LV___	Both: RV___ LV___	RV___ LV___

TACTILE FINGER RECOGNITION

R 1___ 2___ 3___ 4___ 5___ R __0__ / 20
L 1___ 2___ 3___ 4___ 5___ L __0__ / 20

FINGER-TIP NUMBER WRITING

R 1___ 2___ 3 _1_ 4___ 5___ R __1__ / 20
L 1___ 2___ 3___ 4___ 5___ L __0__ / 20

MINNESOTA MULTIPHASIC PERSONALITY INVENTORY

		Hs	54
		D	56
?	50	Hy	58
L	50	Pd	64
F	50	Mf	51
K	70	Pa	62
		Pt	54
		Sc	59
		Ma	63

REITAN-KLØVE LATERAL-DOMINANCE EXAM

Show me how you:
throw a ball	L
hammer a nail	R
cut with a knife	R
turn a door knob	R
use scissors	R
use an eraser	R
write your name	R

Record time used for spontaneous name-writing:
Preferred hand	8 seconds
Non-preferred hand	30 seconds

Show me how you:
kick a football	R
step on a bug	R

NO APHASIC SYMPTOMS.

REITAN-INDIANA APHASIA SCREENING TEST

Form for Adults and Older Children

Name: P. E. (II)   Age: 43

Copy SQUARE	Repeat TRIANGLE
Name SQUARE	Repeat MASSACHUSETTS
Spell SQUARE	Repeat METHODIST EPISCOPAL
Copy CROSS	Write SQUARE
Name CROSS	Read SEVEN
Spell CROSS	Repeat SEVEN
Copy TRIANGLE	Repeat/Explain HE SHOUTED THE WARNING.
Name TRIANGLE	Write HE SHOUTED THE WARNING.
Spell TRIANGLE	Compute 85 – 27 = Initially wrote "78" and then changed to "58".
Name BABY	Compute 17 X 3 =
Write CLOCK	Name KEY
Name FORK	Demonstrate use of KEY
Read 7 SIX 2	Draw KEY
Read MGW	Read PLACE LEFT HAND TO RIGHT EAR.
Reading I	Place LEFT HAND TO RIGHT EAR
Reading II	Place LEFT HAND TO LEFT ELBOW

clock

square

He shouted the warning

85   51
27
—
58

3.37), again we see that clinical interpretation permits a more sensitive evaluation than that provided by a rigid system.

We see that many of P.E.'s scores were within normal limits and represented an able person in terms of general intellectual and cognitive abilities. Nevertheless, the mild deviations from normal expectancy (in terms of both right/left comparisons and specific deficits), coupled with poor performances on other measures (particularly Part B of the Trail Making Test, the Localization component of the Tactual Performance Test, and finger tapping speed with each hand), all indicate the presence of very mild brain-related impairment.

Results on the Minnesota Multiphasic Personality Inventory, suggesting that this man probably needs to be viewed in a favorable light by others, continues to be essentially within normal limits.

Direct comparison of the results of the first examination with the test scores obtained 12 months later generally reflect some improvement as determined in general terms as well as by a reduction of the G-NDS from 33 to 25. The increase of Performance IQ from 109 to 118 is probably somewhat better than might be expected on the basis of positive practice-effect. P.E. performed better particularly on the Digit Symbol subtest, increasing his score from 5 to 9. On Object Assembly the two-point increase may also represent a genuinely better performance. The patient also performed better on Digit Span (from 6 to 9) and Similarities (from 14 to 17), although the five-point increment in Verbal IQ was not particularly striking. P.E. showed no change whatsoever on Picture Arrangement and changes on other measures probably reflected only chance variations.

The patient performed much better in terms of Total Time on the Tactual Performance Test, reducing the time required for completing the task from 17.4 minutes to 5.6 minutes. Although he also showed a substantial improvement on Part B of the Trail Making Test (from 147 seconds to 92 seconds), this result could still be considered impaired with relation to his other scores. On the

second examination he was much quicker with each hand on the Tactile Form Recognition Test. The drawing of the key may have been a little better on the second testing, but this is difficult to judge. However, finger-tip number writing perception on the right hand, which had initially shown impairment (5 errors), was now within the normal range (1 error).

Although there were better performances on a number of variables, there were also mild tendencies toward worse performances. For example, on the Memory component of the Tactual Performance Test P.E. recalled only seven figures (compared with nine on the first examination). In addition, his nearly perfect score of 29 correct on the Seashore Rhythm Test was now reduced to 26. Although absolute finger tapping speed did not change strikingly, the disparity between the two hands was more pronounced on the second examination. The drawing of the cross may also have been a little worse than it was initially. In other respects the test results on the two examinations were about comparable.

In total, we would judge that this man had shown some degree of improvement, but it was not as striking as we might have expected (compared to results of other patients). It is also possible that P.E.'s age (42) was a factor influencing his degree of improvement.

P.E. was again examined 18 months after the initial testing. In summary, the results of the third neuropsychological examination indicate that (1) the general intelligence and overall adaptive abilities of this man were fairly adequate, (2) he showed no significant emotional or affective problems as measured by the MMPI and the Cornell Medical Index Health Questionnaire, and (3) there were certain distinct and definite deviations from normal expectancy concerning both right and left cerebral functioning, manifested particularly by comparative performances on the two sides of the body. We will defer comparison of the specific test findings on the three examinations until we review the results of the third testing.

THE HALSTEAD-REITAN
NEUROPSYCHOLOGICAL TEST BATTERY

Patient __P.E. (III)__ Age __43__ Sex __M__ Education __12__ Handedness __R__

WECHSLER-BELLEVUE SCALE

VIQ	117
PIQ	125
FS IQ	123
Information	15
Comprehension	13
Digit Span	6
Arithmetic	12
Similarities	14
Vocabulary	14
Picture Arrangement	12
Picture Completion	14
Block Design	13
Object Assembly	12
Digit Symbol	10

NEUROPSYCHOLOGICAL DEFICIT SCALE

Level of Performance	18
Pathognomonic Signs	0
Patterns	1
Right-Left Differences	9
Total NDS Score	28

HALSTEAD'S NEUROPSYCHOLOGICAL TEST BATTERY

Category Test		27

Tactual Performance Test

Dominant hand:	5.4	
Non-dominant hand:	3.9	
Both hands:	3.1	
	Total Time	12.4
	Memory	7
	Localization	3

Seashore Rhythm Test

Number Correct	27	3

Speech-sounds Perception Test

Number of Errors	3

Finger Oscillation Test

Dominant hand:	46	46
Non-dominant hand:	39	

Impairment Index	0.3

TRAIL MAKING TEST

Part A: __41__ seconds
Part B: __74__ seconds

STRENGTH OF GRIP

Dominant hand: __48.5__ kilograms
Non-dominant hand: __50.0__ kilograms

REITAN-KLØVE TACTILE FORM RECOGNITION TEST

Dominant hand: __11__ seconds; __0__ errors
Non-dominant hand: __12__ seconds; __0__ errors

MINNESOTA MULTIPHASIC PERSONALITY INVENTORY

		Hs	52
		D	56
?	50	Hy	60
L	56	Pd	60
F	55	Mf	46
K	61	Pa	59
		Pt	44
		Sc	51
		Ma	63

REITAN-KLØVE SENSORY-PERCEPTUAL EXAM

			Error Totals	
RH___ LH___	Both H: RH___ LH___	RH___ LH___		
RH___ LF___	Both H/F: RH___ LF___	RH___ LF___		
LH___ RF___	Both H/F: LH___ RF___	RF___ LH___		
RE___ LE___	Both E: RE___ LE__2_	RE___ LE__2_		
RV___ LV___	Both: RV___ LV___	RV___ LV___		

REITAN-KLØVE LATERAL-DOMINANCE EXAM

Show me how you:

throw a ball	L
hammer a nail	R
cut with a knife	R
turn a door knob	R
use scissors	R
use an eraser	R
write your name	R

Record time used for spontaneous name-writing:

Preferred hand	11 seconds
Non-preferred hand	45 seconds

Show me how you:

kick a football	R
step on a bug	R

TACTILE FINGER RECOGNITION

R 1___ 2___ 3___ 4___ 5___ R __0__ / 20
L 1___ 2___ 3___ 4___ 5___ L __0__ / 20

FINGER-TIP NUMBER WRITING

R 1_2_ 2___ 3_2_ 4___ 5___ R __4__ / 20
L 1___ 2___ 3___ 4___ 5___ L __0__ / 20

NO APHASIC SYMPTOMS.

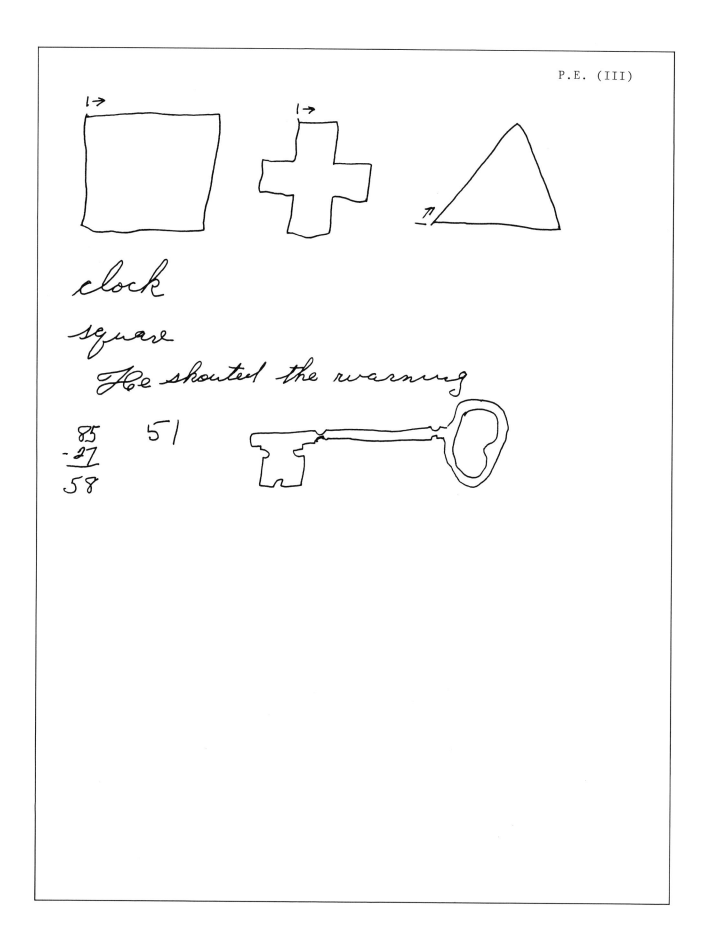

clock

square

He shouted the warning

85
-27

58

51

P.E. earned a Verbal IQ (117) in the upper part of the High Average range and a Performance IQ (125) in the Superior range. Among the Verbal subtests, Digit Span (6) appeared to be particularly low, but there did not seem to be any special significance to the variability among Performance subtests.

P.E. earned an Impairment Index of 0.3 (about 30% of the tests had scores in the brain-damaged range). Although he performed well on the Category Test (27), he was a little slower than might be expected with relation to his IQ values on Part B of the Trail Making Test (74 sec) and earned a definitely deficient score (3) on the Localization component of the Tactual Performance Test. These results might raise a question about cerebral impairment, particularly when considering the subject's relatively high IQ values. In fact, the Level of Performance section of the G-NDS was considerably higher (18) than for control subjects (11.95), despite his high IQ values.

Lateralizing indicators of cerebral dysfunction were fairly definite. Although right-handed, the patient's grip strength was less in his right upper extremity (48.5 kg) than his left (50 kg). This finding could possibly have been due to peripheral dysfunction, but notice that P.E. also showed tactile input impairment on the right side. With his right hand he made four mistakes in 20 trials in finger-tip number writing perception; with his left hand he had no difficulty at all. As noted above, the presence of both input and output deficits complement each other to imply left cerebral dysfunction.

P.E. was somewhat slow in finger tapping speed with his left hand (39) compared with his right (46) and showed a tendency to fail to perceive an auditory stimulus to his left ear when bilateral stimuli were delivered simultaneously. One could also question whether the patient's drawing of the key was an indicator of right cerebral dysfunction, though it was not scored as constructional dyspraxia on the G-NDS. Even though the general

intellectual and cognitive abilities of the patient were well above average, the overall results on the third examination continued to reflect some neuropsychological impairment. He continued to demonstrate deficits on the Right-Left Differences section of the G-NDS with a score of 9 (as compared with 3.37 for control subjects).

Direct comparisons of the results obtained on the second (12-month) and third (18-month) testings provided rather convincing evidence that in general P.E. performed worse on the third examination, even though his G-NDS was unchanged. In other words, instead of showing continued spontaneous improvement (or even some additional positive practice-effect), his scores actually became worse on many measures. For example, his Verbal IQ decreased from 129 to 117; Digit Span dropped from 9 to 6, Arithmetic from 16 to 12, and Similarities from 17 to 14. These would seem to be genuine changes in the direction of poorer performances. The patient did improve his Performance IQ from 118 to 125, but the only subtest showing a significant change was Picture Arrangement, which increased from 8 to 12.

P.E. was much worse in terms of Total Time on the Tactual Performance Test, now requiring 12.4 minutes to complete the three trials (compared with 5.6 minutes on the second examination). His finger tapping speed with the left hand was exactly the same on both examinations (39), but was reduced from 49 to 46 on the right hand. Grip strength showed a comparable change; the score on the left hand was almost identical on both examinations but decreased from 50.5 kg to 48.5 kg with the right hand. The patient's responses were not as quick on the Tactile Form Recognition Test, and on the third examination he required a total of 23 seconds compared with 15 seconds on the second evaluation.

Although he had made no errors in tests of bilateral simultaneous auditory stimulation on the second examination, P.E. now failed to perceive the stimulus to the left ear on two of the four trials. Finally, on the second examination he had an almost perfect performance on the test of finger-tip number writing perception (making only one error on the right hand). Now, although he continued to make no errors with the left hand, he made four errors on the right hand.

Many of the scores were essentially comparable on the two examinations, but when significant changes occurred they were consistently in the direction of worse performances. In general, then, it would appear that this man's abilities deteriorated during the six months between the 12-month examination and 18-month examination. In fact, several of the decremental changes simulated the specific deficits shown on the first examination, including a worse score on Digit Span, lesser grip strength in the right upper extremity than the left, and errors on the right hand but not the left in finger-tip number writing perception. The only other specific deficit observed initially was on the Picture Arrangement subtest, and on the 18-month examination the patient finally showed some improvement on this measure. Also note that the configuration of results suggesting specific involvement of the right anterior temporal lobe was not demonstrated on the 18-month examination.

P.E. was diagnosed as having sustained cerebral contusions, but the specific locations of these lesions were never well documented. In general, patients who have sustained a contusion generally show a pattern of improvement during the interval between the initial testing and the 12-month examination. When these patients are examined for the third time (18 months after the first testing), patients who had experienced a contusion usually demonstrate very little further improvement and, in fact, frequently perform *worse* than they did at the 12-month testing. It would seem clear from these cases that spontaneous recovery of brain functions is not a linearly progressive phenomenon. It tends to occur initially but then often regresses, especially in patients who had originally sustained structural damage to brain tissue.

Finally, it should also be noted that P.E.'s neurological evaluations revealed only a mild right facial weakness at the time of the initial testing and were within normal limits at both the 12-month and 18-month examinations in contrast to the neuropsychological findings of mild though definite impairment.

Case #4

Name: M.P.   Sex: Male

Age: 58   Handedness: Right

Education: 8   Occupation: Construction Worker

Background Information

This 58-year-old man was employed as a construction worker. One day, while walking on a beam at the job site, he lost his balance, fell approximately 50 feet, and landed on his head. He was wearing a hard hat and did not lose consciousness. He was somewhat stuporous and complained of pains in the right shoulder and chest area when admitted to the hospital about 30 minutes later. Blood and cerebral spinal fluid exuded from his right ear canal; it was thought that the tympanic membrane was ruptured even though there was no laceration of the canal.

Neurological Findings

Neurological examination indicated that M.P. tended to drift off to sleep but was easily arousable when questioned verbally. He answered questions with "yes" or "no" responses and followed other commands very poorly. It was apparent that he had severe aphasic deficits and many of his verbal responses were relatively incoherent. He continually repeated words used in card games and repeatedly asked whose turn it was. He did know his name, but seemed completely disoriented concerning time and place. Cranial nerve function was intact except for evidence of decreased hearing, especially on the right side. Motor findings were symmetrical and within normal limits except for increased deep tendon reflexes and a Babinski sign on the right side. Skull films showed a basilar skull fracture. An electroencephalogram on the day of admission showed diffuse slow-wave activity most prominent in the frontal portion of the left cerebral hemisphere. The findings were considered to be compatible with a left frontal-temporal contusion. An echoencephalogram on the day following admission demonstrated a 4-ml shift from left to right that was consistent with swelling secondary to a left cerebral contusion.

The echoencephalogram had returned to normal by the time M.P. was discharged from the hospital 19 days after the injury. His neurological status remained unchanged for the first 11 days following post-injury. He demonstrated a considerable degree of generalized confusion as well as severe aphasic symptoms. During the last five days of hospitalization his mental status and general alertness improved remarkably. However, even though he was fully oriented and showing improvement, he still had significant aphasic deficits. He was amnesic for the events surrounding his accident and for all events that occurred two weeks following the injury.

Neurological examination at the time of discharge indicated that the patient had impairment of right VIIIth cranial nerve function with a loss of auditory acuity. He also had a mild weakness of grip strength on the right, impaired tactile form recognition bilaterally (worse on the right side than the left), and decreased two-point discrimination on the right side. The rest of the neurological examination, including coordination and gait, was normal. The final diagnosis was left cerebral contusion with aphasia and a basilar skull fracture with VIIIth nerve paresis. M.P.'s past history was negative neurologically except for a history of "black-out spells." It was not possible to elicit any further detailed information from him about this problem, and apparently there had been no formal diagnosis or treatment of this condition.

Neuropsychological Examination

Neuropsychological examination was done 41 days after the injury. When questioned directly M.P. had no complaints except to indicate that his memory was poor since sustaining the head injury. However, his responses on the Cornell Medical Index Health Questionnaire revealed many complaints of both a somatic and emotional nature. He indicated that he was hard of hearing, often had severe toothaches, often suffered from an upset stomach and indigestion, was made miserable by pain or pressure in his head, had constant numbness or tingling in parts of his body, had severe pains and aches that made it impossible for him to work, was constantly made miserable by poor health, was always ill and unhappy, and worried continually about his health. He also indicated that he was usually unhappy and depressed, often cried, was always miserable and blue, and felt that life looked entirely hopeless. He said he worried continually, that every little thing got on his nerves and wore him out, that he continually needed someone at his side to advise him, and that he often shakes and trembles.

It was apparent that this man had many complaints when questioned specifically, but did not seem to be able to pull his thoughts together well enough to express them spontaneously. The electroencephalogram was strikingly abnormal at this time, but the findings were more diffuse in nature and demonstrated abnormalities in both temporal regions, more pronounced on the left side than the right side.

As a general summary statement, we can say that the neuropsychological test results showed unequivocal evidence of cerebral damage, involving the left hemisphere to a greater extent than the right hemisphere, in a person who appeared to have developed intellectual functions within the average range. The test results also indicated significant emotional distress.

M.P. earned a Verbal IQ (94) within the lower part of the average distribution, exceeding about 34% of his age peers. His Performance IQ (101) was almost exactly at the average level, exceeding 53%. These values yielded a Full Scale IQ (95) that was in the lower part of the average range, exceeding 37%. Except for a poor score on Digit Span (4), the scores on the individual Verbal subtests showed little variability. It would be difficult to infer the presence of significant brain-related impairment from the distribution of Verbal subtest scores, although it is entirely possible that they were all somewhat depressed.

The Performance subtest scores were somewhat more revealing, with a particularly low score (3) on Picture Arrangement. On the basis of this score one might postulate right anterior temporal lobe damage, but considering the Wechsler results alone the best general conclusion would be equivocal with respect to the possibility of brain damage.

The four most sensitive measures in the Halstead-Reitan Battery all had scores well within the brain-damaged range. M.P. had an Impairment Index of 1.0 (all of Halstead's tests had scores in the brain-damaged range), performed very poorly on Part B of the Trail Making Test (159 sec), was not able to correctly localize any of the shapes in the Tactual Performance Test, and was at about the average level for brain-damaged subjects on the Category Test (64). The score on the Category Test was clearly the best of these four measures, particularly considering the probability that M.P.'s performance may have been mildly impaired by aging effects in addition to the cerebral damage. Research findings have shown that the Category Test is particularly susceptible to aging effects, even in neurologically normal subjects (Reitan, 1967).

THE HALSTEAD-REITAN
NEUROPSYCHOLOGICAL TEST BATTERY

Patient _____ **M.P. (I)** _____ Age __58__ Sex __M__ Education __8__ Handedness __R__

WECHSLER-BELLEVUE SCALE

VIQ	94
PIQ	101
FS IQ	95
Information	7
Comprehension	9
Digit Span	4
Arithmetic	7
Similarities	8
Vocabulary	6
Picture Arrangement	3
Picture Completion	6
Block Design	8
Object Assembly	8
Digit Symbol	6

NEUROPSYCHOLOGICAL DEFICIT SCALE

Level of Performance	39
Pathognomonic Signs	8
Patterns	2
Right-Left Differences	17
Total NDS Score	66

TRAIL MAKING TEST

Part A: __71__ seconds
Part B: __159__ seconds

STRENGTH OF GRIP

Dominant hand: __16.5__ kilograms
Non-dominant hand: __22.0__ kilograms

REITAN-KLØVE TACTILE FORM RECOGNITION TEST

Dominant hand: __15__ seconds; __0__ errors
Non-dominant hand: __14__ seconds; __0__ errors

REITAN-KLØVE SENSORY-PERCEPTUAL EXAM

					Error Totals	
RH___ LH___	Both H:	RH___ LH___	RH___ LH___			
RH___ LF___	Both H/F:	RH___ LF___	RH___ LF___			
LH___ RF___	Both H/F:	LH___ RF___	RF___ LH___			
RE___ LE___	Both E:	RE _3_ LE___	RE _3_ LE___			
RV___ LV___	Both:	RV _1_ LV _1_	RV _1_ LV _1_			

TACTILE FINGER RECOGNITION

R 1___ 2 _3_ 3 _2_ 4 ___ 5 ___   R _5_ / 20
L 1___ 2___ 3 _1_ 4 ___ 5 ___   L _1_ / 20

FINGER-TIP NUMBER WRITING

R 1 _1_ 2___ 3 _1_ 4 ___ 5 ___   R _2_ / 20
L 1___ 2___ 3 ___ 4 ___ 5 ___   L _0_ / 20

HALSTEAD'S NEUROPSYCHOLOGICAL TEST BATTERY

Category Test _____ 64

Tactual Performance Test

Dominant hand:	**15.0 (6 blocks)**
Non-dominant hand:	**15.0 (10 blocks)**
Both hands:	**10.8 (10 blocks)**

Total Time	**40.8 (26 blocks)**
Memory	5
Localization	0

Seashore Rhythm Test

Number Correct __20__ _____ 10

Speech-sounds Perception Test

Number of Errors _____ 24

Finger Oscillation Test

Dominant hand: __24__ _____ 24
Non-dominant hand: __31__

Impairment Index ___ 1.0

MINNESOTA MULTIPHASIC PERSONALITY INVENTORY

		Hs	93
		D	104
?	50	Hy	82
L	73	Pd	86
F	66	Mf	57
K	66	Pa	67
		Pt	97
		Sc	92
		Ma	58

REITAN-KLØVE LATERAL-DOMINANCE EXAM

Show me how you:
throw a ball	R
hammer a nail	R
cut with a knife	R
turn a door knob	R
use scissors	R
use an eraser	R
write your name	R

Record time used for spontaneous name-writing:
Preferred hand	12 seconds
Non-preferred hand	20 seconds

Show me how you:
kick a football	R
step on a bug	R

REITAN-INDIANA APHASIA SCREENING TEST

Form for Adults and Older Children

Name: _____M. P. (I)_____ Age: __58__

Copy SQUARE	Repeat TRIANGLE
Name SQUARE	Repeat MASSACHUSETTS First said, "That's a state." Instructions repeated. Then OK.
Spell SQUARE	Repeat METHODIST EPISCOPAL "Methodis Epistocal"
Copy CROSS After first attempt said, "It's an awful square, I'll tell you."	Write SQUARE
Name CROSS	Read SEVEN
Spell CROSS "S-Q-U-A-R-E." Examiner repeated the item and patient again responded: "S-Q-U-A-R-E."	Repeat SEVEN
Copy TRIANGLE	Repeat/Explain HE SHOUTED THE WARNING. Explanation—"Talked loud." (SEE BELOW *)
Name TRIANGLE Could not think of name. Said "Starts with a T." Patient was finally told.	Write HE SHOUTED THE WARNING.
Spell TRIANGLE	Compute 85 – 27 =
Name BABY	Compute 17 X 3 = Verbalized first and then wrote "53." Given 13x3 and again verbalized first.
Write CLOCK	Name KEY
Name FORK	Demonstrate use of KEY
Read 7 SIX 2	Draw KEY Patient wanted to try a second time.
Read MGW	Read PLACE LEFT HAND TO RIGHT EAR. "Place left hand to right hand." Examiner asked him to read it again. Then OK.
Reading I	Place LEFT HAND TO RIGHT EAR
Reading II	Place LEFT HAND TO LEFT ELBOW

*Examiner questioned further. Patient responded, "Army sergeant."

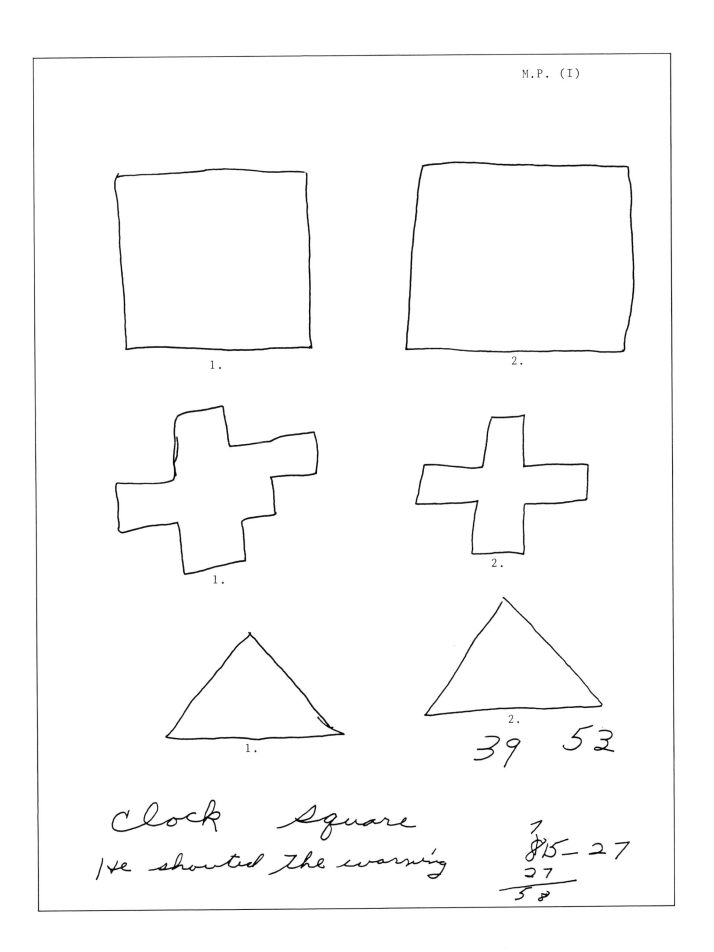

1.

2.

1.

2.

1.

2.

39   53

Clock   Square

He shouted the warning

$$8\overset{1}{5} - 27$$
$$27$$
$$\overline{58}$$

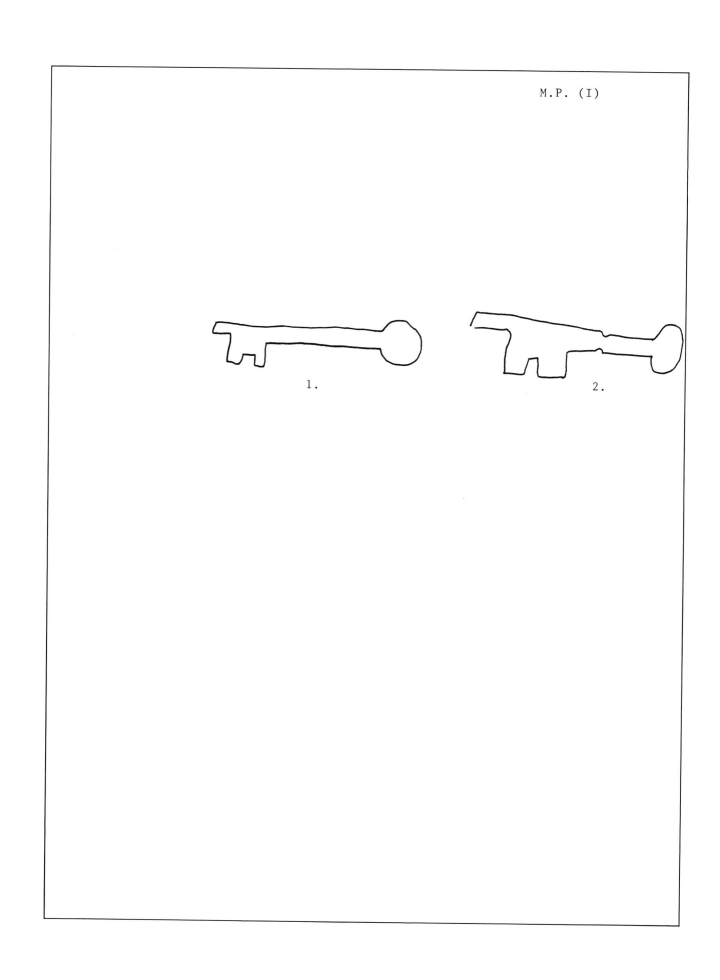

1.

2.

Results on both the Seashore Rhythm Test (20 correct) and the Speech-sounds Perception Test (24 errors) fell in the impaired range. M.P. had particular difficulty with the Speech-sounds Perception Test, suggesting that his problem extended beyond an inability to attend to specific stimulus material; his poor score also reflected his difficulty in dealing with the specific requirements of the task.

The lateralizing indicators quite clearly demonstrated principal impairment of the left cerebral hemisphere. In making a judgment of this type, it is particularly helpful to observe comparative performances on the two sides of the body. Although M.P. was strongly right-handed, he had diminished grip strength in his right arm (16.5 kg) as compared with his left arm (22.0 kg) and reduced finger tapping speed in his right hand (24) compared to his left hand (31). His lateralized motor problems were not limited to measures of primary motor functions, but also were clearly manifested on a test of complex motor problem-solving skills (Tactual Performance Test). Even though direct comparisons usually showed evidence of more difficulty on the right side of his body than the left, it was clear that M.P. had a great deal of difficulty on both his right and left sides, suggesting a generalized component of cerebral damage.

The sensory-perceptual deficits on the right side of the body, in conjunction with the motor deficits, gave credence to the hypothesis of left cerebral damage. M.P. had a distinct tendency to fail to perceive an auditory stimulus to the right ear when an identical stimulus was delivered to both sides simultaneously. It must be noted that the patient had reduced auditory acuity of the right ear, and this is sometimes a complicating factor on this test. However, he also had much more difficulty in tactile finger localization on the right side (5) than on the left side (1) and on finger-tip number writing perception also had more difficulty on the right side (2) than the left (0).

The fact that M.P. performed almost perfectly on both of these tests with his left hand augments the significance of the errors on the right hand. In addition, the right-handed errors in tactile finger localization assume additional validity when considering the fact that the patient was able to perform finger-tip number writing perception (generally a more difficult perceptual task) with fewer errors. Thus, results of both motor and sensory-perceptual measures were quite clear in demonstrating significant impairment of the left cerebral hemisphere. Sometimes such findings can help localize the principal structural damage within the hemisphere. In this case the motor deficits are probably somewhat more pronounced than the sensory-perceptual losses, but the best inference to draw from these findings would be to recognize the lateralized impairment in both areas.

M.P. also demonstrated deficits on the Aphasia Screening Test. He spontaneously showed a naming deficit in his comment after his first attempt to copy a cross. He mistakenly called the figure a square, probably verbally perseverating from his previous copying, naming and spelling of SQUARE. This perseveration was even more prominent when he was asked to spell CROSS. He had just named the figure correctly, but spelled the word S-Q-U-A-R-E. He responded in the same way when the examiner asked him to perform the task again. This is a typical manifestation of verbal perseveration that is seen among dysphasic subjects.

The responses of this man reinforce the importance of following the directions for administration of the test exactly. When the patient is asked to spell, the examiner does not repeat the name of the figure but instead only asks for the spelling. If the examiner had asked M.P. to spell CROSS explicitly, it is entirely possible that he would not have manifested this typical deficit of left cerebral functioning.

M.P. again manifested evidence of dysnomia in his inability to give the name of the TRIANGLE. It was necessary for the examiner to finally tell him the correct name, and he was able to spell the name correctly when given the name explicitly.

M.P. had additional difficulties that indicate the presence of auditory receptive impairment in the language area. He apparently failed to understand the instructions when asked to repeat MASSACHUSETTS (even though he had just repeated TRIANGLE correctly), because he instead provided information about the word. After the instructions were repeated he was able to perform correctly. He had a little difficulty enunciating METHODIST EPISCOPAL, but the type of mistakes M.P. made in this particular attempt are not uncommon among control subjects. Therefore, we would not consider this response to be an indication of left cerebral dysfunction. M.P. had considerable difficulty in explaining HE SHOUTED THE WARNING. It was apparent that he was somewhat confused and did not understand the meaning of the sentence.

It is often difficult to separate the receptive from the expressive aspects of verbal impairment, and in this case both aspects of verbal functioning may have been impaired. Nevertheless, the information communicated by the patient represented a very limited degree of understanding of the meaning of the sentence and is typical of persons with impairment in verbal comprehension (auditory verbal dysgnosia). This type of difficulty implies damage in the posterior part of the language area in the left cerebral hemisphere. Expressive deficits tend to be associated with anterior involvement (anterior left temporal, anterior left parietal and posterior left frontal).

M.P. had additional signs of difficulty in dealing with verbal and symbolic material. Although his error in calculating 17×3 would not necessarily be considered a sign of left cerebral damage (for a person with only an eighth-grade education), the fact that he felt it was necessary to verbalize the response before writing it suggests that he needed this additional cue in order to be able to write the answer. He showed the same tendency when given an additional problem (13×3).

M.P. also made an error in reading PLACE LEFT HAND TO RIGHT EAR. He read the item as, "Place left hand to right hand." The examiner asked him to read it again and he performed the task correctly. On the basis of this single mistake, we would not formally classify the patient as "dyslexic," but it is nevertheless almost certainly another sign of impairment in dealing with language symbols (a manifestation of left cerebral damage). It can be seen, then, that a number of responses on the Aphasia Screening Test were unequivocally indicative of left cerebral damage. Even though the deficits were not pronounced, it is likely that they represented fairly extensive involvement in the language area.

Finally, we should note the evidence of constructional dyspraxia, demonstrated by M.P.'s first attempt to copy a cross and his second attempt to copy the key. There is no doubt that this man was significantly impaired in his ability to deal with simple spatial configurations, a finding that definitely implicates the right cerebral hemisphere.

The lateralizing indicators consistently pointed toward more significant impairment of the left cerebral hemisphere than the right. However, it would not have been possible to have drawn this conclusion except for the results on comparative performances on the two sides of the body. Although the patient showed definitive impairment in the ability to deal with language symbols for communicational purposes (dysphasia), he also showed definite evidence of impairment in dealing with simple spatial configurations (constructional dyspraxia). In cases of head injury (including closed head injury) it is not unusual to find specific indications of damage to both cerebral hemispheres, even though one side of the brain may be clearly more impaired than the other.

M.P. performed many tasks poorly on both sides of the body (and worse on the right side). This indicates significant generalized (rather than strictly lateralized) impairment. For example, his finger tapping speed was quite slow with the left hand (31). He also performed poorly with his left hand on the Tactual Performance Test (15.0 min).

Note, though, that on both of these tasks his performances were significantly worse with his right hand. Thus, there were a number of indications, in addition to evidence of constructional dyspraxia, suggesting that the patient had generalized impairment rather than a specific focal lesion of the left cerebral hemisphere. This case illustrates typical neuropsychological findings of craniocerebral trauma.

On both the MMPI and the Cornell Medical Index Health Questionnaire M.P. indicated significant emotional problems. There is no doubt that he is depressed, feels insecure and anxious, lacks confidence in himself and his ability to meet his problems, and is generally frightened and affectively disturbed. It is not uncommon to encounter results of this kind in persons who have sustained significant impairment from head injury, but from psychological testing it is difficult to determine the extent to which such indications are a direct result of the head injury and which difficulties may represent pre-morbid affective problems. Some evidence is present in the literature which strongly suggests that head injury may precipitate emotional and affective disturbances which were present (although in a lesser degree) before the injury was sustained (Aita & Reitan, 1948). Nevertheless, the emotional distress experienced by many patients following a head injury constitutes a significant clinical problem.

M.P. was re-examined 12 months later. The neurological examination continued to demonstrate various deficits. The patient complained that he was less energetic, had a decreased general interest in events in his environment, and had a bilateral posterior headache that was present most of the time. He showed definite weakness on the right side, had developed a right upper homonymous quadrantanopsia, had diminished hearing bilaterally (no longer with any evidence of more pronounced impairment on the right side), showed truncal ataxia and a Romberg sign, mild bilateral dysdiadochokinesis, and mild nystagmus on lateral gaze.

An electroencephalogram had been done three months after the initial neuropsychological testing and showed moderate but definite improvement. However, a pronounced disturbance of brain function was present in the left frontal and temporal areas, and to a much lesser extent, in the homologous regions of the right cerebral hemisphere. An EEG done at the time of the 12-month examination showed slight deterioration in comparison with the tracings done at three months. In addition to widespread abnormalities there were also marked abnormalities over the left frontal and temporal areas.

Responses on the Cornell Medical Index Health Questionnaire were frequently positive, particularly concerning psychophysiological and emotional complaints. M.P. said that working tired him out completely and he found it impossible to work because of severe aches and pains, that he often gets spells of complete exhaustion or fatigue, that he usually gets up tired and exhausted in the morning, that he is constantly too tired and exhausted even to eat, and that he suffers from severe nervous exhaustion. He indicated that he is always ill and unhappy and constantly made miserable by poor health. He responded that he usually feels unhappy and depressed, often cries, is always miserable and blue, and believes that life is entirely hopeless. He also indicated (as contrasted with his responses 12 months earlier) that he often wished that he were dead and away from it all. He had many other responses that indicated that he was apprehensive, had little self confidence, worried continually, was usually misunderstood by others and easily upset by criticism, constantly keyed up and jittery, etc. These responses definitely suggested that M.P. had become more anxious, apprehensive, depressed, and bewildered by his circumstances and was less able to deal with life now than he had been 12 months earlier.

We will initially consider the test results of the 12-month examination and evaluate their significance for brain-behavior relationships. We will

THE HALSTEAD-REITAN
NEUROPSYCHOLOGICAL TEST BATTERY

Patient **M.P. (II)** Age **59** Sex **M** Education **8** Handedness **R**

WECHSLER-BELLEVUE SCALE

VIQ	98
PIQ	95
FS IQ	98
Information	8
Comprehension	9
Digit Span	6
Arithmetic	7
Similarities	9
Vocabulary	4
Picture Arrangement	4
Picture Completion	4
Block Design	8
Object Assembly	9
Digit Symbol	7

NEUROPSYCHOLOGICAL DEFICIT SCALE

Level of Performance	32
Pathognomonic Signs	4
Patterns	2
Right-Left Differences	15
Total NDS Score	53

HALSTEAD'S NEUROPSYCHOLOGICAL TEST BATTERY

Category Test 61

Tactual Performance Test

Dominant hand:	15.0 (5 blocks)
Non-dominant hand:	15.0 (6 blocks)
Both hands:	15.9 (10 blocks)

Total Time	45.9 (21 blo◖
Memory	7
Localization	2

Seashore Rhythm Test

Number Correct **16** 10

Speech-sounds Perception Test

Number of Errors 22

Finger Oscillation Test

Dominant hand:	30	30
Non-dominant hand:	34	

Impairment Index 0.9

TRAIL MAKING TEST

Part A: **38** seconds
Part B: **84** seconds

STRENGTH OF GRIP

Dominant hand: **29.5** kilograms
Non-dominant hand: **34.5** kilograms

REITAN-KLØVE TACTILE FORM RECOGNITION TEST

Dominant hand: **15** seconds; **1** errors
Non-dominant hand: **10** seconds; **0** errors

MINNESOTA MULTIPHASIC PERSONALITY INVENTORY

		Hs	78
		D	72
?	50	Hy	79
L	53	Pd	83
F	68	Mf	57
K	61	Pa	70
		Pt	89
		Sc	88
		Ma	53

REITAN-KLØVE SENSORY-PERCEPTUAL EXAM

			Error Totals
RH___LH ___	Both H: RH___LH ___	RH___LH ___	
RH___LF ___	Both H/F: RH___LF ___	RH___LF ___	
LH___RF ___	Both H/F: LH___RF ___	RF___LH ___	
RE___LE ___	Both E: RE_1_LE ___	RE_1_LE ___	
RV___LV ___	Both: RV___LV ___	RV___LV ___	

REITAN-KLØVE LATERAL-DOMINANCE EXAM

Show me how you:

throw a ball	R
hammer a nail	R
cut with a knife	R
turn a door knob	R
use scissors	R
use an eraser	R
write your name	R

Record time used for spontaneous name-writing:

Preferred hand	9	seconds
Non-preferred hand	16	seconds

TACTILE FINGER RECOGNITION

R 1___ 2___ 3___ 4 _2_ 5___ R **2** / 20
L 1___ 2 _1_ 3 _2_ 4 _1_ 5___ L **4** / 20

FINGER-TIP NUMBER WRITING

R 1___ 2___ 3___ 4 _1_ 5 _1_ R **2** / 20
L 1 _1_ 2 _1_ 3___ 4___ 5 _1_ L **3** / 20

Show me how you:

kick a football	R
step on a bug	R

REITAN-INDIANA APHASIA SCREENING TEST

Form for Adults and Older Children

Name: _____M. P. (II)_____ Age: __59__

Copy SQUARE	Repeat TRIANGLE
Name SQUARE	Repeat MASSACHUSETTS
Spell SQUARE	Repeat METHODIST EPISCOPAL "Metodist epistical"
Copy CROSS On second attempt, patient wanted to stop and start again.	Write SQUARE
Name CROSS	Read SEVEN
Spell CROSS	Repeat SEVEN
Copy TRIANGLE	Repeat/Explain HE SHOUTED THE WARNING. "Accident." Examiner questioned. "There was an accident." Examiner questioned.
Name TRIANGLE	Write HE SHOUTED THE WARNING "And danger."
Spell TRIANGLE	Compute 85 – 27 =Patient asked, "Is that multiply or subtract?–oh it's subtract. Originally wrote a 5 and corrected to 8.
Name BABY	Compute 17 X 3 = Verbalized before writing answer.
Write CLOCK	Name KEY
Name FORK	Demonstrate use of KEY Patient asked, "Turn to right or left?" Examiner repeated instruction. Then OK.
Read 7 SIX 2 Said "Six." Examiner questioned. See a 7 and a 2." Responded correctly when examiner pointed to each item.	Draw KEY
Read MGW	Read PLACE LEFT HAND TO RIGHT EAR. Read silently and performed movement correctly. Examiner asked him again to read the sentence.
Reading I	Place LEFT HAND TO RIGHT EAR Then OK.
Reading II	Place LEFT HAND TO LEFT ELBOW

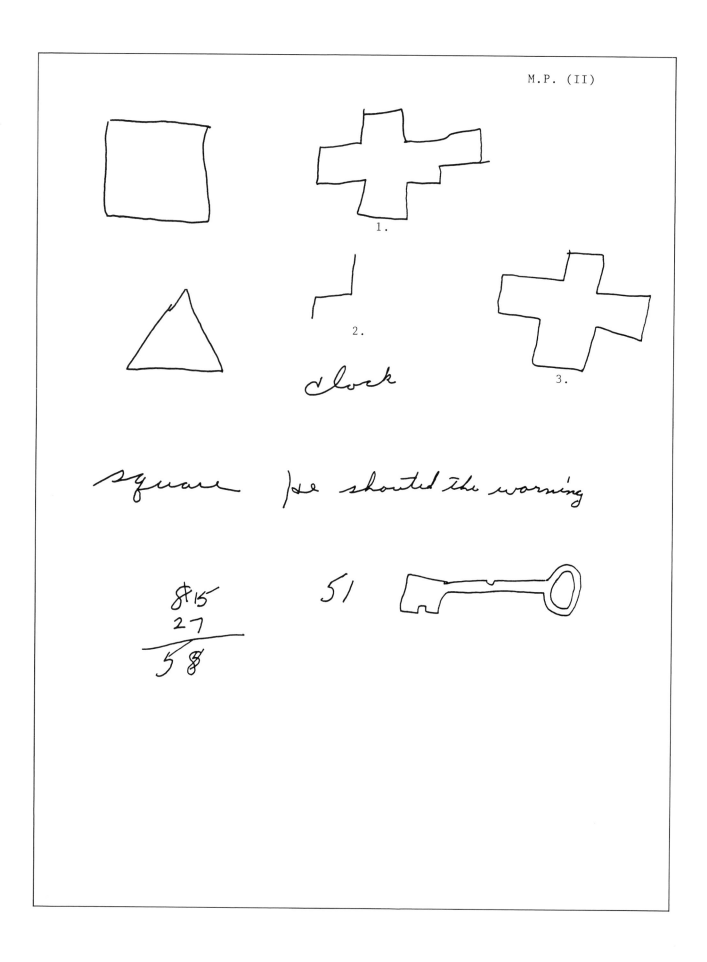

1.

2.

3.

clock

square   He shouted the warning

$\begin{array}{r} 815 \\ 27 \\ \hline 58 \end{array}$

51

then compare the findings of this testing with the results of the first testing (12 months earlier).

M.P. earned both Verbal (98) and Performance (95) IQ values that fell within the lower part of the average range. These values yielded a Full Scale IQ (98) that was nearly at the average level. (The reader may be concerned with the rather low weighted scores in relation to the IQ values. We should note that in the older age ranges the Wechsler-Bellevue Scale had an inordinate adjustment for age, particularly for the Performance IQ.) The Verbal subtest scores were consistently below the average level. Except possibly for the exceptionally low score (4) on the Vocabulary subtest, they were not remarkable in terms of their brain-related significance. On the Performance subtests the Picture Arrangement score was low (4), but there was otherwise no remarkable variability.

In relation to his IQ values M.P. performed very poorly on the four most sensitive indicators. Probably his best score was on Part B of the Trail Making Test (84 sec), a result suggesting that impairment of brain functions had become relatively chronic and static in nature. The patient consistently performed poorly not only on tests that were rather simple in nature and required only close attention to specific stimulus material; he also showed deficits on measures of motor function and complex-problem solving capabilities. Thus, it would appear that M.P.'s neuropsychological impairment was rather generalized in nature.

Lateralizing indicators implicated the left cerebral hemisphere to a greater extent than the right. The Lateral Dominance Examination revealed that M.P. was definitely right-handed. Nevertheless, his finger tapping speed with his right hand (30) was less than his left hand (34) and his grip strength with his right hand (29.5 kg) was less than his left hand (34.5 kg). In addition, on the Tactile Form Recognition Test M.P. showed a degree of deficiency with the right hand (15 sec, 1 error) as compared with the left hand (10 sec, 0 errors).

Finally, he had some difficulty in perceiving bilateral simultaneous auditory stimulation with his right ear.

Other results on the neuropsychological tests definitely implicated the right cerebral hemisphere. M.P. demonstrated distinct constructional dyspraxia in his drawings of simple spatial configurations. His first drawing of the cross showed his confusion about which direction turns had to be made in order to complete the figure. The patient became somewhat confused in his second attempt, was not sure just what to do, and asked if he could start again. He was permitted to do this and his third attempt to draw the cross showed definite disparity in the position of the extremities. Even though this effort was better than his first attempt, the error on the first trial should not be overlooked or excused; its implications for right cerebral damage are definite and significant.

M.P. also had some difficulty in copying the triangle. He drew the first line on the left side quite satisfactorily but then drew the bottom line too long and had to compensate in order to complete the figure. Finally, although the patient drew a rather skeletal representation of the key, which provides us little data to evaluate, it should be noted that the indentation in the stem not only was placed toward the middle but that there was no corresponding indentation on the bottom side.

These results make it quite clear that M.P. had a significant problem in dealing with simple spatial configurations, severe enough to be classified as "constructional dyspraxia." Other findings implicating the right hemisphere include more difficulty in tactile finger recognition on his left hand (4 errors) than his right hand (2 errors), but it is difficult to be certain that such a difference has specific significance for lateralizing the location of the cerebral damage.

The overall configuration of the neuropsychological test results indicated the presence of cerebral damage of a generalized nature with the left cerebral hemisphere somewhat more involved than the right. Findings of the kind shown by this man are quite consistent with an interpretation of a traumatic insult to the brain. The current results represent chronic and probably permanent residual deficits.

Specific comparisons of the test results obtained on the initial examination and the testing done 12 months post-injury indicated that M.P. performed somewhat better on a number of tests and slightly worse on others. Finger tapping speed and grip strength were increased in both upper extremities, probably as a result of being up and around and getting more physical exercise. Note, though, that the impairment of the right (preferred) hand as compared with the left hand was still present. M.P. showed some improvement in his aphasic deficits and in his perception of bilateral simultaneous auditory stimuli. He was also able to remember two of the locations of the shapes on the Tactual Performance Test. He improved slightly on the Digit Span subtest of the Wechsler Scale (from 4 to 6) and showed a significant improvement on Part B of the Trail Making Test (from 159 sec to 84 sec). In all probability, some of these indications of improvement relate to a stabilization of his brain functions.

Nevertheless, M.P. seemed to perform worse on certain tests. His Performance IQ fell from 101 to 95 (instead of improving from positive practice-effect). The major change probably occurred on the Picture Completion subtest (from 6 to 4). M.P. also showed a comparable decrease on the Vocabulary subtest. He performed significantly worse in terms of the Total Time required on the Tactual Performance Test (40.8 min and 26 blocks placed compared to 45.9 min and 21 blocks placed). This decrement in performance was largely attributable to a poorer performance with the left hand (15.0 min and 10 blocks placed compared to 15.0 min and 6 blocks placed) and the performance with both hands (10.8 min and 10 blocks placed compared to 15.9 min and 10 blocks placed).

It would appear that M.P. did not have the intellectual energy or capability to do as well as he had on the first examination. His number of correct answers on the Seashore Rhythm Test decreased from 20 to 16. He also showed a change in finger-tip number writing perception; although he still made two errors on his right hand, the number of errors increased from 0 to 3 on his left hand.

In an overall sense, these results are subject to an interpretation similar to the one initially obtained. However, M.P. did not improve as consistently as many head-injured persons; he clearly deteriorated in his performances on as many tests as showed improvement. Considering the tests involved, the improvement probably was related to development of chronicity of the injury and stability of brain functions in a biological sense. The decrement in performances may very well have been related to speed of response and ability to sustain concentrated effort directed toward the task. A pattern of this kind, in which improvements are counterbalanced by poorer performances, is rarely seen among younger head-injured patients. It is very likely that the age of this man was a substantial factor in his failure to show consistent and definite neuropsychological improvement. It should also be noted that the neurological examination and results of electroencephalography did not show any remarkable change in a positive direction.

M.P. was again examined 18 months after the initial neuropsychological evaluation. He still complained of occasional headaches, although he said that they were less frequent and less severe than previously. However, he reported that six weeks prior to this examination he was taking a nap at home and the next thing he recalled was waking up in the hospital having a major motor seizure. He says that he has generally felt very tired and has noticed that his memory is significantly impaired. For example, although he has been a carpenter, he said that he couldn't remember the measurements of a door or how it opened long enough to get to the lumber yard to buy a new

THE HALSTEAD-REITAN
NEUROPSYCHOLOGICAL TEST BATTERY

Patient __M.P. (III)__ Age __60__ Sex __M__ Education __8__ Handedness __R__

WECHSLER-BELLEVUE SCALE

VIQ	94
PIQ	107
FS IQ	97
Information	11
Comprehension	4
Digit Span	7
Arithmetic	7
Similarities	5
Vocabulary	7
Picture Arrangement	4
Picture Completion	7
Block Design	5
Object Assembly	11
Digit Symbol	7

NEUROPSYCHOLOGICAL DEFICIT SCALE

Level of Performance	37
Pathognomonic Signs	2
Patterns	4
Right-Left Differences	9
Total NDS Score	52

HALSTEAD'S NEUROPSYCHOLOGICAL TEST BATTERY

Category Test __69__

Tactual Performance Test

Dominant hand:	17.8
Non-dominant hand:	15.0 (3 blocks)
Both hands:	7.3

Total Time	40.1 (23 blocks)
Memory	4
Localization	1

Seashore Rhythm Test

Number Correct __17__ __10__

Speech-sounds Perception Test

Number of Errors __20__

Finger Oscillation Test

Dominant hand:	30	30
Non-dominant hand:	35	

Impairment Index __1.0__

TRAIL MAKING TEST

Part A: __39__ seconds
Part B: __72__ seconds

STRENGTH OF GRIP

Dominant hand: __37.0__ kilograms
Non-dominant hand: __34.5__ kilograms

REITAN-KLØVE TACTILE FORM RECOGNITION TEST

Dominant hand: __18__ seconds; __1__ errors
Non-dominant hand: __14__ seconds; __2__ errors

MINNESOTA MULTIPHASIC PERSONALITY INVENTORY

		Hs	88
		D	89
?	50	Hy	78
L	66	Pd	76
F	80+	Mf	65
K	57	Pa	73
		Pt	83
		Sc	90
		Ma	48

REITAN-KLØVE SENSORY-PERCEPTUAL EXAM

			Error Totals
RH ___ LH ___	Both H:	RH ___ LH ___	RH ___ LH ___
RH ___ LF ___	Both H/F:	RH ___ LF ___	RH ___ LF ___
LH ___ RF ___	Both H/F:	LH _1_ RF ___	RF ___ LH _1_
RE ___ LE ___	Both E:	RE ___ LE _1_	RE ___ LE _1_
RV ___ LV ___	Both:	RV ___ LV ___	RV ___ LV ___

REITAN-KLØVE LATERAL-DOMINANCE EXAM

Show me how you:

throw a ball	R
hammer a nail	R
cut with a knife	R
turn a door knob	R
use scissors	R
use an eraser	R
write your name	R

Record time used for spontaneous name-writing:

Preferred hand	9 seconds
Non-preferred hand	35 seconds

Show me how you:

kick a football	R
step on a bug	R

TACTILE FINGER RECOGNITION

R 1___ 2___ 3 _2_ 4 _2_ 5 _1_   R _5_ / 20
L 1___ 2___ 3 _1_ 4 _2_ 5 _3_   L _6_ / 20

FINGER-TIP NUMBER WRITING

R 1 _1_ 2 _1_ 3 _1_ 4 ___ 5 _1_   R _4_ / 20
L 1 _3_ 2 ___ 3 ___ 4 _1_ 5 _1_   L _5_ / 20

REITAN-INDIANA APHASIA SCREENING TEST
Form for Adults and Older Children

Name: _____M. P. (III)_____ Age: __60__

Copy SQUARE	Repeat TRIANGLE
Name SQUARE	Repeat MASSACHUSETTS
Spell SQUARE	Repeat METHODIST EPISCOPAL "Methodist Epistical"
Copy CROSS	Write SQUARE
Name CROSS	Read SEVEN
Spell CROSS	Repeat SEVEN
Copy TRIANGLE	Repeat/Explain HE SHOUTED THE WARNING. "A signal." Examiner questioned. "Of danger.
Name TRIANGLE	Write HE SHOUTED THE WARNING.
Spell TRIANGLE	Compute 85 – 27 ="48." Also given 96–38.
Name BABY	Compute 17 X 3 = Verbalized answer before writing.
Write CLOCK	Name KEY
Name FORK	Demonstrate use of KEY
Read 7 SIX 2 "6" – pause – then responded correctly.	Draw KEY
Read MGW	Read PLACE LEFT HAND TO RIGHT EAR.
Reading I	Place LEFT HAND TO RIGHT EAR
Reading II	Place LEFT HAND TO LEFT ELBOW

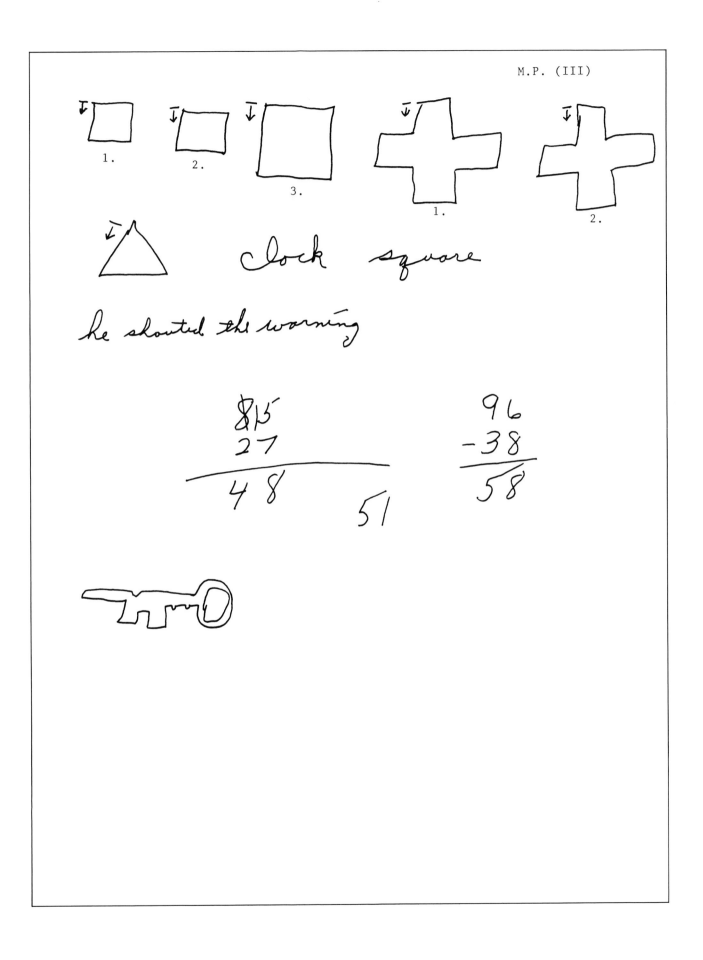

clock   square

he shouted the warning

$$\begin{array}{r} 8\!\!\!/15 \\ 27 \\ \hline 48 \end{array}$$ 51

$$\begin{array}{r} 96 \\ -38 \\ \hline 58 \end{array}$$

one. In general, he felt that he had deteriorated and was not capable of performing as well as he should.

Neurological examination showed evidence of moderate to mild truncal ataxia, although there was some improvement from the examination six months earlier. He showed some improvement in strength of the right upper extremity compared to the previous examination and did not demonstrate any aphasic manifestations in his verbal communications. Nevertheless, he showed a slight hyperreflexia of his right upper extremity, bilateral mild dysdiadochokinesia, a bilateral hearing loss, and bilateral decrement in visual acuity. He also showed a mild nystagmus which the neurologist thought might possibly be due to anti-epileptic medication. At this time the electroencephalogram showed a slight degree of improvement from results obtained six months earlier, although some evidence of a generalized disturbance of brain functions was still present and there were definite abnormalities of the left frontal-temporal area.

M.P.'s answers on the Cornell Medical Index Health Questionnaire were essentially similar to those obtained earlier. He had relatively few definite somatic complaints, but he did complain of spells of complete exhaustion, being worn out by every little effort, being too tired and exhausted even to eat, suffering from severe nervous exhaustion, constantly being made miserable by poor health, feelings of depression and anxiety, feeling very inadequate with respect to meeting his problems, being easily upset and irritated and misunderstood by others, etc.

A brief summary of the neuropsychological test results obtained 18 months after the injury continued to reflect evidence of cerebral damage, with certain findings pointing toward involvement of the left cerebral hemisphere and other results implicating the right cerebral hemisphere. M.P. continued to have IQ values that were in the normal range, although positive practice-effect may have been a factor. The apparent increment in Performance IQ (from 95 to 107) was largely a function of M.P. having reached 60 years of age and use of the recommended adjustment in determining the IQ value. Except for a relatively good score on Part B on the Trail Making Test (72 sec), he also performed poorly on the four most sensitive measures in the Halstead-Reitan Battery.

Lateralizing indicators were also present. Although definitely right-handed, M.P. was slow in finger tapping speed with his right hand (30) as compared with his left hand (35) and somewhat slow on the same side in tactile form recognition with his right hand (18 sec compared with 14 sec).

Results on the Aphasia Screening Test also showed certain deficits. In attempting to read 7 SIX 2 M.P. first responded by saying "six." He then paused for a moment and finally responded correctly. His enunciation of METHODIST EPISCOPAL was not perfect but the kind of mistake he made is not uncommon among control subjects with relatively poor educational levels. He performed somewhat better than he had previously in explaining the sentence HE SHOUTED THE WARNING, although his first response still failed to include a recognition of danger. His error in computing $85 - 27 =$ may possibly be explained on the basis of his limited education, but this is less likely considering the fact that he was able to write the answer to 17×3 correctly. Except for the key, M.P. did not make gross errors in his copying of simple spatial configurations. Nevertheless, the errors on the key (particularly the elongated "nose" and the notches on the stem) clearly indicate the presence of constructional dyspraxia.

On the sensory-perceptual examination M.P. failed to perceive a tactile stimulus to the left hand when it was given simultaneously with a stimulus to the right face, and made a similar mistake on auditory perception on the left side. However, these were single errors and cannot be counted heavily as indicators of impaired brain functions.

On tactile finger localization and finger-tip number writing perception M.P. made a considerable number of errors on each hand. The overall results are strongly indicative of impaired brain functions, although the lateralizing findings are considerably less pronounced than they were previously. In fact, at this point one would question whether one cerebral hemisphere was more significantly involved than the other.

Results of this kind are quite typical of long-term effects of cerebral damage; in time the specificity of deficits and the distinctness of lateralizing signs gradually decrease. The chronicity indicators (e.g., Part B of the Trail Making Test) show some gradual improvement, although other indicators of significant impairment are still present. In terms of the overall comparison, it would appear that M.P. had performed just about as poorly as he had performed before, even though the specific deficits and lateralizing signs were not as pronounced.

In summary, it is clear that M.P. did not make the degree of improvement following brain injury that is frequently seen. Very probably this outcome was due to his age at the time that the injury was sustained and may also have been a long-term reaction to the left cerebral contusion. In addition, the reader will recall that the patient was reported to have had "blackout spells" before the injury occurred. Even though no basis for these spells was established, they may have represented some degree of impairment of brain functions upon which the craniocerebral trauma was imposed. Thus, aging effects, the nature of brain damage, and prior brain involvement may have been factors in limiting the potential for recovery. In any case, the results for this patient suggest that injury of a previously compromised brain, either by some prior type of pathological involvement or aging effects, may constitute an adverse circumstance that limits recovery potential.

Case #5

Name: K.C.

Age: 25

Education: 16

Sex: Female

Handedness: Right

Occupation: Financial
              Counselor

Background Information

K.C., a 25-year-old college graduate, was employed as a financial counselor for a large metropolitan hospital when she was involved in an automobile accident and suffered a severe head injury. She was unconscious for about two months and had many difficulties after she regained consciousness.

In the hospital emergency room it was determined that K.C.'s left middle meningeal artery was lacerated in the accident. She was taken to surgery and a large epidural hematoma was evacuated. Although she initially showed some improvement following this procedure, she gradually became less responsive; on the right side her movements were less purposeful and on the left side she demonstrated a complete decerebrate response. A left percutaneous carotid arteriogram demonstrated a 3 mm–4 mm left-to-right shift of the pericallosal arteries and the internal cerebral vein.

Gradually, K.C. began to show improvement and after five and one-half months of hospitalization she was transferred to an extended care facility. At this time she had a dense and spastic left hemiparesis, slow and deliberate speech, impairment in verbal communicational skills (for which speech therapy was given), urinary frequency with a spastic bladder, and significant impairment in the ability to care for herself. Serial electroencephalograms done during her hospitalization showed a gradual improvement, but at the time of discharge the patient still had a persistent indication of severe right cerebral hemisphere damage. In the hospital K.C. had been given three months of intensive rehabilitation, oriented principally toward physical therapy and gait training. She made some improvement but appeared to have reached a plateau and was transferred to an extended care facility where her rehabilitation and speech therapy would be continued.

After four and one-half months at the extended care facility K.C. was re-admitted to the hospital for further evaluation. She had made some progress in the extended care facility but continued to have a dense spastic hemiparesis on the left side, urinary incontinence and a spastic bladder, impaired ambulation, minimal self-care ability, and intellectual impairment. A treatment plan was developed that focused on continued physical rehabilitation and speech therapy and the patient was discharged to a nursing home.

Follow-up reports were available for more than three years after the injury. K.C. was reported to spend most of the day in a wheelchair, but with assistance was able to walk with a four-pronged walker. She continued to have a left hemiparesis, speech defects, and obvious intellectual impairment. The medical staff reported that K.C. complained constantly and had frequent temper tantrums characterized by loud shouting, stamping her foot, and banging on any available surface.

Neuropsychological Examination

The first comprehensive neuropsychological examination was done 10 months after the injury. The neurological examination at that time demonstrated a spastic left hemiplegia and left hemihypesthesia, hyperactive reflexes and a Babinski sign on the left side, nystagmus on right lateral gaze, slowed and deliberate speech, and evidence of decreased intellectual functioning. The electroencephalogram showed marked abnormalities in the temporal areas of both cerebral hemispheres with variable spread to the adjacent frontal or parietal-occipital regions. The tracings were interpreted as being compatible with prior cortical contusions.

K.C.'s responses on the Cornell Medical Index Health Questionnaire included a number of somatic complaints, such as a constantly running nose, constant stomach trouble, sensitive or tender skin, frequent severe headaches, numbness or tingling in parts of the body, problems with bladder control and urinary frequency, and spells of complete exhaustion or fatigue. She also indicated that she worries continually, must constantly attempt to control herself in order to avoid going to pieces, has frightening thoughts that keep coming back to her mind, that life looked entirely hopeless, and that she often wishes that she were dead and away from it all.

K.C. earned a Verbal IQ (101) that fell almost exactly at the Average level (exceeding 53% of her age peers). Her Performance IQ (66) was in the range of Mild Mental Retardation (exceeding only about 1%). The scaled scores on Comprehension (11), Similarities (11), Information (10), and Vocabulary (10) subtests were at the Average level, indicating that in the past K.C. had been able to achieve at least average intellectual development. Thus, the striking disparity between her Verbal and Performance IQ values would suggest that she had suffered impairment in performance intelligence.

Except for Digit Span (7), the scores on the Verbal subtests showed relatively little variability.

Considering her significant neuropsychological impairment (which will be described later), it is possible that K.C. had experienced a generalized loss of verbal intelligence; however, it would not be possible to draw such a conclusion solely from the results on the Wechsler Scale.

The distribution of scores on the Performance subtests was fairly typical of right cerebral damage. The Picture Completion subtest had the highest score (8), and tended to approach the level of the Verbal subtest scores; this is not an uncommon finding in persons with right cerebral damage. Nevertheless, it is always advisable to obtain information regarding the general aspects of brain functions before proceeding to secondary questions, such as the comparative status of the two cerebral hemispheres. The significance of the low Performance IQ is substantially enhanced when we consider K.C.'s performances on the four most sensitive general indicators in the Halstead-Reitan Battery. In addition, she had a G-NDS score of 77, which falls in the range of severe impairment. On these measures her scores consistently fell in the brain-damaged range, clearly indicating impairment of brain-related abilities. This finding provides a neuropsychological framework within which to make comparisons of K.C.'s verbal and performance intelligence.

K.C. earned an Impairment Index of 0.9 (about 90% of Halstead's tests had scores in the brain-impaired range). The only measure that had a score in the normal range was the Seashore Rhythm Test (27 correct). The patient showed evidence of significant impairment on the Category Test (71 errors), suggesting that she has difficulty understanding the nature of complex relationships and formulating hypotheses based on her observations. She also did very poorly on the Localization component of the Tactual Performance Test (2). On the Trail Making Test K.C. demonstrated her confusion and inflexible thinking. She was able to

THE HALSTEAD-REITAN
NEUROPSYCHOLOGICAL TEST BATTERY

Patient ___**K.C. (I)**___ Age __**25**__ Sex __**F**__ Education __**16**__ Handedness __**R**__

WECHSLER-BELLEVUE SCALE

VIQ	101
PIQ	66
FS IQ	84
Information	10
Comprehension	11
Digit Span	7
Arithmetic	9
Similarities	11
Vocabulary	10
Picture Arrangement	4
Picture Completion	8
Block Design	3
Object Assembly	5
Digit Symbol	3

NEUROPSYCHOLOGICAL DEFICIT SCALE

Level of Performance	48
Pathognomonic Signs	5
Patterns	3
Right-Left Differences	21
Total NDS Score	77

HALSTEAD'S NEUROPSYCHOLOGICAL TEST BATTERY

Category Test _____71_____

Tactual Performance Test

Right hand: __**15.0 (3 blocks)**__

Right hand: __**9.4 (2 blocks)**__

Right hand: _____   Pt. tore off blindfold; test discontinued

Total Time	24.4 (5 blocks)
Memory	3
Localization	2

Seashore Rhythm Test

Number Correct __**27**__   __**3**__

Speech-sounds Perception Test

Number of Errors   __**12**__

Finger Oscillation Test

Dominant hand: __**40**__   __**40**__

Non-dominant hand: __**—**__

Impairment Index __**0.9**__

MINNESOTA MULTIPHASIC PERSONALITY INVENTORY

		Hs	60
		D	57
?	50	Hy	66
L	53	Pd	86
F	60	Mf	33
K	53	Pa	59
		Pt	56
		Sc	58
		Ma	70

TRAIL MAKING TEST

Part A: __**145**__ seconds
Part B: __**330**__ seconds
Discontinued at G (Circle #14)

STRENGTH OF GRIP

Dominant hand: __**23.0**__ kilograms

Non-dominant hand: __**—**__ kilograms

REITAN-KLØVE TACTILE FORM RECOGNITION TEST

Dominant hand: __**72**__ seconds; __**0**__ errors

Non-dominant hand: __**—**__ seconds; __**—**__ errors

REITAN-KLØVE SENSORY-PERCEPTUAL EXAM

			Error Totals	
RH ___ LH ___	Both H:	RH ___ LH **2**	RH ___ LH **2**	
RH ___ LF ___	Both H/F:	RH **2** LF **2**	RH **2** LF **2**	
LH ___ RF ___	Both H/F:	LH **2** RF ___	RF ___ LH **2**	
RE ___ LE ___	Both E:	RE ___ LE **3**	RE ___ LE **3**	
RV ___ LV ___	Both:	RV ___ LV ___	RV ___ LV ___	
___ ___		___ ___		
___ ___		___ ___		

TACTILE FINGER RECOGNITION

R 1___ 2___ 3 **1** 4___ 5 **1**   R **2** / **20**

L 1 **1** 2___ 3___ 2 **4** 4 **5** 1   L **8** / **20**

FINGER-TIP NUMBER WRITING

R 1___ 2___ 3___ 4___ 5 **2**   R **2** / **20**

L 1 **4** 2 **4** 3 **4** 4 **4** 5 **4**   L **20** / **20**

REITAN-KLØVE LATERAL-DOMINANCE EXAM

Show me how you:	
throw a ball	R
hammer a nail	R
cut with a knife	R
turn a door knob	R
use scissors	R
use an eraser	R
write your name	R

Record time used for spontaneous name-writing:

Preferred hand	__**17**__ seconds
Non-preferred hand	__**—**__ seconds

Show me how you:	
kick a football	R
step on a bug	R

REITAN-INDIANA APHASIA SCREENING TEST

Form for Adults and Older Children

Name: _____K. C. (I)_____ Age: _25_ Date: _____ Examiner: _____

Copy SQUARE	Repeat TRIANGLE
Name SQUARE	Repeat MASSACHUSETTS
Spell SQUARE	Repeat METHODIST EPISCOPAL
Copy CROSS	Write SQUARE
Name CROSS	Read SEVEN
Spell CROSS	Repeat SEVEN
Copy TRIANGLE	Repeat/Explain HE SHOUTED THE WARNING.
Name TRIANGLE	Write HE SHOUTED THE WARNING.
Spell TRIANGLE	Compute 85 – 27 =Initial response: 8x5=40. Second trial:8x5-27. Then said, I don't know whether they are adding-(SEE BELOW)*
Name BABY	Compute 17 X 3 =
Write CLOCK	Name KEY
Name FORK	Demonstrate use of KEY
Read 7 SIX 2 " 7 S-I-X - 6 - 2 "	Draw KEY
Read MGW	Read PLACE LEFT HAND TO RIGHT EAR.
Reading I	Place ~~LEFT~~ HAND TO ~~RIGHT~~ EAR RIGHT LEFT Placed right hand to right ear.
Reading II	Place ~~LEFT~~ HAND TO ~~LEFT~~ ELBOW RIGHT RIGHT Placed right hand to right shoulder.

* or subtracting." Examiner pointed to minus sign. Then patient performed correctly.

1.

2.

1.

2.

1.

2.

1. $8 \times 5 = 40$

2. $8 \times 5 - 27$

$$\begin{array}{r} 85 \\ -27 \\ \hline 58 \end{array}$$

a clock   square

He shouted a warning.

51

complete Part A in 145 seconds, but became entirely bewildered on Part B and the test was discontinued at the fourteenth circle (about 60% of the way through the 25 circles).

On the Tactual Performance Test K.C. demonstrated an equally striking indication of generalized deficit in dealing with relatively complex tasks that require mental alertness and immediate problem-solving capability. Since she was not able to use her left hand for this task, the examiner attempted to have K.C. do the test three times with her right hand. On the first trial the patient made very little progress and was able to place only three blocks in 15 minutes. She was able to do no better on the second trial and finally, in anger and frustration, tore off the blindfold and the test was discontinued. At that time it was taking her approximately five minutes to place each block. Results on this test indicate not only the problems K.C. experienced in dealing with complex and difficult tasks, but also her inability to continue working at the problem even though the task was difficult and frustrating.

The reader might be surprised to see that K.C. was able to perform so well on the Seashore Rhythm Test (27 of 30 items correct) when she demonstrated such significant impairment on other tests. It is possible that her good score on this test represented a selective retention of premorbid abilities, much as would be true for the Verbal subtests of the Wechsler Scale. However, the good score on the Rhythm Test adds more to our understanding of K.C.'s neuropsychological functions than the mere fact that she was able to differentiate pairs of rhythmic beats. The pairs of rhythmic beats represent well-defined and rather simple stimulus material and a fundamental requirement of the task is that the patient can pay close attention and maintain concentration through the series of 30 items. The fact that K.C. was able to do this task suggests that her brain is relatively stabilized in a biological sense. This observation, considered with relation to the indications of significant and serious deficits on other

tasks, strongly suggests that she will continue to have significant and serious impairment in the future because many aspects of spontaneous recovery of brain functions have probably been completed and her remaining deficits largely represent chronic residuals. Thus, even though K.C. may continue to improve to some degree, it is likely that her areas of deficit will continue to be pronounced.

Although lateralizing findings were present to implicate both cerebral hemispheres, they were much more pronounced for the right cerebral hemisphere. K.C. had very definite motor and sensory-perceptual deficits on the left side of her body. Her primary motor functions (grip strength and finger tapping speed) were not obviously or grossly impaired on the right side, but she was not able to perform these tasks at all with her left upper extremity. Although she was quite slow and unsure of herself with her right hand, with her left hand she was completely unable to hold and identify the forms used in the Tactile Form Recognition Test. On the Tactual Performance Test she was not able to use her left hand with any degree of effectiveness and, as noted above, the examiner asked her to perform this task only with her right hand.

Findings on tests of bilateral simultaneous tactile stimulation yielded evidence of much more difficulty on the left side of the body than the right side, but K.C. made some mistakes on the right hand when it was in competition with the left face. This finding tends to generalize the significance of the results regarding lateralization of cerebral damage and suggests that left cerebral functions are also implicated. On the test of bilateral simultaneous auditory stimulation K.C. had definite difficulty on the left side. Similar results were present on measures of tactile finger localization and finger-tip number writing perception; the patient had much more difficulty on the left hand than the right hand.

These lateralized motor and sensory-perceptual deficits support the diminished Performance IQ as an indicator of right cerebral damage. K.C.'s drawings on the Aphasia Screening Test also suggest that she has specific difficulties in dealing with simple spatial configurations. Thus, the lateralizing indicators which implicate the right cerebral hemisphere include both higher level skills (intellectual and visual-spatial abilities) and lower level functions (primary motor and sensory-perceptual skills) that depend principally upon the status of the right cerebral hemisphere.

Although the specific indications of left cerebral damage (which appeared primarily on the Aphasia Screening Test) were definite, they were not as pronounced as the findings implicating the right cerebral hemisphere. Note that K.C. failed to recognize that the letters "S-I-X" represented a word. In her first attempt she read them as individual letters; then, after a brief pause, she said the word "six." This response, which occurs very rarely among control subjects, is almost definitely an indication of left cerebral damage.

In her attempt to do simple arithmetic K.C. also had difficulty that extends beyond a state of general confusion. When initially given the problem "$85 - 27 =$" she wrote "$8 \times 5 = 40$." The examiner asked her to look at the problem more carefully and to do it again. This time she wrote "$8 \times 5 - 27$" and finally said, "I don't know whether they're adding or subtracting." Finally, the examiner pointed to the minus sign and this cue was sufficient to enable K.C. to proceed with the correct solution. However, the overall responses made it quite obvious that she was clearly confused by arithmetical processes and probably also by the symbolic significance and relationships of numbers. This type of deficit occurs about four times more frequently in persons with left cerebral damage than in patients with right cerebral damage (Wheeler & Reitan, 1962).

One may wonder how a patient can perform almost at the average level on the Arithmetic subtest on the Wechsler Scale and still demonstrate such a degree of confusion in performing simple arithmetical procedures. Despite the fact that this disparity occurs often in persons with left cerebral lesions, its exact biological basis has never been clearly demonstrated. Thus, in practical terms, the Arithmetic score on the Wechsler Scale is not a good lateralizing indicator (even though it is of some value as a general indicator of brain dysfunction), whereas specific confusion in solving the arithmetic problems on the Aphasia Screening Test occurs much more commonly in persons with left cerebral damage than right cerebral damage. K.C. also demonstrated evidence of right-left confusion, another deficit that occurs much more commonly in persons with left cerebral damage than right cerebral damage (Wheeler & Reitan, 1962).

Finally, when asked to place her right hand to her right elbow, K.C. placed her right hand to her right shoulder. One may question whether this response was due to a failure in auditory verbal comprehension (a manifestation of auditory verbal dysgnosia) or a confusion of body parts (body dysgnosia). Since she had shown no other specific difficulties on the Aphasia Screening Test in understanding instructions given by the examiner, in all probability this error reflected body dysgnosia. In either case, however, both of these deficits occur much more commonly in persons with left cerebral damage than right cerebral damage (Wheeler & Reitan, 1962).

Thus, although the indicators of right cerebral damage were much more pronounced (especially because they include comparisons of performances on the two sides of the body), specific indications of left cerebral damage were also clearly present. Specific deficits involving both cerebral hemispheres, in the context of indications of generalized impairment (even though one hemisphere is clearly more involved than the other), are to be expected in instances in which craniocerebral trauma causes severe cognitive impairment.

Results on the Minnesota Multiphasic Personality Inventory (MMPI) suggest that this woman has a number of difficulties in terms of affective reactions and adjustments to her environmental circumstances. However, her principal problems clearly center on motor, sensory-perceptual, and intellectual and cognitive deficits.

A neurological examination and electroencephalogram done three months after the initial neuropsychological testing showed essentially the same abnormalities that were previously found, except that there may have been very slight improvement. Twelve months after the initial examination the EEG showed striking abnormalities involving the left temporal area and, to a lesser extent, the homologous areas of the right cerebral hemisphere. Compared with the EEG done nine months earlier, this tracing showed no significant improvement. Conversely, the neurological examination showed that K.C.'s self-care abilities were improved, especially the skills relating to bladder control and urinary continence.

The neurologist also felt that K.C.'s memory for past events had continued to improve during the 12-month period since the first neuropsychological examination. In other respects, however, she continued to show neurological deficits, including a dense left hemiplegia with spasticity on the left side, hypalgesia of the left arm with hyperalgesia of the left leg, decreased facial sensitivity on the left side, mild ataxia on the right side, hyperreflexia and a Babinski sign on the left, and a mild left lower motor neuron facial weakness. K.C.'s answers on the Cornell Medical Index Health Questionnaire were positive much less frequently. She did indicate that she suffers from constant stomach trouble, frequently has severe headaches, and worries continually. The MMPI was not given because of the patient's impaired reading ability.

The pattern of results on the neuropsychological testing done 12 months after the first evaluation continues to indicate that K.C. had developed within the range of normal intellectual functions but had sustained significant impairment of abilities dependent upon brain functions. She still demonstrated specific evidence of right cerebral damage.

K.C.'s Verbal IQ (102) exceeded 55% of her age peers and her Performance IQ (84) exceeded 14%. Except for Digit Span (6), she scored at the average level or above on each of the Verbal subtests. On the Performance subtests she scored below the average level on four of the five subtests, including the two subtests that are particularly sensitive to right cerebral damage (Picture Arrangement, 8 and Block Design, 6) as well as the subtest that is most sensitive to cerebral involvement regardless of location (Digit Symbol, 5). Comparison of the distribution of Verbal and Performance subtest scores, together with the comparative IQ values, suggests that K.C. may have a depression of performance intelligence as a result of right cerebral damage.

K.C. continued to do poorly on each of the four most sensitive measures in the Halstead-Reitan Battery, although her score on the G-NDS had fallen into the range of Moderate Impairment. Her best performance occurred on the Category Test (65 errors), but even this score exceeded the average for a heterogeneous group of persons with cerebral damage. K.C. became quite confused on Part A of the Trail Making Test and had trouble finding the numbers. On Part B she became confused about the sequence of numbers and letters as well as the visual searching problem. This pattern of significant impairment in dealing with the spatial requirements of the Trail Making Test, in addition to the general requirements related to alertness and flexibility in thought processes, is fairly characteristic of persons with severe right cerebral damage.

The patient also had a great deal of difficulty on the Tactual Performance Test (especially the first trial). She performed much better on tasks that required only alertness to well-defined and specifically identified stimulus material (such as the Seashore Rhythm Test [25 correct] and the Speech-sounds Perception Test [9 errors]), indicating that she has basic attentional capabilities and that the first level of central processing is relatively intact.

THE HALSTEAD-REITAN
NEUROPSYCHOLOGICAL TEST BATTERY

Patient **K.C. (II)** Age **26** Sex **F** Education **16** Handedness **R**

WECHSLER-BELLEVUE SCALE

VIQ	102
PIQ	84
FS IQ	93
Information	10
Comprehension	12
Digit Span	6
Arithmetic	10
Similarities	11
Vocabulary	12
Picture Arrangement	8
Picture Completion	13
Block Design	6
Object Assembly	4
Digit Symbol	5

NEUROPSYCHOLOGICAL DEFICIT SCALE

Level of Performance	35
Pathognomonic Signs	3
Patterns	3
Right-Left Differences	17
Total NDS Score	58

TRAIL MAKING TEST

Part A: **223** seconds
Part B: **210** seconds
Discontinued at 6 (Circle #11)

STRENGTH OF GRIP

Dominant hand: **36.5** kilograms

Non-dominant hand: **2.5** kilograms

REITAN-KLØVE TACTILE FORM RECOGNITION TEST

Dominant hand: **65** seconds; **0** errors

Non-dominant hand: **—** seconds; **—** errors

REITAN-KLØVE SENSORY-PERCEPTUAL EXAM

			Error Totals	
RH___ LH___	Both H:	RH___ LH **2**	RH___ LH **2**	
RH___ LF___	Both H/F:	RH___ LF___	RH___ LF___	
LH___ RF___	Both H/F:	LH___ RF___	RF___ LH___	
RE___ LE___	Both E:	RE___ LE___	RE___ LE___	
RV___ LV___	Both:	RV___ LV___	RV___ LV___	

TACTILE FINGER RECOGNITION

R 1___ 2___ 3___ 4___ 5___ R **0** / **20**

L 1___ 2___ 3 **1** 4 **3** 5 **1** L **5** / **20**

FINGER-TIP NUMBER WRITING

R 1___ 2___ 3___ 4___ 5___ R **0** / **20**

L 1 **1** 2___ 3 **1** 4___ 5 **1** L **3** / **20**

HALSTEAD'S NEUROPSYCHOLOGICAL TEST BATTERY

Category Test   **65**

Tactual Performance Test

Right hand: **15.0 (4 blocks)**

Right hand: **9.5**

Right hand: **10.6**

Total Time	**35.1 (24 blocks)**
Memory	**5**
Localization	**0**

Seashore Rhythm Test

Number Correct **25**   **6**

Speech-sounds Perception Test

Number of Errors   **9**

Finger Oscillation Test

Dominant hand: **44**   **44**

Non-dominant hand: **—**

Impairment Index **1.0**

MINNESOTA MULTIPHASIC PERSONALITY INVENTORY } NOT GIVEN; IMPAIRED READING ABILITY

		Hs	___
		D	___
?	___	Hy	___
L	___	Pd	___
F	___	Mf	___
K	___	Pa	___
		Pt	___
		Sc	___
		Ma	___

REITAN-KLØVE LATERAL-DOMINANCE EXAM

Show me how you:

throw a ball	**R**
hammer a nail	**R**
cut with a knife	**R**
turn a door knob	**R**
use scissors	**R**
use an eraser	**R**
write your name	**R**

Record time used for spontaneous name-writing:

Preferred hand	**16** seconds
Non-preferred hand	**—** seconds

Show me how you:

kick a football	**R**
step on a bug	**R**

REITAN-INDIANA APHASIA SCREENING TEST

Form for Adults and Older Children

Name: _____ K. C. (II) _____ Age: __26__

Copy SQUARE	Repeat TRIANGLE
Name SQUARE	Repeat MASSACHUSETTS
Spell SQUARE	Repeat METHODIST EPISCOPAL
Copy CROSS	Write SQUARE
Name CROSS	Read SEVEN
Spell CROSS	Repeat SEVEN
Copy TRIANGLE	Repeat/Explain HE SHOUTED THE WARNING.
Name TRIANGLE	Write HE SHOUTED THE WARNING.
Spell TRIANGLE	Compute 85 – 27 =
Name BABY	Compute 17 X 3 =
Write CLOCK	Name KEY
Name FORK	Demonstrate use of KEY
Read 7 SIX 2	Draw KEY
Read MGW	Read PLACE LEFT HAND TO RIGHT EAR.
Reading I	Place LEFT HAND TO RIGHT EAR
Reading II	Place LEFT HAND TO LEFT ELBOW With aid of her right hand, she lifted left hand to left shoulder, realized her mistake, and said she couldn't do it.

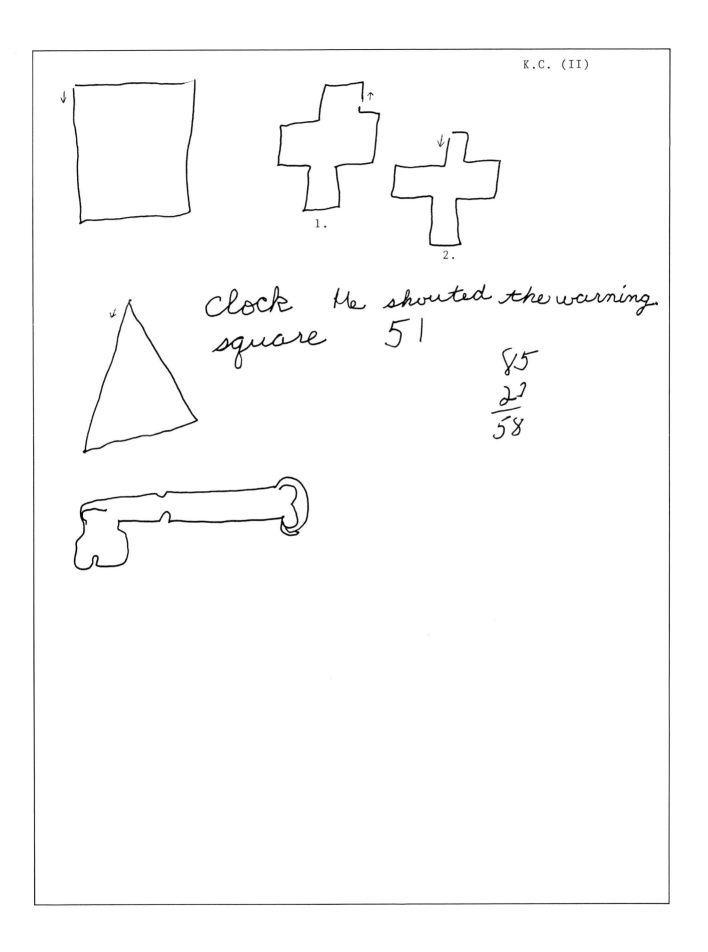

1.

2.

clock   He shouted the warning.

square   51

85
23
58

As in the initial examination, the lateralizing results implicated principally the right cerebral hemisphere. On the left side of the body K.C. had marked motor deficits (finger tapping speed and grip strength) and definite tactile-perceptual losses. These deficits were manifested on the Tactile Form Recognition Test, by impaired perception on the left hand in tests of bilateral simultaneous tactile stimulation, and evidence of impairment on the left hand in tactile finger localization and finger-tip number writing perception.

These deficits would hardly be considered to be induced by peripheral involvement, considering the fact that peripheral involvement alone would be unlikely to account for (1) both motor and tactile-perceptual losses, (2) significant impairment on generalized tests of brain function, and (3) higher-level indicators of right cerebral dysfunction that included mild constructional dyspraxia and a clearly lower Performance than Verbal IQ.

The patient also showed a definite indication of left cerebral dysfunction (body dysgnosia) when she was asked to place her left hand to her left elbow. She confused her shoulder with her elbow, realized her mistake, and then said she was not able to do the task.

Direct comparisons of the neuropsychological test results obtained at the initial examination with the findings obtained 12 months later indicates that improvement occurred in a number of areas: (1) The Performance IQ had risen from 66 to 84, (2) Part B of the Trail Making Test was somewhat improved, (3) On the Tactual Performance Test only about 1.5 minutes per block were required (compared to five minutes per block on the first testing), (4) Grip strength had increased with the right upper extremity from 23.0 kg to 36.5 kg, (5) There were fewer instances of failure to perceive a stimulus with bilateral simultaneous stimulation, (6) On the left hand there was a striking reduction in the number of errors on finger-tip number writing perception (from 20 errors to 3

errors), (7) There was no evidence of dyscalculia, right-left confusion, or difficulty in perceiving the symbolic significance of verbal material. As shown by the G-NDS (which decreased from 77 to 58), the improvement occurred principally on level of performance.

In many respects K.C.'s scores on the second testing were approximately the same as her scores on the initial examination and the difference in scores demonstrated only chance variation. The Localization score on the Tactual Performance Test (0) was reduced from a score of 2 on the first testing, but this single measure would scarcely be a basis for presuming any significant deterioration of brain functions. In summary, K.C. showed significant improvement on a number of tests, had unchanged scores on others, and did not show evidence of significant deterioration. A direct comparison of the two examinations substantiates the contention that when there is improvement, it occurs principally in the area of initial deficit, indicating once again that spontaneous or natural recovery is a process in which the initial wound (impairment) is repaired.

Formal rehabilitation efforts for K.C. had focused principally on physical therapy, an area in which she showed probably the least recovery (judging from comparison of the two sets of neuropsychological test results). It is possible, of course, that the lesion involving motor functions was too extensive or pronounced to permit recovery in this area, regardless of the rehabilitational effort expended. The possibility of a distinct dissociation occurring between the degree of recovery of motor functions and recovery of higher-level neuropsychological abilities is clearly indicated by the patient's test results.

A neurological examination performed 18 months after the initial neuropsychological testing showed findings which were very similar to those obtained 6 months earlier. K.C. may have shown some mild improvement in strength and movement of the left extremities, but she did not demonstrate any improvement in coordination. In addition to noting essentially the same neurological deficits, the neurologist also remarked that K.C. appeared to be depressed, tearful, and angry regarding her physical handicaps. The electroencephalogram continued to show marked disturbances of brain functions, principally involving the left temporal area. Compared with the EEG obtained six months earlier, the most recent EEG showed evidence of slight, if any, improvement.

K.C. had great difficulty reading any material, such as the Minnesota Multiphasic Personality Inventory or Cornell Medical Index Health Questionnaire items; she would position her head strangely and move her head in short jerks as she tried to read successive material. She also had poor visual acuity which antedated the head injury. Since this combination of factors appeared to impair their validity, these tests were not administered. Upon direct questioning the patient had no particular complaints and said that there had been no changes since the time of the examination six months before. This statement was made despite her angry, tearful, and depressed comments made to the neurologists.

Results of the 18-month examination continued to show certain indications of mild improvement; however, compared with the examination done six months earlier, there was also deterioration on some of the tests. The general pattern of deficits was very similar to the pattern on the two previous testings. The G-NDS score increased from 58 to 66.

K.C. earned a Verbal IQ of 108, a Performance IQ of 84, and a Full Scale IQ of 96. Considering the changes in one direction or another on the various subtests, it would be difficult to support a contention of any reliable ability changes on the Wechsler Scale. Except for the reappearance of arithmetical confusion and an increased number of errors on the Sensory-perceptual Examination,

K.C. showed relatively mild changes on the rest of the Battery.

The four general indicators were still significantly impaired, but on this examination the patient was able to complete the Trail Making Test (even though it took her 510 seconds). Although she was quite slow (with a Total Time of 52.2 min), she was also able to complete all three trials of the Tactual Performance Test using her right hand. Grip strength showed no change with the right hand; however, K.C. was probably gaining a little strength in her left upper extremity even though it was still strikingly impaired.

The major indications of increased deficit centered on simple sensory-perceptual tasks. On the 12-month examination K.C. had relatively little difficulty on tests of bilateral simultaneous sensory stimulation (two errors), but on the 18-month examination she made many more errors (11). It was particularly striking that her inability to perceive an auditory stimulus to the left ear when a stimulus was given simultaneously to the right ear was just as profound (if not even more so) as at the time of the initial examination. She also had much more difficulty perceiving bilateral simultaneous tactile stimuli. Although she had essentially recovered her ability to perceive numbers written on her finger-tips, on this examination she clearly had more difficulty on the left hand than she had on the 12-month testing.

Finally, K.C. again demonstrated significant difficulties in solving simple arithmetical problems. She became confused when subtracting 27 from 85, giving an answer of "28." She was able to mentally multiply 17 × 3 satisfactorily, but, in recording the answer, caught herself just as she was writing a "0" after her answer of "51." Because of these instances of obvious confusion, the examiner asked the patient to multiply 6 × 4. As can be observed, K.C. responded by writing "64."

It does not seem likely that these additional deficits can be explained by a hypothesis of any

THE HALSTEAD-REITAN
NEUROPSYCHOLOGICAL TEST BATTERY

Patient ___K.C. (III)___ Age __27__ Sex __F__ Education __16__ Handedness __R__

WECHSLER-BELLEVUE SCALE

VIQ	108
PIQ	84
FS IQ	96
Information	10
Comprehension	11
Digit Span	9
Arithmetic	10
Similarities	14
Vocabulary	13
Picture Arrangement	11
Picture Completion	9
Block Design	5
Object Assembly	7
Digit Symbol	4

NEUROPSYCHOLOGICAL DEFICIT SCALE	
Level of Performance	40
Pathognomonic Signs	2
Patterns	5
Right-Left Differences	19
Total NDS Score	66

HALSTEAD'S NEUROPSYCHOLOGICAL TEST BATTERY

Category Test   57

Tactual Performance Test

Right hand: __19.0__

Right hand: __21.1__

Right hand: __12.1__

Total Time	52.2
Memory	5
Localization	1

Seashore Rhythm Test

Number Correct __26__   5

Speech-sounds Perception Test

Number of Errors   13

Finger Oscillation Test

Dominant hand: __47__   47

Non-dominant hand: __—__

Impairment Index   0.9

TRAIL MAKING TEST

Part A: __131__ seconds

Part B: __510__ seconds

STRENGTH OF GRIP

Dominant hand: __35.5__ kilograms

Non-dominant hand: __5.5__ kilograms

REITAN-KLØVE TACTILE FORM RECOGNITION TEST

Dominant hand: __61__ seconds; __0__ errors

Non-dominant hand: __—__ seconds; __—__ errors

REITAN-KLØVE SENSORY-PERCEPTUAL EXAM

				Error Totals	
RH___ LH___	Both H:	RH _1_ LH _2_	RH _1_ LH _2_
RH___ LF___	Both H/F:	RH _3_ LF___	RH _3_ LF___
LH___ RF___	Both H/F:	LH _1_ RF___	RF___ LH _1_
RE___ LE___	Both E:	RE___ LE _4_	RE___ LE _4_
RV___ LV___	Both:	RV___ LV___	RV___ LV___
___ ___		___ ___	
___ ___		___ ___	

TACTILE FINGER RECOGNITION

R 1___ 2___ 3___ 4___ 5 _1_   R _1_ / 20

L 1 _1_ 2 _2_ 3 _3_ 4 _1_ 5 _2_   L _9_ / 20

FINGER-TIP NUMBER WRITING

R 1 _1_ 2___ 3___ 4___ 5___   R _1_ / 20

L 1 _1_ 2___ 3___ 4___ 5___   L _1_ / 20

MINNESOTA MULTIPHASIC PERSONALITY INVENTORY

NOT GIVEN; IMPAIRED READING ABIL.

		Hs	___
		D	___
?	___	Hy	___
L	___	Pd	___
F	___	Mf	___
K	___	Pa	___
		Pt	___
NOT GIVEN. IMPAIRED		Sc	___
READING ABILITY.		Ma	___

REITAN-KLØVE LATERAL-DOMINANCE EXAM

Show me how you:

throw a ball	R
hammer a nail	R
cut with a knife	R
turn a door knob	R
use scissors	R
use an eraser	R
write your name	R

Record time used for spontaneous name-writing:

Preferred hand	__14__ seconds
Non-preferred hand	__—__ seconds

Show me how you:

kick a football	R
step on a bug	R

REITAN-INDIANA APHASIA SCREENING TEST

Form for Adults and Older Children

Name: _____ K. C. (III) _____ Age: ___27___

Copy SQUARE	Repeat TRIANGLE
Name SQUARE	Repeat MASSACHUSETTS
Spell SQUARE	Repeat METHODIST EPISCOPAL
Copy CROSS	Write SQUARE
Name CROSS	Read SEVEN
Spell CROSS	Repeat SEVEN
Copy TRIANGLE	Repeat/Explain HE SHOUTED THE WARNING.
Name TRIANGLE	Write HE SHOUTED THE WARNING.
Spell TRIANGLE	Compute 85 – 27 = "28." Given 96 – 38 and done correctly.
Name BABY	Compute 17 X 3 = Started to write a "0" after "51", but said, "A boo-boo," and examiner permitted her to erase. Gave 6x4 and she answered
Write CLOCK	Name KEY "64."
Name FORK	Demonstrate use of KEY
Read 7 SIX 2	Draw KEY
Read MGW	Read PLACE LEFT HAND TO RIGHT EAR.
Reading I	Place LEFT HAND TO RIGHT EAR
Reading II	Place LEFT HAND TO LEFT ELBOW

clock   square

He shouted the warning.

85
-27
28

96
-38   51 64
58

progression in general confusion. In fact, K.C. continued to be quite alert and able to focus her attention to specific stimulus material (as demonstrated by a Seashore Rhythm Test score of 26) and had general intelligence levels that were a little higher than at the 12-month examination. Her Category Test score was slightly better (although the improvement may have reflected only positive practice-effect), and on this examination she was somewhat more capable on both the Tactual Performance Test and the Trail Making Test than she had been at the 12-month testing.

From these neuropsychological test results it would appear that the patient must have had some progressive deterioration of the brain, probably in fairly focal areas, that was the basis for the rather specific additional deficits that were present. Although other patients with evidence of initial structural cerebral damage often show more striking evidence of deterioration during the 12th to 18th months post-injury, K.C. also demonstrated the same general pattern.

CASE #6

Name: J.B.

Age: 68

Education: 11

Sex: Male

Handedness: Right

Occupation: Shopkeeper

Background Information

J.B. was a 68-year-old man who had owned and operated the same second-hand store for many years. One evening, as he was putting some items on shelves in the back of the store, a robber entered through the front door. He approached J.B. from behind and hit him on the head several times with a blunt object. A neighbor who heard the commotion came over to investigate and found J.B. lying on the floor, holding his head and moaning. The neighbor immediately called an ambulance.

On the way to the hospital J.B. was reportedly confused and disoriented but probably unconscious only for a brief period of time. In the hospital emergency room he was very disoriented and started to vomit. He had several scalp lacerations, particularly on the posterior part of his head. X-rays showed multiple compound linear skull fractures but no evidence of depressed bone fragments.

Neurological Examination

Physical examination at the time of admission revealed nystagmus on left lateral gaze. There was no evidence of dysphasia or lateralizing focal signs. J.B. was alert and oriented by the time he was seen by a neurosurgeon, shortly after being admitted to the hospital. The neurological examination demonstrated mild impairment of extraocular movements, paresis of the fourth cranial nerve without diplopia, and increased nystagmus on left lateral gaze. On the basis of these findings a diagnosis of brain stem contusion was made. The

patient had no signs of contusion or focal damage involving the cerebral hemispheres.

J.B.'s condition was somewhat improved the day following the injury; the nystagmus had resolved and cranial nerve functions were normal. He continued to show steady improvement up to the time of discharge from the hospital on the sixth day post-injury.

Neuropsychological Examination

Neuropsychological examination was done 16 days after the injury. An electroencephalogram done at that time suggested a marked disturbance of brain functions, primarily involving the right frontal area. The homologous area of the left hemisphere was also affected, but to a much lesser extent. On the Cornell Medical Index Health Questionnaire J.B. offered absolutely no complaints except that he was hard of hearing.

In a person this age (68) it is sometimes difficult to differentiate neuropsychologically between the adverse effects of normal aging and the effects of brain trauma. The cognitive consequences of aging on the Halstead-Reitan Battery have been studied in detail (Reitan, 1967; Reitan & Wolfson, 1986a). However, a problem exists when interpreting test results for an older individual who has sustained a head injury. There may be some confusion because the effects are adverse in each instance and may cause changes that deviate from normality in the same direction. We will use the case of J.B. to differentiate test findings

THE HALSTEAD-REITAN
NEUROPSYCHOLOGICAL TEST BATTERY

Patient _____ **J.B. (I)** _____ Age __**68**__ Sex __**M**__ Education __**11**__ Handedness __**R**__

WECHSLER-BELLEVUE SCALE
VIQ	104
PIQ	98
FS IQ	102
Information	9
Comprehension	9
Digit Span	9
Arithmetic	10
Similarities	6
Vocabulary	8
Picture Arrangement	6
Picture Completion	6
Block Design	7
Object Assembly	6
Digit Symbol	3

NEUROPSYCHOLOGICAL DEFICIT SCALE
Level of Performance	41
Pathognomonic Signs	6
Patterns	4
Right-Left Differences	11
Total NDS Score	62

HALSTEAD'S NEUROPSYCHOLOGICAL TEST BATTERY
Category Test _____ 79

Tactual Performance Test

Dominant hand:	15.0 (3 blocks)
Non-dominant hand:	15.0 (3 blocks)
Both hands:	15.0 (7 blocks)

Total Time	45.0 (13 block
Memory	3
Localization	1

Seashore Rhythm Test

Number Correct __**21**__ _____ **10**

Speech-sounds Perception Test

Number of Errors _____ **30**

Finger Oscillation Test

Dominant hand:	41	41
Non-dominant hand:	33	

Impairment Index __**1.0**__

TRAIL MAKING TEST
Part A: __**105**__ seconds
Part B: __**235**__ seconds

STRENGTH OF GRIP
Dominant hand:	31.5	kilograms
Non-dominant hand:	28.5	kilograms

REITAN-KLØVE TACTILE FORM RECOGNITION TEST
Dominant hand:	23	seconds;	0	errors
Non-dominant hand:	18	seconds;	0	errors

MINNESOTA MULTIPHASIC PERSONALITY INVENTORY

			Hs	65
			D	63
?	50		Hy	67
L	70		Pd	64
F	50		Mf	51
K	77		Pa	56
			Pt	62
			Sc	61
			Ma	45

REITAN-KLØVE SENSORY-PERCEPTUAL EXAM

		Error Totals	
RH___LH___	Both H: RH___LH___	RH___LH___	
RH___LF___	Both H/F: RH___LF___	RH___LF___	
LH___RF___	Both H/F: LH___RF___	RF___LH___	
RE___LE___	Both E: RE___LE _1_	RE___LE _1_	
RV___LV___	Both: RV___LV___	RV___LV___	
___ ___	___ ___		
___ ___	___ ___		

REITAN-KLØVE LATERAL-DOMINANCE EXAM

Show me how you:
throw a ball	R
hammer a nail	R
cut with a knife	R
turn a door knob	R
use scissors	R
use an eraser	R
write your name	R

Record time used for spontaneous name-writing:
Preferred hand	7	seconds
Non-preferred hand	27	seconds

Show me how you:
kick a football	R
step on a bug	R

TACTILE FINGER RECOGNITION
R 1__ 2__ 3__ 4 _2_ 5 _1_   R _3_ / 20

L 1__ 2 _4_ 3 _2_ 4__ 5__   L _6_ / 20

FINGER-TIP NUMBER WRITING
R 1 _1_ 2 _1_ 3 _1_ 4 _2_ 5 _1_   R _6_ / 20

L 1 _2_ 2 _1_ 3 _2_ 4 _1_ 5 _1_   L _7_ / 20

REITAN-INDIANA APHASIA SCREENING TEST

Form for Adults and Older Children

Name: _____ J. B. (I) _____ Age: __68__

Copy SQUARE	Repeat TRIANGLE
Name SQUARE "One." Examiner questioned. "Well, it's a square."	Repeat MASSACHUSETTS
Spell SQUARE	Repeat METHODIST EPISCOPAL "Methodist Apiscopull"
Copy CROSS	Write SQUARE
Name CROSS "Two." Examiner questioned. "Is it a cross?"	Read SEVEN
Spell CROSS	Repeat SEVEN
Copy TRIANGLE	Repeat/Explain HE SHOUTED THE WARNING Repeat –"He shouted the word." Then, self-corrected. Explain – SEE BELOW *
Name TRIANGLE "Is that a four?" Examiner repeated instructions. "Is it a rectangle?"	Write HE SHOUTED THE WARNING.
Spell TRIANGLE	Compute 85 – 27 =
Name BABY	Compute 17 X 3 =
Write CLOCK	Name KEY
Name FORK	Demonstrate use of KEY
Read 7 SIX 2	Draw KEY
Read MGW	Read PLACE LEFT HAND TO RIGHT EAR.
Reading I	Place LEFT HAND TO RIGHT EAR
Reading II	Place LEFT HAND TO LEFT ELBOW

*"Some little thing came about in the Revolutionary War and a warning was given." Examiner asked for further explanation. "Oh, in time of danger."

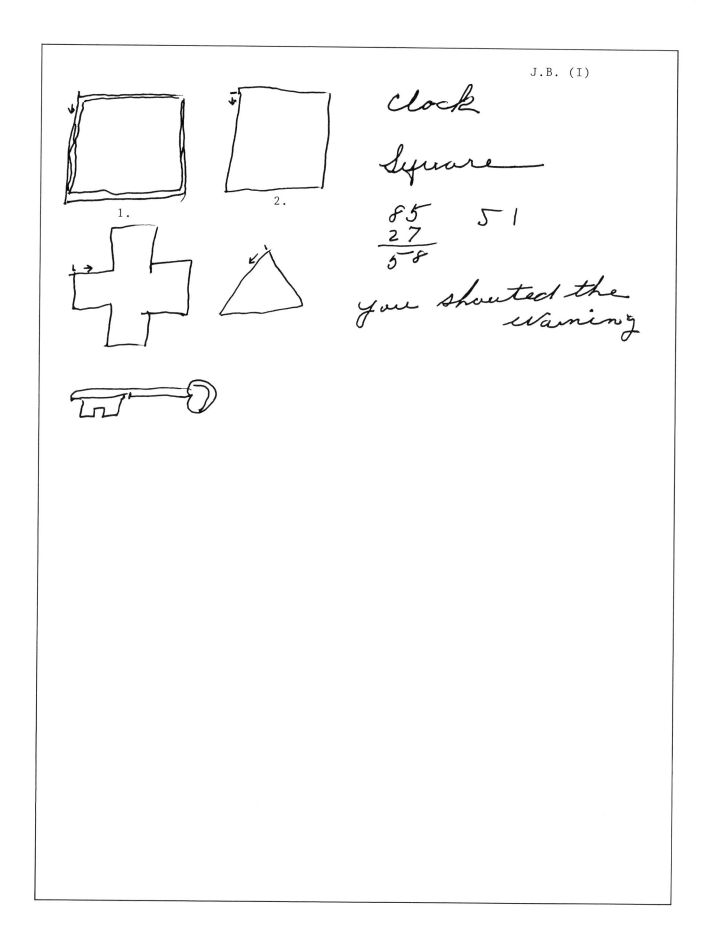

1.

2.

clock

square

$$\begin{array}{r} 85 \\ 27 \\ \hline 5\;8 \end{array}$$
51

you shouted the
warning

due to aging from those resulting from a head injury.

The principal changes caused by aging are reflected by the tests most specifically sensitive to the status of the brain (e.g., the Category Test). The effects of aging also tend to impair the level of performance rather generally on brain-sensitive tests, and aging by itself does not usually generate specific focal or lateralized signs. Of course, neuropsychological deficits due to head injury are also reflected principally by the tests most sensitive to brain damage; however, in most instances of brain trauma, certain specific or lateralizing indicators are also present, even though they may involve both cerebral hemispheres concurrently.

J.B. earned a Verbal IQ (104) in the upper part of the average range, exceeding about 61% of his age peers. Although he did poorly on Similarities (6), most of his Verbal subtest scores were just below or near the average level. Even though the Similarities subtest has been identified as the most sensitive of the Verbal subtests to cerebral damage, it would be difficult to attribute the poor performance on this test to cerebral damage because other factors, including chance, could have played a role.

In terms of the weighted scores, the Performance subtests were consistently performed as poorly as the Verbal subtests or worse. Except for an especially low score on Digit Symbol (3), the Performance subtests showed little variability. In older persons it is not at all unusual to see lower weighted scores on the Performance subtests than on the Verbal subtests; therefore, J.B.'s results probably suggest only some generalized deterioration of Performance intelligence skills. It is possible, though, that the low score on Digit Symbol may be due to more than the effects of aging and may reflect actual cerebral damage.

J.B. performed poorly on all four of the most sensitive measures in the Halstead-Reitan Battery. The Impairment Index of 1.0 indicates that all of his scores on Halstead's tests were in the brain-damaged range. Compared to normal subjects J.B.

performed poorly on the Category Test (79) and was very slow on Part B of the Trail Making Test (235 sec). On his drawing of the Tactual Performance Test board he could localize only one block. Considering his age, the best of J.B.'s scores was on the Category Test. Of all of the tests in the Battery, the Category Test is generally the most sensitive to aging effects among normal subjects. While 79 errors is worse than would be expected from most 68-year-old normal subjects, it is not indicative of severe impairment for persons that age. Among these four most sensitive measures, Part B of the Trail Making Test was most suggestive of significant impairment due to brain trauma. Thus, in accordance with recovery from the effects of the recent traumatic insult, on future examinations one might expect J.B. to show some improvement on Part B of the Trail Making Test.

J.B. also performed poorly on other measures of generalized cerebral functions. He was very slow in placing the blocks on the Tactual Performance Test and was unable to complete the test in 15.0 minutes on any of the trials. In fact, across the three trials he required an average of 3.46 minutes to place each block, which would have averaged 34.60 minutes for *each* of the three trials (if he had been able to place all of the blocks on each trial). J.B. remembered the shapes of only three of the 10 blocks, and as noted earlier, was able to localize only one of the figures in his drawing.

The patient also performed poorly on the Seashore Rhythm Test (21 correct) and the Speech-sounds Perception Test (30 errors). In fact, considering his Verbal IQ of 104, his score on the Speech-sounds Perception Test (which indicates special impairment of receptive language abilities) might raise a question of specific damage of the left cerebral hemisphere. The slow performance with each hand on the Tactile Form Recognition Test and the number of errors on each hand in finger-tip number writing perception also suggested generalized impairment of cognitive functions. Therefore, considering J.B.'s poor performances on the tests sensitive to generalized brain functions with relation to his IQ values, the results indicate generalized damage involving each cerebral hemisphere.

Note also that J.B. showed definite evidence of lateralized dysfunction. Although the results on the Aphasia Screening Test implicated the left cerebral hemisphere, one would be reluctant to identify the patient's defective responses as representing actual dysphasia.

J.B.'s naming problems (dysnomia) were clearly demonstrated when he was asked to name the square, cross, and triangle. He showed a tendency toward numbering his responses rather than naming the figure. One might wonder whether this represented generalized confusion, but such a hypothesis is scarcely consistent with a Verbal IQ of 104. We see that when J.B. was asked to respond in a highly specific way to well-identified stimulus material he used very inappropriate verbalizations. In fact, when questioned by the examiner, he finally identified the first figure as a square but did not seem quite sure of his response. After he called the cross a "two" the examiner questioned J.B. further and then he was even less sure of the appropriate word to use to identify the figure. This kind of naming confusion continued when he was asked to give the name of the triangle. Responses of this kind are definitely not within the normal range (even for older persons) and probably represent a mild degree of dysphasia manifested by dysnomia.

J.B. performed correctly on the next items until he was asked to repeat METHODIST EPISCO-PAL. The type of error he made is seen among many normal subjects and is not significant with respect to brain damage.

Notice, though, that his confusion in dealing with simple verbal material for communicational purposes was again demonstrated when he was asked to repeat and then explain the sentence HE SHOUTED THE WARNING. J.B. first responded, "He shouted the word," then realized he had made a mistake and corrected himself. This kind of error

rarely occurs among normal subjects and almost certainly reflects confusion in registering the sentence after hearing it spoken by the examiner and then attempting to repeat it.

When asked to give the meaning of the sentence, the patient resorted to a statement that was scarcely relevant, and in effect managed only to repeat that a warning was given. Only after he was asked for further explanation was he able to evoke the concept of danger. This latter result suggests that his initial failure to repeat the sentence was probably related to limited registration and poor understanding (an impairment in the area of auditory verbal comprehension) and that the total response, including the explanation, most likely indicates the presence of auditory verbal dysgnosia.

J.B.'s difficulty in using verbal symbols for communicational purposes (and his tendency toward confusion in this respect) was also demonstrated when he was asked to write HE SHOUTED THE WARNING. It can be seen that he wrote quite legibly but substituted "you" for "He."

Finally, certain responses on the Aphasia Screening Test were also quite definite in suggesting right cerebral dysfunction. The patient's drawing of the cross showed confusion concerning the spatial configuration as well as dyssymmetry of the lateral extremity on the right side of the figure. Although the general configuration was almost within normal limits, the details and types of errors J.B. made are strongly suggestive of right cerebral dysfunction.

The patient had comparable difficulties copying the key. He was confused about the handle of the key as it joined the stem, the drawing of the inside part of the handle, and the notches in the stem near the teeth of the key. Mistakes of this kind are strongly indicative of cerebral damage rather than limited drawing ability.

In summary, then, the Aphasia Screening Test revealed definite deviations from normal expectancy (even for a 68-year-old person) and identified deficits that were probably caused by craniocerebral trauma. If this presumption is correct, one would expect these signs of deficit to improve as recovery from brain damage progressed.

Further review of lateralizing indicators (the right hand compared with the left on the Tactile Form Recognition Test) showed only possible left hemisphere impairment. However, the very poor performance on the Speech-sounds Perception Test with relation to Verbal IQ and the impairment shown on the Aphasia Screening Test in dealing with verbal symbols for communicational purposes rather definitely implicate the left cerebral hemisphere.

In addition to demonstrating mild drawing difficulties of the type shown by persons with cerebral damage (if not specifically called constructional dyspraxia), J.B. showed slow finger tapping speed with his left hand (33) as compared with his right (41), impaired ability to identify fingers touched on the left hand (6 errors) as compared with the right hand (3 errors), no improvement on the second trial of the Tactual Performance Test (three blocks placed in 15 minutes), and a very mild tendency to fail to perceive an auditory stimulus to the left ear when given simultaneously to both ears. (Note that although the performance with the left hand on the TPT was particularly poor, the most outstanding implication of this test relates to generalized impairment.)

Results on the Minnesota Multiphasic Personality Inventory suggest that J.B. has a number of emotional and affective problems. He seems to want to give a very good impression of himself, has some anxiety and concern about his physical functioning, and experiences feelings of general anxiety. In most respects, however, the MMPI profile was not strikingly deviant.

The G-NDS was distinctly elevated with a score of 62 (compared to the average of 17.20 points for control subjects). This value falls well into the range of moderate impairment and exceeds the expected increment for older persons. In addition, the section of Pathognomonic Signs had a score of 6, and even among normal older persons deficits of the kind are minimal (Reitan & Wolfson, 1986b).

In summary, the results of the first neuropsychological examination demonstrated significant impairment of brain-related abilities, with some specific indicators implicating left cerebral damage and other findings suggesting right cerebral involvement. It is difficult to differentiate perfectly between the indicators of generalized impairment related to aging and the deficits caused by the head injury. However, it is likely that the very poor performance on Part B of the Trail Making Test is due to the immediate effects of brain trauma and probably will show improvement on future testings.

As noted above, J.B. was extremely impaired on the Tactual Performance Test. Even though his performance is probably partially due to brain injury and some improvement can also be expected to occur as the brain recovers, it is likely that future performances on this test will continue to demonstrate some impairment. The "dysphasic" deficits are probably due to the recent head injury and will most likely show some improvement in time. The right hemisphere lateralizing effects may also be at least partially caused by cerebral trauma. The disparity between the left and right hands on finger tapping speed will probably be less pronounced when the patient is re-examined and the performance with the left hand on the Tactual Performance Test may improve.

Two factors operating concurrently make it difficult to predict how much change or improvement will be seen on later examinations: (1) The patient should be showing some degree of improvement from the recent impairing effects of the head injury, but (2) he may also show progressive deterioration as a result of normal aging. In addition, one should remember that the brain of an older person does not have the same capacity for spontaneous recovery as the brain of a younger person. Although the lateralizing findings should be less pronounced on future testings, we would predict that relatively little overall improvement will be seen.

J.B. was re-examined neurologically three months after the first evaluation. The neurological examination indicated the following: (1) Both the upper and lower right extremities were weaker than the left extremities, (2) a terminal tremor on finger-to-finger testing was worse with the right hand than the left, (3) the right ankle jerk reflex was weaker on the left side, (4) when the tongue was protruded it deviated slightly to the right side, (5) tandem gait was done poorly (with a tendency to veer either to the left or right), (6) rapid alternating movements were slow and performed poorly on each side, (7) the snout reflex was present; and (8) hearing was diminished bilaterally. EEG tracings showed improvement compared to the previous examination, but moderate abnormalities were still present over the frontal-temporal areas of both cerebral hemispheres.

When questioned directly, J.B. said that his memory was about the same as it had been previous to the accident. He remembered being in his store and checking an item on the shelf when someone approached him from behind and struck him on the head. His next recollection was of being in the hospital and being transported from the emergency room to x-ray.

Twelve months after the initial neuropsychological testing J.B. was re-evaluated. The neurological examination indicated that his strength was improved and no apparent difference existed on the two sides. The snout reflex was still present and his hearing was diminished bilaterally. The EEG showed marked disturbances over the right frontal areas and, to a lesser extent, the homologous regions of the left hemisphere. The patient's responses on the Cornell Medical Index Health Questionnaire indicated that he was frequently ill but he offered no specific complaints.

The test results, initially considered without reference to the previous neuropsychological findings, indicate significant impairment of brain-related abilities in a person who apparently had developed approximately average intelligence levels previously. J.B. earned a Verbal IQ (105) in the upper part of the average range (exceeding about 63% of his age peers) and a Performance IQ (103) just two points lower, exceeding 58%. These values yielded a Full Scale IQ (101) almost exactly at the the average level, exceeding 53%. The Verbal subtest scores showed relatively little variability. It is unusual for a brain-damaged person to have his best score on the Arithmetic subtest (10), but this might have been related to J.B.'s activities as a storekeeper.

J.B. consistently performed worse on the Performance subtests than on the Verbal subtests, a finding that is not unusual for a person his age. From the results of the Wechsler Scale alone it would be difficult to conclude that this man had sustained any cerebral damage.

J.B. performed quite poorly on the four most sensitive measures in the Halstead-Reitan Battery. His Impairment Index (1.0) indicated that all of Halstead's tests had scores in the brain-damaged range. He also did poorly on the Category Test (86) and the Localization component (1) of the Tactual Performance Test. He was much slower than we would expect on Part B of the Trail Making Test (201 sec). The results on these measures, especially when considered with relation to the IQ values, suggest that J.B. is more significantly impaired than the normal 69-year-old person.

Other indicators of the generalized aspects of brain functions also demonstrated serious impairment. J.B. was somewhat able to concentrate his attention on specific stimulus material (22 correct on the Seashore Rhythm Test), but he performed extremely poorly on tasks that were more difficult and required adaptability to relatively novel circumstances (e.g., the Tactual Performance Test). His Total Time on the TPT (38.6 min with only 26 rather than all 30 blocks placed) represented one of his worst performances.

Lateralizing signs, which principally implicated the left cerebral hemisphere, were also present on the second examination but were not particularly striking. Although right-handed, J.B. was

THE HALSTEAD-REITAN
NEUROPSYCHOLOGICAL TEST BATTERY

Patient __J.B. (II)__ Age __69__ Sex __M__ Education __11__ Handedness __R__

WECHSLER-BELLEVUE SCALE

VIQ	105
PIQ	103
FS IQ	101
Information	8
Comprehension	9
Digit Span	9
Arithmetic	10
Similarities	8
Vocabulary	6
Picture Arrangement	4
Picture Completion	4
Block Design	7
Object Assembly	5
Digit Symbol	5

NEUROPSYCHOLOGICAL DEFICIT SCALE

Level of Performance	36
Pathognomonic Signs	5
Patterns	3
Right-Left Differences	11
Total NDS Score	55

TRAIL MAKING TEST

Part A: __115__ seconds
Part B: __201__ seconds

STRENGTH OF GRIP

Dominant hand: __30.0__ kilograms

Non-dominant hand: __25.0__ kilograms

REITAN-KLØVE TACTILE FORM RECOGNITION TEST

Dominant hand: __18__ seconds; __0__ errors

Non-dominant hand: __14__ seconds; __0__ errors

REITAN-KLØVE SENSORY-PERCEPTUAL EXAM — No errors

Error Totals

RH___LH___	Both H:	RH___LH___		RH___LH___	
RH___LF___	Both H/F:	RH___LF___		RH___LF___	
LH___RF___	Both H/F:	LH___RF___		RF___LH___	
RE___LE___	Both E:	RE___LE___		RE___LE___	
RV___LV___	Both:	RV___LV___		RV___LV___	

TACTILE FINGER RECOGNITION

R 1___ 2___ 3___ 4 __2__ 5___   R __2 / 20__

L 1___ 2___ 3___ 4___ 5___   L __0 / 20__

FINGER-TIP NUMBER WRITING

R 1 __4__ 2 __1__ 3 __2__ 4 __2__ 5 __1__   R __10 / 20__

L 1 __1__ 2 __2__ 3 2 4___ 5 __2__   L __7 / 20__

HALSTEAD'S NEUROPSYCHOLOGICAL TEST BATTERY

Category Test	86

Tactual Performance Test

Dominant hand:	15.0 (7 blocks)
Non-dominant hand:	15.0 (9 blocks)
Both hands:	8.6

Total Time	38.6 (26 blocks)
Memory	5
Localization	1

Seashore Rhythm Test

Number Correct	22	10

Speech-sounds Perception Test

Number of Errors	23

Finger Oscillation Test

Dominant hand:	36	36
Non-dominant hand:	36	

Impairment Index __1.0__

MINNESOTA MULTIPHASIC PERSONALITY INVENTORY

			Hs	65
			D	70
?	50		Hy	69
L	75		Pd	60
F	48		Mf	51
K	74		Pa	56
			Pt	62
			Sc	57
			Ma	40

REITAN-KLØVE LATERAL-DOMINANCE EXAM

Show me how you:

throw a ball	R
hammer a nail	R
cut with a knife	R
turn a door knob	R
use scissors	R
use an eraser	R
write your name	R

Record time used for spontaneous name-writing:

Preferred hand	__8__ seconds
Non-preferred hand	__20__ seconds

Show me how you:

kick a football	R
step on a bug	R

REITAN-INDIANA APHASIA SCREENING TEST

Form for Adults and Older Children

Name: _____ J. B. (II) _____ Age: __69__

Copy SQUARE Examiner asked him to draw it again, disregarding the double line.	Repeat TRIANGLE Had difficulty understanding instructions.
Name SQUARE	Repeat MASSACHUSETTS Still had difficulty understanding what he was supposed to do.
Spell SQUARE	Repeat METHODIST EPISCOPAL "Methodist Epistical"
Copy CROSS	Write SQUARE
Name CROSS	Read SEVEN
Spell CROSS	Repeat SEVEN
Copy TRIANGLE Patient wanted to try it again.	Repeat/Explain HE SHOUTED THE WARNING. Repeat – "Who shouted the word." Examiner repeated the test item – then, OK. Explain*
Name TRIANGLE	Write HE SHOUTED THE WARNING.
Spell TRIANGLE	Compute 85 – 27 =
Name BABY	Compute 17 X 3 =
Write CLOCK	Name KEY
Name FORK	Demonstrate use of KEY
Read 7 SIX 2	Draw KEY
Read MGW	Read PLACE LEFT HAND TO RIGHT EAR.
Reading I	Place LEFT HAND TO RIGHT EAR
Reading II	Place LEFT HAND TO LEFT ELBOW

* Revolutionary War. Examiner asked for further explanation. "A warning was given to beware to be careful or to look for."

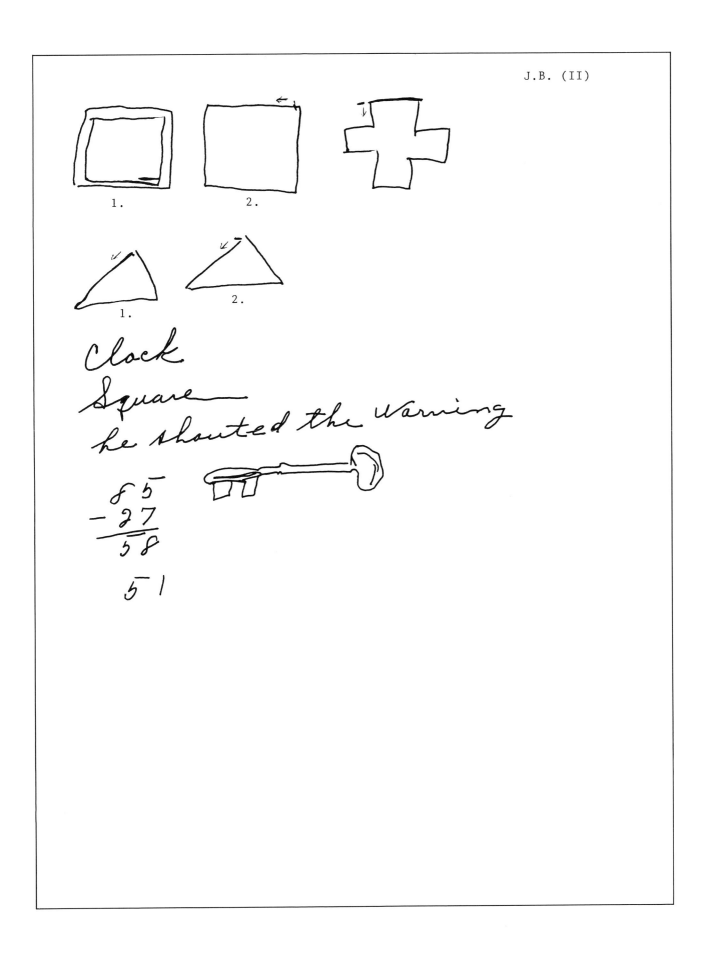

1.   2.

1.   2.

Clock

Square

he shouted the warning

$$\begin{array}{r} 8\,\overline{5} \\ -\ 2\,7 \\ \hline \overline{5}\,8 \end{array}$$

$\overline{5}\ 1$

not able to tap any faster with his right hand than his left (36). He also had some difficulty on tactile finger localization on the right hand (2 errors) but no problems on his left hand. On finger-tip number writing perception he made more errors on his right hand (10) than his left hand (7) and on the Tactile Form Recognition Test he was slower with his right hand (18 sec) than his left hand (14 sec).

The relatively poor performance on the Speech-sounds Perception Test (23 errors) appears to represent a specific deficit associated with left cerebral involvement. Among Halstead's tests this measure has the highest correlation with Verbal IQ. Therefore, the disparity between the Verbal IQ of 105 and the 23 errors on the Speech-sounds Perception Test suggests that J.B. had specific difficulty processing verbal information which was perceived almost simultaneously via the auditory and visual avenues. In fact, results from the Aphasia Screening Test indicate that the patient had impairment of auditory verbal comprehension.

The examiner noted that J.B. had difficulty understanding the instructions when he was told to repeat words after the examiner. In addition, when asked to repeat HE SHOUTED THE WARNING, J.B. said "Who shouted the word?" The examiner repeated the test item and then the subject was able to repeat the sentence correctly. However, his response was initially quite tangential when asked to explain what the sentence might mean. Although he became more specific when requested to elaborate on his explanation, the concept of danger was never explicitly invoked and toward the end of his explanation J.B. became somewhat confused in his verbal expression. Findings of this kind are sufficient evidence to conclude that the patient had an auditory verbal dysgnosia, a definite sign of involvement of the posterior part of the language area in the left cerebral hemisphere.

Although the indications of damage to the left cerebral hemisphere were more pronounced, J.B. also showed mild evidence of right cerebral involvement. His drawings of the square, cross, triangle, and key indicate that he had at least mild

difficulties, even though one would be hesitant to label the deficits constructional dyspraxia. J.B. also had a slightly reduced grip strength with his left upper extremity (25 kg) compared with his right (30 kg), but this finding can hardly be considered sufficient to merit specific attention.

The G-NDS score was 55, falling in the range of moderate impairment. In addition to performing much more poorly than control subjects (Level of Performance section), J.B. also had deficits that were shown in the Pathognomonic Sign and Left-Right sections, and these types of deficits are usually minimally related to aging effects.

In conclusion, the results of the second neuropsychological examination strongly suggest that J.B. had probably developed within the range of normal intelligence premorbidly and now demonstrates significant impairment in various areas of brain function. The lateralizing indicators implicated the left cerebral hemisphere to a greater extent than the right in a context of generalized impairment of brain functions.

Results on the Minnesota Multiphasic Personality Inventory showed some elevation of the neurotic triad (Hypochondriasis, Depression, and Hysteria). Considering the problems that he apparently was having, though, it is not surprising that J.B. would show an elevation on these scales.

A direct comparison of the initial test results with findings obtained 12 months later indicates that J.B. showed about a comparable degree of impairment in many respects. These aspects of the test results probably represent deterioration attributable to both aging and residual effects of brain damage. However, as noted earlier, we would expect some degree of improvement, particularly in the lateralizing signs.

On the second neuropsychological testing J.B. showed some improvement on Part B of the Trail Making Test and on the Total Time and Memory components of the Tactual Performance Test. On the Tactile Form Recognition Test he was also a little quicker and more alert with each hand. He also was considerably better in tactile finger localization. His dysphasia (dysnomia) was clearly improved, although he continued to have some problems with auditory verbal comprehension. The changes in finger tapping speed are difficult to understand. On the first examination J.B. had been slow with his left hand compared with his right hand; on the 12-month examination the relationship was reversed. He continued to have significant difficulty in finger-tip number writing perception with his left hand and his right hand had actually become somewhat worse (from 6 errors to 10 errors).

In certain respects, then, J.B. showed a degree of improvement, but in other areas of functioning his scores were at least somewhat worse. Nevertheless, the overall interpretation of the second testing was essentially similar to the interpretation for the initial examination: evidence of generalized impairment of adaptive abilities dependent on brain functions with lateralizing indications implicating each cerebral hemisphere.

J.B. was re-examined 18 months after the original evaluation. The neurological examination showed improvement in strength and steadiness of gait. It was not possible to detect any ataxia, although the patient still had a slight terminal tremor when placing his index fingers together. His hopping skill was still not quite normal but was definitely better than at the time of the previous examination. The snout reflex was barely perceptible. J.B. still had markedly diminished hearing bilaterally. EEG recordings were somewhat different from the previous examination but were still judged to show no significant change in the overall degree of disturbance. At this time, the abnormal tracings were generally distributed but most prominent over the frontal-temporal areas on each side. (Recall that the EEG done at the time of the 12-month examination had shown irregularities principally implicating the right cerebral hemisphere but the neuropsychological test results did not support this conclusion.)

On direct questioning the patient said that he continues to feel as if he has an abnormal weight on his head, that the muscles of his neck "act up" and are not quite normal, that he has a sore back, and that the upper part of the left side of his face "kind of twinges." However, his responses on the Cornell Medical Index Health Questionnaire revealed no complaints whatsoever.

J.B.'s initial neurological evaluation had suggested the diagnosis of a brain stem contusion, but there were no findings to indicate contusion at the cerebral level. Nevertheless, cerebral involvement would also be expected when brain stem signs were present (Reitan & Wolfson, 1986b), and many of the neuropsychological test findings at the time of both the initial and 12-month examinations showed impairment of cerebral cortical functioning, including both general and more specific lateralized indicators. If J.B. had suffered a cerebral contusion initially, one might expect him to perform considerably worse in some respects than he had at the 12-month examination. However, in this instance we would expect him to have some potential for continued improvement of higher-level brain functions, much as if he had suffered only a concussion of the cerebral hemispheres. In addition, we would expect the specific signs of lateralized involvement to diminish even more than they had at the time of the 12-month examination.

The results for the third neuropsychological testing continue to indicate that for his age J.B. did relatively well on the Wechsler Scale, earning a Full Scale IQ of 106 (exceeding about 66% of his age peers). It must be remembered that the entire test battery was being administered for the third time within an 18-month period. Considering the patient's age, the distribution of subtest scores was not remarkable.

The four most sensitive indicators in the Halstead-Reitan Battery continued to have scores in the brain-damaged range. For a 70-year-old man, J.B.'s best performance was probably on the Category Test (68). Nevertheless, his scores on the

THE HALSTEAD-REITAN
NEUROPSYCHOLOGICAL TEST BATTERY

Patient __J.B. (III)__ Age __70__ Sex __M__ Education __11__ Handedness __R__

WECHSLER-BELLEVUE SCALE

VIQ	109
PIQ	110
FS IQ	106
Information	10
Comprehension	13
Digit Span	7
Arithmetic	9
Similarities	8
Vocabulary	9
Picture Arrangement	7
Picture Completion	8
Block Design	5
Object Assembly	5
Digit Symbol	5

NEUROPSYCHOLOGICAL DEFICIT SCALE

Level of Performance	38
Pathognomonic Signs	2
Patterns	3
Right-Left Differences	6
Total NDS Score	49

HALSTEAD'S NEUROPSYCHOLOGICAL TEST BATTERY

Category Test		68

Tactual Performance Test

Dominant hand:	11.5
Non-dominant hand:	15.3
Both hands:	11.3

Total Time	38.1
Memory	5
Localization	2

Seashore Rhythm Test

Number Correct	24	8

Speech-sounds Perception Test

Number of Errors		22

Finger Oscillation Test

Dominant hand:	33	33
Non-dominant hand:	33	

TRAIL MAKING TEST

Part A: __76__ seconds
Part B: __161__ seconds

Impairment Index	1.0

MINNESOTA MULTIPHASIC PERSONALITY INVENTORY

		Hs	62
		D	70
?	58	Hy	69
L	66	Pd	53
F	53	Mf	47
K	64	Pa	47
		Pt	48
		Sc	53
		Ma	45

STRENGTH OF GRIP

Dominant hand:	32.0	kilograms
Non-dominant hand:	28.0	kilograms

REITAN-KLØVE TACTILE FORM RECOGNITION TEST

Dominant hand:	18	seconds;	0	errors
Non-dominant hand:	20	seconds;	0	errors

REITAN-KLØVE SENSORY-PERCEPTUAL EXAM — No errors

				Error Totals		
RH ___ LH ___	Both H:	RH ___ LH ___		RH ___ LH ___		
RH ___ LF ___	Both H/F:	RH ___ LF ___		RH ___ LF ___		
LH ___ RF ___	Both H/F:	LH ___ RF ___		RF ___ LH ___		
RE ___ LE ___	Both E:	RE ___ LE ___		RE ___ LE ___		
RV ___ LV ___	Both:	RV ___ LV ___		RV ___ LV ___		

REITAN-KLØVE LATERAL-DOMINANCE EXAM

Show me how you:

throw a ball	R
hammer a nail	R
cut with a knife	R
turn a door knob	R
use scissors	R
use an eraser	R
write your name	R

Record time used for spontaneous name-writing:

Preferred hand	9	seconds
Non-preferred hand	25	seconds

TACTILE FINGER RECOGNITION

R 1 ___ 2 ___ 3 ___ 4 _1_ 5 _1_   R __2__ / 20
L 1 ___ 2 ___ 3 _2_ 4 ___ 5 ___   L __2__ / 20

FINGER-TIP NUMBER WRITING

R 1 _2_ 2 _3_ 2 _4_ 2 _5_ 2   R __10__ / 20
L 1 _3_ 2 _2_ 3 _2_ 4 _1_ 5 _3_   L __11__ / 20

Show me how you:

kick a football	R
step on a bug	L

REITAN-INDIANA APHASIA SCREENING TEST

Form for Adults and Older Children

Name: _____ J. B. (III) _____ Age: __70__

Copy SQUARE	Repeat TRIANGLE
Name SQUARE	Repeat MASSACHUSETTS
Spell SQUARE	Repeat METHODIST EPISCOPAL "Methodist Epis...Epis...Episcopol"
Copy CROSS	Write SQUARE
Name CROSS	Read SEVEN
Spell CROSS	Repeat SEVEN
Copy TRIANGLE	Repeat/Explain HE SHOUTED THE WARNING.
Name TRIANGLE	Write HE SHOUTED THE WARNING.
Spell TRIANGLE	Compute 85 – 27 =
Name BABY	Compute 17 X 3 =
Write CLOCK	Name KEY
Name FORK	Demonstrate use of KEY
Read 7 SIX 2	Draw KEY
Read MGW	Read PLACE LEFT HAND TO RIGHT EAR.
Reading I	Place LEFT HAND TO RIGHT EAR
Reading II	Place LEFT HAND TO LEFT ELBOW

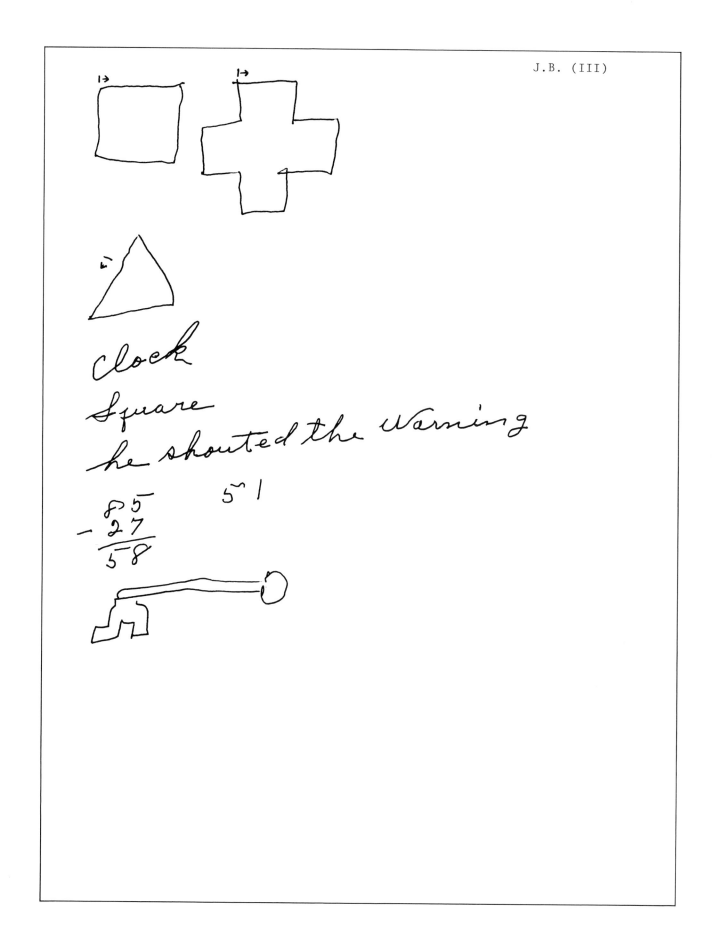

clock

square

he shouted the warning

$5^{\sim}1$

$$
\begin{array}{r}
8\,5^{-} \\
-\ 2\,7 \\
\hline
5^{-}8
\end{array}
$$

four most sensitive measures demonstrated considerable impairment of brain-related adaptive abilities, especially when considered with relation to his IQ levels. As the Impairment Index of 1.0 implies, J.B. performed at least somewhat poorly on all of the general indicators. However, the score on the Seashore Rhythm Test (24 correct) indicates that he had sufficient basic central processing capabilities to be able to pay attention to stimulus material fairly well and maintain his attention at least briefly over time.

It should be noted that J.B. continued to perform poorly on the Speech-sounds Perception Test (22 errors), which also requires close and continued attention to specific stimulus material. However, when considered with relation to the Verbal IQ (109), this score, as noted above, probably suggests some specific deficit related to the content of the test and its particular requirements. Thus, in this instance the Speech-sounds Perception Test may very well reflect a degree of left cerebral damage.

Other lateralizing findings implicating the left cerebral hemisphere were relatively minimal. As in the second examination, the patient was able to tap no faster with his right hand (33) than his left (33). The Aphasia Screening Test did not show any significant impairment in the ability to use specific language symbols for communicational purposes. The mild stuttering J.B. manifested when he repeated METHODIST EPISCOPAL is not in its own right a sign of cerebral damage.

Certain findings were also present to implicate the right cerebral hemisphere. Although J.B. did not perform well in terms of the Total Time score on the Tactual Performance Test (38.1 min.), his left-hand performance (15.3 min) was poor compared to the right (11.5 min). In addition, he demonstrated mild constructional dyspraxia, particularly by his confusion in dealing with the spatial configurations of the teeth of the key. Despite the fact that the general shape was correct, his drawing of the cross also represented a significant problem in dealing with simple spatial configurations. One might raise a question about the difference score between the two hands on the Tactile Form Recognition Test, but considering the fact that there were eight trials for each hand, requiring 20 seconds with the left hand and 18 seconds with the right hand is probably of no significance.

The G-NDS continued to show improvement (from an initial score of 62 to 55 on the second testing and to 49 currently), but the pattern of change should be noted. The major change from the initial to the 12-month testing occurred on the Level of Performance section, even though we had also anticipated improvement on the Pathognomonic Signs and Right-Left Difference sections. On the 18-month examination there was no further improvement on the Level of Performance section, but the expected improvement on Pathognomonic Signs and Right-Left Differences was finally realized. The delay in recovery in these areas may well have been due to J.B.'s age and the fact that recovery occurred at all, even though late, to the absence of demonstrable tissue damage on neurological evaluation following the injury.

In summarizing the results of the third neuropsychological examination, we find evidence that appeared to validly implicate the left cerebral hemisphere (the poor score on the Speech-sounds Perception Test and the relatively slow finger tapping speed with the right hand compared with the left hand). Results suggesting right cerebral hemisphere dysfunction included constructional dyspraxia and a somewhat poor performance with the non-dominant left hand (15.3 min) compared with the dominant right hand (11.5) on the Tactual Performance Test. These results are not particularly striking or pronounced as lateralizing indicators and would certainly not suggest the presence of specific, identifiable focal lesions in either cerebral hemisphere. Instead, in the context of evidence of generalized impairment, they are quite typical of residual deficits associated with significant traumatic brain injury.

A direct comparison of the test results obtained on the 12-month and 18-month examinations indicates that J.B. continued to show some degree of improvement on some of the general indicators but seemed to demonstrate a mild degree of deterioration of ability with the left (non-preferred) hand. He improved his Verbal IQ by four points and increased his Performance IQ by seven points. The comparative weighted scores for the individual subtests suggests that there may in fact have been some improvement on certain subtests, such as Comprehension (from 9 to 13) and Picture Arrangement (from 4 to 7).

J.B. showed definite improvement that probably went beyond positive practice-effect on the Category Test (from 86 errors to 68 errors) and on Part B of the Trail Making Test (from 201 sec to 161 sec). In addition, he no longer had any particular difficulty in understanding the verbal directions of the Aphasia Screening Test and did not demonstrate any auditory verbal dysgnosia. There was no doubt of his improvement on the Total Time on the Tactual Performance Test (38.6 min and only 26 blocks placed compared with 38.1 min and all 30 blocks placed).

Note, though, that J.B. also performed somewhat worse on certain tests. His finger tapping speed was slightly reduced for each hand. On the Tactile Form Recognition Test his left hand performance increased from 14 seconds to 20 seconds. On the third testing he continued to make two mistakes in twenty trials with the right hand in tactile finger localization, and on the left hand his number of errors increased from 0 to 2. On both the 12-month examination and the 18-month examination the patient had made 10 mistakes on his right hand in finger-tip number writing perception. However, the number of errors on the left hand increased from 7 to 11. J.B. definitely showed more evidence of confusion about spatial configurations in his drawing of the key on the 18-month examination than on the examination six months earlier. Finally, although his general performance was better in terms of the Total Time score on the Tactual Performance Test, the comparative results with the two hands indicated a poor performance with the left hand compared with the right.

Although the overall results did not point strongly toward lateralizing findings, a direct comparison of the performances on the 12-month and 18-month examinations shows consistently worse performances with the left hand. This finding certainly suggests that the patient has experienced a mild degree of deterioration in the right cerebral hemisphere, probably fairly focal in nature, and perhaps centering in the right parietal area.

In summary, findings on the 18-month examination showed definite continued improvement in terms of general alertness and certain aspects of higher-level brain functions. Other test results pointed toward mild but very consistent changes in the direction of worse performances with the left upper extremity, implying a mild progression of fairly focal damage in the right cerebral hemisphere.

Case #7

Name: L.W.

Age: 24

Education: 11

Sex: Female

Handedness: Right

Occupation: Unemployed

Background Information

L.W. was injured in an automobile accident when she was 24 years old. The ambulance drivers who were first to arrive at the scene of the accident found L.W. lying on the floor of the passenger side of the car. They reported that she was conscious but confused and disoriented. She had a severely comminuted open fracture of the left leg and her eyes deviated to the right.

Neurological Findings

When examined in the emergency room L.W. was conscious and oriented but in acute distress. She had multiple facial lacerations, including a deep laceration across the brow. Her eyes were fixed in right lateral gaze and her pupils were dilated and non-reactive to light. She was not able to move her eyes to the left past the midline. Although L.W. was initially able to move all four extremities, it was later noted that she had a left hemiparesis.

L.W. was immediately taken to surgery and underwent exploratory laparotomy for closure of her lacerations, drainage around the liver, and a cholecystostomy. The facial lacerations were repaired and the left femoral fracture was reduced and set. Multiple x-ray examinations were done but no skull fracture was identified. An electroencephalogram done the day following admission showed very severe diffuse abnormalities, particularly in the temporal, frontal, and occipital areas of the right cerebral hemisphere. The tracings suggested a right-sided subdural hematoma, or even more likely, a cerebral contusion.

Immediately after surgery L.W. was reported to be obtunded, but this may have been related to recently having undergone major surgery. By 11:30 PM, approximately 16 hours post-injury, she appeared to be relatively alert but was amnesic for a period of about 24 hours preceding the injury.

Eight days after the injury the EEG was repeated and continued to show marked abnormalities involving essentially the entire right cerebral hemisphere, principally located in the temporal area. Compared with the EEG taken one week earlier, though, this EEG showed some improvement. The patient was diagnosed as having a contusion involving the middle part of the right cerebral hemisphere, manifested particularly by a left hemiparesis and hemihypesthesia.

Neuropsychological Examination

Neuropsychological examination was done approximately 12 weeks after the injury. At this time L.W. still had a left hemiparesis. Her left leg was in a cast and her left arm was in a sling. An EEG done at this time continued to show mild widespread abnormalities; the most prominent disturbances occurred in the middle portion of the right cerebral hemisphere, including the parietal and posterior temporal areas. The tracings were suggestive of a cortical contusion.

On the Cornell Medical Index Health Questionnaire L.W. had very few somatic complaints.

THE HALSTEAD-REITAN
NEUROPSYCHOLOGICAL TEST BATTERY

Patient ___L.W. (I)___ Age __24__ Sex __F__ Education __11__ Handedness __R__

WECHSLER-BELLEVUE SCALE

VIQ	99
PIQ	84
FS IQ	91
Information	10
Comprehension	11
Digit Span	10
Arithmetic	1
Similarities	14
Vocabulary	9
Picture Arrangement	6
Picture Completion	9
Block Design	6
Object Assembly	11
Digit Symbol	7

NEUROPSYCHOLOGICAL DEFICIT SCALE

Level of Performance	32
Pathognomonic Signs	2
Patterns	3
Right-Left Differences	16
Total NDS Score	53

HALSTEAD'S NEUROPSYCHOLOGICAL TEST BATTERY

Category Test	96

Tactual Performance Test

Right hand:	13.2
Right hand:	15.1
Right hand:	12.6

Total Time	40.9
Memory	9
Localization	3

Seashore Rhythm Test

Number Correct ___23___   9

Speech-sounds Perception Test

Number of Errors   8

Finger Oscillation Test

Dominant hand:	42	42
Non-dominant hand:	—	

Impairment Index   0.9

TRAIL MAKING TEST

Part A: __55__ seconds
Part B: __102__ seconds

STRENGTH OF GRIP

Dominant hand: __24.0__ kilograms
Non-dominant hand: __3.0__ kilograms

MINNESOTA MULTIPHASIC PERSONALITY INVENTORY

		Hs	48
		D	55
?	50	Hy	52
L	50	Pd	64
F	48	Mf	52
K	51	Pa	56
		Pt	56
		Sc	64
		Ma	38

REITAN-KLØVE TACTILE FORM RECOGNITION TEST

Dominant hand: _____ seconds; _____ errors } NOT
Non-dominant hand: _____ seconds; _____ errors } DONE

REITAN-KLØVE SENSORY-PERCEPTUAL EXAM — No errors

Error Totals

RH___ LH___	Both H:	RH___ LH___	RH___ LH___
RH___ LF___	Both H/F:	RH___ LF___	RH___ LF___
LH___ RF___	Both H/F:	LH___ RF___	RF___ LH___
RE___ LE___	Both E:	RE___ LE___	RE___ LE___
RV___ LV___	Both:	RV___ LV___	RV___ LV___

REITAN-KLØVE LATERAL-DOMINANCE EXAM

Show me how you:
throw a ball	R
hammer a nail	R
cut with a knife	R
turn a door knob	R
use scissors	R
use an eraser	R
write your name	R

Record time used for spontaneous name-writing:
Preferred hand	12 seconds
Non-preferred hand	— seconds

TACTILE FINGER RECOGNITION

R 1___ 2___ 3___ 4 _2_ 5___   R _2_ / 20
L 1___ 2 _1_ 3 _1_ 4 _2_ 5___   L _4_ / 20

FINGER-TIP NUMBER WRITING

R 1___ 2___ 3 _1_ 4___ 5___   R _1_ / 20
L 1 _2_ 2 _3_ 3 _3_ 4 _3_ 5 _3_   L _14_ / 20

Show me how you:
kick a football	R
step on a bug	R

REITAN-INDIANA APHASIA SCREENING TEST

Form for Adults and Older Children

Name: _____ L. W. (I) _____ Age: __24__

Copy SQUARE	Repeat TRIANGLE
Name SQUARE	Repeat MASSACHUSETTS

Spell SQUARE
   "S–Q–U–R–E"
	Repeat METHODIST EPISCOPAL
	   "Methodist Epicobol"

Copy CROSS	Write SQUARE
Name CROSS	Read SEVEN
Spell CROSS	Repeat SEVEN
Copy TRIANGLE	Repeat/Explain HE SHOUTED THE WARNING.
Name TRIANGLE	Write HE SHOUTED THE WARNING.
Spell TRIANGLE	Compute 85 – 27 =
Name BABY	Compute 17 X 3 = "39." Examiner gave 6x4 and patient responded correctly.
Write CLOCK	Name KEY
Name FORK	Demonstrate use of KEY
Read 7 SIX 2	Draw KEY
Read MGW	Read PLACE LEFT HAND TO RIGHT EAR.
Reading I	Place ~~LEFT~~ HAND TO RIGHT EAR RIGHT Responded correctly.

Reading II	Place ~~LEFT~~ HAND TO ~~LEFT~~ ELBOW
	   RIGHT RIGHT
	                     Responded correctly.

Clock

He shouted the warning

Square

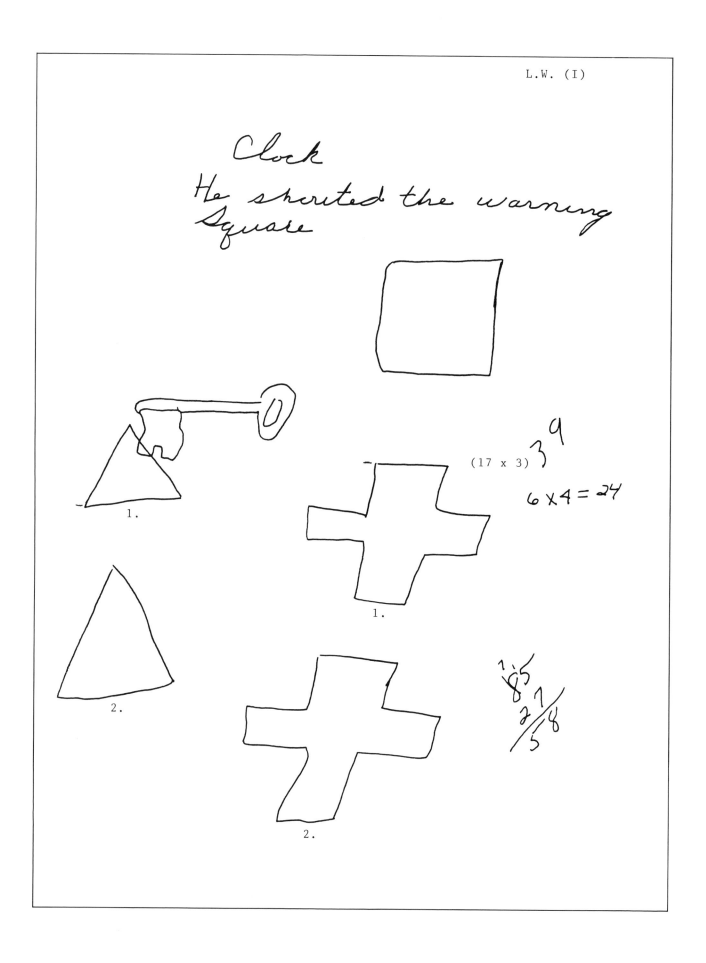

(17 x 3) 3⁹

6 × 4 = 24

1.

1.

2.

2.

However, she said that she often cried, considered herself to be extremely shy or sensitive, was always upset by criticism and had her feelings easily hurt, was usually misunderstood by others, easily became upset or irritated, often did things on sudden impulse, became angry when anyone told her what to do, became frightened at sudden movements or noises that occurred at night, and often jumped or shaked badly in response to sudden noises.

L.W. earned a Verbal IQ (99) that was nearly at the Average level and a Performance IQ (84) in the Low Average range. However, her Impairment Index was 0.9, indicating that about 90% of Halstead's tests had scores in the brain-damaged range. Despite the relatively low Performance IQ value, this relationship is an initial indicator that the patient's immediate adaptive abilities closely dependent upon brain functions are more significantly impaired than the abilities that are acquired over the years (e.g., verbal intelligence). Thus, even a brief inspection of the test results suggests that L.W. has experienced significant impairment of brain-related abilities.

Although her Verbal IQ exceeded 47% of her age peers, we see that L.W. performed very poorly on the Arithmetic subtest (1). She was able to solve the first two very simple items, but she could not figure out how much change she would get back from 25 cents if she were to buy eight cents worth of stamps. In fact, she was able to get no further credit on any of the remaining items in the Arithmetic subtest. It is possible that L.W. had always had a striking deficiency in dealing with simple arithmetical problems, but considering the deficits shown on the rest of the neuropsychological examination, it is more likely that she sustained serious impairment of abilities in the area of arithmetical reasoning as a result of the accident. Scores on all of the other Verbal subtests were nearly at the average level or above.

L.W.'s performances on the Performance subtests yielded an IQ value (84) that exceeded only 14% of her age peers. She performed rather poorly on the Digit Symbol subtest (7), a measure that is sensitive to cerebral damage regardless of its lateralization or localization. However, her two lowest Performance subtest scores were on Picture Arrangement (6) and Block Design (6), the two subtests among the Performance subtests that are the most sensitive to right cerebral damage. Thus, one might postulate the presence of cerebral damage on the basis of the Wechsler results alone.

The Arithmetic subtest is probably the most sensitive of the Verbal subtests of the WAIS to brain damage generally considered. The low scores on the Arithmetic and Digit Symbol subtests implicate brain dysfunction in general terms and the low scores on Picture Arrangement and Block Design point more specifically to right cerebral hemisphere damage.

L.W. did not perform well on any of the four most sensitive indicators in the Halstead-Reitan Battery, earning especially poor scores on the Impairment Index (0.9) and the Category Test (96). Although her score on Part B of the Trail Making Test (102 sec) fell in the range characteristic of brain-damaged persons, it was considerably better than the Impairment Index or Category Test score.

In developing a conceptualization of impaired brain functions for this woman, the score on the Trail Making Test contra-indicates any presumption that cerebral damage was rapidly progressive in nature and, in a biological sense, may even reflect a relatively stabilized condition. This latter inference would be supported by the comparatively good score on the Speech-sounds Perception Test (8 errors). This score also indicates that L.W. had the basic attentional capability to concentrate on the 60 items of this test. A fairly good score on the Speech-sounds Perception Test in the context of other scores indicating significant impairment is often seen in persons on a recovery gradient or persons with a relatively stabilized brain.

Although L.W.'s score on the Seashore Rhythm Test (23 correct) was not as good, it is not as significant; the patient had already demonstrated her ability to pay attention to specific stimuli on the Speech-sounds Perception Test.

Before referring to lateralizing indicators, it is worth noting that L.W. was able to perform relatively simple tasks fairly well but her ability decreased very sharply when the task became more complex in nature. More specifically, she did quite well on the Memory component (9) of the Tactual Performance Test (a task of remembering a limited number of specific shapes), on the Speech-sounds Perception Test (a task requiring correlation of defined and highly specific verbal stimulus material), and the Trail Making Test (a task dealing only with numbers and letters, albeit under rather complex and demanding conditions). L.W. had much more difficulty in more open-ended situations which required defining the nature of the task before proceeding to a solution (e.g., the Category Test and Total Time score on the Tactual Performance Test). Comparisons of results on these measures strongly suggest that the patient is generally able to perform much better on well-defined and simple tasks than on tasks that require initiative, analysis, and a definition of the problem.

L.W. used her right hand on all three trials of the Tactual Performance Test. It is interesting to note that she showed very little improvement on successive trials, which demonstrates that she had little capability to learn from her exposure to the task. This type of dysfunction (inability to learn how to learn or profit from experience) is a frequent manifestation of impaired cerebral functions and is seen particularly in persons who perform poorly on the Category Test. In other words, it is likely that this woman's failure to show substantial improvement on successive trials on the Tactual Performance Test is another demonstration of her significant impairment in dealing with more complex tasks (as compared with relatively simple tasks).

Considering the fact that the realistic problems one encounters in everyday living are relatively complex in nature and require definition by the person dealing with them, it would be safe to predict that the impairment shown by L.W. would be quite disabling. She probably has little capability for taking initiative in planning her activities and will be grossly inefficient in defining a course of action and following through successfully to its completion.

Lateralizing findings for left cerebral damage were not prominent. The patient did omit the "A" in spelling SQUARE and this error almost certainly is a reflection of impaired cerebral functions. She also became confused in multiplying 17 × 3 and gave "39" as the answer. These results would be highly unusual for a person with normal brain functions, but considered by themselves — and especially in the context of a relatively normal Verbal IQ and a good score on the Speech-sounds Perception Test — they can hardly be considered definite indications of specific left cerebral damage.

Note, however, that the lateralizing indicators for right cerebral damage were unequivocal in their significance. As demonstrated on the Finger Oscillation Test and measurement of grip strength, L.W. had a pronounced motor deficit involving her left upper extremity. She was not able to perform the Tactual Performance Test at all with her left hand and all three trials were done with the right hand. L.W. also demonstrated tactile-perceptual deficits on the left side. Impairment of ability in tactile finger localization was relatively mild, although more significant on the left hand (4 errors) than the right (2 errors). The patient had a great deal of difficulty on the left hand in finger-tip number writing perception (14 errors), but with her right hand made only one error.

In addition, L.W. demonstrated some difficulties in her drawings of simple spatial configurations. She had a particular problem drawing the cross; she was not able to maintain symmetry of the extensions. Although she did not have specific difficulty drawing the key, note that it ran over into the drawing of the triangle because L.W. did not plan well and failed to leave enough space for the drawing. This kind of difficulty suggests a specific problem in dealing with spatial relationships. We see that in addition to motor dysfunction, L.W. had clearly lateralized tactile-perceptual (input) losses and higher-level difficulties in dealing with spatial relationships. These findings all complement the distribution of Performance subtest scores on the Wechsler Scale, as described above.

Although the results on the individual scales of the Minnesota Multiphasic Personality Inventory were essentially within the normal range, the elevated scores on the Psychopathic Deviate and Schizophrenia scales and the low score on the Hypomania scale may have some clinical significance. L.W. probably has a tendency to feel that she has been treated unfairly in life and has some reactions of anger and resentment. She probably is insecure and anxious in interpersonal relationships and may tend to isolate herself somewhat. It is likely also that she feels somewhat apathetic, out of energy, and lacking the motivation necessary to change her situation. Of course, results of this kind may be a reaction to the circumstances and problems that have occurred during the 12 weeks that have elapsed since the time of her injury.

The neurological examination and EEG were repeated three months after the initial neuropsychological testing (six months post-injury). The physical examination continued to demonstrate a left hemiparesis that involved the distal aspects of the extremities more than the proximal muscles. There was also a mild hemisensory loss on the left side and increased reflex responses. The EEG still showed abnormalities, particularly involving the middle part of the right cerebral hemisphere. In addition, there were rare epileptiform discharges involving this area that had not been observed previously. There was less evidence of slow-wave disturbances on this examination than on previous examinations.

The neurologic examination done 12 months after the initial neuropsychological testing continued to show similar findings. There was a left hemiparesis with decreased muscle tone on the left side,

impaired position sense, and a mild degree of dysstereognosis. Reflexes were increased more on the left side than on the right and the neurologist noted that the right side of L.W.'s face moved better than the left side. The EEG showed definite improvement, with only slightly abnormal activity in the middle part of the right cerebral hemisphere.

At this time the Cornell Medical Index Health Questionnaire revealed no somatic complaints whatsoever, although L.W. did accurately identify her past illnesses and injuries. She also noted that she was extremely shy or sensitive, was a "touchy" person whose feelings were easily hurt, was easily upset or irritated, became angry if anyone told her what to do, was usually misunderstood by others, was bothered by eating anywhere except in her own home, and often became frightened at sudden movements or noises at night. Except for impairment on the left side of the body, L.W. had no specific complaints directly related to her head injury.

Although the test results obtained 12 months after the initial neuropsychological examination showed considerable improvement in a number of respects, they continued to indicate right cerebral dysfunction.

We will briefly review the test results and then consider the changes that occurred between the first and second neuropsychological examinations. L.W. earned a Verbal IQ (99) almost exactly at the Average level, exceeding about 47% of her age peers. Her Performance IQ (105) was a few points higher, exceeding 63%. These values yielded a Full Scale IQ (102) that exceeded 55%. The Verbal subtests showed relatively little significant variability except for a very poor performance on the Arithmetic subtest (1). This specific and selective deficit almost certainly reflects impairment of previously acquired abilities.

The Performance subtests demonstrated a greater degree of variability, with the lowest scores occurring on Picture Arrangement (8), Block Design (9), and Object Assembly (9). The good score

THE HALSTEAD-REITAN
NEUROPSYCHOLOGICAL TEST BATTERY

Patient **L.W. (II)** Age **25** Sex **F** Education **11** Handedness **R**

WECHSLER-BELLEVUE SCALE

VIQ	99
PIQ	105
FS IQ	102
Information	11
Comprehension	10
Digit Span	10
Arithmetic	1
Similarities	14
Vocabulary	9
Picture Arrangement	8
Picture Completion	13
Block Design	9
Object Assembly	9
Digit Symbol	13

NEUROPSYCHOLOGICAL DEFICIT SCALE

Level of Performance	13
Pathognomonic Signs	0
Patterns	1
Right-Left Differences	16
Total NDS Score	30

TRAIL MAKING TEST

Part A: **26** seconds
Part B: **60** seconds

STRENGTH OF GRIP

Dominant hand: **28.5** kilograms
Non-dominant hand: **6.0** kilograms

REITAN-KLØVE TACTILE FORM RECOGNITION TEST

Dominant hand: **10** seconds; **0** errors
Non-dominant hand: **—** seconds; **—** errors

REITAN-KLØVE SENSORY-PERCEPTUAL EXAM — No errors

				Error Totals	
RH___LH___	Both H:	RH___LH___	RH___LH___	
RH___LF___	Both H/F:	RH___LF___	RH___LF___	
LH___RF___	Both H/F:	LH___RF___	RF___LH___	
RE___LE___	Both E:	RE___LE___	RE___LE___	
RV___LV___	Both:	RV___LV___	RV___LV___	

TACTILE FINGER RECOGNITION

R 1___2___3___4 _1_ 5___   R _1_ / 20
L 1___2 _1_ 3 _1_ 4___5 _1_   L _3_ / 20

FINGER-TIP NUMBER WRITING

R 1 _1_ 2___3___4___5___   R _1_ / 20
L 1 _1_ 2 _1_ 3 _1_ 4 _1_ 5 _3_   L _7_ / 20

HALSTEAD'S NEUROPSYCHOLOGICAL TEST BATTERY

Category Test	59

Tactual Performance Test

Right hand:	6.7
Right hand:	3.6
Right hand:	2.8
Total Time	13.1
Memory	9
Localization	8

Seashore Rhythm Test

Number Correct	25	6

Speech-sounds Perception Test

Number of Errors	3

Finger Oscillation Test

Dominant hand:	46	46
Non-dominant hand:	—	

Impairment Index **0.4**

MINNESOTA MULTIPHASIC PERSONALITY INVENTORY

		Hs	50
		D	73
?	50	Hy	56
L	43	Pd	86
F	55	Mf	47
K	48	Pa	59
		Pt	55
		Sc	54
		Ma	35

REITAN-KLØVE LATERAL-DOMINANCE EXAM

Show me how you:

throw a ball	R
hammer a nail	R
cut with a knife	R
turn a door knob	R
use scissors	R
use an eraser	R
write your name	R

Record time used for spontaneous name-writing:

Preferred hand	**7** seconds
Non-preferred hand	**—** seconds

Show me how you:

kick a football	R
step on a bug	R

REITAN-INDIANA APHASIA SCREENING TEST

Form for Adults and Older Children

Name: _____ L. W. (II) _____ Age: _25_

Copy SQUARE	Repeat TRIANGLE
Name SQUARE	Repeat MASSACHUSETTS
Spell SQUARE	Repeat METHODIST EPISCOPAL
Copy CROSS	Write SQUARE
Name CROSS	Read SEVEN
Spell CROSS	Repeat SEVEN
Copy TRIANGLE	Repeat/Explain HE SHOUTED THE WARNING.
Name TRIANGLE	Write HE SHOUTED THE WARNING.
Spell TRIANGLE	Compute 85 – 27 =
Name BABY	Compute 17 X 3 ="41"
Write CLOCK	Name KEY OK. Then," The answer should have been 51." Referring to 17 x 3.
Name FORK	Demonstrate use of KEY
Read 7 SIX 2	Draw KEY
Read MGW	Read PLACE LEFT HAND TO RIGHT EAR.
Reading I	Place LEFT HAND TO RIGHT EAR
Reading II	Place ~~LEFT~~ HAND TO ~~LEFT~~ ELBOW RIGHT RIGHT Responded correctly.

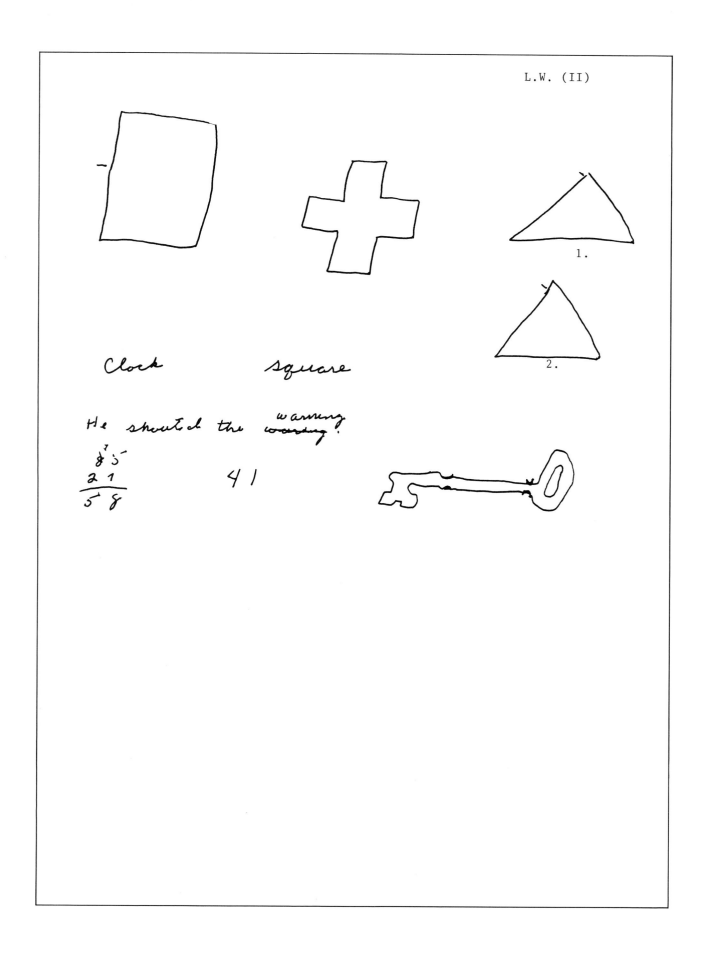

1.

2.

Clock   square

He should the ~~wording~~ warning.

$\frac{\overset{.}{8}\overset{.}{5}}{5\ 8}$ $\begin{array}{c}2\ 1\end{array}$

41

on the Digit Symbol subtest (13) is not typical or even characteristic of instances of cerebral damage, although the relatively low scores on Picture Arrangement and Block Design might possibly reflect right cerebral damage. Using the results of the Wechsler Scale alone, it would be difficult to draw confident conclusions concerning cerebral damage. However, the overall distribution, particularly the Arithmetic subtest score, must be viewed as a meaningful deviation from normality.

L.W. performed relatively well overall on the four most sensitive indicators in the Halstead-Reitan Battery. Although the Impairment Index of 0.4 was a borderline value and the Category Test (59) was done rather poorly, the score on Part B of the Trail Making Test (60 sec) and the Localization component of the Tactual Performance Test (8) were both well within the normal range. Thus, results on these four measures were somewhat equivocal with respect to indicating the presence of cerebral damage.

Lateralizing indicators, particularly those implicating the right cerebral hemisphere, were of unequivocal significance. L.W. showed few signs of left cerebral hemisphere damage, but her error in writing WARNING (even though self-corrected) is the type of mistake that is characteristic of left cerebral involvement. However, L.W. performed quite well on other verbal tests, showing no other signs of dysphasia, and did particularly well on the Speech-sounds Perception Test (3 errors).

The low score (1) on the Arithmetic subtest of the Wechsler Scale cannot be considered to have specific significance for left cerebral damage; instead, it should be viewed as a general indicator of cerebral functions. Specific deficits on the arithmetic problems of the Aphasia Screening Test occur about four times more frequently among persons with left cerebral damage than among persons with right cerebral lesions, and the difference in lateralizing significance appears to relate to the specific arithmetical problem-solving procedures

required on the Aphasia Screening Test. In contrast, the types of problems on the Arithmetic subtest of the Wechsler Scale seem to involve more arithmetical reasoning.

Although L.W. did have some difficulty drawing the key (suggesting mild constructional dyspraxia), lateralizing findings that implicated the right cerebral hemisphere were based mainly upon comparisons of performances on the two sides of the body. The patient was not able to register any score at all in finger tapping with her left hand and had a strikingly reduced grip strength with her left hand. It is important to note that these deficits were not limited to motor impairment; there were also definite tactile-perceptual deficits on the left side. When using her left hand L.W. was completely unable to recognize the forms used in the Tactile Form Recognition Test. She had minimal (but probably definite) difficulty in tactile finger localization on her left hand (3 errors) and was clearly deficient in finger-tip number writing perception (7 errors) with her left hand. The fact that both motor (expressive) and tactile-perceptual (receptive) deficits were present on the same side leans the interpretation toward central (cerebral) damage rather than peripheral dysfunction.

The MMPI continued to show elevated scores on the Depression and Psychopathic Deviate scales and a low score on the Hypomania scale. The results suggest that the patient is depressed, angry, resentful of her circumstances and would like to strike back, but has a feeling of hopelessness.

Direct comparison of the initial test results with those obtained 12 months later rather consistently showed at least some degree of improvement on measures of intellectual and cognitive functions, as manifested by a reduction of the G-NDS score from 53 (moderate impairment) to 30 (mild impairment). The pattern of results on the MMPI was generally similar but considerably more pronounced on the second testing. Thus, the findings suggest that L.W.'s neuropsychological functions had improved but that her emotional distress had worsened.

It is interesting to note that L.W. made the greatest improvement on the neuropsychological tests that initially appeared to be the most impaired. Her Performance IQ rose from 84 to 105, a 21-point increase; the Verbal IQ values were essentially unchanged. We must also note, however, that the subtest with the most striking indication of initial impairment — Arithmetic — showed no change whatsoever. The patient's Impairment Index improved from 0.9 to 0.4 and her Category Test score was reduced from 96 to 59. She showed a great deal of improvement in Total Time on the Tactual Performance Test (40.9 min to 13.1 min), on Part B of the Trail Making Test (102 sec to 60 sec), and the Localization component of the Tactual Performance Test (from three figures localized to eight). Obviously, L.W. continued to be quite alert in a general sense, making only three errors on the Speech-sounds Perception Test (compared with eight errors on the first examination). Although relatively minimal changes occurred on the test of tactile finger recognition, the patient made a striking improvement on the left hand (which had initially performed poorly) in fingertip number writing perception. These changes support the conclusion that spontaneous recovery is principally manifested on measures that initially showed the most deficit.

Only a minor degree of improvement was demonstrated on the Seashore Rhythm Test and on measures of finger tapping speed and grip strength. We would have expected L.W. to show substantial improvement with her impaired (left) hand in finger tapping speed and grip strength, but there was only the slightest change. The potential for improvement may depend upon the severity and totality of damage of relevant neural tissue. In this case, it is possible that the tissue involved in motor functions of the left upper extremity may have been so extensively damaged that there was no longer any potential for improvement. This did not seem to be true for tissue subserving tactile-perceptual functions, but the deficits of this type were not complete on the initial examination.

The patient may have shown a minor degree of improvement in the adequacy of her drawings, particularly on the cross and the use of space on the page, but the improvement was not particularly striking. Finally, as noted above, the pattern of scores on the MMPI remained the same but were more pronounced on the 12-month examination and suggested that L.W. has increasingly severe reactive affective problems.

Eighteen months after the initial testing L.W. returned for a neurological examination, EEG, and neuropsychological evaluation. The neurologist noted that the patient's left hemiparesis was possibly slightly improved since the 12-month examination. She also demonstrated hyperreflexia and a Babinski sign on the left side and impaired stereognosis and graphesthesia on the left hand. The muscles on the right side of her face appeared to move better than those of the left side. At this time the EEG was entirely within normal limits.

When questioned directly about problems resulting from the brain injury, the patient noted her partial paralysis on the left side and said that she also continued to feel a tingling sensation in her left hand. On the Cornell Medical Index Health Questionnaire she denied having any somatic difficulties but responded to questions concerned with emotional aspects of adjustment similarly to the way she had answered previously. She said that she often cries, is extremely sensitive and her feelings are easily hurt, is always upset by criticism and misunderstood by others, must be on guard even with her friends, is easily upset or irritated, becomes angry when anyone tells her what to do, and is frightened by sudden noises or movements at night. In addition, she felt that her efficiency of performance falls apart when under pressure and

THE HALSTEAD-REITAN
NEUROPSYCHOLOGICAL TEST BATTERY

Patient __L.W. (III)__ Age __26__ Sex __F__ Education __11__ Handedness __R__

WECHSLER-BELLEVUE SCALE

VIQ	101
PIQ	104
FS IQ	103
Information	10
Comprehension	11
Digit Span	9
Arithmetic	4
Similarities	14
Vocabulary	11
Picture Arrangement	8
Picture Completion	14
Block Design	9
Object Assembly	8
Digit Symbol	12

NEUROPSYCHOLOGICAL DEFICIT SCALE

Level of Performance	14
Pathognomonic Signs	3
Patterns	0
Right-Left Differences	15
Total NDS Score	32

TRAIL MAKING TEST

Part A: __19__ seconds
Part B: __46__ seconds

STRENGTH OF GRIP

Dominant hand: __29.0__ kilograms
Non-dominant hand: __10.5__ kilograms

REITAN-KLØVE TACTILE FORM RECOGNITION TEST

Dominant hand: __10__ seconds; __0__ errors
Non-dominant hand: __—__ seconds; __—__ errors

REITAN-KLØVE SENSORY-PERCEPTUAL EXAM — No errors

			Error Totals	
RH___ LH ___	Both H:	RH___ LH ___	RH___ LH ___	
RH___ LF ___	Both H/F:	RH___ LF ___	RH___ LF ___	
LH___ RF ___	Both H/F:	LH___ RF ___	RF___ LH ___	
RE___ LE ___	Both E:	RE___ LE ___	RE___ LE ___	
RV___ LV ___	Both:	RV___ LV ___	RV___ LV ___	

TACTILE FINGER RECOGNITION

R 1___ 2___ 3___ 4 _1_ 5___   R _1_ / 20
L 1___ 2___ 3 _2_ 4 _1_ 5___ L _3_ / 20

FINGER-TIP NUMBER WRITING

R 1 _1_ 2___ 3___ 4___ 5___   R _1_ / 20
L 1 _3_ 2 _1_ 3 _3_ 4___ 5 _1_ L _8_ / 20

HALSTEAD'S NEUROPSYCHOLOGICAL TEST BATTERY

Category Test		92

Tactual Performance Test

Right hand:	3.7	
Right hand:	3.1	
Right hand:	2.2	
	Total Time	9.0
	Memory	9
	Localization	6

Seashore Rhythm Test

Number Correct	25	6

Speech-sounds Perception Test

Number of Errors		7

Finger Oscillation Test

Dominant hand:	51	51
Non-dominant hand:	4	

Impairment Index __0.3__

MINNESOTA MULTIPHASIC PERSONALITY INVENTORY

			Hs	48
			D	73
?	50		Hy	47
L	46		Pd	79
F	60		Mf	45
K	42		Pa	62
			Pt	63
			Sc	61
			Ma	45

REITAN-KLØVE LATERAL-DOMINANCE EXAM

Show me how you:

throw a ball	R
hammer a nail	R
cut with a knife	R
turn a door knob	R
use scissors	R
use an eraser	R
write your name	R

Record time used for spontaneous name-writing:

Preferred hand	9	seconds
Non-preferred hand	—	seconds

Show me how you:

kick a football	R
step on a bug	R

REITAN-INDIANA APHASIA SCREENING TEST

Form for Adults and Older Children

Name: _____L. W. (III)_____ Age: __26__

Copy SQUARE	Repeat TRIANGLE
Name SQUARE	Repeat MASSACHUSETTS
Spell SQUARE	Repeat METHODIST EPISCOPAL
Copy CROSS	Write SQUARE
Name CROSS	Read SEVEN
Spell CROSS	Repeat SEVEN
Copy TRIANGLE	Repeat/Explain HE SHOUTED THE WARNING.
Name TRIANGLE	Write HE SHOUTED THE WARNING. "He shoted the warning."
Spell TRIANGLE	Compute 85 – 27 = "56." Given 96 – 58 and responded correctly.
Name BABY	Compute 17 X 3 = "41." 16x4="54." 12x5="50." 7x8="42." 5x7="35."
Write CLOCK	Name KEY
Name FORK	Demonstrate use of KEY
Read 7 SIX 2	Draw KEY
Read MGW	Read PLACE LEFT HAND TO RIGHT EAR.
Reading I	Place LEFT HAND TO RIGHT EAR
Reading II	Place LEFT HAND TO LEFT ELBOW

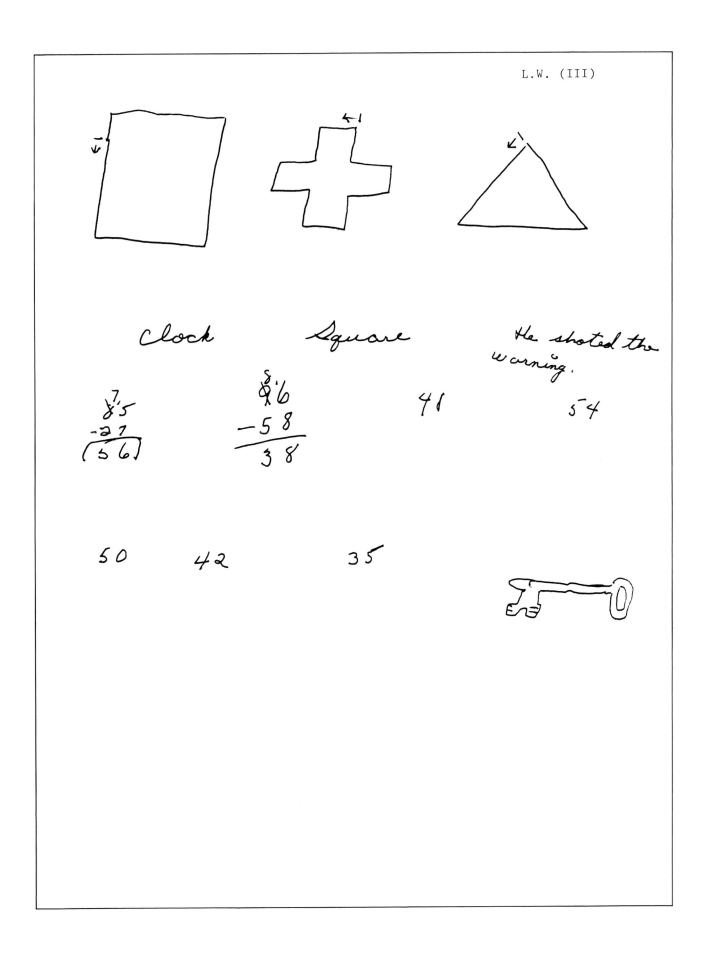

Clock   Square   He shoted the
                                           warning.

$$\begin{array}{r} 7 \\ \cancel{8}\,5 \\ -2\,7 \\ \hline (5\ 6] \end{array}$$

$$\begin{array}{r} 8 \\ \cancel{9}\cancel{6} \\ -5\ 8 \\ \hline 3\ 8 \end{array}$$

41   5¯4

50   42   35

that she becomes completely mixed up when required to do things quickly. On the 12-month examination she had not responded positively to these latter two questions.

L.W. continued to show scores implicating cerebral damage, particularly involving the right side of the brain. She earned both Verbal (101) and Performance (104) IQ values that were just above the Average level, yielding a Full Scale IQ (103) that exceeded about 58% of her age peers. Among the Verbal subtests, the Arithmetic Score (4) continued to be strikingly depressed. The pattern of results on the Performance subtests was very similar to the one shown on the previous examination; scores on Picture Arrangement (8), Block Design (9), and Object Assembly (8) were the lowest.

Except for a very poor performance on the Category Test (92 errors), the patient performed relatively well on the four most sensitive indicators. Most persons with cerebral damage would not have such a poor score on the Category Test in the presence of normal scores on the other three measures. However, the overall configuration of scores, particularly those that implicate the right cerebral hemisphere, serve as a context for attributing this poor performance to cerebral damage.

It is clear that L.W. was relatively quick and alert, able to pay attention to specific stimulus material and maintain close and accurate work over at least short periods of time, and could adapt to fairly complex tasks (such as the Tactual Performance Test). We would postulate that she had gained some familiarity with the requirements of the Tactual Performance Test and by the time of the third examination it had changed from an unusual type of task that required her to define the problem to a procedure that she could understand and manage. By the third examination she had become accustomed to the shapes of the figures and their locations and as a result was able to make progress toward better performances on successive trials.

The lateralizing indicators continued to implicate the right cerebral hemisphere to a significant extent, although the patient demonstrated an error in writing ("shoted" for SHOUTED) that is often seen among persons with left cerebral damage. Finger tapping speed and grip strength were still markedly reduced in the left upper extremity compared with the right. Tactile-perceptual deficits were also prominent on the left side. The patient was completely unable to recognize and differentiate the shapes of the various plastic forms used in the Tactile Form Recognition Test and she continued to have significantly more difficulty on the left hand than the right hand in tactile finger localization and finger-tip number writing perception.

Finally, although the differences comparing the two hands (in terms of both receptive and expressive performances) constituted the most significant evidence of right cerebral damage, L.W. also showed evidence of difficulty in her drawing of a key that is quite characteristic of persons with right cerebral lesions. First, she failed to achieve symmetry in her representation of the "teeth" of the key. The most significant error was probably the curved line directly above the teeth. Persons who make this type of mistake frequently appear to be drawing the "nose" of the key prematurely, failing to consider the general shape of the figure. We would postulate that the patient started to draw the nose of the key and then decided that additional space was necessary. Thus, it is very likely that she had a significant problem in estimating the overall aspects of the spatial configuration, another sign of right cerebral damage.

Results on the MMPI continued to show elevated scores on the Depression and Psychopathic Deviate scales and a somewhat depressed score on the Hypomania scale.

In summary, the test results obtained on the third neuropsychological examination were quite definite in demonstrating right cerebral hemisphere dysfunction in the context of generalized cognitive impairment.

A direct comparison of the performances on the 12-month and 18-month neuropsychological examinations indicated that L.W. performed better on a number of measures, about the same on some tests, and worse on the Category Test and the Localization component of the Tactual Performance Test. Her scores on the G-NDS were similar for the two examinations.

L.W. had made a considerable degree of improvement on the Total Time score for the Tactual Performance Test, especially when using her right hand on the first trial. As noted above, she probably had become sufficiently familiar with this task to overcome the initial requirement of defining the problem. Therefore, she was able to proceed with the task in terms of its specific stimulus elements and profit from her previous experience. She also showed a slight increase in finger tapping speed with both hands. Grip strength was not improved with the right upper extremity but showed some improvement with the left. In addition, results on the MMPI were not quite as pronounced on certain scales (Psychopathic Deviate and Hypomania) as they had been at the time of the second testing.

L.W.'s IQ values and the results on the Seashore Rhythm Test, Tactile Finger Localization, and Finger-tip Number Writing Perception were very similar on the 12-month and the 18-month examinations. We would question whether the patient was significantly worse on the Speech-sounds Perception Test on the 18-month examination, even though the score changed from three to seven errors on this test. It is necessary to focus attention very closely and make a very deliberate and continued effort to achieve a score of only three errors.

Therefore, a score of seven errors might reflect only a little less intense effort on the part of the patient. However, a decrease from eight blocks to six blocks on the Localization score on the Tactual Performance Test may represent an actual decrease in cognitive capability.

Finally, there is no question that the increase in errors on the Category Test (from 59 to 92) represents significant deterioration of brain-related abilities. This had been one of the patient's particularly poor performances on the initial neuropsychological examination (96 errors). She had shown substantial improvement at the 12-month examination (59 errors), which might have been partially due to positive practice-effect. Even with possible practice-effect operating on the third (18-month) testing, the patient performed much worse. There is no doubt that she is considerably less capable in terms of abstract reasoning and analytical ability to define multidimensional problems than she had been 12 months after the injury. Although she had improved on tasks that were more specifically defined, she showed definite deterioration on a task (Category Test) that was more taxing and had more difficult requirements in the area of the patient's principal initial deficit. Thus, even though L.W. showed continued improvement on a number of tests over the course of the three neuropsychological examinations, clinical evaluation of results on individual tests showed significant deterioration in certain respects, consistent with the general trend manifested by patients with cerebral tissue damage (penetrating brain wounds or cerebral contusion).

Case #8

Name:	R. A.	Sex:	Male
Age:	29	Handedness:	Right
Education:	16	Occupation:	Auditor

Background Information

This 29-year-old man sustained a severe head injury in a moving vehicle accident. He was admitted to a local hospital and transferred to a major medical center three days later. R.A. was completely comatose for two weeks following the injury and remained in an impaired state of consciousness another two weeks. During the second two-week period there were occasions when R.A. appeared to be oriented and recognized other persons, but frequently he appeared to be confused, answered questions inappropriately, occasionally appeared to have hallucinations, and varied widely in terms of his alertness and general orientation. He was later amnesic for this entire one-month period.

Neurological Examination

R.A. sustained multiple injuries in the accident. In the emergency room both of his pupils reacted quickly to light but the left pupil was a little larger than the right. Extraocular muscle function was within normal limits. Deep tendon reflexes were increased, more on the right than the left side. These observations were confirmed during repeated examinations. Skull x-rays were within normal limits. Other x-rays demonstrated three rib fractures on the left side, a fracture of the T-12 vertebra, and dislocation of the L-1 vertebra. The neurologists believed that the vertebral fractures did not have any neurological significance. An electroencephalogram revealed striking generalized abnormalities, most prominent in the temporal and adjacent areas of both hemispheres.

During the third and fourth weeks following the injury R.A. was frequently totally irrational and erratic; sometimes he would shout and curse and at other times he was relatively cooperative. At the time of discharge (eight weeks post-injury) neurological examination was entirely within normal limits except that the patient had some difficulty with concentration. At this time the EEG showed moderate disturbance of brain function that principally involved the left anterior temporal, inferior frontal, and adjacent areas; however, this tracing demonstrated marked improvement compared to the EEG obtained 10 days after the injury.

Neuropsychological Examination

The initial neuropsychological examination was done eight weeks post-injury and three days before R.A. was discharged from the hospital. His neurological diagnosis was cerebral and brain stem contusions. It was believed that the focal signs of cerebral tissue damage were specific but minimal. On the Cornell Medical Index Health Questionnaire R.A. had absolutely no somatic or emotional complaints.

As a general summary statement, we can say that the test results indicate that R.A. had sustained significant impairment of certain aspects of general intelligence and other adaptive abilities. In addition, the findings implicate both cerebral hemispheres and suggest that the condition of the

THE HALSTEAD-REITAN
NEUROPSYCHOLOGICAL TEST BATTERY

Patient **R.A. (I)** Age **29** Sex **M** Education **16** Handedness **R**

WECHSLER-BELLEVUE SCALE

VIQ	105
PIQ	81
FS IQ	93
Information	14
Comprehension	12
Digit Span	10
Arithmetic	4
Similarities	11
Vocabulary	12
Picture Arrangement	7
Picture Completion	10
Block Design	7
Object Assembly	4
Digit Symbol	6

NEUROPSYCHOLOGICAL DEFICIT SCALE

Level of Performance	35
Pathognomonic Signs	2
Patterns	4
Right-Left Differences	13
Total NDS Score	54

HALSTEAD'S NEUROPSYCHOLOGICAL TEST BATTERY

Category Test — 50

Tactile Performance Test

Dominant hand:	9.4
Non-dominant hand:	4.3
Both hands:	5.3

Total Time	19.0
Memory	5
Localization	2

Seashore Rhythm Test

Number Correct **22** — 10

Speech-sounds Perception Test

Number of Errors — 6

Finger Oscillation Test

Dominant hand:	46	46
Non-dominant hand:	31	

Impairment Index 0.7

TRAIL MAKING TEST

Part A: **63** seconds
Part B: **103** seconds

STRENGTH OF GRIP

Dominant hand: **40.5** kilograms
Non-dominant hand: **39.5** kilograms

REITAN-KLØVE TACTILE FORM RECOGNITION TEST

Dominant hand: **16** seconds; **1** errors
Non-dominant hand: **16** seconds; **1** errors

MINNESOTA MULTIPHASIC PERSONALITY INVENTORY

		Hs	62
		D	63
?	50	Hy	60
L	60	Pd	71
F	55	Mf	51
K	69	Pa	62
		Pt	56
		Sc	61
		Ma	60

REITAN-KLØVE SENSORY-PERCEPTUAL EXAM

		Error Totals
RH___ LH ___	Both H: RH **2** LH **1**	RH **2** LH **1**
RH___ LF ___	Both H/F: RH___ LF ___	RH___ LF ___
LH___ RF ___	Both H/F: LH___ RF ___	RF___ LH ___
RE___ LE ___	Both E: RE **1** LE **1**	RE **1** LE **1**
RV___ LV ___	Both: RV___ LV ___	RV___ LV ___

REITAN-KLØVE LATERAL-DOMINANCE EXAM

Show me how you:

throw a ball	R
hammer a nail	R
cut with a knife	R
turn a door knob	R
use scissors	R
use an eraser	R
write your name	R

Record time used for spontaneous name-writing:

Preferred hand	**6** seconds
Non-preferred hand	**11** seconds

Show me how you:

kick a football	L
step on a bug	R

TACTILE FINGER RECOGNITION

R 1___ 2 **1** 3___ 4___ 5___ R **1** / 20
L 1 **1** 2 **1** 3 ___ 4 **1** 5 **1** L **4** / 20

FINGER-TIP NUMBER WRITING

R 1 **1** 2 ___ 3___ 4 **2** 5___ R **3** / 20
L 1 **2** 2 ___ 3 **1** 4 ___ 5 **2** L **5** / 20

NO APHASIC SYMPTOMS.

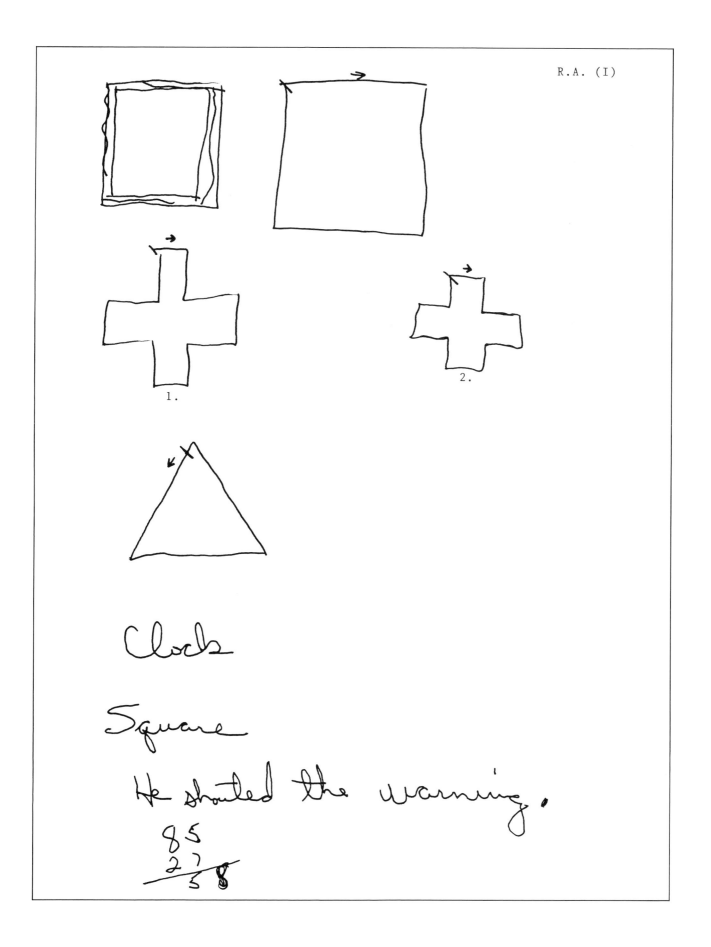

Clock

Square

He shouted the warning.

85
27
5 8

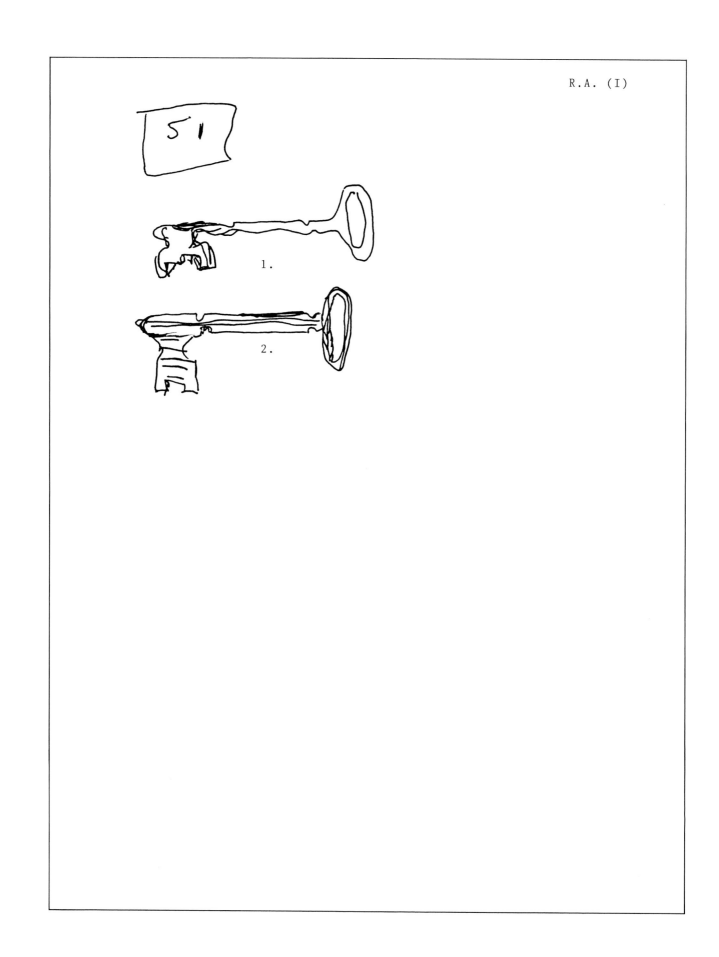

brain is relatively stabilized at this time. His G-NDS score of 54 fell in the range of moderate impairment.

R.A. earned a Verbal IQ (105) in the upper part of the Average range (exceeding about 63% of his age peers). His Performance IQ (81) was 24 points less, falling in the lower part of the Low Average distribution (exceeding only about 10%). Scores on the Information (14), Comprehension (12), Similarities (11), and Vocabulary (12) subtests were above average, suggesting that the patient's premorbid intelligence level was above average. Since R.A. was a college graduate, it is possible that the scores on these measures were somewhat reduced from earlier levels; however, such an inference would be speculative. There is almost no doubt, though, that a score of 4 the Arithmetic subtest (which generally is the most sensitive of the Verbal subtests to brain damage) showed significant impairment.

We would also presume that R.A. demonstrated generalized impairment of performance intelligence. It is not uncommon for the Picture Completion subtest to be less affected by right cerebral damage than the other subtests. However, the distribution of Performance subtest scores does not suggest any specific or focal damage within the right cerebral hemisphere. It seems that the results on the Wechsler Scale were strongly suggestive of brain-related impairment; however, the extent to which they might underestimate the degree of impairment, or fail to show significant areas of deficit, would be unknown at this point because the Wechsler Scale was never designed to provide a full assessment of brain-behavior relationships.

R.A. showed significant evidence of cognitive impairment on the four most sensitive indicators in the Halstead-Reitan Battery. When contrasted with his good scores on the Verbal subtests of the Wechsler Scale, his Impairment Index of 0.7 is almost a certain indicator of loss of brain-related adaptive abilities. The patient also performed quite

poorly on the Localization component of the Tactual Performance Test (2) and showed at least mild impairment on the Category Test (50 errors) and Part B of the Trail Making Test (103 sec). At this point, therefore, it would be possible to conclude that R.A. had had relatively adequate intelligence premorbidly but had suffered significant impairment of higher-level aspects of brain functions (as confirmed by the G-NDS score of 54 as noted above).

Lateralizing indications of neuropsychological impairment were also present. Measures of lateral dominance indicated that R.A. was strongly and definitely right-handed. Nevertheless, his grip strength was barely greater with his right hand (40.5) than with his left hand (39.5). In addition, the pattern of performances on the three trials of the Tactual Performance Test indicated impairment with the right upper extremity as compared with the left. Note, though, that the patient showed no evidence of aphasia and performed quite well on the Speech-sounds Perception Test (6 errors). Findings such as these would argue against a specific, identifiable focal lesion of the left cerebral hemisphere. The good score on the Speech-sounds Perception Test certainly indicates that R.A. has the ability to concentrate his attention to specific stimulus material. Even though he did not do very well on the Seashore Rhythm Test (22 correct), it must be remembered that a person may do poorly on the Rhythm Test for reasons other than an inability to concentrate and maintain continued attention.

Positive findings were also present to implicate the right cerebral hemisphere. Considering R.A.'s right-handedness, his finger tapping speed was quite slow with his left hand (31) compared with his right hand (46). Tests of tactile finger localization and finger-tip number writing perception also demonstrated greater indications of right cerebral dysfunction than left hemisphere dysfunction.

R.A.'s performances in copying simple spatial configurations also suggested right cerebral damage. His first attempt to draw the cross showed no gross evidence of specific difficulty, but the width of the lateral extremities was somewhat unusual in relation to the vertical extremities. The examiner asked R.A. to draw the figure a second time, and although the patient completed the figure fairly well he still demonstrated some disparity in the position of the lateral extremities. However, these drawings probably can be considered to be essentially within normal limits.

R.A. had somewhat more difficulty in his first attempt to copy the key. He tried conscientiously to improve the drawing, but made relatively little progress with the lines he added. It probably is noteworthy that he initially failed to include the "nose" of the key. After his first attempt R.A. was asked to draw the key again. He did somewhat better on the second trial and there are no specific errors on this figure that implicate the right cerebral hemisphere. However, the first drawing suggests that in dealing with simple spatial relationships R.A. has the type of difficulties that are typical of persons with right cerebral damage.

Considering both the general and specific indicators, it is clear that the overall neuropsychological test results point toward generalized cerebral damage and there is no evidence supporting a specific focal lesion involving either cerebral hemisphere. Additional findings of general significance were derived even from measures that frequently identify focal lesions. For example, on the Tactile Form Recognition Test R.A. was somewhat slow as well as inaccurate with both hands. In addition, he showed evidence of impairment on each side of the body on both tactile and auditory tests of bilateral simultaneous stimulation.

The test results also suggest that even though there is evidence of definite impairment, R.A.'s brain is relatively stabilized in a biological sense. The absence of aphasia, the good score on the Speech-sounds Perception Test, and the absence of severe impairment on Part B of the Trail Making Test, considered with relation to the pronounced indications of impairment shown both by general and specific tests, would argue strongly against a focal progressive lesion (such as a stroke or intrinsic tumor). In fact, the test results are quite characteristic of a person with a serious closed head injury.

The Minnesota Multiphasic Personality Inventory (MMPI) suggests that R.A. has certain affectively based deviations in his behavioral pattern. It is likely that on one hand he is somewhat defensive and unconcerned about social conventions, but conversely he is also interested in presenting himself as particularly competent and respectable. There is no strong evidence to suggest that any specific patterns on the MMPI relate particularly to cranial-cerebral trauma. It is more likely that the MMPI results reflect R.A.'s premorbid personality characteristics.

The second examination was performed one year later, when R.A. was 30 years old. The patient himself felt that there were no residual deficits from the injury and on the Cornell Medical Index Health Questionnaire he had absolutely no complaints. The neurological examination also was within normal limits, but the EEG showed mild to moderate focal abnormalities over the left temporal region. Electroencephalograms had been done during the initial hospitalization, three months post-trauma, and at the time of the present examination (12 months after the first neuropsychological testing). Although the deficits continued to be present in the same areas as in the initial tracings, each consecutive EEG examination showed a mild degree of improvement.

Recognizing that a certain degree of positive-practice effect is likely to occur, it is still advantageous to initially review the test results without reference to the original test findings. Of course, the second phase of the interpretation requires a comparison of the two examinations.

THE HALSTEAD-REITAN
NEUROPSYCHOLOGICAL TEST BATTERY

Patient ___R.A. (II)___ Age __30__ Sex __M__ Education __16__ Handedness __R__

WECHSLER-BELLEVUE SCALE

VIQ	129
PIQ	115
FS IQ	122
Information	14
Comprehension	17
Digit Span	9
Arithmetic	15
Similarities	16
Vocabulary	14
Picture Arrangement	11
Picture Completion	13
Block Design	10
Object Assembly	12
Digit Symbol	11

NEUROPSYCHOLOGICAL DEFICIT SCALE

Level of Performance	12
Pathognomonic Signs	0
Patterns	2
Right-Left Differences	6
Total NDS Score	20

HALSTEAD'S NEUROPSYCHOLOGICAL TEST BATTERY

Category Test	27

Tactual Performance Test

Dominant hand:	4.6
Non-dominant hand:	3.6
Both hands:	2.8
Total Time	11.0
Memory	8
Localization	5

Seashore Rhythm Test

Number Correct	26	5

Speech-sounds Perception Test

Number of Errors		6

Finger Oscillation Test

Dominant hand:	46	46
Non-dominant hand:	36	

Impairment Index __0.1__

TRAIL MAKING TEST

Part A: __27__ seconds
Part B: __69__ seconds

MINNESOTA MULTIPHASIC PERSONALITY INVENTORY

		Hs	41
		D	48
?	50	Hy	53
L	50	Pd	69
F	53	Mf	62
K	57	Pa	67
		Pt	52
		Sc	51
		Ma	70

STRENGTH OF GRIP

Dominant hand: __59.0__ kilograms
Non-dominant hand: __54.0__ kilograms

REITAN-KLØVE TACTILE FORM RECOGNITION TEST

Dominant hand: __8__ seconds; __0__ errors
Non-dominant hand: __8__ seconds; __1__ errors

REITAN-KLØVE SENSORY-PERCEPTUAL EXAM — No errors

			Error Totals
RH___ LH ___	Both H: RH ___ LH ___	RH ___ LH ___	
RH___ LF ___	Both H/F: RH ___ LF ___	RH ___ LF ___	
LH ___ RF ___	Both H/F: LH ___ RF ___	RF ___ LH ___	
RE ___ LE ___	Both E: RE ___ LE ___	RE ___ LE ___	
RV ___ LV ___	Both: RV ___ LV ___	RV ___ LV ___	

REITAN-KLØVE LATERAL-DOMINANCE EXAM

Show me how you:

throw a ball	R
hammer a nail	R
cut with a knife	R
turn a door knob	R
use scissors	R
use an eraser	R
write your name	R

Record time used for spontaneous name-writing:

Preferred hand	6 seconds
Non-preferred hand	14 seconds

TACTILE FINGER RECOGNITION

R 1__ 2__ 3__ 4__ 5__   R _0_ / _20_
L 1__ 2__ 3__ 2 4__ 5__   L _2_ / _20_

FINGER-TIP NUMBER WRITING

R 1__ 2__ 3__ 4__ 5__   R _0_ / _20_
L 1 1 2__ 3__ 4__ 5__   L _1_ / _20_

Show me how you:

kick a football	R
step on a bug	R

NO APHASIC SYMPTOMS.

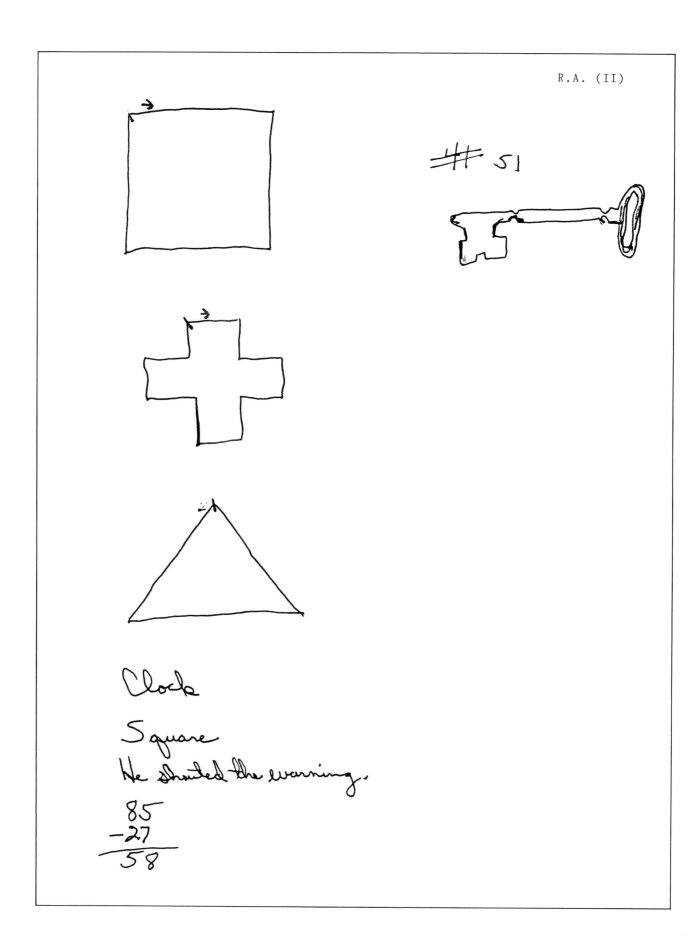

51

Clock

Square

He shouted the warning.

85
−27
‾‾‾
58

R.A. earned a Verbal IQ (129) in the Superior range (exceeding 97% of his age peers) and a Performance IQ (115) in the middle part of the High Average range (exceeding 84%). These values yielded a Full Scale IQ (122) that was within the lower part of the Superior range (exceeding 93%). The distribution of individual subtest scores revealed no significant information. The patient did somewhat poorly on the Digit Span subtest (9), but this is not an uncommon occurrence among many patients (including persons who have no evidence of brain damage).

Scores on the four most sensitive indicators in the Halstead-Reitan Battery all fell within the normal range. The only test that contributed to the Impairment Index of 0.1 was the Finger Oscillation Test. On tasks that required more complex and demanding cognitive functions the patient's scores were in the normal range. His G-NDS score of 20 was also within normal limits, but the section on Right-Left Differences was mildly deviant because of slow finger tapping with the left hand as well as two errors in finger localization. It would appear that R.A.'s adaptive abilities, in addition to his general intellectual skills, were quite adequate.

There were no lateralizing indicators present to implicate the left cerebral hemisphere. R.A. made an error when asked to mentally compute 17 × 3 (responding "41"), but he recognized the error immediately and corrected it spontaneously.

There were some indications of right cerebral dysfunction. Probably the strongest of these indicators related to finger tapping speed with the left hand (36) as compared with the right hand (46). R.A. also had some difficulty in tactile finger localization on his left hand (2 errors) but made no errors on the right hand. Even though he responded quickly on the Tactile Form Recognition Test, he made an error with his left hand that is rarely seen in control subjects; although he corrected his mistake, he initially identified the circle as a square. Finally, on the Tactual Performance

Test he did not improve quite as much as would normally be expected on the second trial (using his left hand), but this deviation from normality was so mild that it cannot be attributed much significance.

In conclusion, the neuropsychological test results obtained one year after the first examination (14 months post-injury) were within normal limits in terms of level of performance. However, there were very mild indications of right cerebral dysfunction. We would not question the validity of the consistent EEG findings of left cerebral dysfunction, but it should be noted that in this instance the EEG and the neuropsychological findings differ with regard to their lateralization significance.

Comparisons of the first and second examinations indicate that almost every measure in the Battery demonstrates a substantial improvement that goes well beyond expected practice-effect. R.A.'s Verbal IQ rose 24 points and his Performance IQ, which had been quite low initially, rose 34 points. In this case it is interesting to note the confirmation that the greatest initial deficit shows the largest subsequent improvement. However, the patient improved so consistently that it is difficult to evaluate the differential improvement on individual tests. The G-NDS improved from 54 (moderate impairment) to 20 (normal range).

Each of the four most sensitive measures demonstrated some improvement: the Impairment Index was reduced from 0.7 to 0.1, the number of errors on the Category Test decreased from 50 to 27, the score on Trails B was reduced from 103 seconds to 69 seconds, and the number of shapes correctly localized on the Tactual Performance Test increased from two to five. We would judge that the greatest improvement among these measures occurred on the Impairment Index; Trails B and the Localization score were secondary. It is not unusual to see a fairly substantial improvement on the Category Test due to practice-effect; however, R.A. clearly improved his Total Time score on the Tactual Performance Test (from 19.0

min to 11.0 min) and also demonstrated his improved ability on the Seashore Rhythm Test (from 22 correct to 26 correct).

On the Tactile Form Recognition Test R.A. reduced the time required to the normal range. He also showed substantial improvement on both Tactile Finger Recognition and Finger-tip Number Writing Perception (especially on the left hand, where there had initially been more errors). R.A.'s Finger tapping speed did not increase with his right hand but was definitely faster with his left hand (which initially was more impaired). However, on grip strength, where the right hand had initially been more impaired, the improvement was substantial on both sides but greater on the right side.

Thus, all of the measures that permit a direct comparison of intraindividual performances with relation to lateralized impairment — Verbal IQ vs. Performance IQ, dominant vs. non-dominant hand on the Tactual Performance Test, dominant vs. non-dominant hand on finger tapping speed, dominant vs. non-dominant hand on grip strength, right vs. left hand on tactile finger localization, and right vs. left hand on finger-tip number writing perception — all showed greater improvement on the measure that initially was more seriously impaired.

R.A. also improved his drawings. Although the Speech-sounds Perception Test score remained the same (6 errors), that test had not demonstrated any deficit initially. There can be little doubt that this man improved greatly during the time between the first and second examinations. It would also appear that his most substantial improvement occurred on the measures that initially showed the greatest deficit, with the pattern of improvement essentially being of such a nature that on the second examination the overall configuration of test results was nearly within normal limits.

R.A. was re-examined 18 months after the initial evaluation (20 months post-injury). At this time he again had no complaints and the neurological examination was within normal limits. Although the EEG continued to demonstrate residual abnormalities, there was a slight degree of improvement.

First, we will independently evaluate the results of this third examination. Later we will compare the present findings with the results of the first two examinations.

R.A. earned a Verbal IQ (121) in the lower part of the Superior range (exceeding 92% of his age peers) and a Performance IQ (114) that was in the middle part of the High Average range (exceeding 82%). His poor score (4) on the Digit Span subtest suggests that he may have been distractible or had difficulty focusing his attention to the test. (Note, however, that he had no difficulty whatsoever focusing his attention to the stimulus material on Speech-sounds Perception Test.) It would not be possible to interpret the results on the Wechsler Scale as providing any definite or unequivocal evidence of cerebral disease or damage.

Among the four most sensitive indicators in the Halstead-Reitan Battery, R.A. earned a borderline Impairment Index score of 0.4, did very well on the Category Test (11), performed adequately on Part B of the Trail Making Test (62 sec), and did somewhat poorly on the Localization component of the Tactual Performance Test (4). Even though his performances were not quite as good on these measures as might be expected with relation to his IQ values, these results certainly would not suggest that R.A. had any significant or serious impairment of brain functions. The G-NDS score was 23, falling within the normal range but perhaps a little poor with relation to the IQ values. Again, the section of Right-Left Differences deviated from the normal range.

Lateralizing indicators were present only for the right cerebral hemisphere. (R.A. answered "41" to the problem 17 × 3, but this is not an unusual response among normal subjects.) Impaired performances with the left hand as compared with the

THE HALSTEAD-REITAN
NEUROPSYCHOLOGICAL TEST BATTERY

Patient __R.A. (III)__ Age __31__ Sex __M__ Education __16__ Handedness __R__

WECHSLER-BELLEVUE SCALE

VIQ	121
PIQ	114
FS IQ	119
Information	14
Comprehension	14
Digit Span	4
Arithmetic	16
Similarities	16
Vocabulary	14
Picture Arrangement	9
Picture Completion	14
Block Design	11
Object Assembly	12
Digit Symbol	10

NEUROPSYCHOLOGICAL DEFICIT SCALE

Level of Performance	15
Pathognomonic Signs	0
Patterns	1
Right-Left Differences	7
Total NDS Score	23

TRAIL MAKING TEST

Part A: __36__ seconds
Part B: __62__ seconds

STRENGTH OF GRIP

Dominant hand: __59.0__ kilograms

Non-dominant hand: __54.0__ kilograms

REITAN-KLØVE TACTILE FORM RECOGNITION TEST

Dominant hand: __11__ seconds; __0__ errors

Non-dominant hand: __13__ seconds; __0__ errors

REITAN-KLØVE SENSORY-PERCEPTUAL EXAM — No errors

Error Totals

RH___LH___	Both H:	RH___LH___	RH___LH___	
RH___LF___	Both H/F:	RH___LF___	RH___LF___	
LH___RF___	Both H/F:	LH___RF___	RF___LH___	
RE___LE___	Both E:	RE___LE___	RE___LE___	
RV___LV___	Both:	RV___LV___	RV___LV___	

TACTILE FINGER RECOGNITION

R 1___2___3___4___5___ R __0__ / 20

L 1___2___3___4___5___ L __0__ / 20

FINGER-TIP NUMBER WRITING

R 1___2___3_1_4_1_5___ R __2__ / 20

L 1_1_2___3_1_4_1_5___ L __3__ / 20

HALSTEAD'S NEUROPSYCHOLOGICAL TEST BATTERY

Category Test	11

Tactual Performance Test

Dominant hand:	4.2
Non-dominant hand:	4.6
Both hands:	2.1

Total Time	10.9
Memory	8
Localization	4

Seashore Rhythm Test

Number Correct __21__   10

Speech-sounds Perception Test

Number of Errors   2

Finger Oscillation Test

Dominant hand:	41	41
Non-dominant hand:	33	

Impairment Index   0.4

MINNESOTA MULTIPHASIC PERSONALITY INVENTORY

		Hs	47
		D	58
?	50	Hy	58
L	50	Pd	57
F	55	Mf	55
K	55	Pa	59
		Pt	56
		Sc	55
		Ma	63

REITAN-KLØVE LATERAL-DOMINANCE EXAM

Show me how you:

throw a ball	R
hammer a nail	R
cut with a knife	R
turn a door knob	R
use scissors	R
use an eraser	R
write your name	R

Record time used for spontaneous name-writing:

Preferred hand	5 seconds
Non-preferred hand	14 seconds

Show me how you:

kick a football	R
step on a bug	R

NO APHASIC SYMPTOMS.

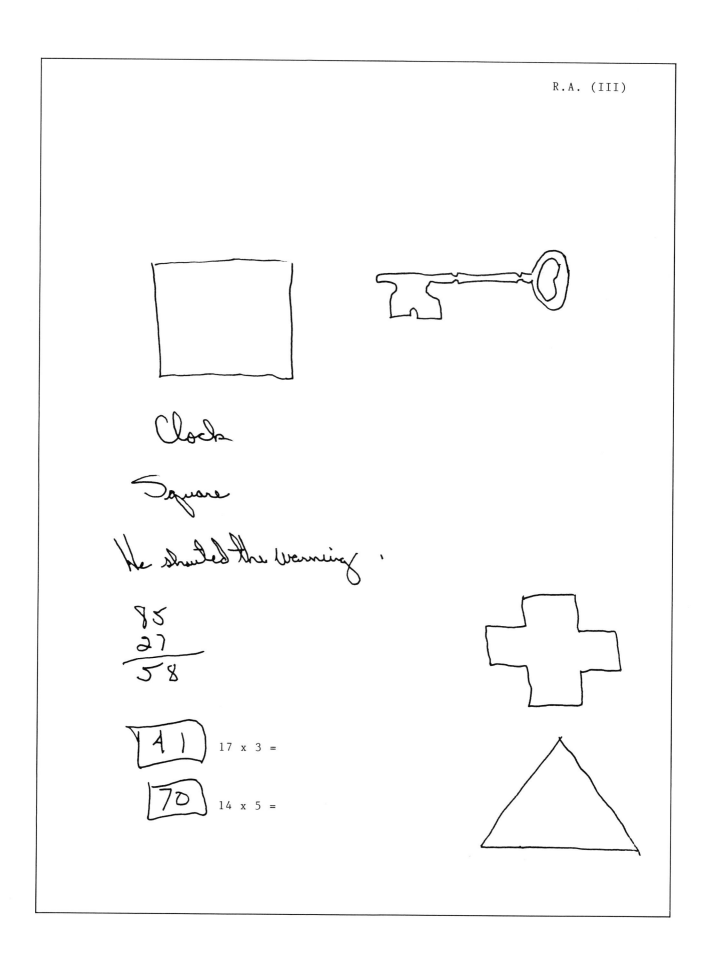

Clock

Square

He shouted the warning .

85
27
___
58

41   17 x 3 =

70   14 x 5 =

right hand constituted evidence of some right cerebral dysfunction. For example, the patient's finger tapping speed, while relatively slow with both hands, was clearly slower than expected with the left hand (33) compared to the right hand (41). On the Tactual Performance Test R.A. also performed worse with his left hand (4.6 min) than with his right hand (4.2 min). He was somewhat slow with both hands on the Tactile Form Recognition Test, but the two-second difference was probably not of significance in implicating the right cerebral hemisphere. The patient's drawings were probably within normal limits, although a question could be raised about loss of symmetry of the "teeth" of the key.

Although they do not have any lateralizing significance, the Seashore Rhythm Test score (21 correct) and results on test of finger-tip number writing perception add to the impression that R.A. may have a mild degree of impairment of neuropsychological functions.

In summary, the findings obtained on the third examination deviated mildly from normal expectations, suggesting that there was evidence of some cognitive impairment. These results contrast rather sharply with the findings obtained on the second examination (six months earlier). Direct comparisons indicate that a number of the scores showed no significant changes, although even these measures may have been expected to show some "improvement" on the basis of practice-effect. On Part B of the Trail Making Test it is possible that the change from 69 seconds to 62 seconds represents a mild genuine improvement, but our informal experiments with this test have indicated that some degree of practice-effect operates through a number of successive trials.

In identifying differences in results of the examinations, nearly all of the changes that appear to be significant were demonstrated as poorer performances on the third examination. For example, R.A.'s Verbal IQ dropped from 129 to 121 and he showed a very significant change on Digit Span (from 9 to 4). He might possibly have shown a mild decrement on Picture Arrangement with the score decreasing from 11 to 9. He definitely performed worse on the Seashore Rhythm Test (from 26 to 21 correct responses) and his drawing of the key might possibly be slightly worse.

R.A. also demonstrated rather definite decrements in motor and sensory functions. His finger tapping speed dropped from 46 to 41 taps with his preferred hand and from 36 to 33 taps with his non-preferred hand. (Notice that he showed no change on either hand in grip strength.) On the Tactile Form Recognition Test he required more time with each hand (although he did not repeat the error he made with the left hand on the prior examination). Finally, R.A. made a total of five errors in finger-tip number writing perception (as compared with one error on the previous examination).

It would be difficult to attribute any particular focus of biological disorder in the brain responsible for these neuropsychological changes, but when compared to the results obtained six months earlier they would nevertheless seem to represent genuine decrements in performance. Although there was no specific and compelling evidence of cerebral contusion (the diagnosis reached on the basis of neurological evaluation during the initial hospitalization), this case follows the pattern that we have seen in many instances of patients with cerebral contusions. The pattern is one of substantial improvement during the first 12 months post-injury followed six months later by retention of improvement on some measures but definite evidence of regression on others. From comparative results on the Minnesota Multiphasic Personality Inventory it would not appear that underlying emotional or affective changes were responsible for the poorer scores. In fact, the MMPI profile appears to be more within normal limits on the third examination than it was on the second.

Case #9

Name: J.W.

Age: 19

Education: 11

Sex: Male

Handedness: Right

Occupation: Laborer

Background Information

This 19-year-old man fell when the bicycle he was riding skidded on some loose gravel. As he fell he struck the left side of his head on a metal pipe. A friend who observed the accident reported that J.W. was motionless for 20 to 30 seconds after hitting his head and was lethargic and confused for 10 to 20 minutes.

Neurological Examination

J.W. was immediately taken to the emergency room of a medical center and was reportedly alert, fully oriented, and in no acute distress. Some bleeding from his left ear was initially observed but appeared to have stopped by the time he reached the emergency room. X-rays showed basilar and left parietal linear skull fractures and J.W. was admitted to the hospital. He showed no significant deficits on the neurological examination, although it was noted that his deep tendon reflexes were slightly increased on the right side. He was fully alert and appropriate in his behavior and was discharged from the hospital two days after admission. An electroencephalogram done the day following the injury showed moderate abnormality over the posterior part of the left cerebral hemisphere, centering particularly in the posterior temporal region. J.W. was diagnosed as having a cerebral concussion.

Neuropsychological Examination

The first neuropsychological examination was performed eight days after the injury. The Cornell Medical Index Health Questionnaire was administered at that time and the patient had essentially no complaints.

J.W. earned both Verbal (109) and Performance (106) IQ values that fell in the upper part of the average range, yielding a Full Scale IQ (109) that also was in the upper part of the average range and exceeded about 73% of the his age peers. The Verbal subtest scores indicate that J.W. performed quite poorly on Digit Span (6) and that the Arithmetic subtest (10) was next lowest. Judging from the higher scores on Information (13), Similarities (14), and Vocabulary (14), we would postulate that in practice the verbal intelligence of this subject probably was somewhat higher than indicated by the IQ value of 109. It would appear that the Digit Span score is somewhat reduced, although it is not possible to conclude that cerebral damage was necessarily the cause. It is also possible that the Arithmetic score is a little lower than it might normally have been, but the Wechsler results alone certainly are not sufficient to postulate that J.W. has sustained brain damage. Variability on the Performance subtests did not appear to be meaningful in terms of brain damage.

J.W. performed relatively well on the four most sensitive indicators in the Halstead-Reitan Battery; each score was within the normal range. Two of Halstead's seven tests had impaired scores, which translated into an Impairment Index of 0.3. His

THE HALSTEAD-REITAN
NEUROPSYCHOLOGICAL TEST BATTERY

Patient __J.W. (I)__ Age __19__ Sex __M__ Education __11__ Handedness __R__

WECHSLER-BELLEVUE SCALE

VIQ	109
PIQ	106
FS IQ	109
Information	13
Comprehension	11
Digit Span	6
Arithmetic	10
Similarities	14
Vocabulary	14
Picture Arrangement	13
Picture Completion	13
Block Design	10
Object Assembly	10
Digit Symbol	10

NEUROPSYCHOLOGICAL DEFICIT SCALE

Level of Performance	22
Pathognomonic Signs	2
Patterns	0
Right-Left Differences	14
Total NDS Score	38

TRAIL MAKING TEST

Part A: __70__ seconds
Part B: __81__ seconds

STRENGTH OF GRIP

Dominant hand: __52.5__ kilograms
Non-dominant hand: __54.5__ kilograms

REITAN-KLØVE TACTILE FORM RECOGNITION TEST

Dominant hand: __18__ seconds; __0__ errors
Non-dominant hand: __10__ seconds; __0__ errors

REITAN-KLØVE SENSORY-PERCEPTUAL EXAM

Error Totals

RH ___ LH ___	Both H:	RH ___ LH ___		RH ___ LH ___	
RH ___ LF ___	Both H/F:	RH ___ LF ___		RH ___ LF ___	
LH ___ RF ___	Both H/F:	LH ___ RF ___		RF ___ LH ___	
RE ___ LE ___	Both E:	RE ___ LE __3__		RE ___ LE __3__	
RV ___ LV ___	Both:	RV ___ LV ___		RV ___ LV ___	

TACTILE FINGER RECOGNITION

R 1___ 2 _1_ 3 ___ 4 _2_ 5 ___   R _3_ / 20
L 1___ 2 _1_ 3 ___ 4 _1_ 5 ___   L _2_ / 20

FINGER-TIP NUMBER WRITING

R 1 _1_ 2 ___ 3 ___ 4 ___ 5 ___   R _1_ / 20
L 1___ 2 ___ 3 ___ 4 ___ 5 ___   L _0_ / 20

HALSTEAD'S NEUROPSYCHOLOGICAL TEST BATTERY

Category Test	47

Tactual Performance Test

Dominant hand:	5.2
Non-dominant hand:	4.4
Both hands:	1.9

Total Time	11.5
Memory	7
Localization	6

Seashore Rhythm Test

Number Correct	25	6

Speech-sounds Perception Test

Number of Errors	6

Finger Oscillation Test

Dominant hand:	43	43
Non-dominant hand:	44	

Impairment Index __0.3__

MINNESOTA MULTIPHASIC PERSONALITY INVENTORY

		Hs	57
		D	56
?	50	Hy	71
L	50	Pd	67
F	58	Mf	76
K	64	Pa	53
		Pt	60
		Sc	61
		Ma	55

REITAN-KLØVE LATERAL-DOMINANCE EXAM

Show me how you:

throw a ball	R
hammer a nail	R
cut with a knife	R
turn a door knob	R
use scissors	R
use an eraser	R
write your name	R

Record time used for spontaneous name-writing:

Preferred hand	4 seconds
Non-preferred hand	11 seconds

Show me how you:

kick a football	R
step on a bug	R

REITAN-INDIANA APHASIA SCREENING TEST

Form for Adults and Older Children

Name: _____ J. W. (I) _____ Age: __19__

Copy SQUARE	Repeat TRIANGLE
Name SQUARE	Repeat MASSACHUSETTS
Spell SQUARE	Repeat METHODIST EPISCOPAL
Copy CROSS	Write SQUARE Had diffuculty forming "q". Initially wrote "g".
Name CROSS	Read SEVEN
Spell CROSS	Repeat SEVEN
Copy TRIANGLE	Repeat/Explain HE SHOUTED THE WARNING. "He voiced louded a caution or something."
Name TRIANGLE	Write HE SHOUTED THE WARNING. Had difficulty with "the."
Spell TRIANGLE	Compute 85 – 27 =
Name BABY	Compute 17 X 3 =
Write CLOCK Printed, and examiner asked him to write. Had difficulty and asked to start over.	Name KEY
Name FORK	Demonstrate use of KEY
Read 7 SIX 2	Draw KEY
Read MGW	Read PLACE LEFT HAND TO RIGHT EAR.
Reading I	Place LEFT HAND TO RIGHT EAR
Reading II	Place LEFT HAND TO LEFT ELBOW

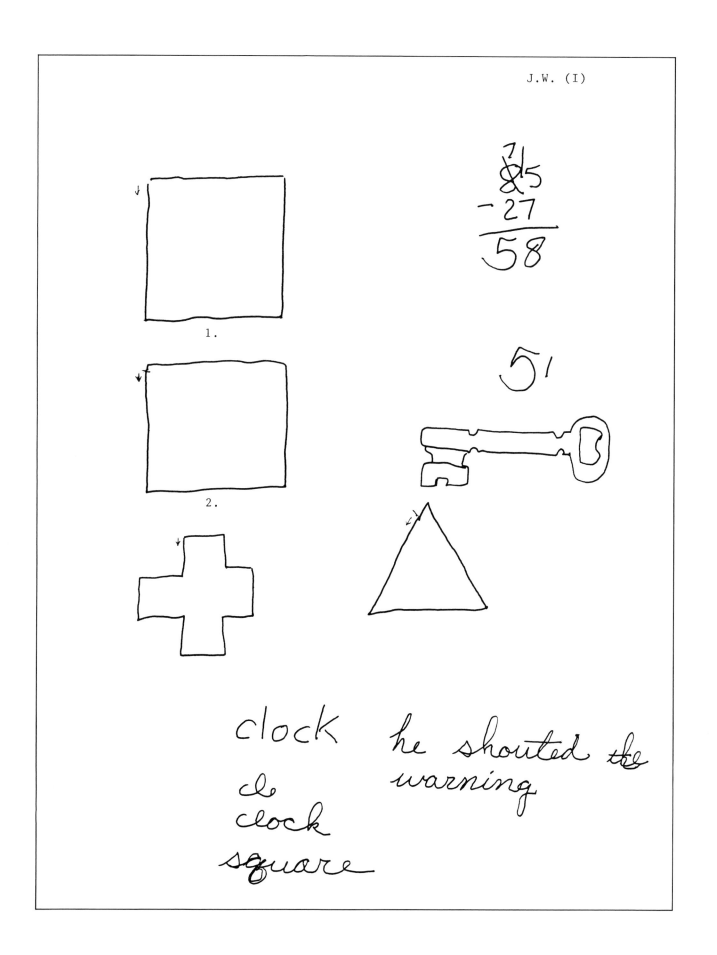

1.

2.

$$\begin{array}{r} \overset{7}{\cancel{8}}5 \\ -\ 27 \\ \hline 58 \end{array}$$

5'

clock

cl

clock

square

he shouted the
warning

finger tapping speed with the preferred (right) hand was significantly slow (43) and the score for the Seashore Rhythm Test (25 correct) was just within the impaired range. In terms of complexity, neither of these measures is among the more demanding tests that contribute to the Impairment Index. We should note, however, that neither the Category Test (47) nor Part B of the Trail Making Test (81 sec) was performed very well even though both scores were in or near the normal range.

In terms of level of performance, a cursory review of J.W.'s scores indicates that they were generally in the normal range or only mildly impaired and one might be inclined to conclude that they were essentially within the range of normal variability and did not demonstrate any definite evidence of cerebral damage. In a case like this the G-NDS is helpful in providing a standardized overall score. In fact, J.W. had a G-NDS score of 38, a value that falls in the range of mild neuropsychological impairment. (Not a single person among 41 control subjects earned a G-NDS score that exceeded 35.)

Nevertheless, a number of findings particularly indicated involvement of the left cerebral hemisphere. Although definitely right-handed, J.W.'s finger tapping speed was less on the right hand (43) than the left (44) and his grip strength was less on the right side (52.5 kg) than the left (54.5 kg). On tactile form recognition he required considerably more time with his right hand (18 sec) than his left (10 sec), suggesting that his right-sided deficits involved tactile-receptive abilities as well as motor functions.

Finally, on the Aphasia Screening Test J.W. had a number of difficulties, particularly involving writing. When asked to look at a picture of a clock and identify it by writing its name, he first printed his answer (which is not uncommon). He was then asked to write rather than print and had difficulty forming the word on the first attempt. He also had a problem writing SQUARE. He was able to read the word when the stimulus figure was presented to him, but in his

attempt to write the word he became somewhat confused in trying to form a "Q." Finally, in writing HE SHOUTED THE WARNING, he became confused in making the "H" in "the."

One might observe that these difficulties were relatively minor in nature; however, using the same items and stimulus material with thousands of patients has demonstrated that the type of errors that J.W. made occur rarely among control subjects whose verbal intelligence scores are in the average range or higher. Although these kinds of problems would not indicate that the patient should be considered dysgraphic, they occur much more frequently in persons with left cerebral damage than in control subjects.

J.W. also had some difficulty in his verbal explanation of HE SHOUTED THE WARNING. When asked what the sentence might mean, he said, "He voiced louded a caution or something." Apparently the subject meant to indicate that someone had raised his voice loudly in order to offer a caution; however, his confusion in verbal expression is also suspicious of left cerebral dysfunction. Despite his apparently good scores with respect to level of performance (although the Level of Performance section of the G-NDS shows that even these scores are somewhat poor compared to control subjects), these indications of mild language difficulty, in conjunction with the lateralized motor and tactile-perceptual difficulties on the right side, almost certainly constitute a basis for concluding that J.W. had mild cerebral dysfunction.

The patient also showed certain indications of right cerebral impairment. The most striking of these signs was his failure to be able to perceive an auditory stimulus to his left ear in three of four trials when stimuli were presented on both sides simultaneously. This particular sign is rarely seen in persons with relatively mild effects of head injuries, but it cannot be neglected. J.W.'s drawing of a cross showed a definite asymmetry of the lateral extremities. While one would not use this finding as a basis for concluding that he had constructional dyspraxia, the deviation from normal expectancy certainly should be noted. J.W. was a little slow with his left hand (4.4 min) as compared with his right hand (5.2 min) on the Tactual Performance Test. He also had some evidence of impairment of tactile finger recognition on both hands, an unusual finding in normal control subjects. Thus, the test results pointed without question toward some degree of dysfunction of both the left and right cerebral hemispheres, in a context of relatively good performances on many of the measures.

Results on the Minnesota Multiphasic Personality Inventory deviated somewhat from normal expectancy, suggesting that J.W. tended to be rather anxious and perhaps apprehensive. We cannot be sure that these results were not influenced by the recent head blow, but it seems more likely that the MMPI results reflected pre-injury aspects of personality adjustment.

In summary, J.W. presented a total configuration of neuropsychological test results that definitely deviated from normal. The neuropsychologist needs experience in clinical interpretation in order to be able to recognize these types of deficits as definitely deviating from normal expectancy, but the G-NDS may prove to be of value as a guide to those who are less experienced. The difficulties in writing and verbal communication, coupled with consistent motor and tactile-perceptual difficulties on the right side, overrule any tendency to conclude that the patient was normal (based on his general intelligence values and other adequate scores).

The indications of right cerebral dysfunction were not as strong, but almost certainly have validity in the context of the rest of the test results. In fact, a retrospective analysis of the test results suggests the possibility that both the Digit Span and Arithmetic scores on the Wechsler Scale reflected a mild degree of impairment and that a similar interpretation was justified with respect to scores on the Category Test and Part B of the Trail Making Test. Even though in this case there were

no previous results available for comparative purposes, we can use the various methods of inference in an integrated manner to infer that J.W. had mild generalized impairment of brain functions. If these deficits were a result of the head blow sustained eight days before the neuropsychological examination, we would expect to see improvement both in level of performance as well as in patterns and relationships of the test results on the examination performed 12 months later.

Another neurological examination was done three months after the injury. The neurologist felt that J.W. demonstrated a mild fine tremor when his hands were outstretched and that his deep tendon reflexes were slightly more active on the left side than the right. However, the overall examination was judged to be within normal limits. An EEG was also done at this time and the tracings showed a degree of improvement compared with the initial EEG. Nevertheless, the recording was suggestive of a slight generalized disturbance of brain function.

Twelve months after the injury the neurological examination was essentially normal. However, the EEG continued to show mild left-sided abnormalities with resolution of the more widespread abnormalities that had been seen previously. These mild abnormalities (which centered over the posterior temporal and parietal regions) were supported by changes induced by activation procedures (hyperventilation and photic stimulation).

The neuropsychological examination was repeated 12 months after the initial testing. Responses on the Cornell Medical Index Health Questionnaire indicated that the patient had essentially no complaints.

The results for the testing done 12 months after the initial examination indicated that J.W. had good abilities and very few of the test results deviated from the normal range. He earned both Verbal and Performance IQ values in the lower part of the high average range (113), yielding a Full Scale IQ (114) that exceeded about 82% of his age

THE HALSTEAD-REITAN
NEUROPSYCHOLOGICAL TEST BATTERY

Patient __J.W. (II)__ Age __20__ Sex __M__ Education __13__ Handedness __R__

WECHSLER-BELLEVUE SCALE

VIQ	113
PIQ	113
FS IQ	114
Information	13
Comprehension	11
Digit Span	10
Arithmetic	9
Similarities	15
Vocabulary	14
Picture Arrangement	14
Picture Completion	13
Block Design	10
Object Assembly	11
Digit Symbol	12

NEUROPSYCHOLOGICAL DEFICIT SCALE

Level of Performance	6
Pathognomonic Signs	0
Patterns	0
Right-Left Differences	7
Total NDS Score	13

TRAIL MAKING TEST

Part A: __25__ seconds
Part B: __112__ seconds

STRENGTH OF GRIP

Dominant hand: __53.5__ kilograms
Non-dominant hand: __51.0__ kilograms

REITAN-KLØVE TACTILE FORM RECOGNITION TEST

Dominant hand: __9__ seconds; __0__ errors
Non-dominant hand: __8__ seconds; __0__ errors

REITAN-KLØVE SENSORY-PERCEPTUAL EXAM — No errors

						Error Totals
RH ___ LH ___	Both H:	RH ___ LH ___		RH ___ LH ___		
RH ___ LF ___	Both H/F:	RH ___ LF ___		RH ___ LF ___		
LH ___ RF ___	Both H/F:	LH ___ RF ___		RF ___ LH ___		
RE ___ LE ___	Both E:	RE ___ LE ___		RE ___ LE ___		
RV ___ LV ___	Both:	RV ___ LV ___		RV ___ LV ___		

TACTILE FINGER RECOGNITION

R 1___ 2___ 3___ 4___ 5___   R __0__ / 20
L 1___ 2___ 3___ 4 _1_ 5___   L __1__ / 20

FINGER-TIP NUMBER WRITING

R 1 _1_ 2___ 3___ 4___ 5___   R __1__ / 20
L 1 _1_ 2___ 3___ 4___ 5___   L __1__ / 20

NO APHASIC SYMPTOMS.

HALSTEAD'S NEUROPSYCHOLOGICAL TEST BATTERY

Category Test	8

Tactual Performance Test

Dominant hand:	4.0
Non-dominant hand:	3.5
Both hands:	2.0

Total Time	9.5
Memory	9
Localization	7

Seashore Rhythm Test

Number Correct	28	2

Speech-sounds Perception Test

Number of Errors	4

Finger Oscillation Test

Dominant hand:	49	49
Non-dominant hand:	49	

Impairment Index __0.1__

MINNESOTA MULTIPHASIC PERSONALITY INVENTORY

		Hs	47
		D	46
?	50	Hy	60
L	46	Pd	74
F	62	Mf	69
K	61	Pa	56
		Pt	54
		Sc	63
		Ma	70

REITAN-KLØVE LATERAL-DOMINANCE EXAM

Show me how you:

throw a ball	R
hammer a nail	R
cut with a knife	R
turn a door knob	R
use scissors	R
use an eraser	R
write your name	R

Record time used for spontaneous name-writing:

Preferred hand	4 seconds
Non-preferred hand	8 seconds

Show me how you:

kick a football	R
step on a bug	R

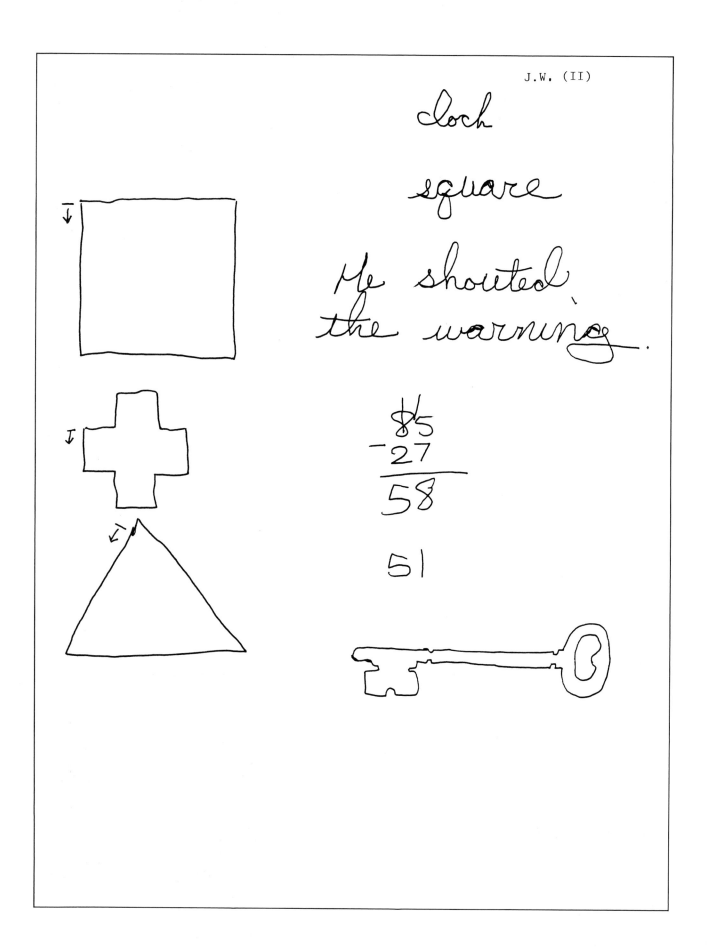

loch

square

He shouted
the warning.

$$\begin{array}{r} \cancel{8}5 \\ -27 \\ \hline 58 \end{array}$$

51

peers. The distribution of subtests was generally unremarkable, although the lowest score (9) among all 11 subtests occurred on Arithmetic and might possibly suggest some degree of impairment.

The patient performed quite well on measures in the Halstead-Reitan Battery, earning an Impairment Index of 0.1 and a G-NDS score of only 13. The only test contributing to the Impairment Index was his finger tapping speed (49). It should also be noted, however, that J.W. also performed poorly on Part B of the Trail Making Test (112 sec). His slow performance was due to the fact that he was somewhat careless, making three errors and requiring additional time to correct these mistakes.

The lateralizing indicators on this examination were not particularly strong, even though the Right-Left Difference section of the G-NDS totalled seven points (as compared with the average 3.37 points for control subjects). J.W. showed no evidence of aphasia. Although he was strongly right-handed, both his grip strength and finger tapping speed were somewhat reduced on the right side as compared with the left side. However, since he had no difficulty on any of the items on the Aphasia Screening Test and showed no significant sensory-perceptual deficits, it would be difficult to use the indications of right-sided motor dysfunction as a basis for a definite conclusion of left cerebral damage.

A similar paucity of significant lateralizing findings was present to implicate the right cerebral hemisphere. J.W. was a little slow with his left hand (3.5 min) as compared with his right hand (4.0 min) on the Tactual Performance Test, but his drawings were within normal limits and he showed no other indications of right cerebral dysfunction.

Results on the Minnesota Multiphasic Personality Inventory suggest that J.W. may have certain difficulties in his environmental adjustment, but problems of this kind also occur with many persons who have never sustained any significant head injury or cerebral damage. Thus, on the basis of test results alone it would be difficult to relate the MMPI findings to the head injury.

Considering the fact that the first set of test results rather clearly indicated that J.W. had sustained some degree of impairment of brain functions, it is likely that the residual deviations continue to be a reflection of some mild degree of impairment. The left cerebral indicators previously had included deficits on the right side as compared with left side in finger tapping speed and grip strength and had also been complemented by right-sided impairment in tactile form recognition and verbal difficulties. At present, however, the patient made no mistakes on the Aphasia Screening Test and had shown a definite improvement in tactile form recognition with his right hand. Previously J.W. had shown evidence of imperception of bilateral simultaneous auditory stimulation on the left side and had difficulty achieving symmetry of the lateral extremities in his drawing of the cross. Thus, these findings were available to complement the slightly poor performance with the left hand as compared with the right hand on the Tactual Performance Test. In fact, it would appear that the subject's performances have improved to the extent that residual lateralized indicators are so mild in nature that they can be recognized only by comparison with results of the first examination.

Direct comparison of the results of the two examinations does not indicate any deterioration in performance. Major improvements occurred on the right-left comparisons that reflected lateralized deficits as noted above. J.W.'s IQ values were somewhat better, but this may have been due in large part to positive practice-effect. The greatest change (an increase of four points) occurred on Digit Span, a test which we had originally postulated to be impaired. However, we also had noted the relatively low score on Arithmetic and this test, in fact, was one point lower (9) on the second examination.

A striking improvement occurred on the Category Test (from 47 errors to 8 errors), which goes well beyond expected practice-effect. However, on Part B of the Trail Making Test J.W. now required 112 seconds (as compared with 81 seconds on the initial testing). There was a genuine reduction in errors in tactile finger localization, and as noted, the patient performed much better with his right hand in tactile form recognition and no longer showed evidence of auditory imperception on the left side with bilateral simultaneous stimulation. In total, there can be no doubt that J.W. performed better on the second examination, and the changes document the deficits and their brain-related interpretation shown on the first examination. Comparison of the G-NDS scores (38 and 13) for the initial and 12-month examinations also clearly document the improvement that had occurred.

J.W. was re-examined 18 months after the initial testing. At this time the neurological examination was within normal limits and the subject offered no complaints of any kind on the Cornell Medical Index Health Questionnaire. However, there were still slight abnormalities in the posterior areas of the left temporal and parietal regions on the electroencephalogram, even though the tracings showed continued improvement.

The test findings obtained 18 months after the initial examination were similar in most respects to those previously obtained. However, J.W. appeared to show some genuine improvement on a few tests and to manifest some difficulties which were initially present but not seen on the 12-month examination.

Some positive practice-effect would be expected since the patient was taking the same battery of tests for the third time in an 18-month period. The Verbal IQ increased from 113 to 120 and the Performance IQ increased from 113 to 125; these are somewhat larger increases than would normally be expected on the basis of practice-effect alone. J.W. also performed considerably better on Part B of the Trail Making Test (63 sec), but it is possible that his poor performance on the second examination and the resulting errors that were made were due to carelessness. In most respects

the scores were essentially similar to those previously obtained. It should be noted that on the Tactual Performance Test the patient was somewhat slow with his right hand (4.5 min) as compared with his left hand (2.6 min), whereas the opposite relationship had prevailed on the two previous examinations. However, his finger tapping speed and grip strength continued to be mildly impaired with the right extremity as compared with the left.

In some respects J.W. seemed to perform worse than he had six months earlier (on the second examination). He again had difficulty writing, making mistakes that were similar to those on the first examination and which did not occur at the 12-month examination. The patient persisted in writing a "G" instead of a "Q" when attempting to write the word SQUARE, but was not able to correct his mistake and finally quit in disgust. He also had difficulty writing "SHOUTED." Confusion in formation of letters (dysgraphia), as manifested by this subject, is distinctly unusual in a person with his educational background and general intelligence levels. Almost certainly these difficulties were a manifestation of left cerebral dysfunction.

The patient also showed a slight reduction in grip strength with his right upper extremity, reinstituting a pattern in which his right side (51.5 kg) actually was slightly weaker than his left side (53.5 kg). We also would postulate that J.W. was a little less able in drawing figures than he had been at the time of the second examination. This may be observed by carefully inspecting the handle and teeth of the key. The disparities in the "notches" on the handle and assymmetry of the "teeth" are sufficient to conclude that the performance was abnormal (constructional dyspraxia).

J.W. required more time to identify shapes through touch (Tactile Form Recognition Test) than he had on the second examination, but this may possibly have been due to expenditure of less effort to perform well. However, the writing, the drawing, and grip strength of the right upper extremity seem to represent a recurrence of the types

THE HALSTEAD-REITAN
NEUROPSYCHOLOGICAL TEST BATTERY

Patient __J.W. (III)__ Age __21__ Sex __M__ Education __13__ Handedness __R__

WECHSLER-BELLEVUE SCALE

VIQ	120
PIQ	125
FS IQ	125
Information	14
Comprehension	15
Digit Span	9
Arithmetic	10
Similarities	16
Vocabulary	15
Picture Arrangement	17
Picture Completion	14
Block Design	10
Object Assembly	15
Digit Symbol	13

NEUROPSYCHOLOGICAL DEFICIT SCALE

Level of Performance	6
Pathognomonic Signs	4
Patterns	0
Right-Left Differences	6
Total NDS Score	16

HALSTEAD'S NEUROPSYCHOLOGICAL TEST BATTERY

Category Test — 9

Tactual Performance Test

Dominant hand:	4.5	
Non-dominant hand:	2.6	
Both hands:	1.0	
	Total Time	8.1
	Memory	9
	Localization	8

Seashore Rhythm Test

Number Correct __27__ — 3

Speech-sounds Perception Test

Number of Errors — 4

Finger Oscillation Test

Dominant hand:	53	53
Non-dominant hand:	51	

Impairment Index __0.0__

TRAIL MAKING TEST

Part A: __44__ seconds
Part B: __63__ seconds

STRENGTH OF GRIP

Dominant hand: __51.5__ kilograms
Non-dominant hand: __53.5__ kilograms

REITAN-KLØVE TACTILE FORM RECOGNITION TEST

Dominant hand: __13__ seconds; __0__ errors
Non-dominant hand: __13__ seconds; __0__ errors

MINNESOTA MULTIPHASIC PERSONALITY INVENTORY

		Hs	41
		D	48
?	50	Hy	56
L	43	Pd	53
F	66	Mf	69
K	55	Pa	47
		Pt	52
		Sc	59
		Ma	65

REITAN-KLØVE SENSORY-PERCEPTUAL EXAM — No errors

Error Totals

RH___ LH___	Both H:	RH___ LH___		RH___ LH___	
RH___ LF___	Both H/F:	RH___ LF___		RH___ LF___	
LH___ RF___	Both H/F:	LH___ RF___		RF___ LH___	
RE___ LE___	Both E:	RE___ LE___		RE___ LE___	
RV___ LV___	Both:	RV___ LV___		RV___ LV___	

REITAN-KLØVE LATERAL-DOMINANCE EXAM

Show me how you:

throw a ball	R
hammer a nail	R
cut with a knife	R
turn a door knob	R
use scissors	R
use an eraser	R
write your name	R

Record time used for spontaneous name-writing:

Preferred hand	3	seconds
Non-preferred hand	9	seconds

TACTILE FINGER RECOGNITION

R 1___ 2___ 3___ 4___ 5___ R __0__ / __20__
L 1___ 2___ 3___ 4___ 5___ L __0__ / __20__

FINGER-TIP NUMBER WRITING

R 1___ 2___ 3___ 4___ 5___ R __0__ / __20__
L 1___ 2___ 3___ 4___ 5___ L __0__ / __20__

Show me how you:

kick a football	R
step on a bug	R

REITAN-INDIANA APHASIA SCREENING TEST

Form for Adults and Older Children

Name: _____ J. W. (III) _____ Age: __21__

Copy SQUARE	Repeat TRIANGLE
Name SQUARE	Repeat MASSACHUSETTS
Spell SQUARE	Repeat METHODIST EPISCOPAL
Copy CROSS	Write SQUARE Had difficulty making a "q" on repeated attempts.
Name CROSS	Read SEVEN
Spell CROSS	Repeat SEVEN
Copy TRIANGLE	Repeat/Explain HE SHOUTED THE WARNING.
Name TRIANGLE	Write HE SHOUTED THE WARNING. Had difficulty writing "shouted."
Spell TRIANGLE	Compute 85 – 27 =
Name BABY	Compute 17 X 3 = First wrote "17"; then crossed it out and wrote "51."
Write CLOCK	Name KEY
Name FORK	Demonstrate use of KEY
Read 7 SIX 2	Draw KEY
Read MGW	Read PLACE LEFT HAND TO RIGHT EAR.
Reading I	Place LEFT HAND TO RIGHT EAR
Reading II	Place LEFT HAND TO LEFT ELBOW

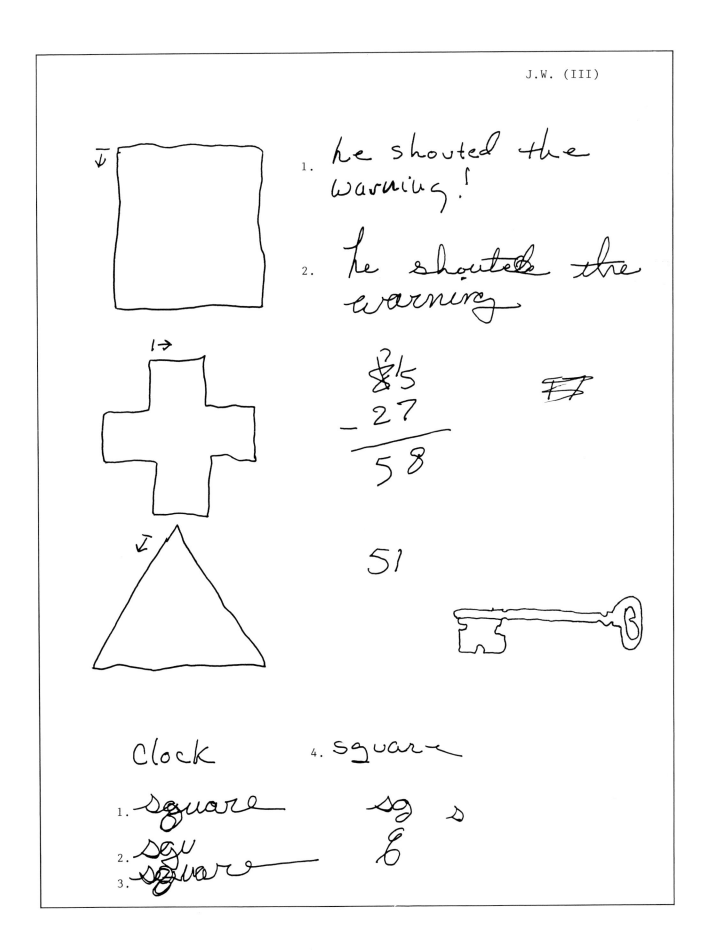

1. he shouted the warning!

2. he shouted the warning

$$\begin{array}{r} 8\!\!\!/5 \\ -\ 27 \\ \hline 58 \end{array}$$

51

Clock

4. square

1. square

2. squ

3. square

of deficits that were present on the first examination and from which the patient apparently had improved on the 12-month examination.

Finally, it should be noted that J.W. also became confused in dealing with numerical relationships. When asked to mentally multiply 17×3 his first response was to write "17." He noticed his error, crossed it out, and then wrote the correct answer. In total it would appear that during the interval between the 12-month and 18-month examinations this man had shown some degree of deterioration of brain functions, probably involving the left hemisphere to a greater extent than the right, even though his IQ values appeared to show some genuine improvement. The G-NDS recapitulates these comparisons showing that the results on the 18-month examination were certainly no better than on the 12-month examination (scores of 16 and 13, respectively), even though they may not have been generally worse.

Case #10

Name: R.P.

Age: 25

Education: 12

Sex: Male

Handedness: Right

Occupation: Student

Background Information

R.P. was a 25-year-old university student who took a severe blow to his head and right shoulder when he fell off his bicycle while performing acrobatics. He was unconscious for one to two minutes and confused and disoriented for about the next hour. He indicated that he had no memory of events up until about five hours before the injury. He was able to remember taking a test in one of his courses at that time, but said that he recalled nothing further until the time of admission to the hospital about one hour after the injury. He complained only of a headache and pain in his right ear and right shoulder.

Neurological Examination

At the time of examination in the emergency room R.P. appeared to be alert and oriented to person, partially oriented to place, and not oriented to time. His behavior and affect seemed appropriate and he recalled remote events quite well and was able to perform arithmetical calculations. He had a minor contusion of the right side of his head, a swollen and very tender right mastoid area, and a laceration of the right ear. The external auditory canal was filled with bright red blood which appeared to be coming from within the canal. The neurological examination was within normal limits except for a bilateral nystagmus on lateral gaze which was greater on the right side than the left. Skull films demonstrated that R.P. had sustained a basilar skull fracture.

R.P.'s hospital course was uneventful. The morning following the injury he seemed more alert than at the time of admission but his retrograde amnesia had not cleared. He could still only vaguely remember the events occurring on the morning before the accident. His bilateral nystagmus resolved and he was discharged from the hospital four days after admission.

Neuropsychological Examination

Neuropsychological examination was performed the day after R.P. was discharged from the hospital (five days after the injury). He offered no complaints during the interview and his responses to the Cornell Medical Index Health Questionnaire revealed no problems. An EEG done the day before R.P. was discharged showed marked disturbances of cerebral functioning, primarily involving the posterior areas of the right hemisphere. The EEG was repeated the day after neuropsychological testing was done and showed no improvement from the original tracing. At that time the EEG abnormalities were most prominent in the right frontal-temporal areas.

It is apparent that R.P.'s general intelligence is well above average. Both his Verbal IQ (127) and Performance IQ (121) values are in the Superior range and yield a Full Scale IQ (126) that exceeds about 96% of his age peers. Nevertheless, the individual subtest scores suggest that R.P. may have experienced some losses from his previous cognitive ability levels. Although his Digit Span score

THE HALSTEAD-REITAN
NEUROPSYCHOLOGICAL TEST BATTERY

Patient __R.P. (I)__ Age __25__ Sex __M__ Education __12__ Handedness __R__

WECHSLER-BELLEVUE SCALE

VIQ	127
PIQ	121
FS IQ	126
Information	14
Comprehension	13
Digit Span	9
Arithmetic	16
Similarities	18
Vocabulary	14
Picture Arrangement	8
Picture Completion	15
Block Design	14
Object Assembly	16
Digit Symbol	11

NEUROPSYCHOLOGICAL DEFICIT SCALE

Level of Performance	9
Pathognomonic Signs	0
Patterns	1
Right-Left Differences	8
Total NDS Score	18

HALSTEAD'S NEUROPSYCHOLOGICAL TEST BATTERY

Category Test — 10

Tactual Performance Test

Dominant hand:	1.8
Non-dominant hand:	2.4
Both hands:	1.7

Total Time	5.9
Memory	8
Localization	4

Seashore Rhythm Test

Number Correct __27__ — 3

Speech-sounds Perception Test

Number of Errors — 2

Finger Oscillation Test

Dominant hand:	53 — 53
Non-dominant hand:	43

Impairment Index __0.1__

MINNESOTA MULTIPHASIC PERSONALITY INVENTORY

		Hs	41
		D	51
?	50	Hy	49
L	40	Pd	57
F	50	Mf	78
K	49	Pa	50
		Pt	56
		Sc	57
		Ma	63

TRAIL MAKING TEST

Part A: __26__ seconds
Part B: __84__ seconds

STRENGTH OF GRIP

Dominant hand: __58.5__ kilograms
Non-dominant hand: __53.0__ kilograms

REITAN-KLØVE TACTILE FORM RECOGNITION TEST

Dominant hand: __10__ seconds; __0__ errors
Non-dominant hand: __12__ seconds; __0__ errors

REITAN-KLØVE SENSORY-PERCEPTUAL EXAM

		Error Totals	
RH___LH___	Both H: RH___LH___	RH___LH___	
RH___LF___	Both H/F: RH___LF___	RH___LF___	
LH___RF___	Both H/F: LH___RF___	RF___LH___	
RE___LE___	Both E: RE_1_LE___	RE_1_LE___	
RV___LV___	Both: RV___LV___	RV___LV___	
___ ___		___ ___	
___ ___		___ ___	

TACTILE FINGER RECOGNITION

R 1___2___3___4___5___ R __0__ / 20
L 1___2___3___4___5___ L __0__ / 20

FINGER-TIP NUMBER WRITING

R 1___2___3___4___5___ R __0__ / 20
L 1___2___3___4___5_1_ L __1__ / 20

REITAN-KLØVE LATERAL-DOMINANCE EXAM

Show me how you:

throw a ball	R
hammer a nail	R
cut with a knife	R
turn a door knob	R
use scissors	R
use an eraser	R
write your name	R

Record time used for spontaneous name-writing:

Preferred hand	5 seconds
Non-preferred hand	13 seconds

Show me how you:

kick a football	R
step on a bug	R

NO APHASIC SYMPTOMS.

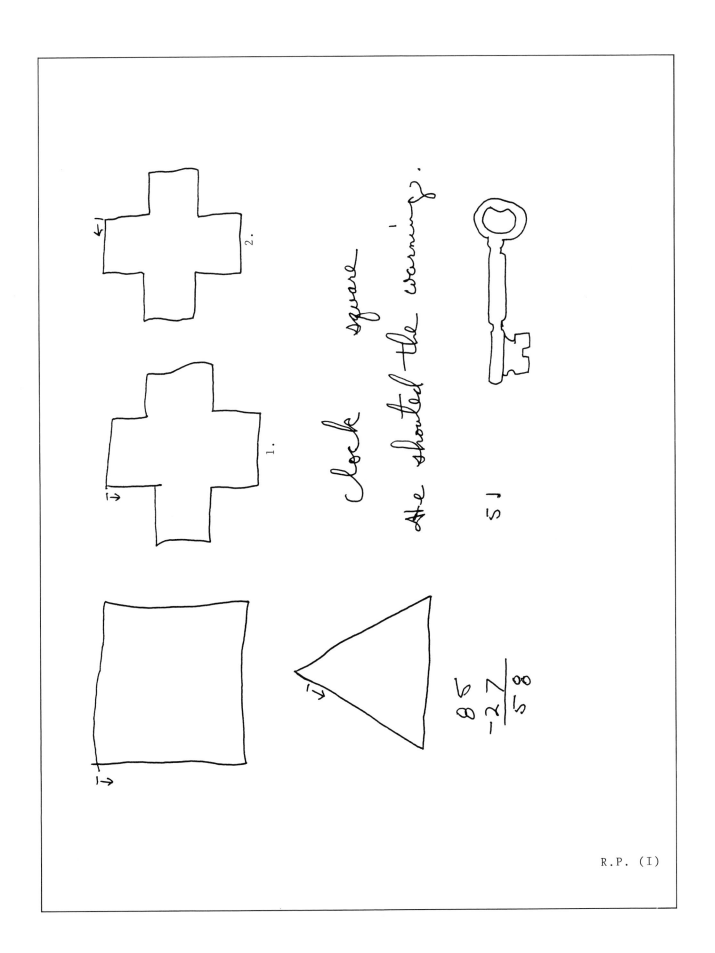

2.

1.

Clock square

Ate shouted the evening.

51

86
−27
58

R.P. (I)

(9) was definitely low, it may or may not have been caused by cerebral damage. His score on Picture Arrangement (8) was distinctly low in relation to the other Performance subtest scores, and it is possible that his score on Digit Symbol (11) may also have been mildly impaired. Thus, while results on the Wechsler Scale were not definitive, they certainly would raise a question of possible cerebral impairment. It should be remembered that a depressed score on Picture Arrangement, occurring in the context of relatively better scores on the other Performance subtests, is sometimes associated with right temporal lobe damage.

R.P. earned adequate scores on the Impairment Index (0.1) and the Category Test (10), but on Part B of the Trail Making Test (84 sec) and the Localization component (4) of the Tactual Performance Test he did not do as well as we would expect from a person with these high general intelligence levels. His G-NDS score was within normal limits, indicating that the overall performance was adequate. He did very well on the Total Time of the Tactual Performance Test (5.9 min), was obviously alert and able to pay close attention to specific stimulus material (as indicated by his scores on the Seashore Rhythm Test [27 correct] and the Speech-sounds Perception Test [2 errors]), and scored within the normal range on other measures. In summary, in terms of level of performance, the test results indicated that R.P.'s basic cognitive skills were excellent and that he had many other abilities that were well above average; however, certain other scores raised a question of impairment of brain functions.

The lateralizing indicators also contributed positive information. Although R.P. made one mistake on the right side in his perception of bilateral simultaneous auditory stimulation, a single error is sometimes related to a peripheral hearing loss rather than to contralateral temporal lobe dysfunction. Since there were no other indicators of left cerebral dysfunction, this error probably does not have any significance.

The indications of right cerebral hemisphere dysfunction were more distinct. For a right-handed person, R.P.'s finger tapping speed was clearly slow with his left hand (43) as compared with his right (53). He also required slightly more time with his left hand (2.4 min) than his right (1.8 min) to complete the Tactual Performance Test. While we must observe that the difference between the two hands amounted to only 0.6 minutes, and that confusion between figures such as the square and the cross could have cost him some time, it still seems that R.P. was less adept when using his left hand. It should also be noted that R.P. did not improve his performance over the first trial when using both hands on the third trial of the TPT, although he possibly would have demonstrated some degree of improvement if he used only his right hand.

R.P.'s first attempt to copy the cross indicated a mild problem in constructing spatial configurations. Even though he performed better on his second attempt, we cannot ignore the definite asymmetry of the lateral extremities in the first drawing. The drawings of other figures, including the key, were within normal limits.

Finally, R.P. required a little more time with his left hand (12 sec) than his right hand (10 sec) to identify shapes on the Tactile Form Recognition Test. However, this indicator was of minimal significance and may not be sufficient to contribute to the rest of the picture.

Results on the Minnesota Multiphasic Personality Inventory (MMPI) distinctly deviated from normality on the Masculine-Feminine scale, but it is highly unlikely that this finding was related to the head injury.

At this point in the interpretation it is necessary to consider the results in somewhat more detail. First, in terms of level of performance, the most significant indicator was probably the score of 84 seconds on Part B of the Trail Making Test (especially considering R.P.'s high IQ levels). The Localization score (4) of the Tactual Performance

Test also seems to be a valid indication of some impairment. On the other hand, whenever an extensive set of tests is administered, obviously the subject will show a range of performances and certain tests will necessarily be lower than others. Thus, at first glance R.P.'s level of performance might be considered to fall within the normal range, but an experienced interpreter would probably raise a question in this regard.

Second, the pattern of lateralizing deficits is quite convincing of impairment of right anterior temporal lobe functions. Over 30 years ago, Reitan (1955c) noted that specific deficits on the Picture Arrangement subtest tended to occur among persons who had chronic, static lesions of the right anterior temporal lobe. We also know that other factors have been associated with this condition: reduced finger tapping speed with the left hand and an impaired performance with the left hand (compared with the right) on the Tactual Performance Test. At least to a degree, R.P.'s scores met all three of these criteria and it would definitely be possible to conclude that he had some right anterior temporal lobe damage in the context of very mild generalized impairment.

Although it is difficult in individual cases to predict recovery potential on the basis of clinical neuropsychological test results, one would postulate that the excellent performances generally shown by this patient and the apparent discreteness of the indications of deficit would permit some spontaneous recovery to occur. In fact, improvement on the tests which originally indicated impairment shortly after the head injury may demonstrate their validity as indicators of cerebral dysfunction and, in addition, substantiate the principal that recovery occurs in the areas of deficit.

A follow-up neurologic examination and electroencephalogram were done three months post-injury. At this time R.P. complained of a constant ringing in his right ear. He stated that he had returned to college and was making normal progress. His retrograde amnesia had improved to the point that he now was able to remember the location of the accident, even though he could not remember the accident itself. The neurologist was able to detect a decreased auditory acuity on the right. The EEG tracings showed marked improvement, although moderate abnormalities were still present over the posterior areas of both cerebral hemispheres and more marked on the right side, particularly in the right temporal region.

The neuropsychological test battery, the neurological examination, and an EEG were repeated 12 months post-injury. The neurological examination was within normal limits, although R.P. still complained of tinnitus and feelings of intermittent pressure in his right ear. However, no hearing loss was discernible. The EEG indicated that more definite abnormalities were present at this time than three months after the injury. The EEG taken at this time showed isolated slow waves over the right temporal area and marked slowing with hyperventilation. However, except for the ringing sensation in his right ear, R.P. had no complaints and continued to make normal academic progress. His responses on the Cornell Medical Health Questionnaire were essentially negative.

The results of the 12-month examination indicated that R.P. was an intelligent man and the findings were essentially within normal limits in terms of their implications regarding brain functions. His IQ values were in the Superior range, none of Halstead's tests contributed to the Impairment Index, the G-NDS score of 3 was well within the normal range, no signs of cerebral damage were present, and comparisons of performances on the two sides of the body were consistently in the normal range (except for mild weakness with the left upper extremity as compared with the right). Considering these test results by themselves, there would be no reason to postulate the presence of cerebral disease or damage. The patient continued to have an elevated score on the Mf scale of the MMPI, but this almost certainly was not related to the head injury.

THE HALSTEAD-REITAN
NEUROPSYCHOLOGICAL TEST BATTERY

Patient ___**R.P. (II)**___ Age __**26**__ Sex __**M**__ Education __**15**__ Handedness __**R**__

WECHSLER-BELLEVUE SCALE

VIQ	138
PIQ	132
FS IQ	138
Information	13
Comprehension	16
Digit Span	17
Arithmetic	16
Similarities	17
Vocabulary	14
Picture Arrangement	13
Picture Completion	14
Block Design	16
Object Assembly	16
Digit Symbol	13

NEUROPSYCHOLOGICAL DEFICIT SCALE

Level of Performance	1
Pathognomonic Signs	0
Patterns	1
Right-Left Differences	1
Total NDS Score	3

TRAIL MAKING TEST

Part A: __19__ seconds
Part B: __40__ seconds

STRENGTH OF GRIP

Dominant hand: __**62.5**__ kilograms
Non-dominant hand: __**53.0**__ kilograms

REITAN-KLØVE TACTILE FORM RECOGNITION TEST

Dominant hand: __**6**__ seconds; __**0**__ errors
Non-dominant hand: __**5**__ seconds; __**0**__ errors

REITAN-KLØVE SENSORY-PERCEPTUAL EXAM — No errors

Error Totals

RH ___ LH ___	Both H: RH ___ LH ___	RH ___ LH ___
RH ___ LF ___	Both H/F: RH ___ LF ___	RH ___ LF ___
LH ___ RF ___	Both H/F: LH ___ RF ___	RF ___ LH ___
RE ___ LE ___	Both E: RE ___ LE ___	RE ___ LE ___
RV ___ LV ___	Both: RV ___ LV ___	RV ___ LV ___
___ ___		___ ___
___ ___		___ ___

TACTILE FINGER RECOGNITION

R 1___ 2___ 3___ 4___ 5___ R **0** / **20**
L 1___ 2___ 3___ 4___ 5___ L **0** / **20**

FINGER-TIP NUMBER WRITING

R 1___ 2___ 3___ 4___ 5___ R **0** / **20**
L 1___ 2___ 3___ 4___ 5___ L **0** / **20**

NO APHASIC SYMPTOMS.

HALSTEAD'S NEUROPSYCHOLOGICAL TEST BATTERY

Category Test	13

Tactual Performance Test

Dominant hand:	**2.7**
Non-dominant hand:	**1.9**
Both hands:	**0.8**

Total Time	**5.4**
Memory	**9**
Localization	**6**

Seashore Rhythm Test

Number Correct __**29**__ ___1___

Speech-sounds Perception Test

Number of Errors ___3___

Finger Oscillation Test

Dominant hand:	**55**	55
Non-dominant hand:	**49**	

Impairment Index __**0.0**__

MINNESOTA MULTIPHASIC PERSONALITY INVENTORY

		Hs	48
		D	47
?	50	Hy	51
L	40	Pd	60
F	53	Mf	73
K	59	Pa	56
		Pt	54
		Sc	59
		Ma	53

REITAN-KLØVE LATERAL-DOMINANCE EXAM

Show me how you:
throw a ball	**R**
hammer a nail	**R**
cut with a knife	**R**
turn a door knob	**R**
use scissors	**R**
use an eraser	**R**
write your name	**R**

Record time used for spontaneous name-writing:
Preferred hand	__**6**__ seconds
Non-preferred hand	__**18**__ seconds

Show me how you:
kick a football	**R**
step on a bug	**R**

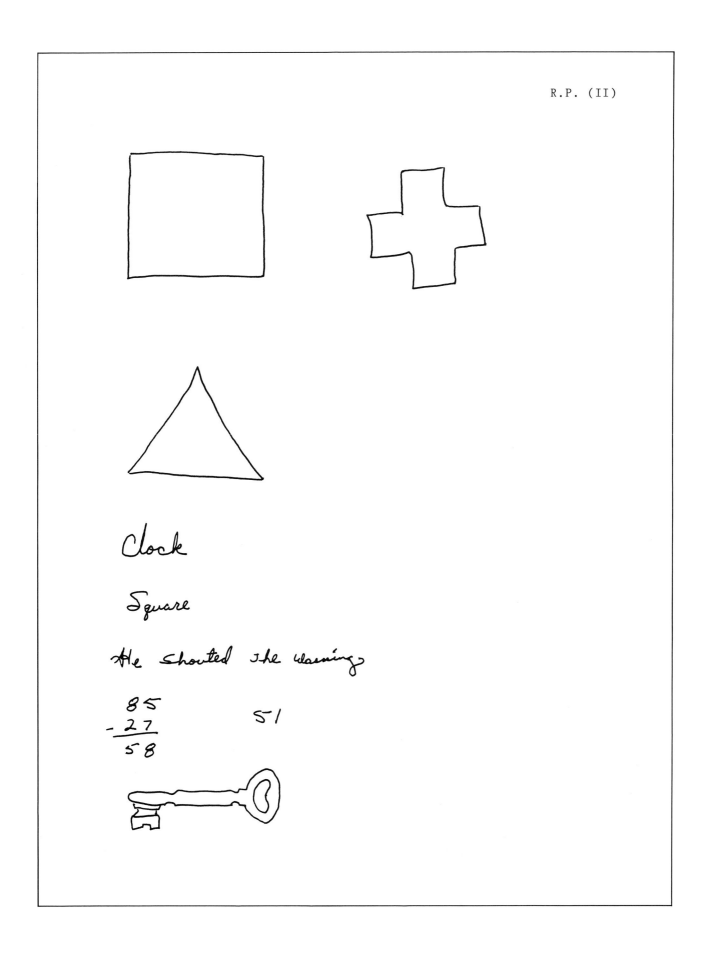

Clock

Square

He shouted the warning

85
- 27
58

51

Attempting to take into account both positive practice-effect and spontaneous improvement following the injury, direct comparison of the scores of the first and second examinations showed evidence of better scores on a number of measures and scarcely any instances of worse performances. Of course, a number of the tests were at essentially the same level on both examinations. R.P. showed an increment of 11 points on both Verbal and Performance IQ values and a 12-point increment on Full Scale IQ. These changes are greater than would normally be expected on the basis of practice-effect. In addition, it is worth noting that substantial gains occurred on Digit Span (from 9 to 17) and Picture Arrangement (from 8 to 13). These were the subtests that had initially been identified as possibly having some implication for brain damage. Although the G-NDS was within the normal range initially, the improvement from 18 to 3 suggests that overall performances were better.

Probably the most striking improvement occurred on Part B of Trail Making Test (from 84 sec to 40 sec). We had initially noted that it was particularly surprising that this man performed as poorly as he did on this test, even though his score was not quite in the "brain-damaged" range. The improved performance almost certainly represented spontaneous recovery.

R.P. was also considerably quicker in his responses in tactile form recognition (from 10 sec to 6 sec with the right hand and from 12 sec to 5 sec with the left hand). His ability to draw the cross had improved, and he probably showed some degree of genuine improvement on the Localization component of the Tactual Performance Test.

R.P.'s finger tapping speed was improved, especially with the left hand (which initially had been considered to be somewhat impaired with relation to the right hand). However, we should note that grip strength was in the normal relationship between the two hands on the first examination and improvement with the right hand established a relationship with the left hand that was the only deviant score in terms of right-left comparisons. While we would be tempted to view the improvement in finger tapping speed with the left hand as spontaneous recovery, such an interpretation would be more difficult to apply to improvement of grip strength with the right upper extremity, and a question could be raised about whether any consistent change in motor functions had actually occurred. In general, however, there can be no doubt that the level of performance shown by this man was better 12 months after the injury than at the time of the initial examination.

The initial neuropsychological test results had been interpreted as showing only selective deficits in terms of level of performance and the major basis for concluding that brain damage was present was derived from the configuration of results pointing toward right cerebral damage. The examination done 12 months after the injury confirms the hypothesis that R.P. had some more impairment in terms of level of performance than had initially been apparent. However, in interpretation of brain-behavior relationships, the more striking finding was the disappearance of the configuration of test results that implicated the right anterior temporal area (a selectively low score on Picture Arrangement with relation to other Performance subtests, a poor performance with the left hand as compared with the right hand on the Tactual Performance Test, and slow finger tapping speed with the left hand as compared with the right hand). Thus, R.P. showed a considerable degree of improvement in neuropsychological findings, even though the EEG done at the same time showed a definite increase in abnormal results.

Eighteen months post-injury R.P. was again seen for a neurological examination, electroencephalogram, and neuropsychological testing. He was making normal progress in college, and except for continued ringing in his right ear, had no complaints either during the clinical interview or in his answers on the Cornell Medical Index Health

THE HALSTEAD-REITAN
NEUROPSYCHOLOGICAL TEST BATTERY

Patient **R.P. (III)** Age **26** Sex **M** Education **15** Handedness **R**

WECHSLER-BELLEVUE SCALE

VIQ	138
PIQ	136
FS IQ	140

Information	15
Comprehension	14
Digit Span	16
Arithmetic	17
Similarities	17
Vocabulary	14

Picture Arrangement	18
Picture Completion	15
Block Design	14
Object Assembly	15
Digit Symbol	13

NEUROPSYCHOLOGICAL DEFICIT SCALE

Level of Performance	2
Pathognomonic Signs	0
Patterns	0
Right-Left Differences	4
Total NDS Score	6

TRAIL MAKING TEST

Part A: **20** seconds
Part B: **39** seconds

STRENGTH OF GRIP

Dominant hand: **59.5** kilograms
Non-dominant hand: **55.0** kilograms

REITAN-KLØVE TACTILE FORM RECOGNITION TEST

Dominant hand: **9** seconds; **0** errors
Non-dominant hand: **8** seconds; **0** errors

REITAN-KLØVE SENSORY-PERCEPTUAL EXAM — No errors

Error Totals

RH ___ LH ___	Both H: RH ___ LH ___	RH ___ LH ___	
RH ___ LF ___	Both H/F: RH ___ LF ___	RH ___ LF ___	
LH ___ RF ___	Both H/F: LH ___ RF ___	RF ___ LH ___	
RE ___ LE ___	Both E: RE ___ LE ___	RE ___ LE ___	
RV ___ LV ___	Both: RV ___ LV ___	RV ___ LV ___	

TACTILE FINGER RECOGNITION

R 1 ___ 2 ___ 3 ___ 4 ___ 5 ___ R **0** / 20
L 1 ___ 2 ___ 3 ___ 4 **1** 5 ___ L **1** / 20

FINGER-TIP NUMBER WRITING

R 1 **1** 2 ___ 3 ___ 4 ___ 5 ___ R **1** / 20
L 1 ___ 2 ___ 3 ___ 4 ___ 5 ___ L **0** / 20

HALSTEAD'S NEUROPSYCHOLOGICAL TEST BATTERY

Category Test **13**

Tactual Performance Test

Dominant hand:	3.1		
Non-dominant hand:	2.2		
Both hands:	1.5		
		Total Time	6.8
		Memory	9
		Localization	7

Seashore Rhythm Test

Number Correct **29** **1**

Speech-sounds Perception Test

Number of Errors **4**

Finger Oscillation Test

Dominant hand: **51** **51**
Non-dominant hand: **49**

Impairment Index **0.0**

MINNESOTA MULTIPHASIC PERSONALITY INVENTORY

		Hs	47
		D	48
?	50	Hy	53
L	36	Pd	55
F	55	Mf	74
K	64	Pa	47
		Pt	52
		Sc	57
		Ma	55

REITAN-KLØVE LATERAL-DOMINANCE EXAM

Show me how you:
throw a ball	R
hammer a nail	R
cut with a knife	R
turn a door knob	R
use scissors	R
use an eraser	R
write your name	R

Record time used for spontaneous name-writing:
Preferred hand	**6** seconds
Non-preferred hand	**11** seconds

Show me how you:
kick a football	R
step on a bug	R

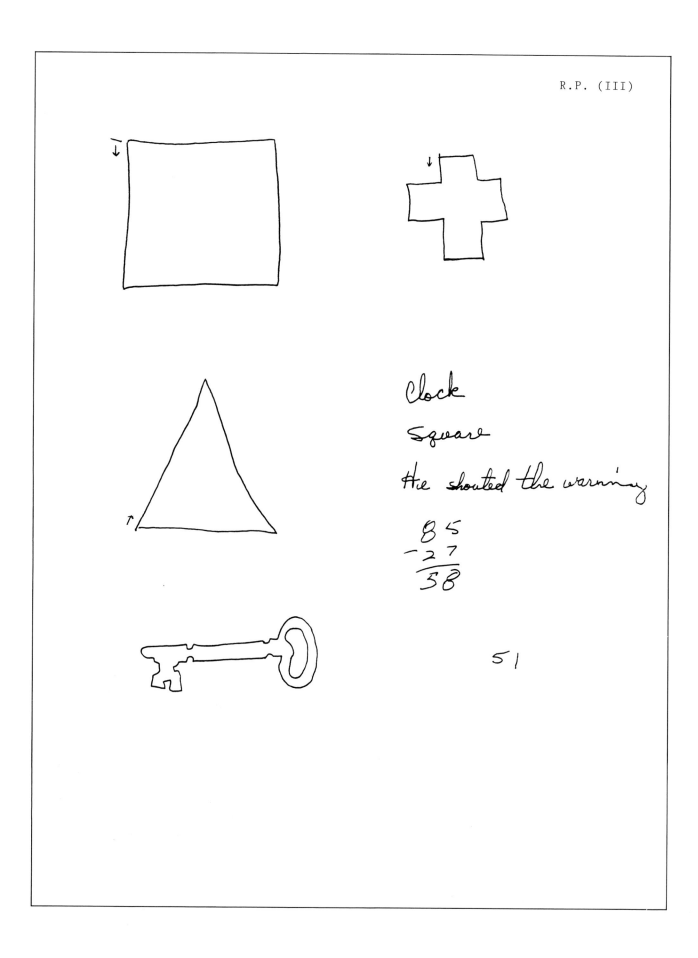

Clock

Square

He shouted the warning

$$\begin{array}{r} 8\,5 \\ -\,2\,7 \\ \hline 3\,8 \end{array}$$

51

Questionnaire. Results of the neurological examination were within normal limits except for decreased auditory acuity of the right ear in comparison with the findings obtained 12 months earlier.

The neurologist indicated that the patient continued to complain of a high-pitch tinnitus and intermittent pressure sensations of the right ear. The EEG continued to show abnormalities which principally involved the right cerebral hemisphere (although some abnormal findings were also demonstrated in the posterior areas of the left cerebral hemisphere). The indications of posterior abnormalities were somewhat less than at the time of the previous examination 12 months earlier but abnormal tracings were slightly more prominent in the temporal and inferior frontal areas, especially of the right hemisphere. Thus, the patient continued to show electroencephalographic findings that were viewed as moderately abnormal. Clinical observations over the years have often identified instances of disparity between EEG results and neuropsychological findings, raising a question about the relationship between the electrical activity of the brain and neuropsychological functioning.

The third set of neuropsychological test results were well within normal limits, yielding a G-NDS score of 6. R.P. continued to demonstrate high IQ values that fell well into the Superior range. Except for the score on Picture Arrangement, the subtest scores on the 12-month examination and 18-month examination were generally similar. None of the tests changed direction by more than two points, except for the five-point increment in Picture Arrangement. Although we cannot be sure that this increase represented continued improvement from the initial deficit, the excellent score on this test 18 months following the initial examination almost certainly documents the validity of the first score (8) as an indicator of impairment.

R.P. continued to perform very well on the four most sensitive indicators in the Halstead-Reitan Battery and also did well on nearly all of the other tests. He showed no patterns or relationships among the test results that were significant as indicators of impaired cerebral functioning. The patient was just a little slow in finger tapping speed with his right hand (51) compared with his left hand (49) and there was a mild degree of imbalance of the extremities in his drawing of the cross. However, considering the excellent scores on most measures, these findings would be considered to be only very mild deviations within the context of an overall normal set of performances.

Direct comparison of the results from the 12-month and the 18-month examinations showed no particular changes in the direction of better performances, except for the Picture Arrangement subtest (from 13 to 18). R.P. was slightly weaker with his right hand in grip strength (from 62.5 kg to 59.5 kg) and slower in finger tapping speed (from 55 to 51). The Total Time score on the Tactual Performance Test increased from 5.4 minutes to 6.8 minutes. Although one might possibly conclude that the patient had shown a mild decrement of ability on tasks that required primary motor skill, it is also possible to postulate that these are essentially chance variations or minor effects of the amount of motivation or effort the patient expended. The increased time required on the Tactile Form Recognition Test (a total of 11 sec compared to 17 sec with both hands) was a function of the testing procedure; on the third examination the examiner did not try to fractionate seconds, using a minimal response-time in scoring of one second.

Finally, a question could be raised regarding R.P.'s drawing of the cross. His first attempt on the initial examination definitely deviated from normal. The second attempt, at the 12-month examination, was a little less adequate than might be expected from such an able person, but was essentially within normal limits. On the third drawing (18-month examination), a slightly more pronounced asymmetry of the lateral extremities was present than on the second testing. In addition, his drawing of the key seemed to lack certain elements of symmetry that might normally have been expected from this man. Although it is difficult to be certain, it seems possible that R.P. may have sustained a very mild degree of further impairment in ability to draw simple spatial configurations, an impairment from which he had not fully recovered 18 months after the injury.

There is no doubt, however, that at 18 months post-injury the overall ability structure of this man was well within the normal range and the results demonstrated 12 months and 18 months after the injury documented the significance of certain deficits that were initially present. Thus, despite the fact that the initial deficits were relatively mild in nature, the patient eventually manifested a degree of spontaneous recovery.

Case #11

Name: W.B.

Age: 19

Education: 12

Sex: Male

Handedness: Right

Occupation: Military Serviceman

Background Information

W.B. had been in the United States Coast Guard for one year when he became involved in a barroom brawl. He was struck on the left side of his head with a bottle and sustained a significant head injury. His medical history included no other illnesses or injuries that would have been likely to cause brain damage.

Neurological Examination

After the incident W.B. was taken to a community hospital in a comatose condition. A significant left hemiparesis was apparent. Plain skull films showed fractures in the left temporal area and base of the skull. The exact duration of unconsciousness was not recorded, but hospital records indicated that W.B. was alert, responsive, and beginning to regain function of his left extremities three days post-injury. A neurological examination performed at this time showed decreased strength, slightly decreased deep tendon reflexes, and a Babinski response on the left side. The patient complained of intermittent dizziness, diplopia, and severe headaches which gradually improved during the next two weeks.

The neurological examination was repeated one week later and indicated that W.B. had no memory for the events immediately preceding the head injury. The examination also documented a slight weakness on the left side of the face, diminished strength of the left arm and leg, slight hyporeflexia and a Babinski sign on the left side, and a fracture involving the left side of the head and the posterior wall of the left orbit. The sensory examination was entirely within normal limits. A radioisotopic brain scan showed increased uptake in the left frontal-parietal area and suggested a cerebral contusion. An electroencephalogram showed moderate abnormalities but had no localizing significance or evidence of epileptiform discharges. W.B. was discharged from the hospital 30 days after the injury with neurological findings essentially the same as those noted above; however, he did seem to be showing definite improvement.

Neuropsychological Examination

The first neuropsychological examination was done 27 days after the injury. Since the neurological evaluation had indicated a cerebral contusion involving the left frontal-parietal area, we would expect W.B. to show neuropsychological deficits consistent with brain damage. It is not uncommon, though, for patients with closed head injuries (even with lateralizing neurological findings) to fail to demonstrate a neuropsychological profile completely consistent with lateralized damage. In fact, we would expect W.B. to show signs of generalized impairment, some indications of left cerebral hemisphere dysfunction, and possibly some manifestations of right cerebral involvement.

To summarize the findings of the first neuropsychological evaluation, W.B. had IQ values in the lower part of the average range, deficits on the

THE HALSTEAD-REITAN
NEUROPSYCHOLOGICAL TEST BATTERY

Patient __W.B. (I)__ Age __19__ Sex __M__ Education __12__ Handedness __R__

WECHSLER-BELLEVUE SCALE

VIQ	95
PIQ	91
FS IQ	93
Information	6
Comprehension	8
Digit Span	9
Arithmetic	9
Similarities	11
Vocabulary	10
Picture Arrangement	7
Picture Completion	7
Block Design	9
Object Assembly	12
Digit Symbol	10

NEUROPSYCHOLOGICAL DEFICIT SCALE

Level of Performance	18
Pathognomonic Signs	6
Patterns	1
Right-Left Differences	7
Total NDS Score	32

TRAIL MAKING TEST

Part A: __42__ seconds
Part B: __77__ seconds

STRENGTH OF GRIP

Dominant hand: __66__ kilograms
Non-dominant hand: __49__ kilograms

REITAN-KLØVE TACTILE FORM RECOGNITION TEST

Dominant hand: __8.5__ seconds; __0__ errors
Non-dominant hand: __8.0__ seconds; __0__ errors

REITAN-KLØVE SENSORY-PERCEPTUAL EXAM — No errors

			Error Totals		
RH___ LH___	Both H:	RH___ LH___	RH___ LH___		
RH___ LF___	Both H/F:	RH___ LF___	RH___ LF___		
LH___ RF___	Both H/F:	LH___ RF___	RF___ LH___		
RE___ LE___	Both E:	RE___ LE___	RE___ LE___		
RV___ LV___	Both:	RV___ LV___	RV___ LV___		
___ ___		___ ___			
___ ___		___ ___			

TACTILE FINGER RECOGNITION

R 1___ 2___ 3 _1_ 4 _5___ R _1_ / 20
L 1___ 2___ 3___ 4___ 5 _1_ L _1_ / 20

FINGER-TIP NUMBER WRITING

R 1___ 2___ 3___ 4___ 5___ R _0_ / 20
L 1___ 2___ 3___ 4 _1_ 5___ L _1_ / 20

HALSTEAD'S NEUROPSYCHOLOGICAL TEST BATTERY

Category Test	52

Tactual Performance Test

Dominant hand:	9.2
Non-dominant hand:	8.6
Both hands:	3.7

Total Time	21.5
Memory	7
Localization	2

Seashore Rhythm Test

Number Correct __27__ | 3

Speech-sounds Perception Test

Number of Errors | 5

Finger Oscillation Test

Dominant hand:	43
Non-dominant hand:	40

43

Impairment Index __0.6__

MINNESOTA MULTIPHASIC PERSONALITY INVENTORY

		Hs	57
		D	56
?	50	Hy	55
L	56	Pd	60
F	62	Mf	45
K	53	Pa	50
		Pt	54
		Sc	63
		Ma	65

REITAN-KLØVE LATERAL-DOMINANCE EXAM

Show me how you:
throw a ball	R
hammer a nail	R
cut with a knife	R
turn a door knob	R
use scissors	R
use an eraser	R
write your name	R

Record time used for spontaneous name-writing:
Preferred hand	__8__ seconds
Non-preferred hand	__17__ seconds

Show me how you:
kick a football	R
step on a bug	R

REITAN-INDIANA APHASIA SCREENING TEST

Form for Adults and Older Children

Name: _____ W. B. (I) _____ Age: __19__

Copy SQUARE	Repeat TRIANGLE
Name SQUARE	Repeat MASSACHUSETTS
Spell SQUARE "S-Q-W-A-R-E"	Repeat METHODIST EPISCOPAL "Methodixt Epixtocal" Tried again, OK.
Copy CROSS	Write SQUARE
Name CROSS " I really don't know. That medical thing or an X. What is it, anyway?"	Read SEVEN
Spell CROSS	Repeat SEVEN
Copy TRIANGLE	Repeat/Explain HE SHOUTED THE WARNING.
Name TRIANGLE	Write HE SHOUTED THE WARNING.
Spell TRIANGLE	Compute 85 – 27 =
Name BABY	Compute 17 X 3 =
Write CLOCK	Name KEY
Name FORK	Demonstrate use of KEY
Read 7 SIX 2	Draw KEY
Read MGW	Read PLACE LEFT HAND TO RIGHT EAR.
Reading I	Place LEFT HAND TO RIGHT EAR Patient started to place right hand to right ear, caught himself, read the card again and performed OK.
Reading II	Place LEFT HAND TO LEFT ELBOW Tried. Then said, "Well, however you do it." Tried again. Said, "I can't do it."

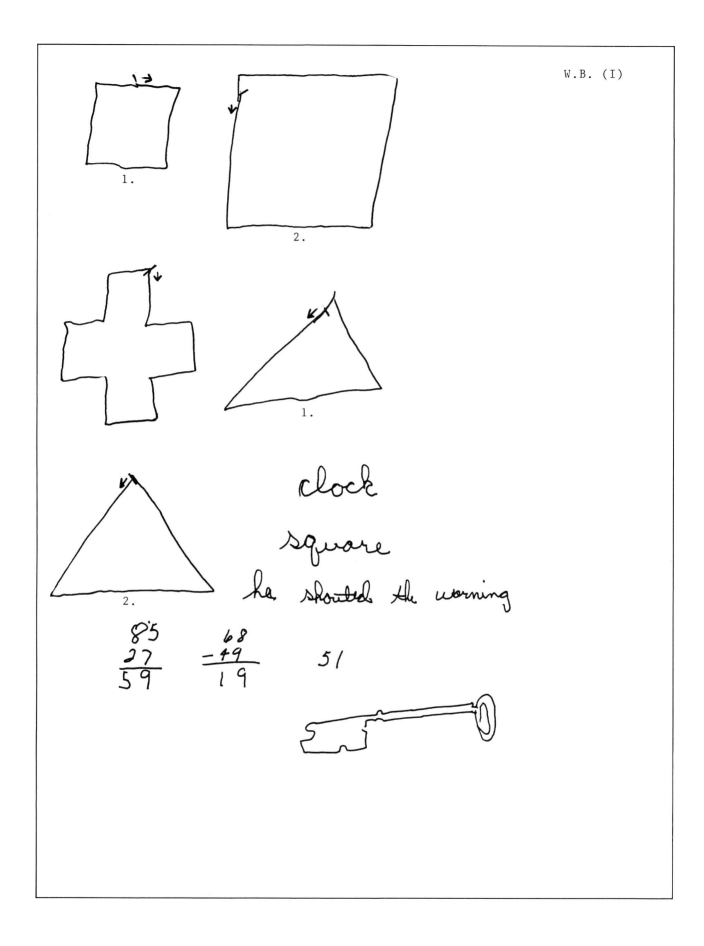

1.

2.

1.

2.

clock

square

he shouted the warning

$$\begin{array}{r} 85 \\ 27 \\ \hline 59 \end{array}$$

$$\begin{array}{r} 68 \\ -49 \\ \hline 19 \end{array}$$

51

more sensitive measures in the Halstead-Reitan Battery, findings suggesting damage of the left cerebral hemisphere, and results indicating that the right cerebral hemisphere was also involved (to a lesser extent).

W.B. earned a Verbal IQ (95) that exceeded about 37% of his age peers, a Performance IQ (91) that exceeded 27%, and a Full Scale IQ (93) that exceeded 32%. Even though W.B. performed rather poorly on the Information subtest (6), it is not possible to infer cerebral impairment from the distribution of Verbal subtest scores. These kinds of results are sometimes seen in persons who are relatively inactive intellectually and do not read very much. The Performance subtests did not provide any definite information regarding cerebral damage.

In contrast, the four most sensitive indicators in the Halstead-Reitan Battery strongly suggested at least mild generalized impairment of neuropsychological functions. The patient earned an Impairment Index of 0.6, indicating that approximately 60% of the scores obtained on Halstead's tests were in the brain-damaged range. The Category Test score (52) indicated mild impairment. W.B. performed even worse on the Localization component (2) of the Tactual Performance Test but his score on Part B of the Trail Making Test (77 sec) was within the normal range. Compared with his average IQ values, these results suggest at least mild generalized impairment of adaptive abilities.

The relatively good scores on the Seashore Rhythm Test (27 correct) and the Speech-sounds Perception Test (5 errors) indicate that W.B. was functioning adequately in terms of general alertness and ability to focus his attention to specific tasks; in other words, according to our model of neuropsychological abilities these scores demonstrate that the first level of central processing was relatively intact. Actually, the good scores on these measures might suggest that in the past W.B. had been more able than most of the scores (including the IQ measures) had implied.

Although the lateralizing findings were not particularly pronounced, W.B. made certain errors on the Aphasia Screening Test that are quite typical of persons with left cerebral damage. For example, his misspelling of SQUARE (S-Q-W-A-R-E) was quite unusual. The neurologist had noticed that W.B. had some difficulty with enunciation and had attributed the problems to IXth cranial nerve dysfunction; however, the patient's enunciation of METHODIST EPISCOPAL (Methodixt Epixtocal) is more characteristic of persons with left cerebral damage than peripheral nerve dysfunction.

W.B. also had some difficulty in calculating $85 - 27 =$. Since he was able to multiply 17×3 correctly, this error suggests another deficit (dyscalculia) more commonly associated with left cerebral damage than right hemisphere dysfunction.

Finally, W.B. showed a mild tendency to become confused when asked to place his left hand to his right ear. He started to place his right hand to his right ear, realized his error, and corrected himself immediately. Although this response occasionally occurs among normal individuals, it is much more commonly seen in persons with left cerebral damage.

Considering the fact that measures of lateral dominance indicated that he was strongly right-handed, W.B. may have been slightly slow in finger tapping speed with his right hand (43) compared with his left (40). However, this finding was minor and could not be considered a significant indicator of left cerebral dysfunction.

The above-mentioned results, particularly in the context of an excellent score on the Speech-sounds Perception Test, practically rule out the presence of a progressive or expanding lesion of the left cerebral hemisphere. Conversely, they are consistent with a type of damage that is not extensive and relatively static.

Findings implicating the right cerebral hemisphere were quite definite. Neurological examination had revealed a left hemiparesis, despite the fact that the cerebral contusion apparently involved the left cerebral hemisphere. Measurement of grip strength indicated that the left upper extremity (49 kg) was deficient compared with the right (66 kg), a finding consistent with residual hemiparesis. W.B. also showed relatively little improvement when using his left hand on the second trial of the Tactual Performance Test. Finally, his drawings of simple figures and a key consistently indicated a mild degree of difficulty dealing with simple spatial configurations. The lateral extremities of the cross were somewhat out of balance and the distortion of the left side of the key was quite apparent. The first attempt to copy an equilateral triangle also demonstrated difficulties dealing with spatial relationships.

The test results are concisely recapitulated by the G-NDS scores. W.B.'s scores on Level of Performance totalled 18 (normal control subjects average 11.95) with the poorest scores on the Impairment Index, the Localization and Total Time components of the Tactual Performance Test, and the Category Test. He was also deficient in finger tapping speed with both hands. W.B. was given six points for the Pathognomonic Signs section (control subjects average 0.54 points), with evidence of dysnomia and right-left confusion strongly suggesting left-cerebral dysfunction and constructional dyspraxia implicating the right cerebral hemisphere. W.B.'s score of seven on the section concerned with left-right differences also contributed to the impression of brain damage (control subjects average 3.37 points), with deficient performances with the left upper extremity occurring on the Tactual Performance Test and grip strength.

Thus, as predicted, W.B. showed generalized impairment, certain findings implicating the left cerebral hemisphere, and other results pointing toward right cerebral damage. Findings of this kind are perfectly compatible with a head injury and it is likely that such a conclusion would have been reached if we had considered the neuropsychological test results independently of the neurological findings.

W.B. was re-examined on two other occasions, 12 months and 18 months after the first examination. Since definite evidence of impairment was present initially, we would expect W.B. to show a considerable degree of improvement on the 12-month examination (more than we would anticipate with practice-effect). However, as you review the test results, recall that a substantial proportion of patients fail to show consistent improvement 18 months after sustaining a contusion and may actually demonstrate deterioration of certain functions that previously had been improving.

The second set of test results, obtained 12 months after the initial examination, showed improvement on nearly every measure. First, we will briefly review the overall configuration of these test scores and then compare them with the initial findings, recognizing that some positive practice-effect may have occurred.

W.B. earned Verbal (99) and Performance (103) IQ values that were both near the 50th percentile, yielding a Full Scale IQ scale of 101. The Verbal subtest scores followed the same general pattern shown previously, with a slightly worse performance on the Arithmetic subtest (6). It is worth noting that the Arithmetic subtest is probably the most sensitive of the Verbal subtests to brain damage, and the pattern of subtest scores on the second examination might be sufficient to raise a question of brain impairment (even though many other factors can cause a poor Arithmetic subtest score).

The Performance subtest scores were near the average level or above. Digit Symbol is generally the most sensitive of Wechsler's subtests to brain damage and it is unusual to see such a good score (15) from a person with cerebral damage.

W.B. did fairly well on the four most sensitive indicators in the Halstead-Reitan Battery and earned an Impairment Index of 0.3 (only 30% of Halstead's tests had scores in the brain-damaged range). In fact, the only tests contributing to the Impairment Index were finger tapping speed (39) and TPT-Localization (3).

THE HALSTEAD-REITAN
NEUROPSYCHOLOGICAL TEST BATTERY

Patient **W.B. (II)** Age **20** Sex **M** Education **12** Handedness **R**

WECHSLER-BELLEVUE SCALE

VIQ	99
PIQ	103
FS IQ	101
Information	8
Comprehension	11
Digit Span	11
Arithmetic	6
Similarities	10
Vocabulary	11
Picture Arrangement	8
Picture Completion	9
Block Design	9
Object Assembly	12
Digit Symbol	15

NEUROPSYCHOLOGICAL DEFICIT SCALE

Level of Performance	11
Pathognomonic Signs	2
Patterns	0
Right-Left Differences	5
Total NDS Score	18

HALSTEAD'S NEUROPSYCHOLOGICAL TEST BATTERY

Category Test 35

Tactual Performance Test

Dominant hand:	8.2	
Non-dominant hand:	3.6	
Both hands:	1.9	

Total Time	13.7
Memory	8
Localization	3

Seashore Rhythm Test

Number Correct **28** 2

Speech-sounds Perception Test

Number of Errors 4

Finger Oscillation Test

Dominant hand:	39	39
Non-dominant hand:	34	

Impairment Index 0.3

TRAIL MAKING TEST

Part A: **23** seconds
Part B: **58** seconds

STRENGTH OF GRIP

Dominant hand: **66.0** kilograms
Non-dominant hand: **58.0** kilograms

REITAN-KLØVE TACTILE FORM RECOGNITION TEST

Dominant hand: **6.5** seconds; **0** errors
Non-dominant hand: **6.5** seconds; **0** errors

REITAN-KLØVE SENSORY-PERCEPTUAL EXAM — No errors

Error Totals

RH ___ LH ___	Both H:	RH ___ LH ___	RH ___ LH ___		
RH ___ LF ___	Both H/F:	RH ___ LF ___	RH ___ LF ___		
LH ___ RF ___	Both H/F:	LH ___ RF ___	RF ___ LH ___		
RE ___ LE ___	Both E:	RE ___ LE ___	RE ___ LE ___		
RV ___ LV ___	Both:	RV ___ LV ___	RV ___ LV ___		

TACTILE FINGER RECOGNITION

R 1__ 2__ 3__ 4__ 5__ R **0** / 20
L 1__ 2__ 3__ 4 **1** 5__ L **1** / 20

FINGER-TIP NUMBER WRITING

R 1__ 2__ 3__ 4__ 5__ R **0** / 20
L 1__ 2__ 3__ 4__ 5__ L **0** / 20

MINNESOTA MULTIPHASIC PERSONALITY INVENTORY

		Hs	49
		D	60
?	50	Hy	45
L	46	Pd	55
F	44	Mf	43
K	51	Pa	59
		Pt	52
		Sc	57
		Ma	55

REITAN-KLØVE LATERAL-DOMINANCE EXAM

Show me how you:
throw a ball	R
hammer a nail	R
cut with a knife	R
turn a door knob	R
use scissors	R
use an eraser	R
write your name	R

Record time used for spontaneous name-writing:
Preferred hand	**4.5** seconds
Non-preferred hand	**11** seconds

Show me how you:
kick a football	R
step on a bug	R

REITAN-INDIANA APHASIA SCREENING TEST

Form for Adults and Older Children

Name: _____ W. B. (II) _____ Age: __20__

Copy SQUARE	Repeat TRIANGLE
Name SQUARE	Repeat MASSACHUSETTS
Spell SQUARE	Repeat METHODIST EPISCOPAL "Methodist Epistipul"
Copy CROSS	Write SQUARE
Name CROSS	Read SEVEN
Spell CROSS	Repeat SEVEN
Copy TRIANGLE	Repeat/Explain HE SHOUTED THE WARNING.
Name TRIANGLE	Write HE SHOUTED THE WARNING.
Spell TRIANGLE	Compute 85 – 27 =
Name BABY	Compute 17 X 3 = Patient wrote 20. Examiner repeated problem. Patient said,"Oh, times." Wrote 210. "No, that's not right. Wrote "51."
Write CLOCK	Name KEY
Name FORK	Demonstrate use of KEY
Read 7 SIX 2	Draw KEY
Read MGW	Read PLACE LEFT HAND TO RIGHT EAR.
Reading I	Place LEFT HAND TO RIGHT EAR
Reading II	Place LEFT HAND TO LEFT ELBOW

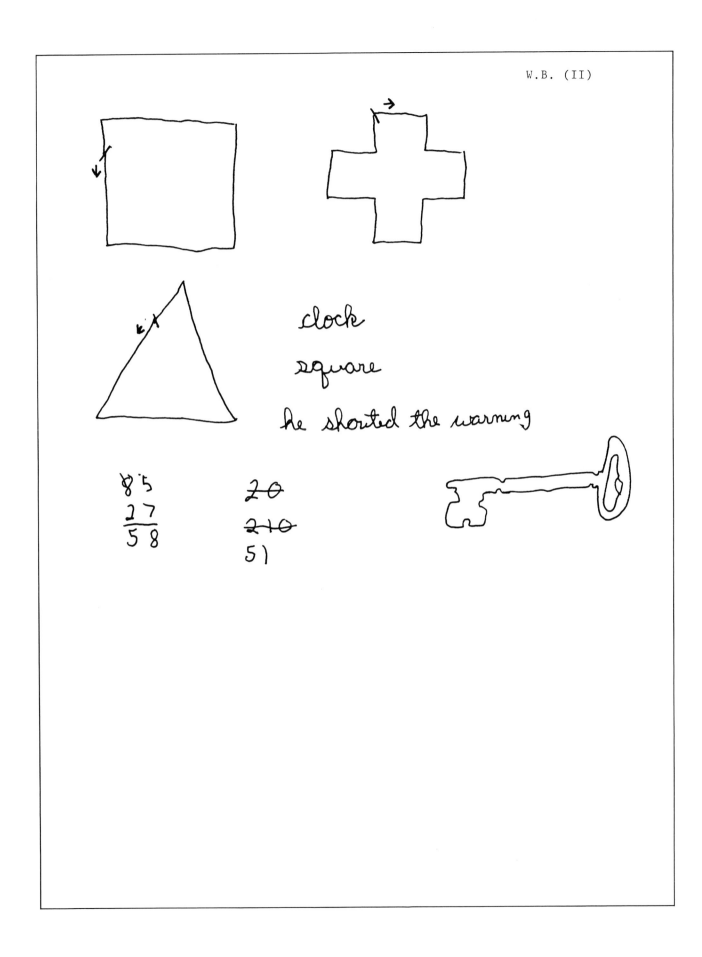

clock

square

he shouted the warning

$$\frac{\begin{array}{r}8\cdot 5\\ 2\,7\end{array}}{5\;8}$$

2 0

2 1 0

5)

W.B. performed fairly well on more complex tests involving abstraction and reasoning and immediate problem-solving abilities (Category Test and Tactual Performance Test). Among the four most sensitive tests, only the Localization component (3) of the Tactual Performance Test was done poorly. The patient continued to do well on the Seashore Rhythm Test (28 correct) and the Speech-sounds Perception Test (4 errors), again demonstrating his basic ability to attend to well-defined and specific stimulus material and maintain concentrated attention over time. His performances on the Reitan-Kløve Sensory-perceptual Examination were entirely within normal limits.

Lateralizing signs of brain damage were relatively minimal. The patient became somewhat confused when asked to multiply 17×3. First, he added the two numbers, then responded "210" (an answer that for some reason is often given by children with learning disabilities), and finally gave the correct answer. This response probably represents a defective performance and may be related to the prior evidence of left cerebral damage. Note, though, that the patient's enunciation of METHODIST EPISCOPAL had improved. He showed a little confusion with EPISCOPAL but gave a response (Epistipul) within the range of normal variation. His finger tapping speed was slow with both hands (RH-39; LH-34), but the difference between the hands was not particularly indicative of lateralized dysfunction. On the Tactual Performance Test W.B. was definitely slow with his right hand (8.2 min) compared with his left (3.6 min), a finding that might suggest some impairment of left cerebral functions.

Indicators of right cerebral damage were not pronounced. The patient had some difficulty copying simple spatial configurations, but the final products of his efforts were within the normal range. It should be noted, however, that W.B. had to effect a considerable compensation in his drawing of the triangle; he drew the second (horizontal) line somewhat long and apparently had to make the figure larger than he had originally intended. One could also question the symmetry of the teeth of the key, but overall the drawing is probably within normal limits.

Grip strength may have been slightly reduced with the left upper extremity (58.0 kg) compared with the right (66.0 kg), but if considered independently this finding would not provide a basis for concluding that right cerebral damage had been sustained. Therefore, although the second set of test results shows some mild deviations from normal expectancy, they are probably within the range of normal variation.

It is clear that in the year intervening between examinations W.B. made some significant improvements that go beyond positive practice-effect expectations. Reduction of the Impairment Index from 0.6 to 0.3 is a significant improvement and indicates that the patient's adaptive abilities were within the normal range rather than in the impaired range. The reduction of errors on the Category Test (from 52 to 35) is not remarkable; improvement on this test due to positive practice-effect is generally quite pronounced. However, the patient probably did demonstrate genuine improvement on Part B of the Trail Making Test (from 77 sec to 58 sec) and certainly improved beyond practice-effect expectations on the Total Time of the Tactual Performance Test (from 21.5 min to 13.7 min).

As noted above, lateralizing indicators were not pronounced on the second examination. W.B. no longer made mistakes in simple spelling, enunciation of words, or right-left orientation. The right hand performance on the Tactual Performance Test on the second examination may reflect some residual deficit of left cerebral functions, even though the TPT results on the first testing had lateralizing significance for the right cerebral hemisphere. At the 12-month evaluation the patient was definitely drawing better figures than at the time of the first examination. Perhaps the most pronounced improvement was in grip strength with the left upper extremity, showing essentially a complete recovery from the hemiparesis that had been noted shortly after the injury.

The Neuropsychological Deficit Scale recapitulates these findings. Level of Performance variables totalled 11 points (average for control subjects is 11.95 points), with only TPT-Localization and finger tapping speed deviating from normal performances. Dyscalculia was the only variable contributing to the section on Pathognomonic signs. Right-left differences totalled 5 points (control subjects: 3.37 points), a finding that might possibly represent very mild residual impairment. However, the G-NDS score of 18 was clearly at the normal level.

In conclusion, one could wonder whether some of the relationships between the test results reflected impaired brain functions, but it appeared that the patient had made a very pronounced recovery and achieved scores that were essentially within the range of normal variation. Probably the two most significant indications of worse performances occurred on the Arithmetic subtest of the Wechsler Scale and finger tapping speed. It is entirely possible that these scores reflect some type of decrement in the subject's capability, but it must also be noted that variability in performances due to chance will occur when an extensive number of tests are given. It is clear that in general this man demonstrated distinct improvement and any evidence of deterioration of performances was clearly outweighed by his good scores.

The final examination of this man was done 18 months after the first testing. Since W.B. had been given exactly the same battery of tests three times, one might expect to see some degree of positive practice-effect. We will first review the test results of the examination performed 18 months after the initial examination. Following this interpretation, we will compare the performances of all three examinations.

W.B. earned a Verbal IQ (104) in the average range and a Performance IQ (118) 14 points higher, in the upper part of the high average range. It would appear that he performed sufficiently well on the subtests of the Wechsler Scale to be expected to do reasonably well on other tests. Note that he had some difficulty with the Arithmetic subtest (6), possibly suggesting left cerebral dysfunction, but he did extremely well on the most sensitive subtest, Digit Symbol (16).

The four most sensitive general indicators raise the question of significant cerebral damage, especially in light of the relatively good scores on the Wechsler Scale. W.B. had an Impairment Index of 0.6 (about 60% of Halstead's tests had scores in the brain-damaged range), earned a score on the Category Test (51) just within the brain-damaged range, and performed somewhat poorly on the Localization component (4) of the Tactual Performance Test. Among the four most sensitive indicators, his only score in the normal range occurred on Part B of the Trail Making Test (54 sec).

Although W.B. did not perform particularly well on the Seashore Rhythm Test (24 correct), his score on the Speech-sounds Perception Test (5 errors) was sufficiently good to indicate that he had adequate ability and concentration to pay attention to specific stimulus material.

Lateralizing indicators were not pronounced, but this right-handed man showed a striking deviation from normal expectancy in finger tapping speed. His right hand (41) was significantly slower than his left (47); along with the poor score on the Arithmetic subtest and the indications of impairment on the general indicators, this may suggest some left cerebral dysfunction. However, there were no signs of defective performances on the Aphasia Screening Test, except for an error in enunciation, to support a hypothesis of left hemisphere damage.

There were essentially no indicators of right cerebral damage. W.B. did not improve quite as much as we might have expected with his left hand (second trial) on the Tactual Performance Test, but his drawings on the Aphasia Screening Test

THE HALSTEAD-REITAN
NEUROPSYCHOLOGICAL TEST BATTERY

Patient __W.B. (III)__ Age __21__ Sex __M__ Education __12__ Handedness __R__

WECHSLER-BELLEVUE SCALE

VIQ	104
PIQ	118
FS IQ	111
Information	8
Comprehension	13
Digit Span	11
Arithmetic	6
Similarities	12
Vocabulary	11
Picture Arrangement	11
Picture Completion	12
Block Design	13
Object Assembly	12
Digit Symbol	16

NEUROPSYCHOLOGICAL DEFICIT SCALE

Level of Performance	14
Pathognomonic Signs	0
Patterns	5
Right-Left Differences	6
Total NDS Score	25

TRAIL MAKING TEST

Part A: __26__ seconds
Part B: __54__ seconds

STRENGTH OF GRIP

Dominant hand: __70.0__ kilograms
Non-dominant hand: __63.5__ kilograms

REITAN-KLØVE TACTILE FORM RECOGNITION TEST

Dominant hand: __8__ seconds; __0__ errors
Non-dominant hand: __9__ seconds; __0__ errors

REITAN-KLØVE SENSORY-PERCEPTUAL EXAM — No errors

			Error Totals	
RH___LH___	Both H: RH___LH___	RH___LH___		
RH___LF___	Both H/F: RH___LF___	RH___LF___		
LH___RF___	Both H/F: LH___RF___	RF___LH___		
RE___LE___	Both E: RE___LE___	RE___LE___		
RV___LV___	Both: RV___LV___	RV___LV___		
___ ___		___ ___		
___ ___		___ ___		

TACTILE FINGER RECOGNITION

R 1___ 2___ 3___ 4___ 5 _1_ R _1_ / 20
L 1___ 2___ 3___ 4___ 5 _2_ L _2_ / 20

FINGER-TIP NUMBER WRITING

R 1 _3_ 2___ 3___ 4___ 5___ R _3_ / 20
L 1 _2_ 2___ 3___ 4___ 5___ L _2_ / 20

HALSTEAD'S NEUROPSYCHOLOGICAL TEST BATTERY

Category Test		51

Tactual Performance Test

Dominant hand:	3.9	
Non-dominant hand:	3.3	
Both hands:	1.7	
	Total Time	8.9
	Memory	8
	Localization	4

Seashore Rhythm Test

Number Correct __24__ 8

Speech-sounds Perception Test

Number of Errors 5

Finger Oscillation Test

Dominant hand:	41	41
Non-dominant hand:	47	

Impairment Index 0.6

MINNESOTA MULTIPHASIC PERSONALITY INVENTORY

			Hs	72
			D	77
?	50		Hy	71
L	63		Pd	79
F	80		Mf	53
K	49		Pa	76
			Pt	69
			Sc	71
			Ma	60

REITAN-KLØVE LATERAL-DOMINANCE EXAM

Show me how you:

throw a ball	R
hammer a nail	R
cut with a knife	R
turn a door knob	R
use scissors	R
use an eraser	R
write your name	R

Record time used for spontaneous name-writing:

Preferred hand	10	seconds
Non-preferred hand	15	seconds

Show me how you:

kick a football	R
step on a bug	R

REITAN-INDIANA APHASIA SCREENING TEST

Form for Adults and Older Children

Name: _____ W. B. (III) _____ Age: __21__

Copy SQUARE	Repeat TRIANGLE
Name SQUARE	Repeat MASSACHUSETTS
Spell SQUARE	Repeat METHODIST EPISCOPAL "Methodist Epilcsapl." Then OK.
Copy CROSS	Write SQUARE
Name CROSS	Read SEVEN
Spell CROSS	Repeat SEVEN
Copy TRIANGLE	Repeat/Explain HE SHOUTED THE WARNING.
Name TRIANGLE	Write HE SHOUTED THE WARNING.
Spell TRIANGLE	Compute 85 – 27 =
Name BABY	Compute 17 X 3 =
Write CLOCK	Name KEY
Name FORK	Demonstrate use of KEY
Read 7 SIX 2	Draw KEY
Read MGW	Read PLACE LEFT HAND TO RIGHT EAR.
Reading I	Place LEFT HAND TO RIGHT EAR
Reading II	Place LEFT HAND TO LEFT ELBOW

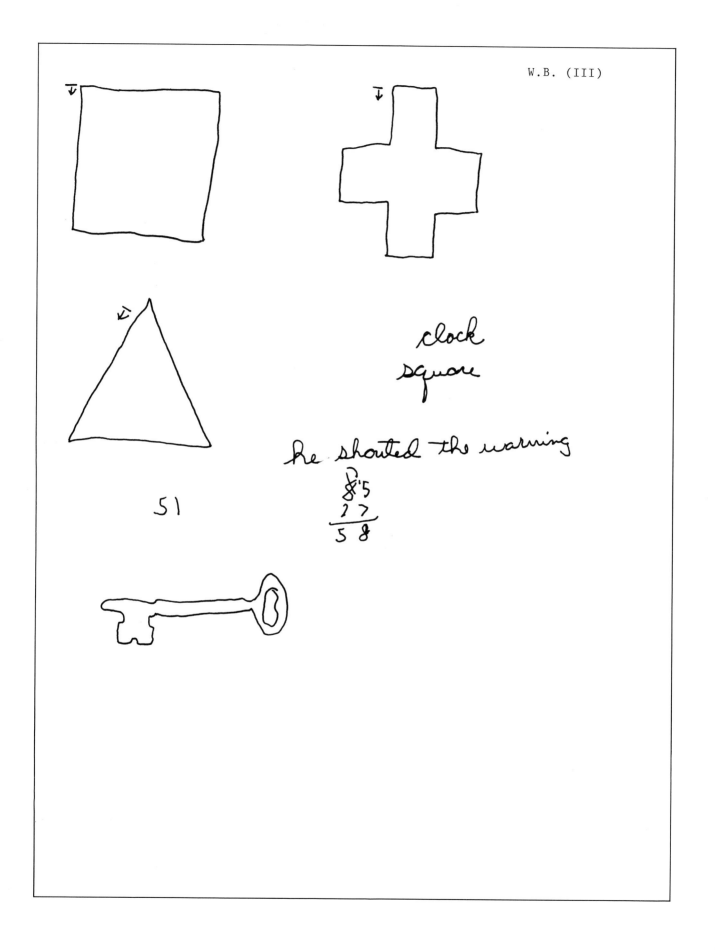

clock

square

he shouted the warning

$$\begin{array}{r} 8\,5 \\ 2\,7 \\ \hline 5\,8 \end{array}$$

51

were essentially within normal limits and no other indicators were present to suggest specific impairment on the left side of the body.

In summary, then, it appears that W.B. did not perform quite as well on the general indicators of brain function as might be expected, and the relatively poor scores on the Arithmetic subtest of the Wechsler Scale and tapping speed with the preferred hand might constitute some evidence of left hemisphere impairment. The mistakes in tactile finger localization and finger-tip number writing perception might also offer mild support to this contention.

In comparing the examinations done at 12 and 18 months, we see that W.B. performed somewhat better on Performance IQ, Total Time on the Tactual Performance Test, and finger tapping speed with the left hand. However, the improvement of the left hand in finger tapping speed on the 18-month examination was a significant factor in the overall interpretation, suggesting a disparity between the two hands that implicated the left cerebral hemisphere. The Impairment Index was worse (0.6) and W.B. did not do as well on the Seashore Rhythm Test (24 correct) and the Category Test (51 errors). He also may have performed somewhat worse on Tactile Finger Localization and Finger-Tip Number Writing Perception.

The G-NDS score for the 18-month testing also reflected these changes. The Level of Performance score changed from 11 to 14, with evidence of mild to moderate impairment on the Impairment Index,

Category Test, TPT-Localization, Seashore Rhythm Test, and finger tapping speed with the right hand. W.B. no longer manifested evidence of confusion in performing simple arithmetic problems, but a 14-point disparity between VIQ and PIQ and an Impairment Index of 0.6 in conjunction with a FSIQ of 111 contributed 5 points to the G-NDS (whereas the section on Patterns had yielded 1 point and 0 points on the two previous testings). Even though no significant right-left differences were present on the 18-month testing, the G-NDS rose from 18 to 25 points.

Generally considered, these results suggest that W.B. had shown a mild but significant degree of deterioration of neuropsychological functions in the period between the 12-month and 18-month examinations. No corresponding findings indicating deterioration were present on physical neurological examination or EEG.

Finally, we should note that the results on the Minnesota Multiphasic Personality Inventory suggest that W.B. is considerably more disturbed emotionally at this time than he was six months ago. It is possible that an interaction of emotional stress and mild residual brain damage could have been responsible for his poorer performances. However, it would seem unlikely that emotional disturbance alone was responsible for the strikingly worse results on the Impairment Index and the Category Test while at the same time permitting somewhat better performances on the Total Time of the Tactual Performance Test and the Performance IQ.

Case #12

Name: L.D.

Age: 23

Education: 13

Sex: Male

Handedness: Right

Occupation: Student

Background Information

L.D. sustained a head injury when he jumped off his bicycle to avoid hitting a truck. He was initially confused and disoriented but did not lose consciousness. In the emergency room it was noted that he was markedly confused, although responsive and oriented to person. A neurological examination performed shortly after admission to the hospital revealed that L.D. appeared to be generally alert and oriented to both person and place but not to time. In other respects the neurological examination was entirely normal.

Neurological Examination

When he was discharged from the hospital the next day L.D. could remember events up to the time of the accident but could not recall any of the details of the accident or anything that occurred for approximately one and one-half hours thereafter. Electroencephalograms done five days after the injury showed slight generalized abnormalities but no focal or epileptiform patterns.

Neurological examinations and electroencephalograms were done at 3-month, 12-month, and 18-month intervals following the injury. Although the neurological examinations were normal in each instance, at the time of the 3-month examination the patient said that it had been somewhat more difficult for him to concentrate than before the injury. However, at 12 months and 18 months post-injury he had no complaints. The EEG was the same at three months as it had been five days

after injury, and entirely normal at the 12-month and 18-month examinations.

In summary, the major manifestations of L.D.'s closed head injury were confusion and disorientation which had totally cleared by the next day. However, even three months after the accident L.D. could not recall the details of the accident.

L.D.'s recovery from his head injury had been uneventful. On the Cornell Medical Health Questionnaire he indicated only that he had experienced difficulty previously in stuttering or stammering, that he became nervous during examinations or questioning, that his feelings were easily hurt, and that sudden movements or noises at night tended to frighten him. In most respects, though, the patient had no complaints. Neuropsychological testing was done 12 days after the injury.

Neuropsychological Examination

In general, this man performed quite well on the first neuropsychological examination. He earned a Verbal IQ (111) in the lower part of the High Average range (exceeding about 77% of his age peers) and a Performance IQ (107) in the upper part of the Average range (exceeding 68%). Except for Digit Span (6), the Verbal subtest scores were consistently above the average level. It is clear that L.D. performed poorly on Digit Span, but the distribution of Verbal subtest scores does not have much specific clinical significance since brain damage is not the only reason for impairment on this test.

THE HALSTEAD-REITAN
NEUROPSYCHOLOGICAL TEST BATTERY

Patient **L.D. (I)**   Age **23**   Sex **M**   Education **13**   Handedness **R**

WECHSLER-BELLEVUE SCALE

VIQ	111
PIQ	107
FS IQ	110
Information	11
Comprehension	13
Digit Span	6
Arithmetic	13
Similarities	13
Vocabulary	13
Picture Arrangement	8
Picture Completion	9
Block Design	14
Object Assembly	14
Digit Symbol	11

NEUROPSYCHOLOGICAL DEFICIT SCALE

Level of Performance	13
Pathognomonic Signs	0
Patterns	0
Right-Left Differences	8
Total NDS Score	21

HALSTEAD'S NEUROPSYCHOLOGICAL TEST BATTERY

Category Test   33

Tactual Performance Test

Dominant hand:	7.3
Non-dominant hand:	3.9
Both hands:	2.4

Total Time	13.6
Memory	9
Localization	6

Seashore Rhythm Test

Number Correct **28**   2

Speech-sounds Perception Test

Number of Errors   7

Finger Oscillation Test

Dominant hand:	51	51
Non-dominant hand:	44	

Impairment Index   0.0

TRAIL MAKING TEST

Part A: **42** seconds
Part B: **88** seconds

STRENGTH OF GRIP

Dominant hand: **51** kilograms
Non-dominant hand: **42.5** kilograms

REITAN-KLØVE TACTILE FORM RECOGNITION TEST

Dominant hand: **7** seconds; **0** errors
Non-dominant hand: **7** seconds; **0** errors

MINNESOTA MULTIPHASIC PERSONALITY INVENTORY

		Hs	47
		D	63
?	50	Hy	55
L	50	Pd	55
F	44	Mf	55
K	55	Pa	56
		Pt	50
		Sc	48
		Ma	50

REITAN-KLØVE SENSORY-PERCEPTUAL EXAM

		Error Totals	
RH___ LH___	Both H: RH___ LH___	RH___ LH___	
RH___ LF___	Both H/F: RH___ LF___	RH___ LF___	
LH___ RF___	Both H/F: LH___ RF___	RF___ LH___	
RE___ LE___	Both E: RE_1_ LE___	RE_1_ LE___	
RV___ LV___	Both: RV___ LV___	RV___ LV___	

REITAN-KLØVE LATERAL-DOMINANCE EXAM

Show me how you:

throw a ball	R
hammer a nail	R
cut with a knife	R
turn a door knob	R
use scissors	R
use an eraser	R
write your name	R

Record time used for spontaneous name-writing:

Preferred hand	**6** seconds
Non-preferred hand	**29** seconds

TACTILE FINGER RECOGNITION

R 1___ 2___ 3___ 4___ 5___   R **0** / 20
L 1___ 2___ 3 _1_ 4___ 5___   L **1** / 20

FINGER-TIP NUMBER WRITING

R 1 _3_ 2___ 3___ 4 _1_ 5___   R **4** / 20
L 1 _2_ 2___ 3___ 4___ 5___   L **2** / 20

Show me how you:

kick a football	R
step on a bug	R

NO APHASIC SYMPTOMS

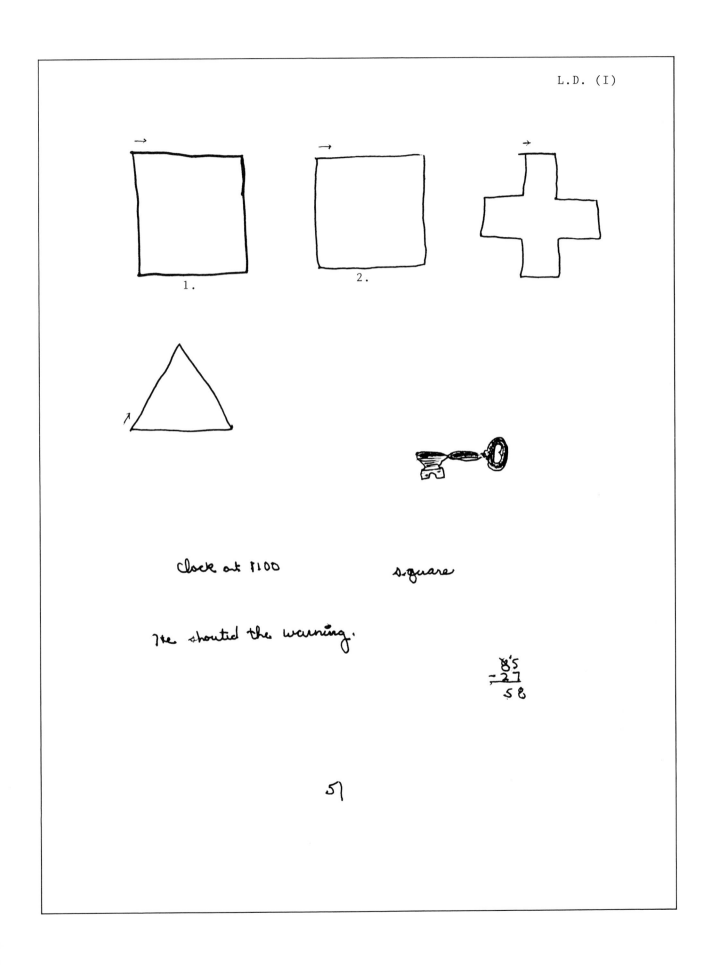

1.

2.

clock at 1100   square

He shouted the warning.

$$\begin{array}{r} 8\rlap{'}5 \\ -27 \\ \hline 58 \end{array}$$

5

The Performance subtests showed somewhat poorer scores on Picture Arrangement (8) and Picture Completion (9). The Picture Arrangement score is often lowered by damage of the right anterior temporal area, but Picture Completion does not have any consistent relationship to cerebral damage. It should also be noted that the Digit Symbol score (11) was not significantly lower than the general level of performance established by this man, and this relatively adequate score would tend to argue against cerebral damage. Thus, results of the Wechsler Scale cannot be interpreted as indicating any significant impairment of cerebral functions. The Picture Arrangement subtest score may have meaning concerning cerebral damage, but it would be difficult to be confident of this at this point in the interpretation.

L.D. also performed relatively well on the four most sensitive indicators in the Halstead-Reitan Battery. His scores on the Impairment Index (0.0), Category Test (33), and Localization component (6) of the Tactual Performance Test were all in the normal range. L.D.'s score on Part B of the Trail Making test was in the range of mild impairment and it is quite unusual for a person with his intelligence levels to require 88 seconds to complete the task. Therefore, this score suggests some mild generalized impairment. The scores on the other tests in the Battery were also adequate. The patient demonstrated good ability to focus his attention to specific stimulus material, as shown by his scores on the Seashore Rhythm Test (28 correct) and Speech-sounds Perception Test (7 errors).

Judging from the level of his performances, we could not conclude that L.D. sustained any significant cerebral damage. However, it is hypothetically possible that his abilities were considerably higher before the head injury and his scores on the neuropsychological examination may actually reflect some degree of cerebral impairment, even though they are still well above average in most instances.

Evaluation of the lateralizing indicators adds additional information. The measures of lateral dominance indicated that L.D. was strongly right-handed; however, on the Tactual Performance Test he performed worse with his right hand (7.3 min) than his left (3.9 min). It must be noted, though, that poor performances on the first trial of the TPT sometimes result from unfamiliarity with the task and difficulty getting started. It is important to also note that L.D. had more difficulty in finger-tip number writing perception on the right hand (4) than the left (2) and made one error on the right side in perceiving bilateral simultaneous auditory stimulation. These findings are certainly not sufficiently strong to imply that the patient has a seriously compromised left cerebral hemisphere; but they do deviate mildly from normal expectancy and may suggest a mild degree of left cerebral dysfunction.

Other findings had about equivalent significance for impairment of the right cerebral hemisphere. The Picture Arrangement score (8) considered by itself would not support a hypothesis of right hemisphere dysfunction, since Picture Arrangement may be lowered for reasons other than right cerebral damage. However, the mild impairment of grip strength and finger tapping speed with the left hand complemented the Picture Arrangement score. Although the finger tapping score was indeed a very mild indication, the grip strength in the left upper extremity was only 83% of the strength registered on the right side.

L.D. demonstrated no aphasic deficits to support the mild left cerebral indicators or any constructional dyspraxia to complement the right hemisphere signs. However, remember that specific deficits of this kind are rarely seen in persons who perform as well as this man did on measures of higher-level intellectual and cognitive tasks; aphasia and constructional dyspraxia are usually seen in persons with more serious cerebral damage. In evaluating the overall configuration of test results, then, it appears that L.D. showed deviations that go slightly beyond normal expectancy and are quite characteristic of mild residual impairment associated with craniocerebral trauma, especially inasmuch as the results implicated each cerebral hemisphere.

The G-NDS (21) was well within the normal range, but L.D. did score higher on the Right-Left Differences section than would have been expected for a person without some impairment of cerebral functions. This case illustrates the importance of avoiding complete dependence on the G-NDS as contrasted with clinical evaluation and interpretation of findings which may deviate only mildly, but consistently, from normality.

L.D. was re-examined 12 months later. At this time he had no complaints regarding his head injury and felt that he had recovered completely. He was again given the Cornell Medical Index Health Questionnaire and complained only of occasional toothaches, difficulty sleeping, and being inclined to have small accidents and injuries.

We will compare the results of the two testings after reviewing the current findings. L.D. earned both Verbal (125) and Performance (125) IQ values in the Superior range and a Full Scale IQ (128) even a few points higher. The patient's Impairment Index was 0.1. The test that contributed to the Impairment Index, the Speech-sounds Perception Test, had just one error above the cut-off point. We have previously noted that Halstead's criterion score for this test (7 errors) was unduly stringent. Therefore, L.D.'s general level of performance appeared to be quite adequate.

Scores on the four most sensitive indicators were well within the normal range, as were the performances on the other tests in the Battery. There is no doubt that L.D. has the ability to pay close and continued attention to specific stimulus material, process verbal material capably, deal well with both simple and more complex visual-spatial tasks, and demonstrate excellent analytical and reasoning skills. In contrast to many persons with limited or impaired brain functions, he showed no tendency to decline in his capability to solve difficult tasks compared with simpler ones. In terms of level of performance, the test results indicate that this man has excellent abilities.

The only deviant results were obtained on measures that compare the performances on each side of his body. L.D.'s grip strength was a little weaker than might be expected with his right hand (54 kg vs. 50 kg), but this difference is so mild that it has limited significance. On the Tactile Form Recognition Test L.D. required eight seconds to complete the four trials with the right hand and six seconds for the left hand, but this difference was also minimal; even some control subjects require an extra small amount of time on the initial trials and the task is always given to the right hand first. The patient also made one mistake in perceiving a tactile stimulus to the right face when it was given simultaneously with a stimulus to the left hand. Finally, he appeared to have more difficulty in finger-tip number writing with his right hand (3 errors) compared with his left (1 error).

These minimal findings suggest that there is probably a very mild degree of residual left cerebral impairment, but in the context of the excellent scores on other measures it is not likely that the deficits have any clinical significance. It is not surprising that L.D. offered no complaints and felt that he had recovered completely from the head injury.

Direct comparison of the initial test results with the findings obtained 12 months later provides unequivocal evidence of improvement in a number of respects. The patient's Verbal IQ had risen from 111 to 125, with a rather consistent improvement among various subtests. His Performance IQ rose from 107 to 125, with substantial increases on two of the subtests most sensitive to cerebral impairment (Picture Arrangement and Digit Symbol). L.D. showed significant improvement on the Category Test (from 33 to 11 errors) even though a considerable degree of positive practice-effect is expected on this test. On the Tactual Performance Test he reduced his time sharply from 13.6 minutes to 6.6 minutes. It is also interesting to note that the major degree of improvement on the TPT occurred on the first trial

THE HALSTEAD-REITAN
NEUROPSYCHOLOGICAL TEST BATTERY

Patient **L.D. (II)** Age **24** Sex **M** Education **13** Handedness **R**

WECHSLER-BELLEVUE SCALE

VIQ	125
PIQ	125
FS IQ	128
Information	13
Comprehension	16
Digit Span	9
Arithmetic	16
Similarities	14
Vocabulary	14
Picture Arrangement	12
Picture Completion	12
Block Design	16
Object Assembly	15
Digit Symbol	14

NEUROPSYCHOLOGICAL DEFICIT SCALE

Level of Performance	6
Pathognomonic Signs	0
Patterns	0
Right-Left Differences	4
Total NDS Score	10

HALSTEAD'S NEUROPSYCHOLOGICAL TEST BATTERY

Category Test	11

Tactual Performance Test

Dominant hand:	3.3
Non-dominant hand:	2.2
Both hands:	1.1

Total Time	6.6
Memory	8
Localization	7

Seashore Rhythm Test

Number Correct	27	3

Speech-sounds Perception Test

Number of Errors	8

Finger Oscillation Test

Dominant hand:	54	54
Non-dominant hand:	48	

Impairment Index 0.1

MINNESOTA MULTIPHASIC PERSONALITY INVENTORY

		Hs	59
		D	48
?	50	Hy	57
L	56	Pd	60
F	53	Mf	49
K	70	Pa	50
		Pt	54
		Sc	59
		Ma	58

TRAIL MAKING TEST

Part A: **24** seconds
Part B: **61** seconds

STRENGTH OF GRIP

Dominant hand: **54.0** kilograms
Non-dominant hand: **50.0** kilograms

REITAN-KLØVE TACTILE FORM RECOGNITION TEST

Dominant hand: **8** seconds; **0** errors
Non-dominant hand: **6** seconds; **0** errors

REITAN-KLØVE SENSORY-PERCEPTUAL EXAM

		Error Totals
RH___ LH___	Both H: RH___ LH___	RH___ LH___
RH___ LF___	Both H/F: RH___ LF___	RH___ LF___
LH___ RF___	Both H/F: LH___ RF **1**	RF **1** LH___
RE___ LE___	Both E: RE___ LE___	RE___ LE___
RV___ LV___	Both: RV___ LV___	RV___ LV___

TACTILE FINGER RECOGNITION

R 1___ 2___ 3___ 4___ 5___   R **0** / 20
L 1___ 2___ 3___ 4___ 5___   L **0** / 20

FINGER-TIP NUMBER WRITING

R 1 **2** 2___ 3___ 4___ 5 **1**   R **3** / 20
L 1 **1** 2___ 3___ 4___ 5___   L **1** / 20

NO APHASIC SYMPTOMS.

REITAN-KLØVE LATERAL-DOMINANCE EXAM

Show me how you:
throw a ball	**R**
hammer a nail	**R**
cut with a knife	**R**
turn a door knob	**R**
use scissors	**R**
use an eraser	**R**
write your name	**R**

Record time used for spontaneous name-writing:
Preferred hand	**7**	seconds
Non-preferred hand	**23**	seconds

Show me how you:
kick a football	**R**
step on a bug	**R**

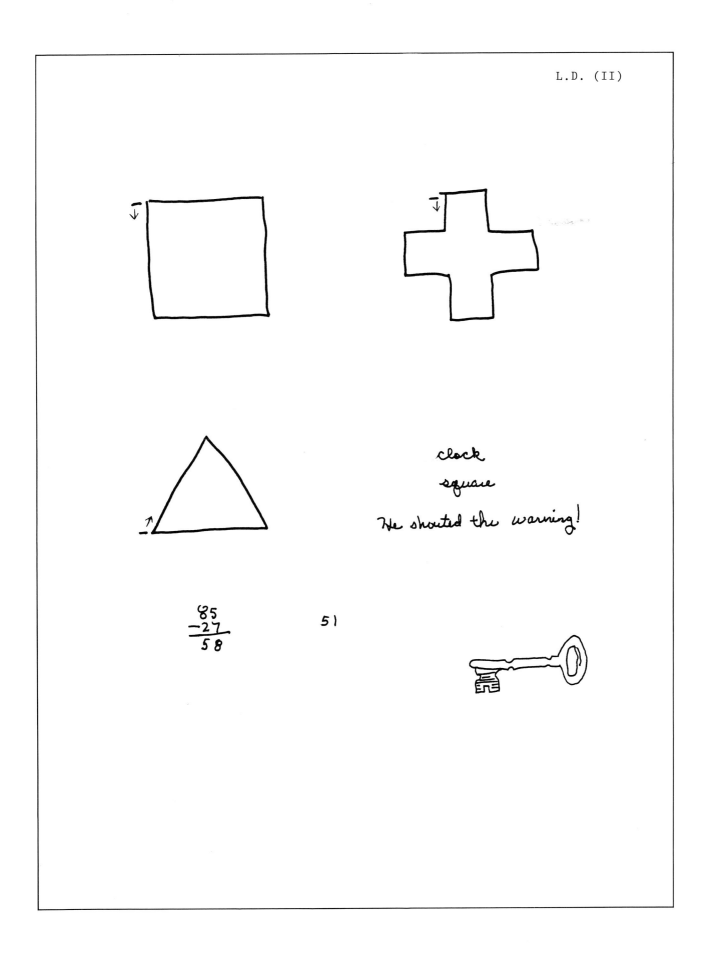

clock

square

He shouted the warning!

$$\begin{array}{r} 85 \\ -27 \\ \hline 58 \end{array}$$

51

(right hand), a performance that was somewhat impaired on the first examination.

Grip strength was increased on both sides, but principally on the left side that had initially been somewhat impaired. Finger tapping speed was also a little faster with each hand. Finally, on Part B of the Trail Making Test L.D. reduced his time from 88 seconds to 61 seconds. Even though the score on the initial examination was not seriously impaired, we considered it to be elevated, especially in light of L.D.'s general indications of ability.

We can see that many of the tests were clearly performed better on the second examination. There was a distinct tendency for improvement to occur on tasks suspected of showing impairment on the first testing. In fact, the better scores on the second examination (which consistently exceeded improvement attributable to positive practice-effect) document quite clearly that L.D. was significantly more impaired shortly after the head injury than it was possible to infer from the first set of test results.

Results on the G-NDS reflect this improvement, decreasing from 21 to 10. The improvement was apparent for both sections on which points had initially been accrued (Level of Performance and Right-Left Differences). Thus, the G-NDS, as well as clinical interpretation of the test results, shows a degree of improvement that extends beyond expected practice-effects and provides a retrospective basis for recognizing the mild deficit that was represented in the first set of test results.

Thus, the overall results for this patient serve as an example of the many instances in which we have found it necessary to infer from later examinations (after recovery had occurred) that significant impairment was present initially, even though the head injury had been relatively mild. On the first set of test results we had observed mild indications of both left and right cerebral dysfunction. The improvements shown on the 12-month examination essentially deleted the right

cerebral indicators, even though indications of mild left cerebral deficits were still present. Based on the results obtained one year after the first examination, we would still conclude that this man has very mild impairment of brain functions, though the overall results on the Halstead-Reitan Battery suggest that they do not have clinical significance.

L.D. was re-examined 18 months after the first testing. At this time he had no complaints, felt that there had been no significant changes in his condition, and acknowledged absolutely no problems on the Cornell Medical Index Health Questionnaire.

The test findings indicate that L.D. has superior intellectual abilities and performed well on the brain-sensitive tests. However, despite his generally good abilities, he demonstrated very mild left cerebral dysfunction.

The patient earned both Verbal (126) and Performance (130) IQ values in the Superior range. He also performed well on the four most sensitive measures in the Halstead-Reitan Battery, although considering his IQ values and good general abilities one might have expected him to perform a little better than 74 seconds on Part B of the Trail Making Test.

Lateralizing indicators, though mild, were present. L.D. required twice as much time to complete the Tactual Performance Test with his right hand (2.6 min) than his left (1.3 min), although one must be reluctant to infer the presence of damage in a cerebral hemisphere when the contralateral hand is able to complete the task so efficiently. L.D. was also a little slower in Tactile Form Recognition with his right hand (11 sec) than his left (9 sec), but a difference of two seconds could be a chance variation. Grip strength was slightly greater with the preferred hand (51.5 kg) than non-preferred hand (49.0 kg), but not as much as one expects to see in normal subjects. Also, the patient definitely had more difficulty in finger-tip writing perception with his right hand

THE HALSTEAD-REITAN
NEUROPSYCHOLOGICAL TEST BATTERY

Patient **L.D. (III)** Age **24** Sex **M** Education **14** Handedness **R**

WECHSLER-BELLEVUE SCALE

VIQ	126
PIQ	130
FS IQ	131
Information	13
Comprehension	13
Digit Span	10
Arithmetic	17
Similarities	16
Vocabulary	13
Picture Arrangement	16
Picture Completion	14
Block Design	15
Object Assembly	14
Digit Symbol	14

NEUROPSYCHOLOGICAL DEFICIT SCALE

Level of Performance	9
Pathognomonic Signs	0
Patterns	0
Right-Left Differences	9
Total NDS Score	18

HALSTEAD'S NEUROPSYCHOLOGICAL TEST BATTERY

Category Test — 10

Tactual Performance Test

Dominant hand:	2.6		
Non-dominant hand:	1.3		
Both hands:	0.8		
		Total Time	4.7
		Memory	8
		Localization	6

Seashore Rhythm Test

Number Correct **27** — 3

Speech-sounds Perception Test

Number of Errors — 4

Finger Oscillation Test

Dominant hand:	51	51
Non-dominant hand:	43	

Impairment Index — 0.0

TRAIL MAKING TEST

Part A: **28** seconds
Part B: **74** seconds

STRENGTH OF GRIP

Dominant hand: **51.5** kilograms
Non-dominant hand: **49.0** kilograms

REITAN-KLØVE TACTILE FORM RECOGNITION TEST

Dominant hand: **11** seconds; **0** errors
Non-dominant hand: **9** seconds; **0** errors

REITAN-KLØVE SENSORY-PERCEPTUAL EXAM — No errors

				Error Totals	
RH___ LH___	Both H:	RH___ LH___	RH___ LH___		
RH___ LF___	Both H/F:	RH___ LF___	RH___ LF___		
LH___ RF___	Both H/F:	LH___ RF___	RF___ LH___		
RE___ LE___	Both E:	RE___ LE___	RE___ LE___		
RV___ LV___	Both:	RV___ LV___	RV___ LV___		

TACTILE FINGER RECOGNITION

R 1___ 2___ 3___ 4___ 5___   R **0** / **20**
L 1___ 2___ 3___ 4___ 5___   L **0** / **20**

FINGER-TIP NUMBER WRITING

R 1___ 2 **1** 3 **2** 4___ 5 **1**   R **4** / **20**
L 1 **1** 2___ 3___ 4___ 5___   L **1** / **20**

MINNESOTA MULTIPHASIC PERSONALITY INVENTORY

		Hs	49
		D	46
?	50	Hy	58
L	46	Pd	55
F	48	Mf	49
K	59	Pa	35
		Pt	38
		Sc	46
		Ma	43

REITAN-KLØVE LATERAL-DOMINANCE EXAM

Show me how you:
throw a ball	R
hammer a nail	R
cut with a knife	R
turn a door knob	R
use scissors	R
use an eraser	R
write your name	R

Record time used for spontaneous name-writing:
Preferred hand	**7** seconds
Non-preferred hand	**13** seconds

Show me how you:
kick a football	R
step on a bug	R

NO APHASIC SYMPTOMS.

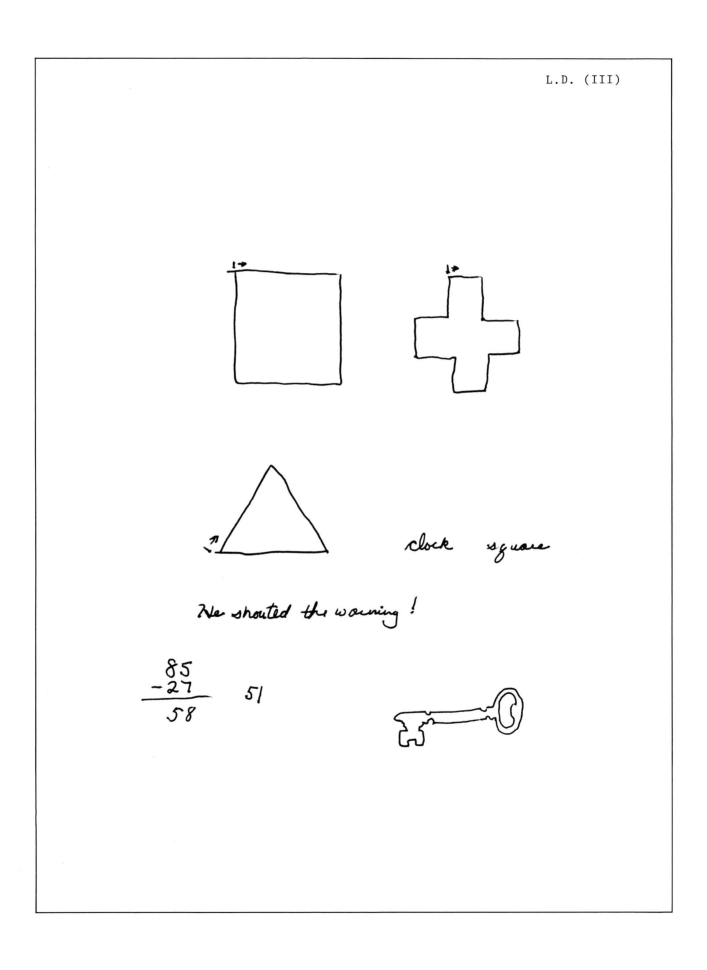

clock   square

We shouted the warning!

$$\begin{array}{r} 85 \\ -27 \\ \hline 58 \end{array}$$ 51

(4 errors) than his left (1 error). All of these deviations from normal expectancy were relatively mild, but in total suggest that L.D.'s left cerebral hemisphere is less capable than his right hemisphere. In this examination there were no indications of right cerebral dysfunction except for a mild reduction in finger tapping speed with the left hand (43) compared with the right (51).

The G-NDS had risen to 18 from a score of 10 on the 12-month examination. While Level of Performance measures determined this change in part (poorer performances especially on Parts A and B of the Trail Making Test, slower responses on the Tactile Form Recognition Test, and slower finger tapping with the left hand), Right-Left Differences were even more important (Grip Strength, Tactile Form Recognition Test, and Finger-tip Number Writing Perception).

In summary, an interpretation of L.D.'s test results obtained 18 months post-injury would necessarily emphasize his many strengths. There is no doubt that his abilities are good and in general his brain functions are within the normal range and better than those of the average person his age. At the same time, it is necessary to note the mild (though consistent) indications of left cerebral dysfunction, even though their clinical significance is questionable.

It is interesting to do a direct comparison of the 18-month test results with those obtained on previous examinations. On the 12-month examination L.D. had shown rather consistent improvement on a number of tests, particularly those that may have been impaired on the initial examination. There were no instances in which a score actually regressed. On the present examination the patient continued to show improvement on the Tactual Performance Test, reducing the Total Time from 6.6 to 4.7 minutes. He also improved on the Speech-sounds Perception Test, reducing his score from 8 errors to 4 errors. Positive practice-effect may have contributed to these better scores or they may be due in part to chance variation.

L.D.'s performances on a number of other measures were essentially at the same level. His Verbal IQ values were practically equal (125 vs. 126) and his scores on the Performance subtests may have improved slightly due to practice-effect (125 to 130). However, note that the greatest change occurred on the Picture Arrangement subtest (from 12 to 16). On the first examination the Picture Arrangement score (8) had been identified as possibly being impaired due to brain damage. On the second testing there was substantial improvement (from 8 to 12) which continued until the 18-month examination (from 12 to 16). The Category Test was still done very well (10), showing no particular change. The patient continued to have difficulties on the right hand in finger-tip number writing perception, with essentially no change from the prior examination (4 errors).

It must also be noted that this man performed somewhat worse on certain tests, even though the decrement was relatively mild. Finger tapping speed was reduced from 54 to 51 taps with the right hand and from 48 to 43 taps with the left hand. Grip strength went down from 54 kg to 51.5 kg with the right hand and from 50 to 49 kg with the left hand, producing a current relationship between the two hands that suggested left cerebral dysfunction a little more strongly than previously. The time required on the Tactile Form Recognition Test increased from 8 seconds to 11 seconds with the right hand and from 6 seconds to 9 seconds with the left hand.

Finally, although the patient's figure drawings were well within the normal range, there can be no doubt that on the 18-month examination he had more trouble achieving symmetry of the four extremities of the cross than he did on the testing done at 12 months. In the drawing done at the 18-month examination the lateral extremities were somewhat uneven in width and the vertical extremities were not in the same plane.

Even though the changes from the 12-month to the 18-month examination were relatively mild, this man actually performed somewhat worse on certain tasks. Although the biological basis remains to be identified, there seems to be no doubt that some patients who have sustained craniocerebral trauma have a long-term recovery process that initially shows a pattern of improvement which is later followed by deterioration of brain-related abilities. As we have noted, this type of change occurs more commonly in persons with neurological evidence of cerebral tissue damage than among persons suffering only concussion, but changes on some measures, in the negative direction, may occur even in the concussion group.

Case #13

Name: W.B.

Age: 23

Education: 12

Sex: Male

Handedness: Right

Occupation: Coast Guard Seaman

Background Information

Until the time of this accident, W.B. had been in good health and had no history of prior head injuries or illnesses that might have caused impaired brain functions. One day, as he was boarding a boat, he slipped and struck his head on the deck. He did not lose consciousness and did not have any anterograde or retrograde amnesia. He was able to leave the boat without assistance and had only a mild headache. He was taken to a community hospital where a frontal laceration was sutured and x-rays revealed a right frontal depressed skull fracture.

W.B. was then transferred to a medical center for further evaluation and treatment. Upon admission to the hospital it was noted that he had remained fully alert and oriented since the injury. Shortly after being admitted the patient was taken to surgery and it was found that a piece of depressed frontal bone, approximately 2.5 cm × 1.5 cm, was indenting the dura mater to a depth of about 1 cm. A small epidural clot was removed, but no bone fragments appeared to lacerate the dura or be driven into the sinus. The dura was then opened surgically. There was no evidence of a subdural hematoma and the cerebral cortex appeared to be entirely intact. Normal dural pulsations were observed. Thus, the surgical procedure involved only debridement of the wound and repair of the skull fracture.

The patient was fully alert the day following the surgery. He complained only of a slight headache and his neurological examination was within

normal limits. He had an uneventful recovery and was discharged from the hospital on the 11th day post-injury.

Neurological Examination

A neurological examination done at the time of the neuropsychological testing (about one week post-trauma) yielded normal results. Electroencephalograms done at the time of neuropsychological examination and at intervals of 3, 12, and 18 months all showed a slight generalized disturbance of brain functions but no lateralized or focal findings. In summary, no cerebral cortical damage was observed at surgery, the patient showed no clinical signs of brain damage at any point following the injury, and the significance of the mild generalized abnormalities on the EEG was equivocal. In this man's case the neurological procedures did not provide any evidence of definite brain damage.

Neuropsychological Examination

W.B. was examined neuropsychologically eight days after sustaining this head injury. On the Cornell Medical Index Health Questionnaire he indicated that he had difficulty breathing and often got out of breath long before anyone else, that it was necessary for him to do things slowly in order to avoid mistakes, and that little annoyances get on his nerves and make him angry. Except for acknowledging his head injury and some prior illnesses, the patient had no additional complaints.

THE HALSTEAD-REITAN
NEUROPSYCHOLOGICAL TEST BATTERY

Patient **W.B. (I)** Age **23** Sex **M** Education **12** Handedness **R**

WECHSLER-BELLEVUE SCALE

VIQ	118
PIQ	118
FS IQ	120
Information	13
Comprehension	15
Digit Span	7
Arithmetic	13
Similarities	14
Vocabulary	13
Picture Arrangement	11
Picture Completion	13
Block Design	14
Object Assembly	15
Digit Symbol	11

NEUROPSYCHOLOGICAL DEFICIT SCALE

Level of Performance	5
Pathognomonic Signs	0
Patterns	0
Right-Left Differences	7
Total NDS Score	12

HALSTEAD'S NEUROPSYCHOLOGICAL TEST BATTERY

Category Test   21

Tactual Performance Test

Dominant hand:	3.6	
Non-dominant hand:	4.9	
Both hands:	2.4	
	Total Time	10.9
	Memory	8
	Localization	5

Seashore Rhythm Test

Number Correct   27   3

Speech-sounds Perception Test

Number of Errors   6

Finger Oscillation Test

Dominant hand:	56	56
Non-dominant hand:	50	

Impairment Index   0.0

TRAIL MAKING TEST

Part A: **25** seconds
Part B: **57** seconds

STRENGTH OF GRIP

Dominant hand: **51.5** kilograms
Non-dominant hand: **50.5** kilograms

REITAN-KLØVE TACTILE FORM RECOGNITION TEST

Dominant hand: **10** seconds; **0** errors
Non-dominant hand: **8** seconds; **0** errors

MINNESOTA MULTIPHASIC PERSONALITY INVENTORY

		Hs	49
		D	48
?	50	Hy	56
L	53	Pd	55
F	53	Mf	53
K	59	Pa	53
		Pt	58
		Sc	51
		Ma	60

REITAN-KLØVE SENSORY-PERCEPTUAL EXAM — No errors

Error Totals

RH ___ LH ___	Both H:	RH ___ LH ___	RH ___ LH ___
RH ___ LF ___	Both H/F:	RH ___ LF ___	RH ___ LF ___
LH ___ RF ___	Both H/F:	LH ___ RF ___	RF ___ LH ___
RE ___ LE ___	Both E:	RE ___ LE ___	RE ___ LE ___
RV ___ LV ___	Both:	RV ___ LV ___	RV ___ LV ___

TACTILE FINGER RECOGNITION

R 1___ 2___ 3___ 4___ 5___   R **0** / 20
L 1___ 2___ 3___ 4 **1** 5___   L **1** / 20

FINGER-TIP NUMBER WRITING

R 1___ 2___ 3___ 4___ 5 **1**   R **1** / 20
L 1___ 2___ 3 **1** 4___ 5___   L **1** / 20

REITAN-KLØVE LATERAL-DOMINANCE EXAM

Show me how you:

throw a ball	R
hammer a nail	R
cut with a knife	R
turn a door knob	R
use scissors	R
use an eraser	R
write your name	R

Record time used for spontaneous name-writing:

Preferred hand	8 seconds
Non-preferred hand	23 seconds

Show me how you:

kick a football	R
step on a bug	R

NO APHASIC SYMPTOMS.

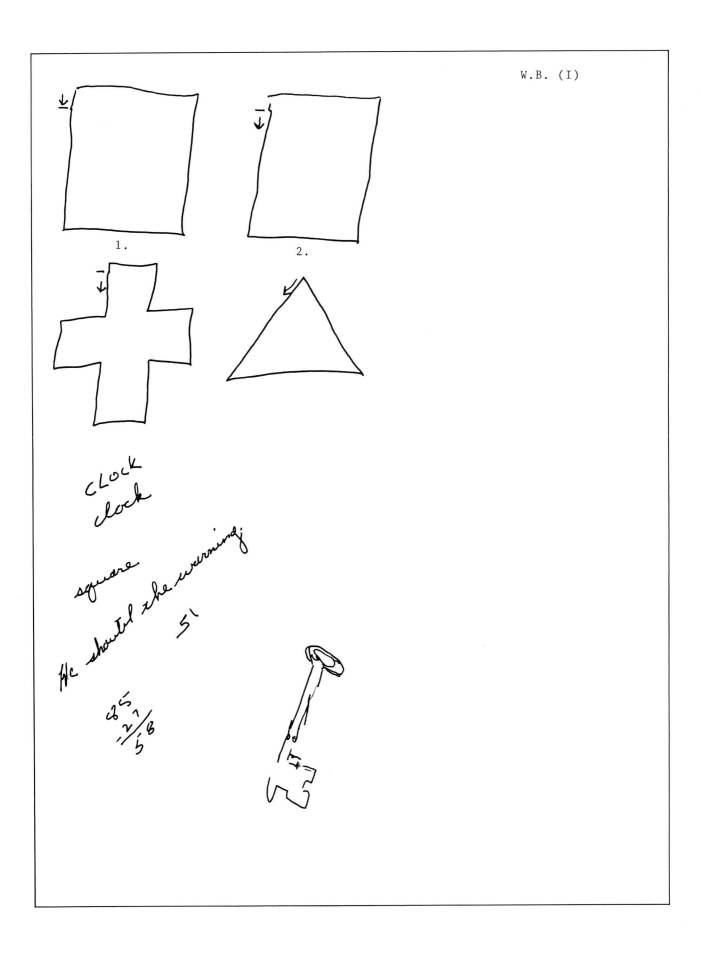

1.

2.

CLOCK

clock

square

the should the warning

51

He believed that he was no different now than before his head injury and felt that he was recovering quite routinely.

W.B.'s Verbal IQ and Performance IQ were both 118, a value in the upper part of the High Average range that exceeds about 89% of his age peers. These values yielded a Full Scale IQ of 120, a score just within the Superior range and exceeding 91%.

Despite these generally good scores, the individual subtests of the Wechsler Scale showed a considerable degree of variability. W.B. did quite poorly on the Digit Span subtest, earning a score of 7. Although this score may not be specific in implicating impaired brain functions (since low scores may also be caused by many other factors), it may possibly indicate some degree of impairment.

The Performance subtests were consistently above the average level, with the poorest performances occurring on Digit Symbol (11) and Picture Arrangement (11). Digit Symbol is frequently impaired as a result of cerebral damage and Picture Arrangement, because of its sensitivity to right anterior temporal lobe damage, often shows impairment in cases of head injury. These scores might be used to suggest that the patient has experienced some impairment, but an experienced neuropsychologist will realize that W.B.'s results on the Wechsler Scale are far from unequivocal in determining brain damage.

W.B. performed extremely well on Halstead's tests. Although the four most sensitive indicators in the Halstead-Reitan Battery all had scores within the range of normal variation, the patient perhaps did not do quite as well on the Localization component of the Tactual Performance Test (5) as he did on the other measures. The level of performance on all of the remaining tests was essentially within the normal range. Using only this method of inference, it would initially appear that this is a bright man whose abilities are essentially uncompromised.

Note, however, that certain results must be considered deviant despite the good scores on many tests. Although definitely right-handed, W.B.'s grip strength was not much greater in his right upper extremity (51.5 kg) than his left (50.5 kg). This obviously could be due to many factors other than left cerebral damage, and considered by itself it is hardly a valid basis for drawing any conclusion about brain impairment.

Notice that W.B. also showed a distinctly deviant result on the Tactual Performance Test. Although he performed very well on the first trial with his right hand (3.6 min), he required considerably more time on the second trial with his left hand (4.9 min). The performance with each hand was well within the normal time limits, but the relationship between the two performances was deviant and may be an indication of right cerebral damage.

W.B.'s finger tapping speed and sensory-perceptual abilities were normal. The excellent scores (in terms of level of performance) on many of the brain-sensitive tests caution against undue emphasis on the limited number of lateralizing signs. Thus, the interpretation of the overall set of test results would be essentially within the normal range; one could not confidently conclude that W.B. had sustained any significant cognitive impairment in association with his head injury. The G-NDS concurred with the clinical interpretation, yielding a total score of 12, which is well within the normal range. In fact, only two of the 42 variables deviated from the normal range (TPT-Localization and the difference between the two hands in Grip Strength).

The same extensive neuropsychological test battery was administered 12 months after the first examination. On the Cornell Medical Index Health Questionnaire W.B. indicated that he sometimes has severe soaking sweats at night, sweats a great deal even in cold weather, and felt that it was necessary for him to do things slowly in order to avoid mistakes. He had essentially no other complaints and did not notice any residual adverse effects from the head injury.

THE HALSTEAD-REITAN
NEUROPSYCHOLOGICAL TEST BATTERY

Patient __W.B. (II)__ Age __24__ Sex __M__ Education __12__ Handedness __R__

WECHSLER-BELLEVUE SCALE

VIQ	118
PIQ	130
FS IQ	126
Information	12
Comprehension	11
Digit Span	14
Arithmetic	10
Similarities	15
Vocabulary	13
Picture Arrangement	18
Picture Completion	14
Block Design	13
Object Assembly	12
Digit Symbol	16

NEUROPSYCHOLOGICAL DEFICIT SCALE

Level of Performance	5
Pathognomonic Signs	0
Patterns	2
Right-Left Differences	11
Total NDS Score	18

TRAIL MAKING TEST

Part A: __25__ seconds
Part B: __47__ seconds

STRENGTH OF GRIP

Dominant hand: __63.0__ kilograms
Non-dominant hand: __60.0__ kilograms

REITAN-KLØVE TACTILE FORM RECOGNITION TEST

Dominant hand: __8__ seconds; __0__ errors
Non-dominant hand: __8__ seconds; __0__ errors

REITAN-KLØVE SENSORY-PERCEPTUAL EXAM — No errors

Error Totals

RH___LH___	Both H:	RH___LH___	RH___LH___		
RH___LF___	Both H/F:	RH___LF___	RH___LF___		
LH___RF___	Both H/F:	LH___RF___	RF___LH___		
RE___LE___	Both E:	RE___LE___	RE___LE___		
RV___LV___	Both:	RV___LV___	RV___LV___		

TACTILE FINGER RECOGNITION

R 1___2___3___4___5___ R __0__ / 20
L 1___2___3_1_4___5___ L __1__ / 20

FINGER-TIP NUMBER WRITING

R 1_1_2___3___4___5___ R __1__ / 20
L 1_3_2___3___4___5___ L __3__ / 20

HALSTEAD'S NEUROPSYCHOLOGICAL TEST BATTERY

Category Test	17

Tactual Performance Test

Dominant hand:	5.4
Non-dominant hand:	2.4
Both hands:	1.7

Total Time	9.5
Memory	9
Localization	5

Seashore Rhythm Test

Number Correct __25__ 6

Speech-sounds Perception Test

Number of Errors 2

Finger Oscillation Test

Dominant hand:	59	59
Non-dominant hand:	62	

Impairment Index __0.1__

MINNESOTA MULTIPHASIC PERSONALITY INVENTORY

		Hs	47
		D	53
?	50	Hy	58
L	53	Pd	55
F	46	Mf	57
K	61	Pa	56
		Pt	56
		Sc	57
		Ma	68

REITAN-KLØVE LATERAL-DOMINANCE EXAM

Show me how you:

throw a ball	R
hammer a nail	R
cut with a knife	R
turn a door knob	R
use scissors	R
use an eraser	R
write your name	R

Record time used for spontaneous name-writing:

Preferred hand	__7__ seconds
Non-preferred hand	__23__ seconds

Show me how you:

kick a football	R
step on a bug	R

NO APHASIC SYMPTOMS.

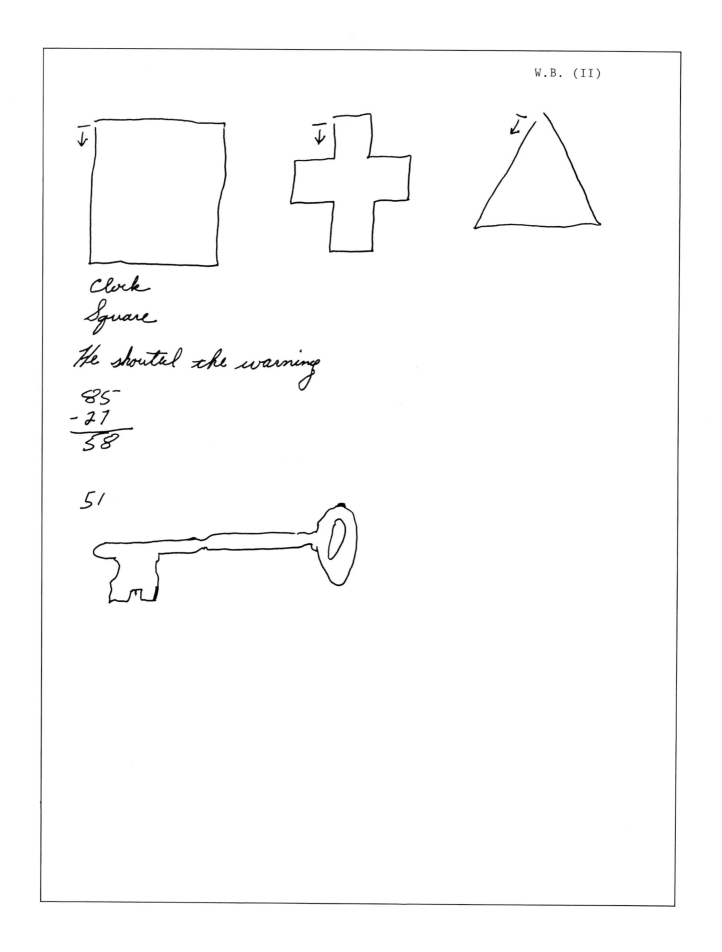

Clerk
Square

He shouted the warning

85
-27

58

51

We will first independently review the findings of the second examination and then compare them with the results of the first examination.

On the second neuropsychological examination W.B. earned IQ values that were well above average, with a Verbal IQ (118) exceeding about 89% of his age peers and a Performance IQ (130) exceeding about 98%. He also performed extremely well on tests in the Halstead-Reitan Battery, earning scores on the four most sensitive indicators well within the normal range. Although the score on the Localization component of the Tactual Performance Test was somewhat low (5), it was still within the range of normal variation. Except for three errors on the left hand in finger-tip number writing perception, the scores for the remaining tests in the Battery were essentially within normal limits.

Despite the generally adequate performances, it should be noted that there were certain variations from normal relationships. Although the Total Time on the Tactual Performance Test was within normal limits, W.B. took somewhat longer with his right hand on the first trial (5.4 min) compared with his left hand on the second trial (2.4 min). Although definitely right-handed, his finger tapping speed was slower with his right hand (59) than his left hand (62). Even though his grip strength with his right upper extremity (63.0 kg) was greater than his left upper extremity (60.0 kg), it was not as much stronger as usually expected. These findings might point toward a very mild degree of left cerebral dysfunction; the greater number of mistakes on the left hand than the right in finger-tip number writing perception might be considered a right cerebral indicator.

Finally, W.B.'s drawing of the key showed a very slight degree of asymmetry of the teeth. Also note the line that he inserted between the teeth; this is sometimes drawn by persons who initially misjudge how wide the space should be.

Considering all of the test results, it is possible that W.B. may have a very mild degree of residual impairment of brain functions, but it would be difficult to conclude that the results deviate significantly from the test findings of normal subjects. The strongest argument for impaired cognitive functioning would probably be derived by contrasting the mild deviations from normality with the excellent performances.

A direct comparison of performances on the two examinations indicates that W.B. performed about comparably, or within expected chance variation, on many of the tests. In some respects it appears that he made genuine improvement. For example, his Performance IQ rose from 118 to 130, with the increment principally due to better scores on Picture Arrangement (11 to 18) and Digit Symbol (11 to 16). These subtests, in addition to Digit Span (which rose from 7 to 14), were the ones that had been noted on the initial examination to possibly indicate impairment.

The patient also showed a definite increase in grip strength (from 51.5 kg to 63.0 kg on the right side and from 50.5 kg to 60.0 kg on the left side); however, the findings on the first examination may have reflected diminished muscular strength due to bedrest following the injury. W.B.'s finger tapping speed was also considerably better, especially in the left hand. Finally, the reduction of errors (from 6 to 2) on the Speech-sounds Perception Test may reflect some genuine improvement.

Many of the test results showed minimal change. On the second examination W.B.'s drawing of the key still showed mild deficiencies similar to the mild deviations from normal expectancy shown on the first examination.

Some of the other tests were performed more poorly on the second examination. On the Wechsler Scale the score on Comprehension fell from 15 to 11; on the Arithmetic subtest it was reduced from 13 to 10. W.B. also performed somewhat worse on the Seashore Rhythm Test (from 27 to 25 correct) and as noted before, had a little more difficulty in finger-tip number writing perception on the left hand.

It would not seem that these changes in test scores relate to any specific hypotheses regarding brain functions, but overall the results would not suggest any striking improvement. It must also be recognized that any expectation of recovery of functions would be limited, because the patient had minimal (if any) impairment on the first examination. Nevertheless, a few of the changes appear to represent genuine improvement.

Some of the apparent improvements in level of performance could scarcely be reflected on the G-NDS because the initial performances were so consistently within the normal range. This observation supports the importance of reliance upon clinical interpretation rather than depending entirely upon the G-NDS score. In addition, however, the section on Right-Left Differences identified some definite changes on the second testing that might have received inadequate emphasis in clinical interpretation. W.B. performed poorly with his right hand compared with his left hand on the TPT and the measurement of grip strength; he performed poorly with his left hand as compared to his right hand in finger-tip number writing perception. The level of performance was still adequate on these measures, but the right-left differences, while noted, may have been slightly attenuated in the clinical interpretation because of the absence of a direct quantitative basis for comparison.

W.B. was re-examined 18 months after the initial testing. He indicated that he had experienced no problems and there had been no changes since the previous examination.

Although positive practice-effect may have influenced the test results to some extent, the scores on the third examination generally fall within normal limits. W.B. continued to demonstrate that his general intelligence was well above average, earning a Verbal IQ (120) just within the lower limits of the Superior range and a Performance IQ (136) in the Superior range. Except for the relatively low Arithmetic (10) and Digit Span (10) scores, the individual subtests of the Wechsler Scale did not show any significant variability. From the results on the Wechsler Scale one would not infer that this man had sustained any significant cerebral damage.

The patient also performed quite well on the four most sensitive indicators, each having a score within the normal range. Other tests in the Battery were also done well. By his scores on the Speech-sounds Perception Test (5 errors) and the Seashore Rhythm Test (25 correct) W. B. demonstrated adequate alertness to specific stimulus material and an ability to concentrate over time. His finger tapping speed was above the average level and most of the sensory-perceptual measures had no errors.

Nevertheless, there were certain findings that were distinctly deviant and hardly ever occur in persons with entirely normal brains. The most outstanding deviation is the fact that on finger-tip number writing perception W.B. made no errors on his left hand and made five mistakes on his right hand. Even though definitely right-handed, his grip strength was scarcely greater in his right upper extremity (57.0 kg) than his left (56.0 kg). His finger tapping speed with the right hand (65) was not as much faster as would normally be expected when compared with the left hand (62).

Finally, W.B. totally omitted the "Q" in his initial attempt to write SQUARE. This error is difficult to understand without inferring at least some temporary degree of left cerebral dysfunction. The examiner noticed the patient's surprise when he made this mistake; W.B. immediately started to write the word again and completed it satisfactorily. One would certainly not label this subject as "aphasic" because of this single mistake, but it did represent an error in dealing with simple language material that is hardly ever seen among normal subjects. This is not to say that a person with a normal brain may not make occasional errors in verbal communication; however, under the controlled circumstances in which the Aphasia

THE HALSTEAD-REITAN
NEUROPSYCHOLOGICAL TEST BATTERY

Patient **W.B. (III)** Age **24** Sex **M** Education **12** Handedness **R**

WECHSLER-BELLEVUE SCALE

VIQ	120
PIQ	136
FS IQ	129
Information	13
Comprehension	15
Digit Span	10
Arithmetic	10
Similarities	16
Vocabulary	14
Picture Arrangement	14
Picture Completion	15
Block Design	15
Object Assembly	15
Digit Symbol	16

NEUROPSYCHOLOGICAL DEFICIT SCALE

Level of Performance	5
Pathognomonic Signs	0
Patterns	2
Right-Left Differences	7
Total NDS Score	14

TRAIL MAKING TEST

Part A: **19** seconds
Part B: **39** seconds

STRENGTH OF GRIP

Dominant hand: **57.0** kilograms
Non-dominant hand: **56.0** kilograms

REITAN-KLØVE TACTILE FORM RECOGNITION TEST

Dominant hand: **9** seconds; **0** errors
Non-dominant hand: **8** seconds; **0** errors

REITAN-KLØVE SENSORY-PERCEPTUAL EXAM — No errors

					Error Totals		
RH___ LH___	Both H:	RH___ LH___		RH___ LH___	
RH___ LF___	Both H/F:	RH___ LF___		RH___ LF___	
LH___ RF___	Both H/F:	LH___ RF___		RF___ LH___	
RE___ LE___	Both E:	RE___ LE___		RE___ LE___	
RV___ LV___	Both:	RV___ LV___		RV___ LV___	

TACTILE FINGER RECOGNITION

R 1___ 2___ 3___ 4___ 5___ R **0** / 20
L 1___ 2___ 3___ 4 **1** 5___ L **1** / 20

FINGER-TIP NUMBER WRITING

R 1 **1** 2___ 3 **1** 4 **1** 5 **2** R **5** / 20
L 1___ 2___ 3___ 4___ 5___ L **0** / 20

HALSTEAD'S NEUROPSYCHOLOGICAL TEST BATTERY

Category Test		17

Tactual Performance Test

Dominant hand:	4.7	
Non-dominant hand:	3.4	
Both hands:	1.5	
	Total Time	9.6
	Memory	9
	Localization	6

Seashore Rhythm Test

Number Correct **25**   **6**

Speech-sounds Perception Test

Number of Errors   **5**

Finger Oscillation Test

Dominant hand: **65**   **65**
Non-dominant hand: **62**

Impairment Index   **0.1**

MINNESOTA MULTIPHASIC PERSONALITY INVENTORY

			Hs	52
			D	44
?	50		Hy	51
L	50		Pd	48
F	48		Mf	55
K	59		Pa	53
			Pt	40
			Sc	48
			Ma	55

REITAN-KLØVE LATERAL-DOMINANCE EXAM

Show me how you:

throw a ball	R
hammer a nail	R
cut with a knife	R
turn a door knob	R
use scissors	R
use an eraser	R
write your name	R

Record time used for spontaneous name-writing:

Preferred hand	**8** seconds
Non-preferred hand	**20** seconds

Show me how you:

kick a football	R
step on a bug	R

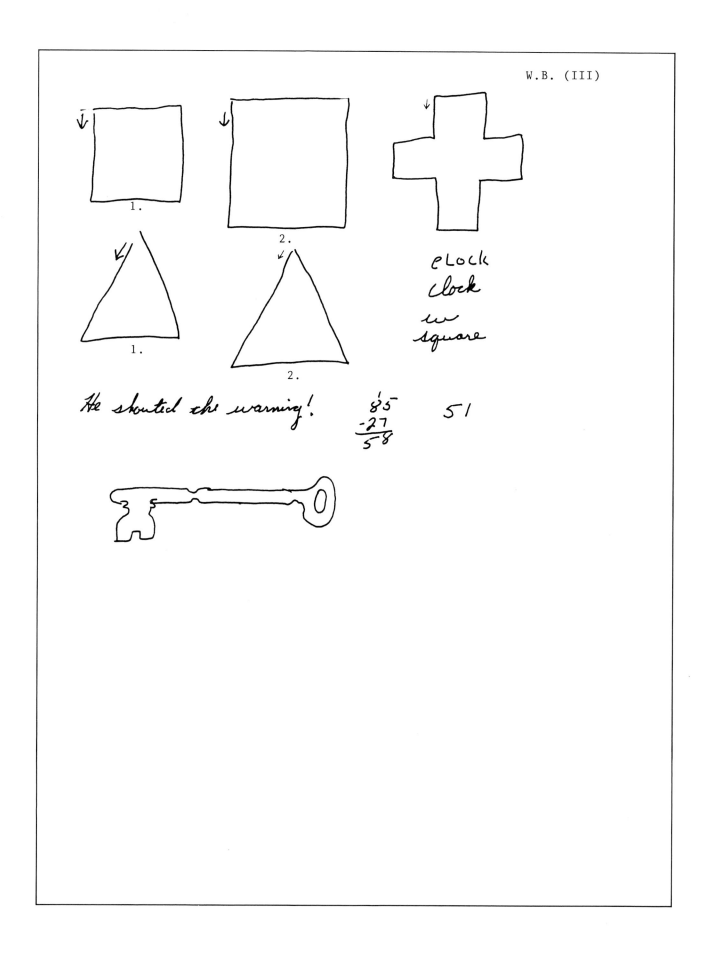

1.

2.

1.

2.

cLock
clock
in
square

He shouted the warning!

$$85$$
$$-27$$
$$58$$

51

Screening Test is administered, hundreds of control subjects (many who were less intelligent than this man) have *never* made this particular mistake.

In summary, mild lateralized signs of primary motor dysfunction were present, at least in the context of comparing the two sides of the subject's own body. A striking deficit was present on the right side in a tactile-receptive function (finger-tip number writing perception) and W.B. made one error dealing with a simple language performance. Even though he performed extremely well on most of the tests, the configuration of W.B.'s results would be sufficient to postulate some type of left cerebral dysfunction.

There is no way to determine whether these deviant results were an eventual manifestation of the head injury sustained 18 months earlier. It is possible, of course, that some other type of lesion was responsible for the present findings. The overall test results are not suggestive of a developing lesion; however, they would be compatible with a relatively discrete, stabilized area of dysfunction in the left cerebral hemisphere. It is entirely possible that the head injury sustained 18 months earlier caused the type of deterioration of brain functions demonstrated at the present examination.

Direct comparisons of the 12-month and 18-month examination results show that there were certain changes, but in most respects the findings were comparable. Even though some substantial changes occurred on individual Performance subtests, some of the scores were better and some were worse, yielding a net gain of six points on the Performance IQ. W.B. did not perform quite as well on the Speech-sounds Perception Test as he had previously (5 errors compared with 2 errors). His finger tapping speed was somewhat faster on the third examination, but his grip strength was mildly reduced. While finger tapping had been a stronger left cerebral indicator on the second examination, grip strength was predominant in this respect on the third examination. The major change, without question, was on finger-tip number writing perception. On the second examination, W.B. made more errors with his left hand; on the third examination he performed perfectly with the left hand and made five errors in 20 trials with the right hand.

It is entirely possible that the complexity of brain-behavior relationships is so great that variability will appear from one examination to another. Even though abnormal results occur (and perhaps be unreliable in a statistical sense), they may still have clinical validity. In this case, for example, it is worth noting that although details of the test results changed from the second to the third testing, both sets of results principally implicated left cerebral hemisphere dysfunction in the context of generally excellent performances.

The G-NDS score continued to be very similar to the score obtained on the 12-month examination, with most scores falling in the normal range except for the differences in performances with the right and left hands noted above. It is apparent that the G-NDS provides a useful guide to use in conjunction with clinical interpretation.

Case #14

Name: T.J.

Age: 21

Education: 14

Sex: Male

Handedness: Right

Occupation: Student

Background Information

T.J. was a junior in college majoring in economics. One day, while riding his bicycle to class, a truck pulled out in front of him and he fell to the side to avoid going under a wheel of the truck. An emergency unit arrived within minutes and found him to be generally alert and walking about, but mildly confused and disoriented. He had extensive abrasions on the right side of his face and complained of shortness of breath and chest pain. He was brought immediately to the emergency room of a medical center and was hospitalized after an initial examination was performed. At the time of examination in the emergency room T.J. was fully alert and oriented and remembered the accident and being brought to the hospital.

Neurological Examination

The neurological examination initially performed in the emergency room appeared to be within normal limits; however, a more comprehensive medical examination revealed a focal area of bleeding in the left retina (resulting in decreased vision), a right pneumohemothorax, a fracture of the right clavicle, and a small basilar skull fracture. T.J. had a deep, irregular laceration that exposed the bone over the lateral portion of the right eyebrow. The right external auditory canal was occluded with bright red blood and the left tympanic membrane had an accumulation of blood behind it. An electroencephalogram done seven days after the injury demonstrated moderate generalized abnormalities more prominent in the left cerebral

hemisphere than the right. T.J. made normal progress and had no complications during his hospitalization. Physical examination also revealed that he had congenital atrophy of the muscles of the right shoulder girdle and right arm.

Neuropsychological Examination

Neuropsychological examination was done 19 days after the injury. An EEG was repeated at that time and showed moderate improvement even though slight generalized disturbances were still present. The neurological examination was within normal limits except for a pericentral scotoma of the left visual field that resulted from the retinal damage.

Three weeks after the injury T.J. had returned to school, was making adequate progress, and had no complaints regarding his injury. On the Cornell Medical Index Health Questionnaire he indicated that he gets out of breath long before anyone else, has difficulty sleeping and gets completely mixed up when he is required to do things quickly. It is important to note, however, that the patient said that he would have given these same answers before the injury.

The test findings indicate that T.J. has abilities that clearly exceed those of the average person. He earned a Verbal IQ (129) that fell in the Superior range (exceeding about 97% of his age peers) and a Performance IQ that was seven points lower (122) but also in the Superior range (exceeding 93%). A question could be raised about whether the patient

THE HALSTEAD-REITAN
NEUROPSYCHOLOGICAL TEST BATTERY

Patient **T.J. (I)** Age **21** Sex **M** Education **14** Handedness **R**

WECHSLER-BELLEVUE SCALE

VIQ	129
PIQ	122
FS IQ	128
Information	14
Comprehension	14
Digit Span	10
Arithmetic	16
Similarities	17
Vocabulary	12
Picture Arrangement	14
Picture Completion	15
Block Design	14
Object Assembly	13
Digit Symbol	11

NEUROPSYCHOLOGICAL DEFICIT SCALE

Level of Performance	7
Pathognomonic Signs	0
Patterns	1
Right-Left Differences	8
Total NDS Score	16

HALSTEAD'S NEUROPSYCHOLOGICAL TEST BATTERY

Category Test 7

Tactual Performance Test

Dominant hand:	7.3
Non-dominant hand:	2.1
Both hands:	1.3

Total Time	10.7
Memory	7
Localization	4

Seashore Rhythm Test

Number Correct **29** 1

Speech-sounds Perception Test

Number of Errors 2

Finger Oscillation Test

Dominant hand:	53	53
Non-dominant hand:	43	

Impairment Index 0.1

TRAIL MAKING TEST

Part A: **26** seconds
Part B: **58** seconds

STRENGTH OF GRIP

Dominant hand: **29.5** kilograms
Non-dominant hand: **40.0** kilograms

REITAN-KLØVE TACTILE FORM RECOGNITION TEST

Dominant hand: **8** seconds; **0** errors
Non-dominant hand: **8** seconds; **0** errors

REITAN-KLØVE SENSORY-PERCEPTUAL EXAM — No errors

Error Totals

RH___ LH___	Both H:	RH___ LH___	RH___ LH___	
RH___ LF___	Both H/F:	RH___ LF___	RH___ LF___	
LH___ RF___	Both H/F:	LH___ RF___	RF___ LH___	
RE___ LE___	Both E:	RE___ LE___	RE___ LE___	
RV___ LV___	Both:	RV___ LV___	RV___ LV___	

TACTILE FINGER RECOGNITION

R 1___ 2___ 3___ 4___ 5___ R **0** / **20**
L 1___ 2___ 3___ 4___ 5___ L **0** / **20**

FINGER-TIP NUMBER WRITING

R 1___ 2___ 3___ 4___ 5___ R **0** / **20**
L 1___ 2___ 3___ 4___ 5___ L **0** / **20**

MINNESOTA MULTIPHASIC PERSONALITY INVENTORY

		Hs	54
		D	53
?	50	Hy	47
L	46	Pd	46
F	55	Mf	65
K	55	Pa	38
		Pt	54
		Sc	51
		Ma	65

REITAN-KLØVE LATERAL-DOMINANCE EXAM

Show me how you:

throw a ball	L
hammer a nail	L
cut with a knife	R
turn a door knob	R
use scissors	R
use an eraser	R
write your name	R

Record time used for spontaneous name-writing:

Preferred hand	**7** seconds
Non-preferred hand	**21** seconds

Show me how you:

kick a football	R
step on a bug	R

NO APHASIC SYMPTOMS.

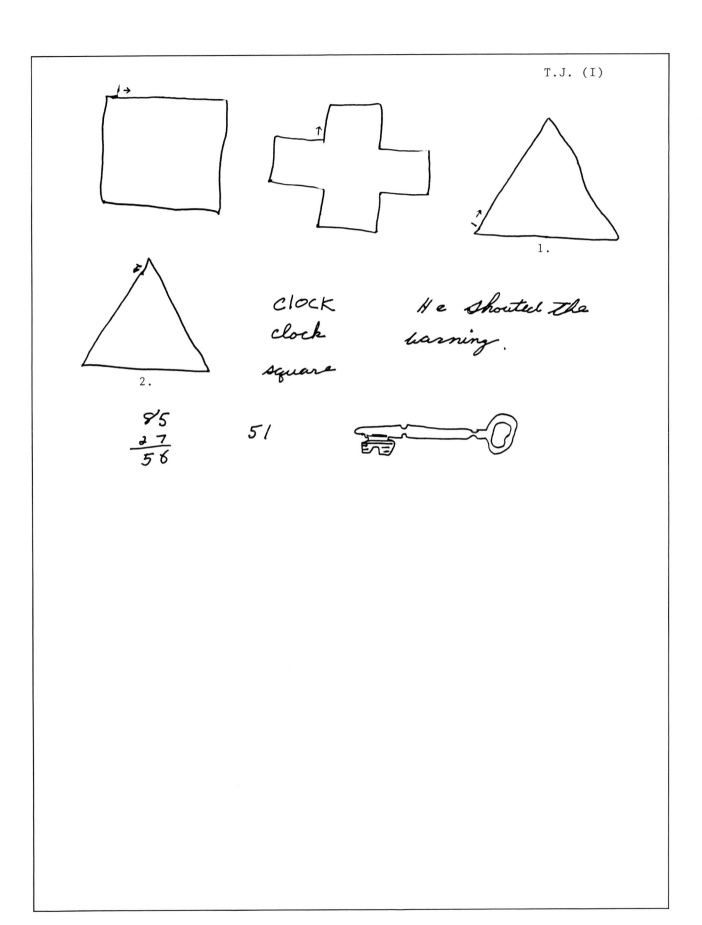

1.

2.

clock
clock
square

He shouted the
warning.

85
27
56

51

had experienced some impairment on the Digit Span subtest (10), since it was the lowest of the Verbal subtests. Similarly, Digit Symbol (11) was the lowest of the Performance subtests. Based on results from the Wechsler Scale alone, it would be difficult to conclude that this patient had experienced any significant impairment; the distribution of subtest results might have reflected only chance variation.

Except for a somewhat low score (4) on the Localization component of the Tactual Performance Test, T.J. performed very well on the four most sensitive indicators in the Halstead-Reitan Battery. There is no doubt that he has excellent attentional capabilities and is able to concentrate on specific stimuli over time: he made only two errors on the Speech-sounds Perception Test and one error on the Seashore Rhythm Test. He performed quite well on tasks that involve visual-spatial analysis and organization (Block Design, 14; Tactual Performance Test — Total Time, 10.7 min). He also did very well on tests that required abstraction, reasoning, logical analysis and flexibility in thought processes (Category Test, 7 errors; Trail Making Test — Part B, 58 sec). Thus, in terms of level of performance, it would appear that T.J. performed well within the normal range and considerably better than the average subject. These observations were confirmed by the Level of Performance section (with a score of 7) and the total G-NDS score (16).

Nevertheless, note that there are some test results which definitely deviated from normal expectancy. On the Tactual Performance Test he performed poorly with the right upper extremity (7.3 min) compared with the left (2.1 min), and on grip strength he was weaker on his right side (29.5 kg) than on his left (40.0 kg). It is important to note that T.J. showed no evidence of dysphasia and performed extremely well on the Speech-sounds Perception Test. These findings, concerned with verbal functions, were reinforced by a Verbal IQ that fell well into the Superior range. It would

be necessary, then, to question whether the lateralized motor deficits on the right side were due to damage of the left cerebral hemisphere or some other factor. As indicated above, this patient had had a congenital condition of atrophy of the muscles of the right shoulder girdle and right arm; in all probability, then, these deficits would be attributable to peripheral rather than central cerebral damage.

Test results that reflect the status of the right cerebral hemisphere were also generally within normal limits. T.J. was somewhat slow in finger tapping speed with his left hand (43) compared with his right (53), but his drawings were fairly adequate and he showed no specific deficits on either the Performance subtests or other lateralizing procedures (such as the tests of bilateral simultaneous sensory stimulation, finger recognition, or finger-tip number writing perception). The only lateralizing finding that was not easily explained is the somewhat slow finger tapping speed with the non-preferred (left) hand. Considered by itself, though, this result would be insufficient to use as a basis for confident implication of the right cerebral hemisphere. The section of the G-NDS concerned with Right-Left Differences yielded a score of 8 (as compared to an average score of 3.37 for control subjects). This finding underscores the importance of assessing differences on the two sides of the body with relation to patterns of higher-level functions in determining whether the findings are due to peripheral or central limitations.

Based on a complete evaluation of the test results, the overall conclusion would be that T.J. had superior general intelligence, excellent adaptive abilities across a broad range of brain-related measures, and no significant evidence of cerebral disease or damage. Results on the Minnesota Multiphasic Personality Inventory were also essentially within the normal range.

A neurological examination was administered three months after the first neuropsychological testing, and except for a continued manifestation of a pericentral scotoma in the left visual field, the results were essentially normal. An EEG done at this time continued to demonstrate mild generalized disturbances, although the neurologist felt that it may have shown some slight improvement over the previous tracings.

Twelve months after the first testing T.J. was re-examined. At this time the results of the neurological examination continued to be essentially normal (except for the visual field loss) and the EEG showed a slight decrease of abnormalities. The patient continued to attend college, make satisfactory progress, and did not feel that the head injury had caused him any significant impairment. On the Cornell Medical Index Health Questionnaire his only complaints were that his work tended to fall to pieces when a superior was watching him, that it was difficult for him to make up his mind, and that he was easily upset by criticism. Despite these rather minimal responses to direct questions concerning aspects of emotional and affective adjustment, the patient had begun to see a psychiatrist because of personal problems in his life.

A review of the test results of the second neuropsychological examination indicates that T.J. continued to perform very well. His Verbal IQ (127) was essentially similar to his score on the first testing, but his Performance IQ (135) increased 13 points. He performed quite adequately on the four most sensitive measures in the Halstead-Reitan Battery, with only the finger tapping score (49) of the right (preferred) hand contributing to the Impairment Index of 0.1. Note, though, that even this score was nearly within normal limits. The patient continued to perform very well on tests that required attention to specific stimulus material (Seashore Rhythm Test, 28 correct and Speech-sounds Perception Test, 1 error).

Lateralizing indicators yielded certain results that reflected dysfunction of the right upper extremity. Grip strength was distinctly reduced in the right upper extremity (35.5 kg) compared with the left (47.0), and finger tapping speed was just a little slower with the right hand (49) than with the left (50). On the Tactual Performance Test T.J. performed somewhat poorly with the right hand (3.6 min) compared with the left (1.9 min). Again, we would presume that these indications of motor dysfunction were related to the congenital atrophy of muscle groups that affected the right upper extremity.

A direct comparison of the results obtained on the initial testing and 12-month examination showed certain changes that appeared to go beyond chance variation. The subject's Verbal IQ remained almost the same, but the score on the Comprehension subtest increased from 14 to 17 and was counterbalanced by a change in the opposite direction on the Similarities subtest (from 17 to 14). On the Performance subtests the major changes were on Picture Arrangement (from 14 to 17) and Digit Symbol (from 11 to 15). These may have been genuine instances of improvement that extend beyond the improvements expected from positive practice-effects.

T.J. also performed better on the Total Time measure of the Tactual Performance Test (from 10.7 min to 7.5 min), a change due principally to an improved performance with the right upper extremity (from 7.3 min to 3.6 min). We had initially been inclined to attribute the relatively poor performance with the right hand on the first trial to peripheral involvement; retrospectively, though, these results suggest that T.J. may have had some impairment of left cerebral functions that was also a contributing factor. The improvement on the Localization component of the TPT (from 4 to 6) may also have reflected genuine improvement of brain functions. The Level of Performance section of the G-NDS had decreased from 7 to 4 points.

The patient showed an unusual change in hand preference. At the time of the first examination he used his right hand to turn a door knob and to manipulate a pair of scissors. However, on the

THE HALSTEAD-REITAN
NEUROPSYCHOLOGICAL TEST BATTERY

Patient **T.J. (II)**   Age **22**   Sex **M**   Education **15**   Handedness **R**

WECHSLER-BELLEVUE SCALE

VIQ	127
PIQ	135
FS IQ	134
Information	13
Comprehension	17
Digit Span	11
Arithmetic	15
Similarities	14
Vocabulary	12
Picture Arrangement	17
Picture Completion	14
Block Design	15
Object Assembly	15
Digit Symbol	15

NEUROPSYCHOLOGICAL DEFICIT SCALE

Level of Performance	4
Pathognomonic Signs	0
Patterns	1
Right-Left Differences	7
Total NDS Score	12

HALSTEAD'S NEUROPSYCHOLOGICAL TEST BATTERY

Category Test   **4**

Tactual Performance Test

Dominant hand:	3.6	
Non-dominant hand:	1.9	
Both hands:	2.0	
	Total Time	7.5
	Memory	7
	Localization	6

Seashore Rhythm Test

Number Correct   28   **2**

Speech-sounds Perception Test

Number of Errors   **1**

Finger Oscillation Test

Dominant hand:	49	49
Non-dominant hand:	50	

Impairment Index   **0.1**

TRAIL MAKING TEST

Part A: **19** seconds
Part B: **63** seconds

STRENGTH OF GRIP

Dominant hand: **35.5**   kilograms
Non-dominant hand: **47.0**   kilograms

REITAN-KLØVE TACTILE FORM RECOGNITION TEST

Dominant hand: **5**   seconds;   **0**   errors
Non-dominant hand: **5**   seconds;   **0**   errors

MINNESOTA MULTIPHASIC PERSONALITY INVENTORY

		Hs	44
		D	77
?	50	Hy	48
L	53	Pd	60
F	62	Mf	61
K	53	Pa	56
		Pt	62
		Sc	53
		Ma	55

REITAN-KLØVE SENSORY-PERCEPTUAL EXAM — No errors

Error Totals

RH___ LH___	Both H:	RH___ LH___		RH___ LH___			
RH___ LF___	Both H/F:	RH___ LF___		RH___ LF___			
LH___ RF___	Both H/F:	LH___ RF___		RF___ LH___			
RE___ LE___	Both E:	RE___ LE___		RE___ LE___			
RV___ LV___	Both:	RV___ LV___		RV___ LV___			

REITAN-KLØVE LATERAL-DOMINANCE EXAM

Show me how you:
throw a ball	L
hammer a nail	L
cut with a knife	R
turn a door knob	L
use scissors	L
use an eraser	R
write your name	R

Record time used for spontaneous name-writing:
Preferred hand	**6** seconds
Non-preferred hand	**20** seconds

Show me how you:
kick a football	R
step on a bug	R

TACTILE FINGER RECOGNITION

R 1___ 2___ 3___ 4___ 5___   R **0** / **20**
L 1___ 2___ 3___ 4___ 5___   L **0** / **20**

FINGER-TIP NUMBER WRITING

R 1___ 2___ 3___ 4___ 5___   R **0** / **20**
L 1___ 2___ 3___ 4___ 5___   L **0** / **20**

NO APHASIC SYMPTOMS.

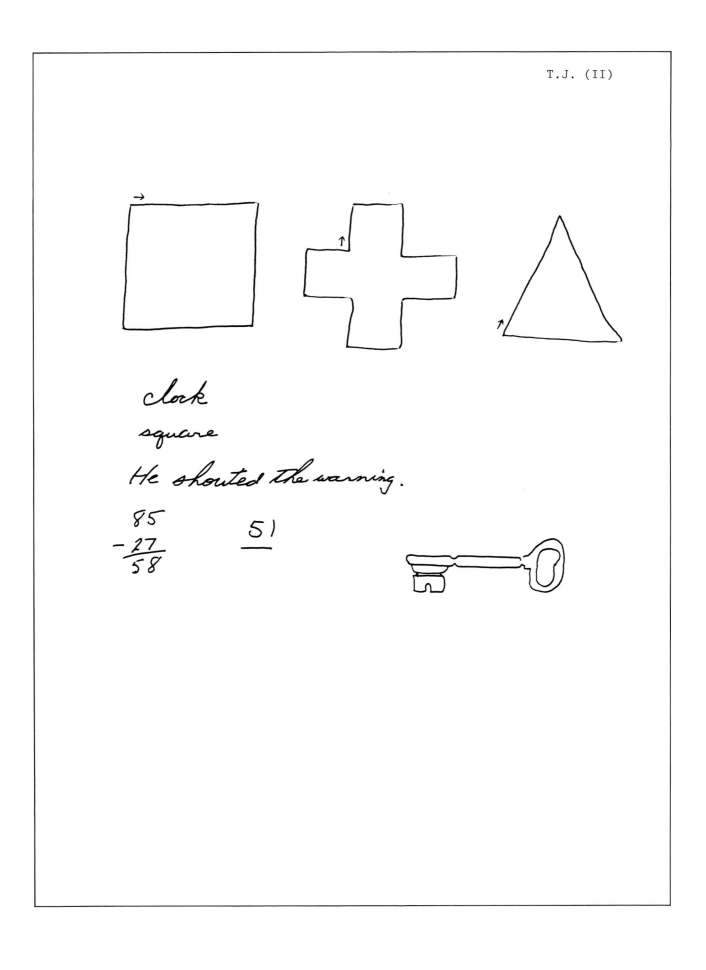

clock

square

He shouted the warning.

$$\begin{array}{r} 85 \\ -27 \\ \hline 58 \end{array}$$

$$\underline{51}$$

present examination (in contrast to the consistency that is usually shown by most persons), he now did these tasks with his left hand. There appears no doubt that this man showed a degree of ambidexterity on the measures of unimanual preference that is rarely seen. In all probability T.J.'s tendency toward left handedness has resulted from congenital atrophy of the muscles involved in the use of the right upper extremity.

On the 12-month examination T.J.'s grip strength was somewhat greater with both the right and left upper extremities (although the disparity indicating impairment of the right upper extremity was still present). Very possibly the lower grip strength results shown on the original examination were due to the fact that the patient was tested only four days after his discharge from the hospital, where he had been essentially bedridden for about two weeks. Limitation of normal activity often leads to a rather significant decrement in muscular strength.

It should be remembered that finger tapping speed is not as much affected by inactivity as muscle strength. On the second examination T.J. showed a mild decrease in finger tapping speed with his right hand and a more pronounced increase with his left hand, and these results are more consistent with expectancy in terms of the other indications of right-sided peripheral dysfunction. The improvement with the left hand, however, may have been representative of spontaneous recovery. The section on Right-Left Differences of the G-NDS stayed almost the same (8 as compared with 7 points).

The patient's drawings of simple geometric figures were within normal limits and no other indications of right cerebral dysfunction were present on the 12-month test results.

Perhaps the most outstanding change in the test results was the increase on the Depression scale of the Minnesota Multiphasic Personality Inventory (from 53 to 77). Personal circumstances were probably responsible for this change and, as noted above, T.J. was being treated psychiatrically because of the problems he was experiencing.

In summary, it would appear that during the interval between the first and second examinations T.J.'s brain-related abilities had shown some degree of improvement over and beyond expected positive practice-effects. Even though the results of the first examination had not been sufficient to support a conclusion of significant impairment, comparison of the two sets of findings does in fact suggest that a mild degree of deficit had been present shortly following the head injury.

T.J. was re-examined 18 months after the original testing. At this time his neurological examination continued to be essentially normal except for an apparently permanent scotoma in the left visual field. Electroencephalographic recordings showed slight abnormalities over the frontal-temporal areas of both cerebral hemispheres, but comparisons with the 12-month EEG showed some improvement.

At this time T.J. had no complaints which he felt were attributable to the head injury. However, on the Cornell Medical Index Health Questionnaire he continued to give responses which were similar to those given at the previous examination. He felt that his work fell to pieces under pressure, that he easily got mixed up in his thinking when he had to do things quickly, and that he was indecisive and upset by criticism. In addition, he indicated that he was a very shy and sensitive person and tended to feel sad and alone at social functions when others were having a good time. During this time T.J. was still being treated by a psychiatrist.

The neuropsychological test results obtained 18 months after the injury were well within the normal range except for somewhat slow finger tapping speed and reduced grip strength in the right upper extremity compared with the left. T.J. continued to have both Verbal (126) and Performance (129) IQ values that fell in the Superior range and he performed quite satisfactorily on the four most sensitive measures in the Halstead-Reitan Battery.

THE HALSTEAD-REITAN
NEUROPSYCHOLOGICAL TEST BATTERY

Patient **T.J. (III)** Age **23** Sex **M** Education **16** Handedness **R**

WECHSLER-BELLEVUE SCALE

VIQ	126
PIQ	129
FS IQ	131
Information	13
Comprehension	13
Digit Span	13
Arithmetic	15
Similarities	15
Vocabulary	13
Picture Arrangement	13
Picture Completion	15
Block Design	16
Object Assembly	15
Digit Symbol	13

NEUROPSYCHOLOGICAL DEFICIT SCALE

Level of Performance	3
Pathognomonic Signs	0
Patterns	0
Right-Left Differences	8
Total NDS Score	11

TRAIL MAKING TEST

Part A: **19** seconds
Part B: **65** seconds

STRENGTH OF GRIP

Dominant hand: **37.5** kilograms
Non-dominant hand: **50.0** kilograms

REITAN-KLØVE TACTILE FORM RECOGNITION TEST

Dominant hand: **8** seconds; **0** errors
Non-dominant hand: **8** seconds; **0** errors

REITAN-KLØVE SENSORY-PERCEPTUAL EXAM — No errors

Error Totals

			Error Totals	
RH___ LH___	Both H: RH___ LH___	RH___ LH___		
RH___ LF___	Both H/F: RH___ LF___	RH___ LF___		
LH___ RF___	Both H/F: LH___ RF___	RF___ LH___		
RE___ LE___	Both E: RE___ LE___	RE___ LE___		
RV___ LV___	Both: RV___ LV___	RV___ LV___		
___ ___	___ ___			
___ ___	___ ___			

TACTILE FINGER RECOGNITION

R 1___ 2___ 3___ 4___ 5___ R **0** / **20**
L 1___ 2___ 3___ 4___ 5___ L **0** / **20**

FINGER-TIP NUMBER WRITING

R 1 **1** 2___ 3___ 4___ 5___ R **1** / **20**
L 1___ 2___ 3___ 4___ 5___ L **0** / **20**

NO APHASIC SYMPTOMS.

HALSTEAD'S NEUROPSYCHOLOGICAL TEST BATTERY

Category Test	7

Tactual Performance Test

Dominant hand:	2.5	
Non-dominant hand:	2.0	
Both hands:	2.0	
	Total Time	6.5
	Memory	9
	Localization	5

Seashore Rhythm Test

Number Correct	29	1

Speech-sounds Perception Test

Number of Errors		2

Finger Oscillation Test

Dominant hand:	51	51
Non-dominant hand:	55	

Impairment Index **0.0**

MINNESOTA MULTIPHASIC PERSONALITY INVENTORY

		Hs	47
		D	70
?	50	Hy	49
L	60	Pd	53
F	60	Mf	65
K	57	Pa	53
		Pt	62
		Sc	59
		Ma	55

REITAN-KLØVE LATERAL-DOMINANCE EXAM

Show me how you:
throw a ball	_____
hammer a nail	_____
cut with a knife	_____
turn a door knob	_____
use scissors	_____
use an eraser	_____
write your name	_____

NOT DONE

Record time used for spontaneous name-writing:
Preferred hand **6** seconds
Non-preferred hand **17** seconds

Show me how you:
kick a football	**R**
step on a bug	**R**

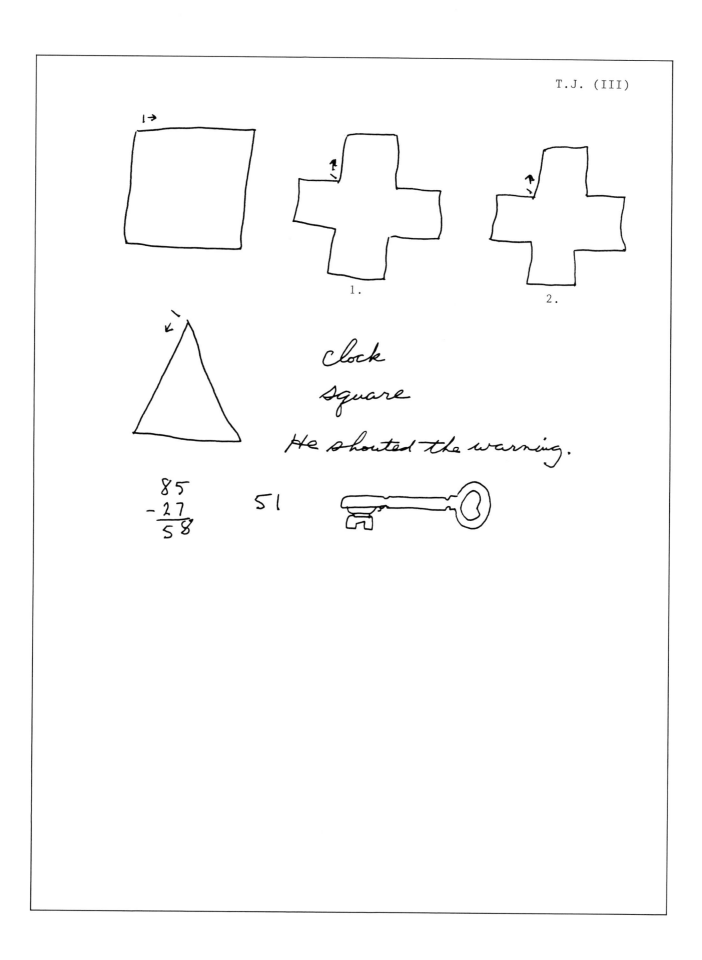

1.

2.

clock

square

He shouted the warning.

85
−27
58

51

In fact, his overall performance was at the average level or above on essentially all tests. His G-NDS score was only 11, even though the section on Right-Left Differences contributed 8 points. He showed no specific signs of cerebral damage and the patterns and relationships of higher-level intellectual and cognitive functions were well within normal limits. As mentioned above, the only deviation from normal expectancy related to finger tapping speed and grip strength of the right upper extremity.

Direct comparisons of the 12-month testing and the 18-month examination is of some interest. T.J.'s Performance IQ dropped from 135 to 129, largely due to a substantial decrease on the Picture Arrangement subtest (from 17 to 13). The patient also showed a comparable decrease on the Comprehension subtest (from 17 to 13). It appears unlikely that these changes are attributable to any progressive deterioration of brain functions; the rest of the test results do not support such an interpretation. In fact, T.J. showed some improvement on the measures that are particularly sensitive to cerebral functions. His performance with the right hand on the Tactual Performance Test was reduced from 3.6 min to 2.5 min; his finger tapping speed was increased slightly on both hands (especially on the left); and his grip strength was also somewhat greater on both sides. The improvement of finger tapping speed with the left hand, which showed a progressive pattern over the three testings (43, 50, and 55), certainly suggests (retrospectively) that the initial measurement showed some degree of impairment. T.J. continued to have an elevated score on the Depression scale of the MMPI. We should note that indicators of affective disturbance of this kind do not appear clinically to affect the neuropsychological test results nor to influence interpretation of neuropsychological data with respect to brain-behavior relationships (Dikmen & Reitan, 1977b).

In summary, it would appear that T.J. showed evidence of spontaneous recovery, even though the initial results were indicative only of mild impairment and considered by themselves were scarcely sufficient to conclude that the patient had any neuropsychological deficits. It would seem probable, however, that the results of the 18-month examination reflected minimal (if any) deficits and that the patient had essentially made a complete recovery.

REFERENCES

Adamovich, B.B., Henderson, J.A., & Auerbach, S. (1985). *Cognitive rehabilitation of closed head injured patients: A dynamic approach.* Boston: College Hill Press.

Adams, J.H., Mitchell, D.E., Graham, D.I., & Doyle, D. (1977). Diffuse brain damage of immediate impact type. Its relationship to "primary brain stem damage" in head injury. *Brain, 100,* 489-502.

Adams, J.H. (1975). The neuropathology of head injuries. In P.J. Vinken & G.S. Bruyn (Eds.), *Handbook of clinical neurology. Vol. 23.* Amsterdam: North Holland Publishing Co.

Adams, K.M., & Brown, G.C. (1986). The role of the computer in neuropsychological assessment. In I. Grant & K.M. Adams (Eds.), *Neuropsychological assessment of neuropsychiatric disorders.* New York: Oxford University Press.

Adams, K.M., & Heaton, R.K. (1985). Automated interpretation of neuropsychological test data. *Journal of Consulting and Clinical Psychology, 53,* 790–802.

Aita, J.A., Armitage, S.G., Reitan, R.M., & Rabinovitz, A. (1947). The use of certain psychological tests in the evaluation of brain injury. *Journal of General Psychology, 37,* 25–44.

Aita, J.A., & Reitan, R.M. (1948). Psychotic reactions in late recovery period following brain injury. *American Journal of Psychiatry, 105,* 161–169.

Aita, J.A., Reitan, R.M., & Ruth, J.M. (1947). Rorschach's Test as a diagnostic aid in brain injury. *American Journal of Psychiatry, 103,* 770–779.

Alfano, D.P., & Finlayson, M.A.J. (1987). Clinical neuropsychology in rehabilitation. *The Clinical Neuropsychologist, 1,* 105–123.

Alfano, A.M., & Meyerink, L.H. (1986). Cognitive retraining with brain-injured adults. *VA Practitioner, 12,* 13.

Alves, W.M., & Jane, J.A. (1985). Mild brain injury: Damage and outcome. In D.P. Becker & J.T. Povlishock (Eds.), *Central nervous system trauma status report 1985.* Prepared for the National Institute of Neurological and Communicative Disorders and Stroke, National Institutes of Health.

Anderson, A.L. (1950). The effect of laterality localization of damage on Wechsler-Bellevue indices of deterioration. *Journal of Clinical Psychology, 6,* 191-194.

Angle, H.V., Ellinwood, E.H., & Carroll, J. (1978). Computer interview problem assessment of psychiatric patients. In F.H. Orthner (Ed.), *Proceedings: The Second Annual Symposium on Computer Application in Medical Care* (pp. 137–148). Washington, DC: Institute of Electrical and Electronics Engineers.

Angle, H.V., Ellinwood, E.H., Hay, W.M., Johnsen, T., & Hay, L.R. (1977). Computer-aided interviewing in comprehensive behavioral assessment. *Behavior Therapy 8,* 747–754.

Bach-y-Rita, P. (Ed.). (1980). *Recovery of function: Theoretical considerations for brain injury rehabilitation.* Bern: Hans Huber Publishers.

Bakker, D.J. (1973). Hemispheric specialization and stages in the learning to read process. *Bulletin of the Orton Society, 23,* 15–27.

Bakker, D.J. (1979). Hemispheric differences and reading strategies: Two dyslexias? *Bulletin of the Orton Society, 29,* 84–100.

Bakker, D.J. (1982a). Cerebral lateralization and reading proficiency. In Y. Lebrun & O. Zangwill (Eds.), *Lateralisation of language in the child.* Lisse: Swets and Zeitlinger.

Bakker, D.J. (1982b). Hemisphere-specific dyslexia models. In R.N. Malatesha, & L.C. Hartlage (Eds.), *Neuropsychology and cognition. Volume 1.* The Hague: Martinus Nijhoff.

Bakker, D.J. (1983). Hemispheric specialization and specific reading retardation. In M. Rutter (Ed.), *Developmental neuropsychiatry.* New York: Guilford.

Barth, J.T., & Boll, T.J. (1981). Rehabilitation and treatment of central nervous system dysfunction: A behavioral medicine perspective. In C.K. Prokop & L.A. Bradley (Eds.), *Medical psychology: Contributions to behavioral medicine.* New York: Academic Press.

Basbaum, A., & Wall, P.D. (1976). Chronic changes in the responsive cells in adult cat dorsal horn following partial deafferentiation. *Brain Research, 116,* 181–204.

Bates, D., Caronna, J.J., Cartlidge, N.E.F., et al. (1977). A prospective study of non-traumatic coma: Methods and results in 310 patients. *Annals of Neurology,* 211–220.

Becker, D.P., Miller, J.D., & Greenberg, R.P. (1982). Prognosis after head injury. In J.R. Youmans (Ed.), *Neurological surgery* (p. 2142). Philadelphia: W.B. Saunders Company.

Becker, D.P., Miller, J.D., Ward, J.D., Greenberg, R.P., Young, H.F., & Sakalas, R. (1977). The outcome from severe head injury with early diagnosis and intensive management. *Journal of Neurosurgery, 47,* 491–502.

Becker, D.P., Miller, J.D., Young, H.F., Selhorst, J.B., Kishore, P.R.S., Greenberg, R.P., Rosner, M.J., & Ward, J.D. (1982). Diagnosis and treatment of head injury in adults. In J.R. Youmans (Ed.), *Neurological surgery.* Philadelphia: W.B. Saunders & Company.

Benson, D.F. (1979). *Aphasia, alexia, and agraphia.* New York: Churchill Livingstone.

Benton, A.L. (1964). Contributions to aphasia before Broca. *Cortex, 1,* 314–327.

Ben-Yishay, Y. (Ed.). (1981). *Working approaches to remediation of cognitive deficits in brain damaged persons.* (Rehabilitation Monograph No. 62). New York: NYU, Institute of Rehabilitation.

Ben-Yishay, Y., & Diller, L. (1983). Cognitive deficits. In M. Rosenthal, E.R. Griffith, M.R. Bond, & J.D. Miller (Eds.), *Rehabilitation of the head injured adult.* Philadelphia: F.A. Davis Company.

Bergman, M., Hirsch, S., & Najenson, T. (1977). Tests of auditory perception in the assessment and management of patients with cerebral cranial injury. *Scandinavian Journal of Rehabilitation Medicine, 9,* 173–177.

Bickford, R.B., & Klass, D.W. (1966). Acute and chronic EEG findings after head injury. In W.F. Caveness & A.E. Walker (Eds.), *Head Injury Conference Proceedings* (pp. 63–88). Philadelphia: J.B. Lippincott Co.

Birch, H.G. (1964). The problem of "brain damage" in children. In H.G. Birch (Ed.), *Brain damage in children: The biological and social aspects.* New York: The Williams & Wilkins Company.

Birch, H.G., & Lefford, A. (1964). Two strategies for studying perception in "brain-damaged" children. In H.G. Birch (Ed.), *Brain damage in children.* New York: The Williams & Wilkins Company.

Boder, E. (1971). Developmental dyslexia: Prevailing diagnostic concepts and a new diagnostic approach.

In H. Myklebust (Ed.), *Progress in Learning Disabilities.* New York: Grune and Stratton.

Boder, E. (1973a). Developmental dyslexia: A diagnostic approach based on three atypical reading-spelling patterns. *Developmental Medicine and Child Neurology, 15,* 663–687.

Boder, E. (1973b). Developmental dyslexia: Prevailing diagnostic concepts and a new approach. *Bulletin of the Orton Society, 23,* 106–118.

Bond, M.R. (1976). Assessment of the psychosocial outcome of severe head injury. *Acta Neurochirurgica, 34,* 57–70.

Boring, E.G. (1929). *A history of experimental psychology.* New York: Century Company.

Bowers, S.A., & Marshall, L.F. (1980). Outcome in 200 consecutive cases of severe head injury treated in San Diego county: A prospective analysis. *Neurosurgery, 6,* 237–242.

Braakman, R., Gelpke, G.J., Habbema, J.D.F., Maas, A.I.R., & Minderhoud, J.M. (1980). Systematic selection of prognostic features in patients with severe head injury. *Neurosurgery, 6,* 362–370.

Brackett, C.E. (1971). Respiratory complications of head injury. In *Head Injuries. Proceedings of an International Symposium* (pp. 255–265). Edinburgh and London: Churchill Livingstone.

Bricolo, A., Turazzi, S., & Feriotti, G. (1980). Prolonged posttraumatic unconsciousness. Therapeutic assets and liabilities. *Journal of Neurosurgery, 52,* 625–634.

Broca, P. (1861). Remarques sur le siege de la faculté du langage articule, suivies d'une observation d'aphemia (perte de la parole). *Bulletin de la Société Anatomique, 36,* 330–357.

Brock, S. (1960). *Injuries of the brain and spinal cord.* New York: Springer Publishing Co.

Brody, H. (1955). Organization of the cerebral cortex. III. A study of aging in the human cerebral cortex. *Journal of Comparative Neurology, 102,* 511–556.

Brooks, D.N. (1983). Disorders of memory. In M. Rosenthal, E.R. Griffith, M.R. Bond, & J.D. Miller (Eds.), *Rehabilitation of the head injured adult.* Philadelphia: F.A. Davis Company.

Bruce, D.A., Langfitt, T.W., Miller, J.D., Shutz, H., Vapalahti, M.P., Stanek, A., & Goldberg, H.I. (1973). Regional cerebral blood flow, intracranial pressure and brain metabolism in comatose patients. *Journal of Neurosurgery, 38,* 131–144.

Bruce, D.A., Schut, L., Bruno, L.A., Wood, J.H., & Sutton, L.N. (1978). Outcome following severe head injuries in children. *Journal of Neurosurgery, 48,* 679–688.

Burns, M.S., Halper, A.S., & Mogil, S.I. (1985). *Clinical management of right hemisphere dysfunction.* Rockville, MD: An Aspen Publication.

Butcher, J.N., Keller, L.S., & Bacon, S.F. (1985). Current developments and future directions in computerized personality assessment. *Journal of Consulting and Clinical Psychology, 53,* 803–815.

Cairns, H., Oldfield, R.C., Pennybacker, J.B., et al. (1941). Akinetic mutism with an epidermoid cyst of the third ventricle. *Brain, 64,* 273–290.

Caplan, B. (Ed.). (1987). *Rehabilitation psychology desk reference.* Rockville, MD: Aspen Publishers.

Carlsson, C.A., von Essen, C., & Lofgren, J. (1968). Factors affecting the clinical course of patients with severe head trauma. Part 1: Influence of biological factors. Part 2: significance of post-traumatic coma. *Journal of Neurosurgery, 29,* 242–251.

Carmon, A., Nachsom, I., & Starinsky, R. (1976). Developmental aspects of visual hemifield differences in perception of verbal material. *Brain and Language, 3,* 463–469.

Chapman, L.F. & Wolff, H.G. (1959). The cerebral hemispheres and the highest integrative functions of man. *A.M.A. Archives of Neurology, 1,* 357–424.

Chatrian, G.E., White, L.E., & Shaw, C.M. (1964). EEG pattern resembling wakefulness in unresponsive decerebrate state following traumatic brain-stem infarct. *Electroencephalography and Clinical Neurophysiology, 16,* 285–289.

Christensen, A.L. (1974). *Luria's neuropsychological investigation.* (2nd ed.). Copenhagen: Munksgaard.

Cooper, P.R., Rovit, R.L., & Ransohoff, J. (1976). Hemicraniectomy in the treatment of acute subdural hematoma: A re-appraisal. *Surgical Neurology, 5,* 25–29.

Corsellis, J.A.N., Bruton, C.J., & Freeman-Browne, D. (1973). The aftermath of boxing. *Psychological Medicine, 3,* 270–303.

Costa, L.D., Vaughan, H.G., Levita, E., & Farber, N. (1963). Purdue Pegboard as a predictor of the presence and laterality of cerebral lesions. *Journal of Consulting Psychology, 27,* 133–137.

Craine, J.F. (1982). Principles of cognitive rehabilitation. In L.E. Trexler (Ed.), *Cognitive rehabilitation: Conceptualization and intervention.* New York: Plenum Press.

Craine, J.F., & Gudeman, H.E. (1981). *The rehabilitation of brain functions — Principles, procedures, and techniques of neuro training.* Springfield, IL: Charles C. Thomas.

Critchley, M. (1953). The parietal lobes. London: Arnold.

Davenport, J.W., & Greenough, W.T. (1976). *Environments as therapy in the treatment of brain dysfunction.* New York: Plenum Press.

Dawson, R.E., Webster, J.E., & Gurdjian, E.S. (1951). Serial electroencephalography in acute head injuries. *Journal of Neurosurgery, 8,* 613–630.

Denckla, M.D., & Rudel, R. (1976). Names of object-drawings by dyslexic and other learning disabled children. *Brain and Language, 3,* 1–15.

Dikmen, S., & Reitan, R.M. (1976). Psychological deficits and recovery of functions after head injury. *Transactions of the American Neurological Association, 101,* 72–77.

Dikmen, S., & Reitan, R.M. (1977a). Emotional sequelae of head injury. *Annals of Neurology, 2,* 492–494.

Dikmen, S., & Reitan, R.M. (1977b). MMPI correlates of adaptive ability deficits in patients with brain lesions. *Journal of Nervous and Mental Disease, 165,* 247–254.

Dikmen, S., Reitan, R.M., & Temkin, N.R. (1983). Neuropsychological recovery in head injury. *Archives of Neurology, 40,* 333–338.

Diller, L., & Gordon, W.A. (1981). Rehabilitation and clinical neuropsychology. In S.B. Filskov & T.J. Boll (Eds.), *Handbook of clinical neuropsychology.* Toronto: John Wiley & Sons.

Doehring, D.G., & Reitan, R.M. (1962). Concept attainment of human adults with lateralized cerebral lesions. *Perceptual and Motor Skills, 14,* 27–33.

Doman, R.J., Spitz, E.B., Zucman, E., Delecato, C.H., & Doman, G. (1960). Children with severe brain injuries. *Journal of the American Medical Association, 174,* 257–262.

Dostrovosky, J.O., Millar, J., & Wall, P.D. (1976). The immediate shift of afferent drive of dorsal column nucleus cells following deafferentation. *Experimental Neurology, 52,* 480– 495.

Dow, R.S., Ulett, G., & Raaf, J. (1943). Electroencephalographic studies immediately following head injury. *American Journal of Psychiatry, 101,* 174–183.

Dresser, A.C., Meirowsky, A.M., Weiss, G.H., McNeel, M.L., Sima, G.A., & Caveness, W.F. (1973). Gainful employment following head injury. Prognostic factors. *Archives of Neurology, 29,* 111–116.

Edelstein, B.A., & Couture, E.T. (Eds.). (1984). *Behavioral assessment and rehabilitation of the traumatically brain-damaged.* New York: Plenum Press.

Editorial: The best yardstick we have. *Lancet, 2,* 1445–1446, 1961.

Eisenberg, H.M. (1985). Outcome after head injury: General considerations and neurobehavioral recovery. Part I: General considerations. D.B. Becker & J.T. Povlishock (Eds.), *Central nervous system trauma status report — 1985.* Prepared for the National Institute of Neurological and Communicative Disorders and Stroke, National Institutes of Health.

Eisenberg, H.M., Cayard, C., Papanicalaou, A.C., Weiner, R.L., et al. (1983). The effects of three potentially preventable complications on outcome after severe closed head injury. In *The Vth International Symposium on Intracranial Pressure* (pp. 549–553). Springer-Verlag, Germany.

Envoldsen, E.M., Cold, G., Jensen, F.T., & Malmros, R. (1976). Dynamic changes in regional CBF, intraventricular pressure, CSF pH and lactate levels during the acute phase of head injury. *Journal of Neurosurgery, 44,* 191–214.

Erdman, H.P., Klein, M., & Greist, J.H. (1985). Direct patient computer interviewing. *Journal of Consulting and Clinical Psychology, 53,* 760–773.

Exner, J.E., Jr. (1974). *The Rorschach: A comprehensive system (Vol. I).* New York: Wiley.

Fell, D.A., Fitzgerald, S., Moiel, R.H., & Caram, P. (1975). Acute subdural hematomas: A review of 144 cases. *Journal of Neurosurgery, 42,* 27–42.

Ferrier, D. (1886). *The functions of the brain.* London: Smith Elder & Company.

Finger, S., & Almli, C.R. (Eds.). (1984). *Early brain damage. Vol. II. Neurobiology and behavior.* Orlando, FL: Academic Press.

Finkelstein, J.N. (1977). BRAIN: A computer program for interpretation of the Halstead-Reitan Neuropsychological Test Battery (Doctoral dissertation, Columbia University, 1976). *Dissertation Abstracts International, 37,* 5349B. (University Microfilms No. 77-8, 8864).

Finlayson, M.A.J., Alfano, D.P., & Sullivan, J.F. (1987). A neuropsychological approach to cognitive remediation: Microcomputer applications. *Canadian Psychology, 28,* 180–190.

Finlayson, M.A.J., Gowland, C., & Basmajian, J.V. (1986). Neuropsychological predictors of treatment response following stroke. *Journal of Clinical and Experimental Neuropsychology, 7,* 647.

Fisher, L.A., Johnson, T.S., Porter, D., Bleich, H.L., & Slack, W.V. (1977). Collection of a clean voided urine specimen: A comparison among spoken, written, and computer-based instructions. *American Journal of Public Health, 67,* 640–644.

Fisk, J.L., & Rourke, B.P. (1983). Neuropsychological subtyping of learning-disabled children: History, methods, implications. *Journal of Learning Disabilities, 16,* 529–531.

Fleiss, J.L., Spitzer, R.L., Cohen, J., & Endicott, J. (1972). Three computer diagnosis methods compared. *Archives of General Psychiatry, 27,* 643–659.

Flourens, P. (1843). *Examen de la phrenologie.* Paris: Paulin.

Fritsch, G., & Hitzig, E. (1870). Uber die electrische Erregbarkeit des Grosshirn. *Arch. f. Anat. u. Physiol, 37,* 300–332.

Froman, C. (1968). Alterations of respiratory functions in patients with severe head injuries. *British Journal of Anesthesiology, 40,* 354–360.

Gallagher, J.P., & Browder, E.J. (1968). Extradural hematoma: Experience with 167 patients. *Journal of Neurosurgery, 29,* 1– 12.

Gazzaniga, M.S. (1974). Determinants of cerebral recovery. In D.G. Stein, J.J. Rose, & N. Butters (Eds.), *Plasticity of function in the central nervous system.* New York: Academic Press.

Gazzaniga, M.S. (1985). *The social brain: Discovering the networks of the mind.* New York: Basic Books.

Gazzaniga, M.S., & Sperry, R.W. (1967). Language after section of the cerebral commisures. *Brain, 90,* 131–148.

Gennarelli, T.A., Spielman, G.M., Langfitt, T.W., Gildenberg, P.L., et al. (1982). Influence of the type of intracranial lesion on outcome from severe head injury. *Journal of Neurosurgery, 56,* 26–33.

Geschwind, N., & Galaburda, A.M. (Eds.). (1984). *Cerebral dominance: The biological foundations.* Cambridge, MA: Harvard University Press.

Gianutsos, R. (1980). What is cognitive rehabilitation. *Journal of Rehabilitation, 23,* 37–40.

Goldberg, E., & Costa, L.D. (1981). Hemisphere differences in the acquisition and use of descriptive systems. *Brain and Language, 14,* 144–173.

Goldstein, G. (1984). Methodological and theoretical issues in neuropsychological assessment. In B.A. Edelstein & E.T. Couture (Eds.), *Behavioral assessment and rehabilitation of the traumatically brain-damaged* (pp. 1-21). New York: Plenum Press.

Goldstein, G. (1986). An overview of similarities and differences between the Halstead-Reitan and Luria-Nebraska Neuropsychological Batteries. In T. Incagnoli, G. Goldstein, & C.J. Golden (Eds.), *Clinical application of neuropsychological test batteries* (pp. 235–275). New York: Plenum Press.

Goldstein, G., & Ruthven, L. (1983). *Rehabilitation of the brain-damaged adult.* New York: Plenum Press.

Goldstein, K.H. (1939). *The organism.* New York: American Book Co.

Goldstein, K. (1936). The significance of the frontal lobes for mental performances. *Journal of Neurology and Psychopathology, 17,* 27–40.

Goltz, F.L. (1881). Uber die Verrichtungen des Grosshirns. Bonn: Gesammette Abhandlungen.

Goodglass, H., & Kaplan, E. (1972). *The assessment of aphasia and related disorders.* Philadelphia: Lea & Febiger.

Goodglass, H., & Kaplan, E. (1979). Assessment of cognitive deficit in the brain-injured patient. In M.S. Gazzaniga (Ed.), *Handbook of behavioral neurobiology* (Vol. 2, Neuropsychology). New York: Plenum Press.

Greenberg, R.P., Becker, D.P., Miller, J.D., & Mayer, D.J. (1977). Evaluation of brain function in severe human head trauma with multimodality evoked potentials: Part II. Localization of brain dysfunction and correlation with post-traumatic neurological conditions. *Journal of Neurosurgery, 47,* 163–177.

Greenberg, R.P., Mayer, D.J., & Becker, D.P. (1976). The prognostic value of evoked potentials in human mechanical brain injury. In R.L. McLaurin (Ed.), *Head injuries: Second Chicago symposium on neural trauma* (pp. 81–88). New York: Grune & Stratton, Inc.

Greenberg, R.P., Mayer, D.J., Becker, D.P., & Miller, J.D. (1977). Evaluation of brain function in severe human head trauma with multimodality evoked potentials, methods, analysis. *Journal of Neurosurgery, 47,* 150–162.

Grimm, B.H., & Bleiberg, J. (1986). Psychological rehabilitation in traumatic brain injury. In S.B. Filskov & T.J. Boll (Eds.), *Handbook of clinical neuropsychology. Vol. II* (pp. 495–560). New York: John Wiley and Sons.

Groher, M. (1983). Communication disorders. In M. Rosenthal, E.R. Griffith, M.R. Bond, & J.D. Miller (Eds.), *Rehabilitation of the head injured adult.* Philadelphia: F.A. Davis Company.

Gronwall, D., & Wrightson, P. (1980). Duration of post-traumatic amnesia after mild head injury. *Journal of Clinical Neuropsychology, 2,* 51–60.

Gudeman, H.E., & Craine, J.F. (1976). *Principles and techniques of neuro training.* Privately published manuscript, Hawaii State Hospital.

Halstead, W.C. (1940). Preliminary analysis of grouping behavior in patients with cerebral injury by the method of equivalent and non-equivalent stimuli. *American Journal of Psychiatry, 96,* 1263–94.

Halstead, W.C. (1947a). *Brain and intelligence. A quantitative study of the frontal lobes.* Chicago: University of Chicago Press.

Halstead, W.C. (1947b). Specialization of behavioral functions and the frontal lobes. *Research Publications of the Association for Research in Nervous and Mental Disease, 27,* 59–66.

Hannay, H.J., Levin, H.S., & Kay, J. (1982). Tachistoscopic visual perception after closed head injury. *Journal of Clinical Neuropsychology, 4,* 117–129.

Harris, P. (1971). Acute traumatic subdural hematomas: Results of neurosurgical care. In *Head Injuries:*

Proceedings of an International Symposium (pp. 321–326). Baltimore, Williams & Wilkins Co.

Head, H. (1926). *Aphasia and kindred disorders of speech. Vol. 1.* Cambridge, England: The University Press.

Hécaen, H., & Albert, M. (1978). *Human neuropsychology.* New York: John Wiley & Sons.

Herring, S. (1983). Neuropsychological performances of male and female subjects with unilateral cerebral lesions. Doctoral dissertation. Tucson, AZ: University of Arizona.

Herring, S., & Reitan, R.M. (1986). Sex similarities in Verbal and Performance IQ deficits following unilateral cerebral lesions. *Journal of Consulting and Clinical Psychology, 54,* 537–541.

Hieskanen, O., & Sipponen, P. (1970). Prognosis of severe brain injury. *Acta Neurologica Skandinavica, 46,* 343–348.

Hofer, P.J., & Green, B.F. (1985). The challenge of competence and creativity in computerized psychological testing. *Journal of Consulting and Clinical Psychology, 53,* 826–838.

Hom, J., & Reitan, R.M. (1982). Effect of lateralized cerebral damage upon contralateral and ipsilateral sensorimotor performances. *Journal of Clinical Neuropsychology, 4,* 249–268.

Hom, J., & Reitan, R.M. (1984). Neuropsychological correlates of rapidly vs. slowly growing intrinsic neoplasms. *Journal of Clinical Neuropsychology, 6,* 309–324.

Hooper, R. (1959). Observations on extradural hemorrhage. *British Journal of Surgery, 47,* 71–87.

Humphrey, M. & Oddy, M. (1981). Return to work after head injury: A review of post-war studies. *Injury, 12,* 107–114.

Incagnoli, T. (1986). Current directions and future trends in clinical neuropsychology. In T. Incagnoli, G. Goldstein, and C.J. Golden (Eds.), *Clinical application of neuropsychological test batteries. New York: Plenum Press.*

James, H.E., Anas, N.G., & Perkin, R.M. (Eds.). (1985). *Brain insults in infants and children: Pathophysiology and management.* Orlando, FL: Grune and Stratton, Inc.

Jamieson, K.G., & Yelland, J.D.N. (1968). Extradural haematoma. Report of 167 cases. *Journal of Neurosurgery, 29,* 13–23.

Jamieson, K.G., & Yelland, J.D.N. (1972). Surgically treated traumatic subdural hematomas. *Journal of Neurosurgery, 37,* 137–149.

Jennett, B. (1962). *Epilepsy after blunt head injuries* (1st ed). London: William Heinemann Ltd.

Jennett, B. (1975). *Epilepsy after non-missile head injury* (1st ed). London: William Heinemann Ltd.

Jennett B., & Bond, M. (1975). Assessment of outcome after severe brain damage. *Lancet, 1,* 480–484.

Jennett, B., & Lewin, W.S. (1960). Traumatic epilepsy after closed head injuries. *Journal of Neurology, Neurosurgery, and Psychiatry, 23,* 295–301.

Jennett, B., & Plum, F. (1972). Persistent vegetative state after brain damage. *Lancet, 1,* 734–737.

Jennett, B., Snoek, J., Bond, M.R., & Brooks, N. (1981). Disability after severe head injury: Observation on the use of the Glasgow Outcome Scale. *Journal of Neurology, Neurosurgery, and Psychiatry, 44,* 285–293.

Jennett, B., & Teasdale, G. (1981). *Management of head injuries.* Philadelphia: F.A. Davis Company.

Jennett, B., Teasdale, G., Braakman, R., Minderhoud, J., Heiden, J., & Kurze, T. (1979). Prognosis of patients with severe head injury. *Neurosurgery, 4,* 283–289.

Jennett, B., Teasdale, G., Braakman, R., Minderhoud, J., & Knill-Jones, R. (1976). Predicting outcome in individual patients after severe head injury. *Lancet, i,* 1031–1035.

Jennett, B., Teasdale, G., Galbraith, S., Pickard, J., Grant, H., Braakman, R., Avezaat, C., Mass, A., Minderhoud, J., Vecht, C.J., Heiden, J., Small, R., Caton,

W., & Kurze, T. (1977). Severe head injuries in three countries. *Journal of Neurology, Neurosurgery, and Psychiatry, 40,* 291–298.

Jennett, B., & van der Sande, J. (1975). EEG prediction of post-traumatic epilepsy. *Epilepsia, 16,* 251–256 (a).

Jennett, S., Ashbridge, K., & North, J.B. (1974). Post-hyperventilation apnoea in patients with brain damage. *Journal of Neurology, Neurosurgery, and Psychiatry, 37,* 288–296.

Johnston, I.H., & Jennett, B. (1973). The place of continuous intracranial pressure monitoring in neurosurgical practice. *Acta Neurochirurgica, 29,* 53–63.

Johnston, I.H., Johnston, J.A., & Jennett, W.B. (1970). Intracranial pressures following head injury. *Lancet, 2,* 433–436.

Karson, S., & O'Dell, J.W. (1975). A new automated interpretation system for the 16 PF. *Journal of Personality Assessment, 39,* 256–260.

Kaufman, H.H., Loyola W.P., Makela, M.E., Frankowski, R.F., et al. (1983). Civilian gunshot wounds: The limits of salvageability. *Acta Neurochirurgica, 67,* 115–125.

Kertesz, A. (1979). *Aphasia and associated disorders.* New York: Grune and Stratton.

Kiresuk, T., & Sherman, R. (1968). Goal-attainment scaling: A general method for evaluating comprehensive mental health programs. *Community Mental Health Journal, 4,* 443–453.

Klatzo, I. (1967). Neuropathological aspects of brain edema. *Journal of Neuropathology and Experimental Neurology, 24,* 1.

Kløve, H., & Cleeland, C.S. (1972). The relationship of neuropsychological impairment to other indices of severity of head injury. *Scandanavian Journal of Rehabilitation Medicine, 4,* 55–60.

Kolb, B., & Whishaw, I.Q. (1980). *Fundamentals of human neuropsychology.* San Francisco: W.H. Freeman.

Lachar, D. (1982). *Personality Inventory for Children revised format manual supplement.* Los Angeles: Western Psychological Services.

Langfitt, T.W., & Gennarelli, T.A. (1982). Can the outcome from head injury be improved? *Journal of Neurosurgery, 56,* 19–25.

Lashley, K.S. (1929). *Brain mechanisms and intelligence.* Chicago: University of Chicago Press.

Laurence, S., & Stein, D.G. (1978). Recovery after brain damage and the concept of localization of function. In S. Finger (Ed.), *Recovery from brain damage: Research and theory.* New York: Plenum Press.

Levati, A., Farina, M.L., Vecchi, G., Rossanda, M., & Marrubini, M.B. (1982). Prognosis of severe head injuries. *Journal of Neurosurgery, 57,* 779–783.

Levin, H.S. (1985). Outcome after head injury: General considerations and neurobehavioral recovery. Part II. Neurobehavioral recovery. In D.P. Becker & J.T. Povlishock (Eds.), *Central nervous system trauma status report 1985* (pp. 281–299). Prepared for the National Institute of Neurological and Communicative Disorders and Stroke, National Institutes of Health.

Levin, H.S., Benton, A.L., & Grossman, R.G. (1982). *Neurobehavioral consequences of closed head injury.* New York: Oxford University Press.

Levin, H.S., Grossman, R.G., & Kelly, P.J. (1977). Impairment of facial recognition after closed head injuries of varying severity. *Cortex, 13,* 119–130.

Levin, H.S., Grossman, R.G., Rose, H.E. & Teasdale, G. (1979). Long- term neuropsychological outcome of closed head injury. *Journal of Neurosurgery, 50,* 412–422.

Levin, H.S., Grossman, R.G., Sarwar, J., & Meyers, C.A. (1981). Linguistic recovery after closed head injury. *Brain and Language, 12,* 360–374.

Levin, H.S., O'Donnell, V.M. & Grossman, R.G. (1979). The Galveston Orientation and Amnesia Test: A practical scale to assess cognition after head injury. *Journal of Nervous and Mental Disease, 167,* 675–684.

Levin, H.S., Papanicolaou, A.C., & Eisenberg, H.M. (1985). Observations on amnesia after nonmissile head injury. In N. Butters & L.R. Squire (Eds.), *The neuropsychology of memory.* New York: The Guilford Press.

Levy, J. (1985). Interhemispheric collaboration: single-mindedness in the asymmetric brain. In C.T. Best (Ed.), *Hemispheric function and collaboration in the child.* Orlando, FL: Academic Press.

Lezak, M.D. (1983). *Neuropsychological assessment.* New York: Oxford University Press.

Loeb, J. (1902). *Comparative physiology of the brain and comparative psychology.* New York: G.P. Putnam and Sons.

Luria, A.R. (1966). *Higher cortical functions in man.* New York: Basic Books.

Luria, A.R. (1970). The functional organization of the brain. *Scientific American, 222,* 66–73.

Luria, A.R. (1973). *The working brain: An introduction to neuropsychology.* (B. Haigh, Trans.). New York: Basic Books.

Lynch, W.J. (1987). Neuropsychological rehabilitation: Description of an established program. In B. Caplan (Ed.), *Rehabilitation psychology desk reference.* Rockville, MD: Aspen Publishers.

Macpherson, P., & Graham, D.I. (1974). Arterial spasm and slowing of the cerebral circulation in ischemia of head injury. *Journal of Neurology, Neurosurgery, and Psychiatry, 37,* 1069–1072.

Mandleberg, I.A., & Brooks, D.N. (1975). Cognitive recovery after severe head injury. I. Serial testing on the Wechsler Adult Intelligence Scale. *Journal of Neurology, Neurosurgery, and Psychiatry, 38,* 1121–1126.

Mandleberg, I.A. (1976). Cognitive recovery after severe head injury. 3. WAIS Verbal and Performance IQ's as a function of post-traumatic amnesia duration and time from injury. *Journal of Neurology, Neurosurgery, and Psychiatry, 39,* 1001–1007.

Marie, P. (1906). La troisieme circonvolution frontale gauche ne joue aucun rôle special dans la function du langage. *Semaine Médicale,* May 23rd, reprinted in P. Marie, 1926, *Travaux et Memoires, Tome I,* Paris: Masson, pp. 3–30. For translation, see M.F. Cole and M. Cole, 1971, *Pierre Marie's papers on speech disorders.* New York: Hafner.

Marks, I.M. (1978). *Living with fear.* New York: McGraw-Hill.

Matarazzo, J.M. (1983). Computerized psychological testing. *Science, 221,* 323.

Matthews, C.G. (1974). Applications of neuropsychological test methods in mentally retarded subjects. In R.M. Reitan & L.A. Davison (Eds.), *Clinical neuropsychology: Current status and applications* (pp. 267–287). New York: Hemisphere Publishing Company.

Mattis, S., French, J.H., & Rapin, I. (1975). Dyslexia in children and young adults: Three independent neuropsychological syndromes. *Developmental Medicine and Child Neurology, 17,* 150–163.

McFie, J., & Piercy, M.F. (1952). The relation of laterality of lesion to performance on Weigl's sorting test. *Journal of Mental Science, 98,* 299–305.

McSweeney, J.J., Grant, I., Heaton, R.K., Prigatano, G.P., & Adams, K.M. (1985). Relationship of neuropsychological status to everyday functioning in healthy and chronically ill persons. *Journal of Clinical and Experimental Neuropsychology, 7,* 281–291.

Meehl, P.E. (1954). *Clinical versus statistical prediction: A theoretical analysis and a review of the evidence.* Minneapolis: University of Minnesota Press.

Meier, M.J. (1974). Some challenges for clinical neuropsychology. In R.M. Reitan & L.A. Davison (Eds.), *Clinical neuropsychology: Current status and applications.* New York: Hemisphere Publishing Corporation.

Meyerink, L.H., Pendleton, M.G., Hughes, R.B., & Thompson, L.L. (1985). Effectiveness of cognitive retraining with brain-impaired adults. *Archives of Physical Medicine and Rehabilitation, 66,* 555.

Millar, J., Basbaum, A.I., & Wall, P.D. (1976). Restructuring of the somatotopic map and appearance of abnormal neuronal activity in the gracile nucleus after partial deafferentation. *Experimental Neurology, 50,* 658–672.

Miller, E. (1984). *Recovery and management of neuropsychological impairments.* New York: John Wiley and Sons.

Miller, J.D., & Becker, D.P. (1982). General principles and pathophysiology of head injury. In J.R. Youmans (Ed.), *Neurological surgery.* Philadelphia: W.B. Saunders Co.

Miller, J.D., Becker, D.P., Ward, J.D., Sullivan, H.G., Adams, W.E., & Rosner, M.J. (1977). Significance of intracranial hypertension in severe head injury. *Journal of Neurosurgery, 47,* 503–516.

Miller, J.D., Sweet, R.C., Narayan, R., & Becker, D.P. (1978). Early insults to the injured brain. *J.A.M.A., 240,* 439–442.

Milner, B. (1962). Laterality effects in audition. In V.B. Mountcastle (Ed.), *Interhemispheric relations and cerebral dominance.* Baltimore: Johns Hopkins University Press.

Milner, B. (1971). Interhemispheric differences in the localization of psychological processes in man. *British Medical Bulletin, 27,* 272–277.

Miner, N.E., & Wagner, K.A. (Eds.). (1986). *Neurotrauma: Treatment, rehabilitation, and related issues.* Boston: Butterworth's.

Mohr, J.P., Weiss, G.H., Caveness, W.F., Dillon, J.D., et al. (1980). Language and motor disorders after penetrating head injury in Viet Nam. *Neurology, 30,* 1273–1278.

Molfese, D.L. (1977). Infant cerebral asymmetry. In S.J. Segalowitz & F.A. Gruber (Eds.), *Language development and neurological theory* (pp. 22–33). New York: Academic Press.

Moruzzi, G., & Magoun, H.W. (1949). Brain stem reticular formation and activation of the EEG. *Electroencephalography and Clinical Neurophysiology, 1,* 455–473.

Mountcastle, V.B. (Ed.) (1962). *Interhemispheric relations and cerebral dominance.* Baltimore: Johns Hopkins University Press.

Mountcastle, V.B. (1979). An organizing principle for cerebral function: The unit module and the distributed system. In F.O. Schmitt & F.O. Worden (Eds.), *The neurosciences: Fourth study program* (pp. 21–42). Cambridge, MA: The MIT Press.

Muizelaar, J.P., & Obrist, W.D. (1985). Cerebral blood flow and brain metabolism with brain injury. In D.P. Becker & J.T. Povlishock (Eds.), *Central nervous system trauma status report 1985.* Prepared for the National Institute of Neurological and Communicative Disorders and Stroke, National Institutes of Health.

Munk, H. (1890). On the visual area of the cerebral cortex, and its relation to eye movements (F.W. Mott, Trans.). *Brain, 13,* 45–67.

Najenson, T., Sazbon, L., Fiselzon, J., Becker, E., & Schechter, I. (1978). Recovery of communicative functions after prolonged traumatic coma. *Scandanavian Journal of Rehabilitation Medicine, 10,* 15–21.

Narayan, R.K., Greenberg, R.P., Miller, J.D., Enas, G.G., et al. (1981). Improved confidence of outcome in severe head injury. *Journal of Neurosurgery, 54,* 751–762.

National Computer Systems. (1984). *1984 catalog.* (Professional Assessment Services Division). Minneapolis, MN: Author.

Newcombe, F. (1985). Neuropsychology qua interface. *Journal of Clinical and Experimental Neuropsychology, 7,* 663–681.

Norrman, B., & Svahn, K. (1961). A follow-up study of severe brain injuries. *Acta Psychiatrica Skandinavica, 37,* 236–264.

North, J.B., & Jennett, S. (1974). Abnormal breathing patterns associated with acute brain damage. *Archives of Neurology, 31,* 338–344.

Obrist, W.D., Langfitt, T.W., terWeeme, C.A., O'Connor, M.J., Gennarelli, T.A., Zimmerman, R.A., & Kuhl, D.E. (1977). Non-invasive, long-term, serial studies of rCBF in acute head injuries. *Acta Neurologica Skandinavica, 56 (Suppl. 64)*, 178–179.

Oddy, M., Humphrey, M., & Uttley, D. (1978). Subjective impairment and social recovery after closed head injury. *Journal of Neurology, Neurosurgery, and Psychiatry, 41*, 611–616.

Oppenheimer, D.R. (1968). Microscopic lesions in the brain following head injury. *Journal of Neurology, Neurosurgery and Psychiatry, 31*, 299–306.

Overgaard, J., Christensen, S., Hvid Jansen, O., Haase, J., Land, A.M., Pederson, K.K., & Tweed, W.A. (1973). Prognosis after head injury based on early clinical examination. *Lancet, 2*, 631–635.

Overgaard, J., & Tweed, W.A. (1974). Cerebral circulation after head injury. Part I: Cerebral blood flow and its regulation after closed head injury with emphasis on clinical correlations. *Journal of Neurosurgery, 41*, 531–541.

Pagni, C.A. (1973). The prognosis of head injured patients in a state of coma with decerebrated posture. *Journal of Neurosurgical Science, 17*, 289–295.

Pazzaglia, P., Frank, G., Frank, F., & Gaist, G. (1975). Clinical course and prognosis of acute post-traumatic coma. *Journal of Neurology, Neurosurgery, and Psychiatry, 38*, 149–154.

Penfield, W., & Roberts, L. (1959). *Speech and brain mechanisms*. Princeton, NJ: Princeton University Press.

Petit, T.L., & Alfano, D.P. (1979). Differential experience following developmental lead exposure: Effects on brain and behaviour. *Pharmacology, Biochemistry and Behaviour, 11*, 165–171.

Piaget, J. (1971). *Biology and knowledge* (B. Walsh, Trans.). Chicago: University of Chicago Press.

Piotrowski, Z.A. (1980). The psychological x-ray in mental disorders. In J.B. Sidowski, J.H. Johnson, & T.A. Williams (Eds.), *Technology in mental health care delivery systems* (pp. 85–108). Norwood, NJ: Ablex.

Pirozzolo, F.J. (1979). *The neuropsychology of developmental reading disorders*. New York: Praeger Publishers.

Pirozzolo, F.J., & Hess, D.W. (1976). A neuropsychological analysis of the ITPA: Two profiles of reading disability. Paper presented to the New York State Orton Society Annual Convention, Rochester, NY.

Plum, F., & Posner, J.B. (1980). *Diagnosis of stupor and coma*. (2nd ed.). Philadelphia: F.A. Davis.

Poole, E.W. (1970). Some aspects of electroencephalographic disturbances following head injury. *Journal of Clinical Pathology, 23 (Suppl), 4*, 187–201.

Porch, B., & Collins, M. (1974). *The rating of patient's independence (ROPI)*. Unpublished manuscript.

Pribram, K.J. (1971). *Languages of the brain: Experimental paradoxes and principles in neuropsychology*. Montery, CA: Brooks/Cole Publishing Company.

Prigatano, G.T. and others (1986). *Neuropsychological rehabilitation after brain injury*. Baltimore: The Johns Hopkins University Press.

Raisman, G., & Field, P.M. (1973). A quantitative investigation of the development of collateral reinnervation of the septal nuclei. *Brain Research, 50*, 241–264.

Ransohoff, J., Vallo, B., Gage, E.J., & Epstein, F. (1971). Hemicraniectomy in the management of acute subdural hematomas. *Journal of Neurosurgery, 34*, 70–76.

Reitan, R.M. (1955a). An investigation of the validity of Halstead's measures of biological intelligence. *AMA Archives of Neurological Psychiatry, 73*, 28–35.

Reitan, R.M. (1955b). Certain differential effects of left and right cerebral lesions in human adults. *Journal of Comparative and Physiological Psychology, 48*, 474–477.

Reitan, R.M. (1955c). Discussion: Symposium on the temporal lobe. *Archives of Neurology and Psychiatry, 74*, 569–570.

Reitan, R.M. (1955d). The distribution according to age of a psychologic measure dependent upon organic brain functions. *Journal of Gerontology, 10*, 338–340.

Reitan, R.M. (1956). Investigation of relationships between "psychometric" and "biological" intelligence. *Journal of Nervous and Mental Disease, 123,* 536–541.

Reitan, R.M. (1958). The validity of the Trail Making Test as an indicator of organic brain damage. *Perceptual and Motor Skills, 8,* 271–276.

Reitan, R.M. (1959a). Effects of brain damage on a psychomotor problem-solving task. *Perceptual and Motor Skills, 9,* 211–215.

Reitan, R.M. (1959b). Impairment of abstraction ability in brain damage: Quantitative versus qualitative changes. *Journal of Psychology, 48,* 97–102.

Reitan, R.M. (1960). The significance of dysphasia for intelligence and adaptive abilities. *Journal of Psychology, 50,* 355–376.

Reitan, R.M. (1964). Psychological deficits resulting from cerebral lesions in man. In J.M. Warren & K.A. Akert (Eds.), *The frontal granular cortex and behavior.* New York: McGraw-Hill.

Reitan, R.M. (1966a). A research program on the psychological effects of brain lesions in human beings. In N.R. Ellis (Ed.), *International review of research in mental retardation: Vol. 1* (pp. 153–218). New York: Academic Press.

Reitan, R.M. (1966b). Problems and prospects in studying the psychological correlates of brain lesions. *Cortex, 2,* 127–154.

Reitan, R.M. (1967). Psychological changes associated with aging and cerebral damage. *Mayo Clinic Proceedings, 42,* 653–673.

Reitan, R.M. (1970). Sensorimotor functions, intelligence and cognition, and emotional status in subjects with cerebral lesions. *Perceptual and Motor Skills, 31,* 275–284.

Reitan, R.M. (1974). Methodological problems in clinical neuropsychology. In R.M. Reitan & L.A. Davison (Eds.), *Clinical neuropsychology: Current status and applications* (pp. 19–46). New York: Hemisphere Publishing Corporation.

Reitan, R.M. (1975). Neuropsychology: The vulgarization Luria always wanted. [Review of A. Christensen, "Luria's neuropsychological investigation"]. *Contemporary Psychology.*

Reitan, R.M. (1976). Neurological and physiological bases of psychopathology. *Annual Review of Psychology, 27,* 189–216.

Reitan, R.M. (1979). *Neuropsychology and rehabilitation.* Tucson, AZ: Neuropsychology Press.

Reitan, R.M. (1980). *Case studies in clinical neuropsychology.* Tucson, AZ: Neuropsychology Press.

Reitan, R.M. (1982). Psychological testing after craniocerebral injury. In J.R. Youmans (Ed.), *Neurological surgery* (pp. 2195–2204). Philadelphia: W.B. Saunders Company.

Reitan, R.M. (1984). *Aphasia and sensory-perceptual deficits in adults.* Tucson, AZ: Neuropsychology Press.

Reitan, R.M. (1985a). Relationships between measures of brain functions and general intelligence. *Journal of Clinical Psychology, 41,* 245–253.

Reitan, R.M. (1985b). *Aphasia and sensory-perceptual deficits in children.* Tucson, AZ: Neuropsychology Press.

Reitan, R.M. (1986). Theoretical and methodological bases of the Halstead-Reitan Neuropsychological Test Battery. In I. Grant & K.M. Adams (Eds.), *Neuropsychological assessment of neuropsychiatric disorders.* New York: Oxford University Press.

Reitan, R.M., & Sena, D.A. (1983, August). The efficacy of the REHABIT technique in remediation of brain-injured people. Paper presented at the meeting of the American Psychological Association, Anaheim, California.

Reitan, R.M., & Tarshes, E.L. (1959). Differential effects of lateralized brain lesions on the Trail Making Test. *Journal of Nervous and Mental Disease, 129,* 257–262.

Reitan, R.M., & Wolfson, D. (1985a). *The Halstead-Reitan Neuropsychological Test Battery: Theory and clinical interpretation.* Tucson, AZ: Neuropsychology Press.

Reitan, R.M., & Wolfson, D. (1985b). *Neuroanatomy and neuropathology: A clinical guide for neuropsychologists.* Tucson, AZ: Neuropsychology Press.

Reitan, R.M., & Wolfson, D. (1986a). The Halstead-Reitan Neuropsychological Test Battery and aging. In T.L. Brink (Ed.), *Clinical gerontology: A guide to assessment and intervention* (pp. 39–61). New York: The Haworth Press.

Reitan, R.M., & Wolfson, D. (1986b). *Traumatic brain injury. Volume I. Pathophysiology and neuropsychological evaluation.* Tucson, AZ: Neuropsychology Press.

Reitan, R.M., & Wolfson, D. (Unpublished manuscript). The Seashore Rhythm Test and brain functions.

Richards, T., & Hoff, J.T. (1974). Factors affecting survival from acute subdural hematoma. *Surgery, 75,* 253–258.

Riese, W. (1959). *A history of neurology.* New York: MD Publications.

Riesen, A.H. (1961). Studying perceptual development using the technique of sensory deprivation. *Journal of Nervous and Mental Disease, 132,* 21–25.

Riesen, A.H., & Aarons, L. (1959). Visual movement and intensity discrimination in cats after deprivation of pattern vision. *Journal of Comparative and Physiological Psychology, 52,* 142–149.

Roberts, A.H. (1969). *Brain damage in boxers; A study of the prevalence of traumatic encephalopathy among professional boxers.* London: Pitman Publishing Ltd.

Roberts, A.H. (1980). *Severe accidental head injuries. An assessment of long-term prognosis.* Baltimore: University Park Press.

Roberts, L. (1958). Functional plasticity in cortical speech areas and the integration of speech. *Research Publications of the Association for Research in Nervous and Mental Diseases, 36,* 449–466.

Roberts, M. (1976). Lesions of the ocular motor nerves (III, IV, and VI). In P.J. Vinken & G.W. Bruyn (Eds.), *Handbook of clinical neurology.* Amsterdam: Elsevier-North Holland Publishing Co.

Robertson, R.C.L., & Pollard, C. (1955). Decerebrate state in children and adolescents. *Journal of Neurosurgery, 12,* 13–17.

Rodin, E.A. (1967). Contribution of the EEG to prognosis after head injury. *Diseases of the Nervous System, 28,* 595–601.

Rodin, E., Whelan, J., Taylor, R., Tomita, T., Grissel, J., Thomas, L.M., & Gurdjian, E.S. (1965). The electroencephalogram in acute head injuries. *Journal of Neurosurgery, 23,* 329–337.

Rose, J., Valtonen, S., & Jennett, B. (1977). Avoidable factors contributing to death after head injury. *British Medical Journal, 2,* 615–618.

Rosen, C.D., & Gerring, J.P. (1986). *Head trauma: Educational reintegration.* San Diego, CA: College-Hill Press.

Rosenthal, M. (1983). Behavioral sequelae. In M. Rosenthal, E.R. Griffith, M.R. Bond, & J.D. Miller (Eds.), *Rehabilitation of the head injured adult.* Philadelphia: F.A. Davis Company.

Rosenthal, M., & Berrol, S. (1986). From the editors. *The Journal of Head Trauma Rehabilitation, 1,* viii.

Rosenthal, M., Griffith, E.R., Bond, N.R., & Miller, J.B. (Eds.). (1983). *Rehabilitation of the head-injured adult.* Philadelphia: F.A. Davis Company.

Rosenzweig, M.R. (1984). Experience, memory and the brain. *American Psychologist, 39,* 365–376.

Rossanda, M., Selenati, A., Villa, C., & Beduschi, A. (1973). Role of automatic ventilation in treatment of severe head injuries. *Journal of Neurosurgical Science, 17,* 265–270.

Rourke, B.P. (1982). Central processing deficiencies in children: Toward a developmental neuropsychological model. *Journal of Clinical Neuropsychology, 4,* 1–18.

Rourke, B.P., Bakker, D.J., Fisk, J.L., & Strang, J.B. (1983). *Child neuropsychology.* New York: The Guilford Press.

Rourke, B.P., & Brown, G.G. (1986). Clinical neuropsychology and behavioral neurology: Similarities and differences. In S.B. Filskov & T.J. Boll (Eds.), *Handbook of clinical neuropsychology. Volume II* (pp. 3–18). New York: John Wiley & Sons.

Rourke, B.P., & Finlayson, M.A.J. (1978). Neuropsychological significance of variations in patterns of academic performance: Verbal and visual-spatial abilities. *Journal of Abnormal Child Psychology, 6,* 121–133.

Rourke, B.P., & Strang, J.D. (1978). Neuropsychological significance of variations in patterns of academic performance: Motor, psychomotor, and tactile-perceptual abilities. *Journal of Pediatric Psychology, 2,* 62–66.

Rourke, B.P., & Strang, J.D. (1983). Subtypes of reading and arithmetical disabilities: A neuropsychological analysis. In M. Rutter (Ed.), *Developmental neuropsychiatry.* New York: Guilford Press.

Russell, E.W. (1981). The chronicity effect. *Journal of Clinical Psychology, 37,* 246–253.

Russell, E.W., Neuringer, C., & Goldstein, G. (1970). *Assessment of brain damage: A neuropsychological key approach.* New York: Wiley Interscience.

Russell, J.R., & Reitan, R.M. (1955). Psychological abnormalities in agenesis of the corpus callosum. *Journal of Nervous and Mental Disease, 121,* 205–214.

Russell, W.R. (1932). Cerebral involvement in head injury. A study based on the examination of 200 cases. *Brain, 55,* 549–603.

Russell, W.R., & Espir, M.L.E. (1961). *Traumatic aphasia. A study of aphasia in war wounds of the brain.* Oxford University Press. New York.

Rylander, G. (1939). Personality changes after operations on the frontal lobes: A clinical study of 32 cases. *Acta Psychiatrica et Neurologica Scandinavica,* (Supplement No. 20), 1–327.

Rylander, G. (1947). Discussion of W.C. Halstead's paper: Specialization of behavioral functions and the frontal lobes. *Association for Research in Nervous and Mental Disease, 27,* 64.

Saul, T.G., & Ducker, T.B. (1982). Effect of intracranial pressure monitoring and aggressive treatment on mortality in severe head injury. *Journal of Neurosurgery, 56,* 498–503.

Scheibel, A.B. (1977). Structural aspects of the aging brain: Spine systems and the dendritic arbor. In R. Katzman, R.D. Terry, & K.L. Bick (Eds.), *Alzheimer's's disease: Senile dementia and related disorders. Aging Vol. VII* (pp. 353–373). New York: Raven Press.

Scialfa, G., & Cristi, G.F. (1973). Prognostic value of cerebral angiography in non-surgical cases of traumatic coma. *Journal of Neurosurgical Science, 17,* 202–204.

Sell, G.H., & Rusk, H.A. (1982). Rehabilitation following central nervous system lesions. In J.R. Youmans (Ed.), *Neurological surgery.* Philadelphia: W.B. Saunders Company.

Selmi, P.M., Klein, M.H., Greist, J.H., Johnson, J.H., & Harris, W.G. (1982). An investigation of computer-assisted cognitive-behavior therapy in the treatment of depression. *Behavior Research Methods and Instrumentation, 14,* 181–185.

Semmes, J. (1968). Hemispheric specialization: A possible clue to mechanism. *Neuropsychologica, 6,* 11–26.

Sena, D.A. (1985). The effectiveness of cognitive retraining for brain-impaired individuals. *The International Journal of Clinical Neuropsychology, 7,* 62.

Sena, D.A. (1986). The effectiveness of cognitive rehabilitation for brain-impaired patients. *Journal of Clinical and Experimental Neuropsychology, 8,* 142.

Sena, D.A., Rakoff Sunde, R., Sena, H.M., & Bracken, D.D. (1987). Cognitive rehabilitation effects on psychobehavioral functioning of brain-impaired patients and family members. *Journal of Clinical and Experimental Neuropsychology, 9,* 270.

Sena, D.A., & Sena, H.M. (1986). Validation of the effectiveness of cognitive retraining. *Journal of Clinical and Experimental Neuropsychology, 8,* 142.

Sena, D.A., Sena, H.M., & Sunde, R.R. (1986a). Changes in cognitive functioning of non-impaired family members. *Archives of Clinical Neuropsychology, 1,* 263.

Sena, D.A., Sena, H.M., & Sunde, R.R. (1986b). Comparison of changes in cognitive functioning of non-impaired family members and brain-impaired patients. *Archives of Clinical Neuropsychology, 1,* 262.

Sena, H.M., & Sena, D.A. (1986a). A comparison of subject characteristics between treatment and non-treatment patients. *Archives of Clinical Neuropsychology, 1,* 74.

Sena, H.M., & Sena, D.A. (1986b). A comparison of treatment and non-treatment patients. *Journal of Clinical and Experimental Neuropsychology, 8,* 142.

Sena, H.M.,, & Sena, D.A. (1986c). A quantitive validation of the effectiveness of cognitive retraining. *Archives of Clinical Neuropsychology, 1,* 74.

Sena, H.M., Sena, D.A., Becker, L.A., & Bracken,, D.D. (1986). A comparison of subject characteristics for a matched sample of cognitive retraining patients with non-treatment patients. *Archives of Clinical Neuropsychology, 1,* 263.

Seron, X. (1979). *Aphasia et neuropsychogie.* Bruxelles: Pierre Mardaga.

Shaywitz, S.E., Shaywitz, B.A., Cohen, D.J., & Young, J.G. (1983). Monoaminergic mechanisms in hyperactivity. In N. Rutter (Ed.), *Developmental neuropsychiatry* (pp. 330–347). New York: The Guilford Press.

Silverberg, R., Bentin, S., Gaziel, T., Obler, L.K., & Albert, M.L. (1979). Shift of visual field preference for English words in native Hebrew speakers. *Brain and Language, 8,* 184–190.

Silverstein, A.B. (1987). Unusual combinations of verbal and performance IQs on Wechsler's intelligence scales. *Journal of Clinical Psychology, 43,* 720–722.

Skinner, B.F. (1950). Are theories of learning necessary? *Psychological Bulletin, 57,* 193–216.

Slack, W.V., & Slack, C.W. (1977). Talking to a computer about emotional problems: A comparative study. *Psychotherapy: Theory, Research and Practice, 14,* 156–164.

Smith, A. (1979). Practices and principles of neuropsychology. *International Journal of Neuroscience, 9,* 233–238.

Smith, A. (1981). Principles underlying human brain functions in neuropsychological sequelae of different neuropathological processes. In S. B. Filskov & T.J. Boll (Eds.), *Handbook of clinical neuropsychology.* New York: Wiley-Interscience.

Sperry, R.W. (1974). Lateral specialization in the surgically separated hemispheres. In F.O. Schmitt & F.G. Worden (Eds.), *The neurosciences. Third Study Program.* Cambridge, MA: Massachusetts Institute of Technology Press.

Sperry, R.W., Gazzaniga, M.S., & Bogen, J.E. (1969). Interhemispheric relationships: The neocortical commissures, syndromes of hemisphere deconnection. In P.J. Vinken & G.W. Bruyn (Eds.), *Handbook of clinical neurology Vol. 4.* Amsterdam: North Holland.

Spradlin, J.E. (1963). Language and communication of mental defectives. In N. Ellis (Ed.), *Handbook of mental deficiency* (pp. 512–556). New York: McGraw-Hill.

Strang, J.D., & Rourke, B.P. (1983). Concept-formation/non-verbal reasoning abilities of children who exhibit specific academic problems with arithmetic. *Journal of Clinical Child Psychology, 12,* 33–39.

Strauss, A.A., & Werner, H. (1941). The mental organization of the brain-injured mentally defective child. *American Journal of Psychiatry, 97,* 1194–1203.

Sweet, R.C., Miller, J.D., Lipper, M., Kishore, P.R. & Becker, D.P. (1978). Significance of bilateral abnormalities on the CT scan in patients with severe head injury. *Neurosurgery, 3,* 16–21.

Swiercinsky, D.P. (1978 August). *Computerized SAINT: System for analysis and interpretation of neuropsychological tests.* Paper presented at the 86th annual convention of the American Psychological Association, Toronto, Ontario, Canada.

Tallala, A., & Morin, M.A. (1971). Acute traumatic subdural hematoma: A review of one hundred consecutive cases. *Journal of Trauma, 11,* 771–777.

Teasdale, G., & Jennett, B. (1976). Assessment and prognosis of coma after head injury. *Acta Neurochirurgica, 34,* 45–55.

Thomsen, I.V. (1974). The patient with severe head injury and his family. *Scandanavian Journal of Rehabilitation Medicine, 6,* 180–183.

Thomsen, I.V. (1975). Evaluation and outcome of aphasia in patients with severe closed head trauma. *Journal of Neurology, Neurosurgery, and Psychiatry, 38,* 713–718.

Trexler, L.E. (1982). *Cognitive rehabilitation: Conceptualization and intervention.* New York: Plenum Press.

von Bonin, G. (1962). Anatomical asymmetries of the cerebral hemispheres. In V.B. Mountcastle (Ed.), *Interhemispheric relations and cerebral dominance.* Baltimore, Johns Hopkins University Press.

von Monakow, C. (1905). *Gehirnpathologie.* Vienna: A. Holder.

Von Zomeren, A.H., & Deelman, B.G. (1978). Long-term recovery of visual reaction time after closed head injury. *Journal of Neurology, Neurosurgery, and Psychiatry, 41,* 452–457.

Wagman, M. (1980). PLATO DCS: An interactive computer system for personal counseling. *Journal of Counseling Psychology, 27,* 16–30.

Wagman, M., & Kerber, K.W. (1980). PLATO DCS, an interactive computer system for personal counseling: Further development and evaluation. *Journal of Counseling Psychology, 27,* 31–39.

Walker, A.E., & Jablon, S. (1959). A follow up of head injured men of World War II. *Journal of Neurosurgery, 16,* 600–610.

Wall, P.D. (1980). Mechanisms of plasticity of connection following damage in adult mammalian nervous systems. In P. Bach-y-Rita (Ed.), *Recovery of function: Theoretical considerations for brain injury rehabilitation* (pp. 91–105). Bern: Hans Huber Publishers.

Wheeler, J., Burke, C.J., & Reitan, R.M. (1963). An application of discriminant functions to the problem of predicting brain damage using behavioral variables. *Perceptual and Motor Skills,* [Monograph supplement], *6,* 417–440.

Wheeler, L., & Reitan, R.M. (1962). The presence and laterality of brain damage predicted from responses to a short aphasia screening test. *Perceptual and Motor Skills, 15,* 783–799.

Williams, D. (1941). The electroencephalogram in acute head injuries. *Journal of Neurology and Psychiatry, 4,* 107–130.

Wirt, R.D., Lachar, D., Klinedinst, J.K., & Seat, P.D. (1984). *Multidimensional description of child personality: A manual for the Personality Inventory for Children* (1984 revision by David Lachar). Los Angeles: Western Psychological Services.

Woodruff, N.L., & Baisden, R.H. (1986). Theories of brain functioning: A brief introduction to the study of the brain and behavior. In D. Wedding, A.M. Horton, Jr., & J. Webster (Eds.), *The neuropsychology handbook: Behavioral and clinical perspectives* (pp. 23–58). New York: Springer Publishing Company.

Ylvisaker, N. (Ed.). (1985). *Head injury rehabilitation: Children and adolescents.* San Diego, CA: College Hill Press.

Zimmerman, R.A., Bilaniuk, L.T., & Gennarelli, T. (1978). Computed tomography of shearing injuries of the cerebral white matter. *Radiology, 127,* 393–396.

SUBJECT INDEX